BIOLOGICAL SCIENCES AND ENVIRONMENTAL HEALTH

The book captures the essence of the First International Conference on Frontiers of Biological Sciences and Environmental Health (FBSEH 2023). It provides a comprehensive roadmap to achieving sovereignty, security and safety of human health by adopting a multi-disciplinary approach to disease diagnosis, mitigation and prevention.

These proceedings contains a repository of unique ideas, cutting edge research methodologies and exhaustive studies by experts, scholars from all over the world. It touches upon a wide array of topics including advances in bioengineering and genetic technologies, nutrition and disease prevention, emerging therapeutic strategies and drug delivery, along with the advent of microfluidics, wearables, and medical devices. It highlights innovative research contributions and practical applications that would prove critical in fighting cancer and genetic disorders in the future.

This is a highly beneficial guide to university professors, research scholars and medical professionals in the rapidly evolving fields such as microbiology, biotechnology, biomedical engineering, molecular medicine, public health and community medicine, and healthcare sciences.

PROCEEDINGS OF THE FIRST INTERNATIONAL CONFERENCE ON FRONTIERS OF BIOLOGICAL SCIENCES AND ENVIRONMENTAL HEALTH (FBSEH 2023), SINGAPORE, 3–5 NOVEMBER 2023

Biological Sciences and Environmental Health

Edited by

Xuan Gao
University College, London, UK

CRC Press
Taylor & Francis Group
Boca Raton London New York Leiden

CRC Press is an imprint of the
Taylor & Francis Group, an **informa** business
A BALKEMA BOOK

First published 2025
by CRC Press/Balkema
4 Park Square, Milton Park, Abingdon, Oxon, OX14 4RN

and by CRC Press/Balkema
2385 NW Executive Center Drive, Suite 320, Boca Raton FL 33431

CRC Press/Balkema is an imprint of the Taylor & Francis Group, an informa business

British Library Cataloguing-in-Publication Data
A catalogue record for this book is available from the British Library

Library of Congress Cataloging-in-Publication Data
A catalog record has been requested for this book

ISBN: 978-1-032-96016-6 (hbk)
ISBN: 978-1-032-96020-3 (pbk)
ISBN: 978-1-003-58759-0 (ebk)

DOI: 10.1201/9781003587590

Typeset in Times New Roman
by MPS Limited, Chennai, India

Biological Sciences and Environmental Health – Gao (Ed.)
© 2025 the Editor(s), ISBN: 978-1-032-96016-6

Table of Contents

Biological Sciences and Environmental Health – Gao (Ed.)
© 2025 the Editor(s), ISBN: 978-1-032-96016-6

Preface

International Conference on Frontiers of Biological Sciences and Environmental Health-Recent Trends in Biological Sciences and Environmental Health (FBSEH 2023) takes place on November 3–5, 2023 in Singapore. The conference aims to bring together the world's top minds, cutting-edge theories, and latest research findings to explore and share the latest developments and future directions in interdisciplinary research in biological sciences and environmental health. The conference provides a platform for scholars and researchers from different fields to exchange and share their latest research findings and experiences, and to promote interdisciplinary cooperation and understanding.

FBSEH 2023 focuses on high-quality presentations and papers with solid theoretical foundations, unique ideas, scientific research methods, in-depth analysis, and abundant research value. We invite scholars, researchers, and experts from all over the world to participate in this conference. The scope of this conference encompasses disciplines within the biological sciences and environmental health. The conference will feature keynote speeches given by renowned scholars, as well as oral/poster presentations covering a broad range of popular topics. Accepted papers will be included in the FBSEH 2023 Conference Proceedings, which will undergo independent peer-review procedures to meet the requirements of international publication standard.

Finally, we would like to express our sincere gratitude to all the authors who, through their insightful presentations and papers, generously contributed to the vibrant exchange of scientific information. Your valuable contributions have significantly enriched the intellectual atmosphere, underscoring the importance of such interactions in ensuring the success and longevity of scientific conferences of this nature.

Biological Sciences and Environmental Health – Gao (Ed.)
 ISBN: 978-1-032-96016-6

Editor Biography

Xuan Gao, PhD, graduated from University College London. His scholarly interests are in 2D materials using MBE and STM techniques, exploring surface and interface phenomena. Gao's academic achievements are notable, having received numerous honors and awards, including the Dean's Prize of UCL, nomination for GRS/ORS scholarships, and various scholarships and awards for his outstanding academic performance and contributions. He has also been recognized for his excellence in extracurricular activities, such as his roles as a student cadre and youth league cadre. Xuan Gao is a talented researcher with a strong academic foundation, excellent research skills, and diverse professional experiences. His contributions to the field of electrochemistry and energy materials, along with his passion for learning and innovation, make him a valuable asset to any academic or research institution.

Biological Sciences and Environmental Health – Gao (Ed.)
© 2025 the Editor(s), ISBN: 978-1-032-96016-6

Organising Committee

Conference Chair
Xuan Gao, *Department of Chemistry, University College London, UK*

Conference Co-Chair
Feng Wang, *School of Environment, Southern University of Science and Technology, China*

Publication Chair
Wei Wei, *Chinese Academy of Sciences (IGGCAS), China*

Conference Organizing Committee
Chongyang Liang, *Jilin University, China*
Junsong Wang, *Tianjin Medical University, China*
Jun Sang, *Chongqing University, China*
Zhigang Liu, *Northwest Agriculture and Forestry University, China*
Binh P. Nguyen, *Victoria University of Wellington, New Zealand*
Xiaohu Luo, *Ningbo University, China*
Hossein Hosseinkhani, *Innovation Center for Advanced Technology, Matrix, Inc, USA*
Parvati Sharma, *Chaudhary Bansi Lal University, India*
Deepika Koundal, *University of Petroleum & Energy Studies, India*
Anna Gaviglio, *University of Milan, Italy*
Anand Mohan, *University of Georgia, USA*
Junyan Liu, *University of Maryland, USA*

Academic Committee
Qingzhu Zeng, *Guangzhou University, China*
Eugenio Demartini, *University of Milan, Italy*
Vajiheh Fadaei, *Islamic Azad University, Iran*
Weirong Hu, *Guangzhou University, China*
Shiyi Ou, *Jinan University, China*
Xinquan Yang, *Yazhouwan Seed Lab, China*
Hongtao Lei, *South China Agricultural University, China*
Feng Wu, *Wuhan University, China*
Riham El Gogary, *Ain Shams University, India*
Lixian Li, *Chongqing University Cancer Hospital, China*
Yujiro Hayashi, *Tohoku University, Japan*
Ewa Dluska, *Warsaw Univeristy of Technology, Poland*
Ho Chee Cheong, *Universiti Tunku Abdul Rahman, Malaysia*
Suriani Mat Jusoh, *Universiti Malaysia Terengganu, Malaysia*
Ozgur Ceylan, *Muğla Sıtkı Koçman University, Turkey*
Pu Chun Ke, *Monash University, Australia*

Chapter 1
Advances in genetic technologies and applications

Biological Sciences and Environmental Health – Gao (Ed.)

Melanoma signaling pathway and suicide gene system

Xinxi Shen
South China Agricultural University, No. Wu Shan Lu, Tianhe District, Guangzhou, China

Tingyu Wang
Nanjing Tech University, Pukou District, Nanjing, China

Xinyue Yu
University of Toronto Mississauga, Mississauga, Canada

ABSTRACT: Melanoma, also known as malignant melanoma, is a life-threatening tumor originating from melanocytes that mainly occurs in the human skin and accounts for a significant proportion of deaths from skin tumors. In recent years, the incidence of malignant melanoma has been the highest among all cancers, showing a year-by-year increase. The standardized incidence, mortality, and disability-adjusted life years (Daly) rates (95% uncertainty interval) of cutaneous malignant melanoma in China in 2019 were 0.92/100000, 0.28/100000, and 7.96/100000, respectively. From 1990 to 2019, the corresponding average annual percent changes (AAPCs) were 3.35%, -0.45%, and -0.56%, respectively. Immunotherapy is currently the most widely used method of treatment, with local resection being the conventional clinical method, but the prognosis remains poor. In addition, melanoma shows low sensitivity to chemotherapy, with a very low response rate. Therefore, finding new therapeutic targets for patients with melanoma is becoming increasingly important. The Hippo signaling pathway plays a critical role in tumor proliferation, invasion, drug resistance, and immunity. One effective way to address the issue of efficacy decay and drug resistance in melanoma is drug therapy targeting the Hippo signaling pathway, which is considered to have great potential. This review introduces the physiological process of the Hippo signaling pathway in melanoma and examines related drugs. At the same time, it explores the oHSV-CD/5-FC suicide gene system.

1 INTRODUCTION

Melanoma is a type of skin cancer caused by the malignant transformation of melanocytes. Since less than half of patients survive for more than five years, it accounts for the majority of skin cancer deaths and is the fifth most common malignancy in the United Kingdom. Moreover, the number of cases has increased in recent years (Emma *et al.* 2022; Weyden *et al.* 2020). Most melanomas occur on the surface of the skin, usually resulting from the proliferation of epidermal melanocytes induced by excessive and strong ultraviolet (UV) radiation (Weyden *et al.* 2020). Intense and prolonged UV exposure tends to induce pre-mutations, which result in a change in a specific base sequence, converting cytosine into uracil. For example, superficial spreading melanoma, the most common type of melanoma usually caused by sunburn, can often be cured by traditional treatments such as surgical removal (Emma *et al.* 2022).

Additionally, the inhibition of the Hippo-YAP signaling pathway can also lead to the occurrence of melanoma (Anwesha *et al.* 2020). The upstream portion of the Hippo signaling pathway is composed of tumor suppressor genes, including SAV1/2, MST1/2, MOB1A, and

DOI: 10.1201/9781003587590-1

LATS1/2, while the downstream portion is composed of YAP/TAZ components. When the skin is damaged due to environmental causes, such as UV exposure, YAP/TAZ overexpression is activated, promoting cell proliferation and the metastasis of cancer cells. Activation of the tumor suppressor gene LATS1/2 is a highly effective way to inhibit the tumor gene YAP/TAZ, but the LATS1/2 activator is still in the development stage (Qi 2022).

Studies have found that the WWC protein activates the Hippo signaling pathway and thus slows down the development of melanoma (Qi 2022; Meng 2020). The WWC protein is present in the MST1/2-SAV1-WWC1/2/3-LATS1/2 signaling module. The first 200 amino acids of WWC protein, defined as Super Hippo, significantly affect the activation of upstream tumor suppressor genes LATS1/2 and SAV1. In addition, WWC protein inhibits tumor cell proliferation in aggressive UVM due to YAP overexpression. Triptonide extracted from Tripterygium Wirelli can activate tumor suppressor genes SAV1 and LATS1 in the Hippo signaling pathway, lyse YAP protein translated by downstream oncogenes, and promote apoptosis in cancer cells. Fenofibrate can inhibit the proliferation and migration of melanoma cells through upregulating tumor suppressor genes MST1 and LATS expression, and its efficacy is dose-dependent.

However, traditional treatments are often ineffective for stage IV melanoma that has metastasized. As the disease progresses, cutaneous melanoma can metastasize to many non-cutaneous sites to form cancer, such as uveal melanoma (UVM) (Emma *et al.* 2022). Due to their inherent fragility, eyes have immune privileges. Compared with other organs and tissues, tumors occurring in the eyes are more likely to evade immune detection, resulting in malignant tumors and tumor metastasis, and can easily spread to vital organs, such as the liver (Liu *et al.* 2023; Weyden *et al.* 2020). Suicide gene therapy using an oncolytic virus as a carrier is an emerging therapy, often used for patients with melanoma who cannot undergo traditional treatments, and has been gradually approved for use in countries such as the United States and Australia (Lundstrom 2023). Suicide genes involve inserting special genes into the genome of cancer cells through specialized vectors and administering non-toxic precursor drugs (Jessica *et al.* 2022). This paper mainly introduces the oHSV-CD/5-FC suicide gene system. In this system, cancer cells express enzymes dependent on the cytosine deaminase (CD) gene that is introduced. The non-toxic precursor drug 5-fluorocytosine (5-FC) is transformed into cytotoxic 5-fluorouracil (5-FU), which directly kills cancer cells (Liu *et al.* 2018, 2020; Jae-Rim *et al.* 2019). In addition, since 5-FU has the characteristics of small molecules, it can produce a bystander effect, spreading to surrounding cancer cells that have not successfully integrated CD genesa and further eliminating tumors. Suicide gene therapy is popular due to its small dosage, selective carrier, minimal side effects, and effectiveness on aggressive tumors.

2 THE FORMATION OF MELANOMA

2.1 *Ultraviolet radiation*

Excessive UV radiation can lead to melanoma. UV radiation can inhibit and destroy normal fibroblasts, causing abnormal proliferation and metastasis of melanoma. Transforming growth factor-b1 (TGF-b1) is secreted autonomously in melanoma, while it requires UV radiation in normal melanocytes. Fibroblast-activating protein-a (FAP-a) is highly expressed in fibroblasts because it activates cancer-associated fibroblasts. Overexpression of this protein induces degradation of the extracellular matrix (ECM). The ECM has the ability to separate different tissues, regulate immune response, and control cell growth; its degradation will enable cancer cells to acquire stronger invasion and metastasis capabilities (Petra *et al.* 2017).

Sunlight-associated melanoma is characterized by a C-T mutation, resulting from UV radiation-induced damage of cyclobutane pyrimidine dimers in DNA. In melanoma, when UV light from the sun hits a specific base-pair sequence (such as CC, TT, TC, and CT), the chemical link becomes unstable, which leads to the problem of pre-mutation. Pre-mutation is the primary cause of melanoma, which involves the normal cell replication process in the occurrence of mutations, resulting in the basic changes in melanoma. The pre-mutation is a persistent chemical instability caused by UV light from sunlight hitting specific base-pair sequences, such as CC, TT, TC, and CT, which results in chemical changes in cytosine, converting it to uracil, a base found in RNA molecules but not present in DNA (Kerryn *et al.* 2018).

2.2 *Abnormality of Hippo-YAP signal pathway*

The Hippo-YAP signaling pathway is a chain of protein kinases and transcription factors that is instrumental in regulating the size of organs, maintaining stability, and regenerating human tissues. Disruption of this pathway can lead to developmental abnormalities or diseases such as tumors (Anwesha *et al.* 2020). The key components of the Hippo-YAP signaling pathway include MST1/2 and its coactivator SAV1, LATS1/2, and its regulatory proteins MOB1, YAP, and TAZ (Jessica *et al.* 2022). The upstream part of the Hippo signaling pathway comprises tumor suppressor genes Sav1/2, MST1/2, MOB1A, and LATS1/2, and the downstream part comprises oncogene YAP/TAZ (Min Hwan and Joon 2017).

The function of the Hippo signaling pathway in melanoma cells is mainly to effectively inhibit the proliferation and metastasis of these cells. The Hippo signaling pathway operates normally, which shows that the upstream tumor suppressor genes Sav1/2, MST1/2, and MOB1A are expressed, and phosphorylated as expected, and then LATS1/2 phosphorylated YAP protein (Zaid *et al.* 2018). As a result, YAP remains located in the cytoplasm and cannot enter the nucleus to activate transcriptional functions, thus regulating organ size and volume and eliminating the tumorigenic role of the oncogene YAP. However, if genes such as LATS1/2, which are upstream of the Hippo signaling pathway, are defective, the oncogene YAP is released and enters the nucleus to bind to TEADs. This interaction promotes the high expression of various oncogenes, thus contributing to the occurrence of melanoma (Floriane *et al.* 2017).

When the body is in a state of UV radiation, chronic inflammatory stimulation, immunosuppression, and oxidative stress for a long time, the steady state of the skin cell population will be disrupted. The upstream signaling factors of the Hippo pathway can be sensitive to changes in the surrounding microenvironment and the release of cell stress signals, leading to a kinase cascade reaction (Min Hwan and Joon 2017). YAP, a downstream effector, is a significant regulator of epidermal stem cell proliferation and tissue growth. When the skin barrier is damaged, keratinocytes can promote abnormal proliferation of YAP/TAZ, activating epidermal stem cells and dermal mesenchymal cells with the potential for heterogeneous differentiation, ultimately leading to the occurrence of cancer (Figure 1) (Kieran *et al.* 2013).

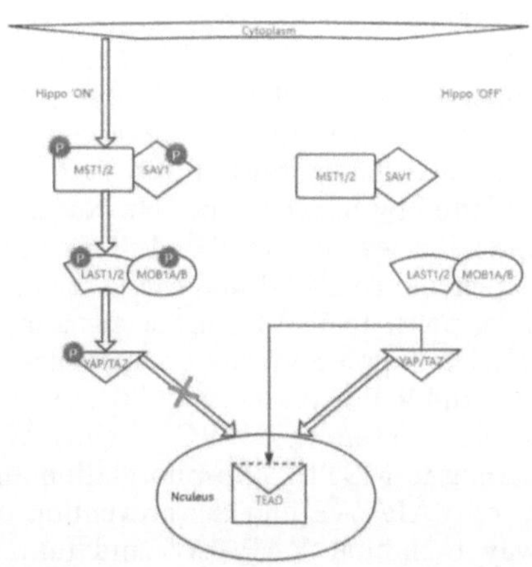

Figure 1. Normality and abnormality of the Hippo-YAP signal pathway (Photo/Picture credit: Original).

The Hippo pathway genes YAP1 and TEAD are linked to melanoma-specific survival. Genetic variation in Hippo pathway genes may serve as an independent predictor of survival in melanoma, with the risk of death increasing with the number of patients carrying these genes (Floriane *et al.* 2017). Studies have shown that Yap overexpression can significantly improve the clonal potential and in vitro invasive ability of melanoma cells. Endogenous YAP/TAZ AIDS melanoma cell metastasis, while knockdown of YAP/TAZ could inhibit lung metastasis of melanoma. These results indicate that the Hippo pathway effector molecule YAP/TAZ plays a vital role in regulating melanoma cell invasion and metastasis, suggesting that YAP/TAZ could become an important target for therapeutic intervention (Li *et al.* 2010).

3 TREATING MELANOMA BY MODULATING THE HIPPO SIGNALING PATHWAY

3.1 *WCC protein activates LATS1/2*

Current scientific research indicates that within the Hippo signaling pathway, there exists the MST1/2-SAV1-WWC1/2/3-LATS1/2 signaling module. As shown in Figure 2, the WWC protein (WCC1/2/3) can organize this signaling module by interacting with LATS1/2 and SAV1, thereby promoting the phosphorylation of LATS1/2 by MST1/2. Ectopic expression of WWC proteins activates LATS1/2.

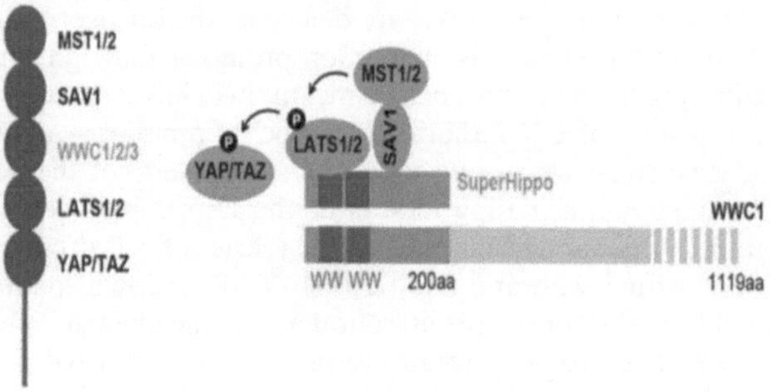

Figure 2. Mechanism of action of WWC proteins in the hippo signaling pathway (Qi 2022).

In WWC proteins, the first 200 amino acids (referred to as Super Hippo) are crucial and sufficient for WWC-induced phosphorylation of LATS1/2 and YAP/TAZ (Qi 2022). A study investigating the effect of Super Hippo on the proliferation of UVM cells with different mutations found that in all cell lines, Super Hippo expression promoted the phosphorylation of LATS1/2 and YAP and inhibited the expression of CYR61. The proliferation of YAP-dependent UVM cells was inhibited by Super Hippo. However, in the absence of LATS1/2 and MOB1A/B, CYR61 expression was not inhibited. This suggests that WWC proteins operate in a manner that is dependent on SAV1 and MST1/2 but not NF2 and MAP4K1-7. Consequently, based on their response to WWC1 in the signaling pathway, it is possible to categorize the upstream LATS1/2 Hippo pathway components into two groups. The first group includes MST1/2, SAV1, and WWC proteins, and the second group includes NF2 and MAP4K1-7, as shown in Figure 3. To sum up, WWC proteins (WWC1/2/3) directly interact with LATS1/2 and SAV1, leading to MST1/2 phosphorylation and activation of LATS1/2. This results in the inhibition of YAP/TAZ and the prevention of melanoma genesis. The most direct and effective way to inhibit YAP/TAZ and tumorigenesis is by activating LATS1/2, but the development of LATS1/2 activators has not yet been successful.

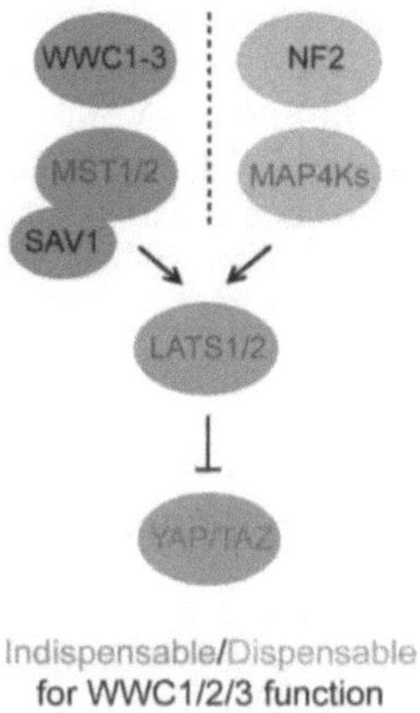

Figure 3. Grouping of LATS1/2 upstream signaling pathway components (Qi 2022).

3.2 *Triptonide triggers activation of SAV1 and LATS1*

Triptonide exhibits a strong and selective anti-metastatic effect against melanoma. It can make melanoma cell cytosol bigger, reduce cell proliferation, increase apoptosis, and effectively inhibit melanoma metastasis in mice. The effect of Triptonide could activate SAV1 and LATS1, the oncogenic components of the Hippo signaling pathway, and promote the lysosomal degradation of its downstream YAP protein. Additionally, it reduces the protein level of p-AKT, inhibits the expression of downstream metastasis-related genes, and finally achieves the purpose of inhibiting the metastasis of melanoma.

3.3 *Fenofibrates upregulate phosphorylation levels of MST1, LATS, and YAP*

Fenofibrate significantly inhibits the proliferation and migration rate of mouse melanoma cells in a concentration-dependent manner (Meng 2020). Transcriptome sequencing revealed that fenofibrate treatment induced changes in the expression of genes within the Hippo signaling pathway. This pathway functions to inhibit the transcription of genes regulated by YAP/TAZ into the nucleus, which has been reported to play an important role in the maintenance of tumor stem cells and tumorigenesis. Western blotting showed that fenofibrate treatment significantly upregulated the phosphorylation levels of MST1, LATS, and YAP in the Hippo signaling pathway in mouse melanoma cells (B16F10), suggesting that fenofibrate exerts an oncostatic effect by activating the Hippo signaling pathway.

4 TUMOR SUICIDE GENE THERAPY

Suicide gene therapy refers to the introduction of certain suicide genes from viruses or bacteria that target tumor cells based on the characteristics of vectors. By translating these genes to produce specific enzymes, which catalyze the conversion of non-toxic drug precursors into cytotoxic substances, the recipient cells carrying these genes are destroyed. Among them, the oHSV-CD/5-FC suicide gene system has shown a significant efficacy in the treatment of melanoma.

This system requires the construction of the oHSV (oncolytic herpes simplex virus) vector by inserting the cytosine deaminase (CD) gene at specific sites and deleting genes associated with virus growth. The oHSV vector integrates the CD gene into the host cell genome. The non-toxic precursor drug 5-fluorocytosine (5-FC) is converted into strongly cytotoxic

5-fluorouracil (5-FU) through the enzyme produced from the expression of CD, which then directly kills tumor cells and reduces their volume (Ashraf *et al.* 2022; Jae-Rim *et al.* 2019; Liu *et al.* 2018; Lv *et al.* 2022; Su-Nam and So Young 2020). This system not only treats common cutaneous melanoma but also UVM, the most common and aggressive form of intraocular melanoma, which often becomes resistant to chemotherapy.

4.1 *oHSV vector*

Oncolytic viruses (OV) can replicate within tumor cells, leading to their lyses. They have been utilized in cancer treatments, especially for cancers that are difficult to cure with conventional therapies (Lundstrom 2023; Su-Nam and So Young 2020). The herpes simplex virus-1 (HSV-1) was genetically engineered into the DNA-based oncolytic virus, oHSV-1, which possesses replication and tumor-killing capabilities. The oHSV-1 vector serves as a carrier for the suicide gene system. It is selective and convergent to tumor cells rather than normal tissues. It also has excellent gene delivery capacity and can replicate in tumor cells. The oHSV-1 vector has been widely used in the clinical treatment of various tumors, and some countries, such as the United States, have approved its use in the treatment of advanced melanoma (Kevin *et al.* 2019; Lundstrom 2023; Liu *et al.* 2020; Su-Nam and So Young 2020).

4.1.1 *Inhibition of IL-6/STAT3 signaling pathway and EMT*

Since the HSV vector retains certain pathogenic abilities, the genome of oHSV-1 must be modified to attenuate the antiviral immune response of the body and reduce the pathogenicity of the virus by definite steps (Lundstrom 2023).

First, the γ134.5 and ICP47 genes are deleted, and the CD gene is inserted into the site of γ134.5 on the oHSV vector to form HSV-CD. The ICP47 gene encodes an antigen-presenting inhibitor, whose expression blocks transporters associated with antigen processing, preventing tumor cells from presenting antigens to CD8+T cells, leading to immune escape (Liu *et al.* 2023). The deletion of ICP47 promotes the presentation of viral antigen and the expression of granulocyte-macrophage colony-stimulating factor (GM-CSF), which improves patients' immune response (Kevin *et al.* 2019).

Second, the US11 gene is modified to inhibit the activation of protein kinase R (PKR) and the expression of interleukin-6 (IL-6). IL-6 activates STAT3 (signal transducer and activator of transcription 3), which is involved in the invasion of tumor cells. When the IL-6/STAT3 signaling pathway is inhibited, tumor cell growth and cancer progression are slowed. Moreover, the inhibiting and reversing of the epithelial–mesenchymal transition (EMT) are also achieved. EMT refers to the transformation of epithelial cells into mesenchymal cells, enabling them to metastasize and invade, promoting the formation of an immunosuppressive microenvironment. This, in turn, leads to increased cell aggressiveness, resulting in chemotherapy resistance (LV *et al.* 2022; Yoav *et al.* 2014). These operations reduce side effects and allow the virus to efficiently translate the proteins it needs (Lundstrom 2023).

4.1.2 *Decrease expression of dihydropyrimidine dehydrogenase*

By expressing the CD gene, target cells convert the precursor drug 5-FC into 5-FU, which is a thymidylate synthase inhibitor that interdicts the DNA synthesis in target cells by competing for nucleotide binding sites, resulting in tumor death (Jae-Rim *et al.* 2019). It is a small molecule that can diffuse inside and outside the cell, which can produce a bystander effect and inhibit cellular thymidylate synthase, thereby preventing DNA replication (Ashraf *et al.* 2022). The bystander effect refers to the ability of cytotoxic drugs transformed by tumor cells that have introduced the CD gene to not only kill the tumor cells they inhabit, but also attack nearby tumor cells that have not introduced the CD gene (Liu *et al.* 2018). This mitigates the off-target effects to a certain extent.

Dihydropyrimidine dehydrogenase (DPYD) is the rate-limiting enzyme of the strongly cytotoxic drug 5-FU. The DPYD expression promotes the degradation of 5-FU into dihydrofluorouracil (DHFU). In addition, the accumulation of its degradative products induces EMT, weakening the cytotoxic effect on cancer cells (Yoav *et al.* 2014). Reducing DPYD expression helps restore the lethality of this suicidal gene system against cancer cells.

As an immune-privileged organ, eyes are more likely to evade immune surveillance and suppress immune response than other tissues, making chemotherapy resistance a major obstacle in the treatment of UVM (Liu *et al.* 2023; LV *et al.* 2022). The oHSV-CD/5-FC suicide gene system can be targeted to treat UVM, and synergistically enhance the anti-tumor effect through DPYD downregulation and EMT inhibition (Liu *et al.* 2018, 2020). In addition, 5-FU is a non-selective chemotherapy drug, and its dosage in suicide gene therapy is lower than that in conventional chemotherapy, reducing side effects and showing no obvious toxicity to normal cells (Jae-Rim *et al* 2019; Su-Nam and So Young 2020). Although UVM, which is prone to drug resistance, has low sensitivity to 5-FU, the reduced efficacy can be compensated by oHSV-1 in the oHSV-CD/5-FC suicide gene system (Ashraf *et al.* 2022; Yoav *et al.* 2014). Since UVM is sensitive to oHSV-1, and the gene editing of the oHSV vector does not affect the function of oHSV-1, the oHSV-CD/5-FC suicide gene system has a more comprehensive effect on melanoma (Liu *et al.* 2018).

5 CONCLUSION

Since abnormalities in the Hippo-YAP signaling pathway can lead to melanoma, modulation of the Hippo-YAP signaling pathway combined with suicide gene therapy can be an efficient treatment for melanoma. There are three ways of modulating the Hippo-YAP signaling pathway: activation by WWC protein, modulation by Triptonide (medicine), and treatment with fenofibrate. Suicide gene therapy involves the insertion of the CD gene at specific sites, the deletion of genes associated with viral growth, and the construction of the oHSV vector, which integrates the CD gene into the host cell genome and converts the nontoxic precursor drug, 5-FC, into the highly cytotoxic 5-FU, which directly kills tumor cells by expressing CD. Both treatments are effective in treating melanoma, though suicide gene therapy is relatively more advanced, while Hippo-YAP modulation is still in the research phase. Our research suggests that treating melanoma through gene regulation could be clinically realized in the near future, leading to more diverse and precise cancer treatments. This approach could potentially be applied to other highly lethal cancers, such as pancreatic cancer, through future research.

AUTHOR CONTRIBUTIONS

All authors contributed equally, and their names are listed in alphabetical order.

REFERENCES

Anwesha D., Varelas X. and Guan KL., (2020). *Nature Reviews Drug Discovery* 19, 480–494.

Ashraf S.A.E., Nabil Z.M., Marwa A.Y., Mahmoud M.A., Reyad El., Nesma E., Mostafa G.A., (2022). *Heliyon* 8, e10660–e10660.

Emma J.D., Terlizzo M. and Andrew J.H., (2022). *Surgery (Oxford)* 40, 46–52.

Floriane G., Manon S., Fabrice B., Patricia M., Philippe C., *Journal of Medicinal Chemistry* 61, 5057–5072 (2017).

Jae-Rim H., Kyung A.H., Seung U.K. and Kyung-Chul C., (2019). *Cancer Research and Treatment*, 51, 797–811.

Jessica B.A., Liliana M.E.F. and Gerardo C.G., (2022). *Veterinary & Comparative Oncology* 20, 372–380.
Kerryn E., Martin B., Stefan F., Markus L., Jimmy V.E., Anders S., Anders R.C. and Erik L., (2018). *PLoS Genetics* 14, e1007849-e1007849.
Kevin H., Daniel J.F., Beth K., James H., Jean-Charles S., (2019). *Nature Reviews. Drug Discovery* 18, 689–706.
Kieran F.H., Zhang XM. and David M.T., (2013). *Nature Reviews Cancer* 13, 246–257.
Li Z., Bin Z., Ping W., Fei C., Dong ZH., Yang HR., Guan KL. and Xu YH., (2010). *Genes & Development* 24, 235–240.
Liu S., Fang S., Su X., Zhang Q., Zhu G., Zhu L., Zhao M. and Liu F., (2020). *Cancer Letters*, 495 123–134.
Liu S., Li M., Sun F., Zhang J. and Liu F., (2023). *Journal of Cancer Research and Clinical Oncology* 149, 901–912.
Liu S., Song W., Liu F., Zhang J. and Zhu S., (2018). *Experimental Eye Research* 172, 144–151.
Lundstrom K. (2023). *Viruses* 15, 698.
LV YF., He LX., Jin MY., Sun WX., Tan G. and ZG. L. (2022). *Journal of Oncology* 2022, 1–19.
Meng H., (2020). *Chinese Journal of Biochemistry and Molecular Biology* 36, 647–679.
Min Hwan K. and Joon K., (2017). *Cell Mol Life Sci* 74, 1457–1474.
Petra W., Kyriakos O., Ida E., Inger R., Oliver S., Karin Ö., (2017). *British Journal of Cancer* 117, 535–544.
Su-Nam J., So Young Y. (2020). *Cancers*, 12, 1070.
SX. Qi, (2022). *Molecular Cell* 82, 1850–1864.
Van der Weyden, L., Brenn, T., Patton, E.E., Wood, G.A. and Adams, D.J. (2020). *The Journal of Pathology* 252, 4–21.
Yoav D.S., Elizaveta F., William C.C., Jason R.C., Wai Leong T., Prathapan T., Dohoon K., Naama K., Michael E.P., Walter W.C., Brian B., Richard P., Ferenc R., Robert A.W., Michael B.Y., David M.S., (2014). *Cell* 158, 1094–1109.
Zaid T., Janse van Rensburg H.J. and Yang XL., (2018). *Cancers* 10, 94.

Biological Sciences and Environmental Health – Gao (Ed.)
© 2025 the Author(s), ISBN: 978-1-032-96016-6

CRISPR/Cas9 gene editing technology and its application in tumor research

Sifan Wang
School of Chemistry and Chemical Engineering, North University of China, Shanxi, China

ABSTRACT: According to the latest public health data, neoplasms are widespread worldwide. As per the World Health Organization (WHO) statistics, over 10,000,000 individuals worldwide are diagnosed with malignant tumors annually. Furthermore, cancer ranks among the primary causes of mortality globally, imposing significant health burdens in certain regions. Tumor treatment presents a profound challenge in contemporary medicine, owing to its intricate initiation and progression, commonly accompanied by immune evasion and the establishment of an immunosuppressive tumor microenvironment. Additionally, tumor cells exhibit a high propensity for metastasis and migration. Therefore, it is imperative to address the challenge of immune evasion in tumor cells as a critical task in tumor treatment. With the advent of gene-editing technology, CRISPR/Cas9 system functions by the sgRNA for target and Cas protein for cleavage to delete or insert DNA sequence. Due to its precise and efficient gene editing, it has shown great potential in tumor research, providing new means for CAR-T cell therapy and TCR-T cell therapy, and is expected to improve tumor treatment effects and promote the development of personalized medicine. This review systematically introduces the background, development, principle, and application of CRISPR/Cas9 gene editing technology in CAR-T cell therapy and TCR-T cell therapy and explores the utilization of CRISPR-Cas9 system in tumor treatment therapies.

1 INTRODUCTION

1.1 *CRISPR technology and tumor therapy*

In the field of disease research and treatment, particularly in relation to cancer, the CRISPR-Cas system has gained increased notoriety in recent years. Genetic alterations and dysregulation in cancer genesis and progression have been strongly associated with various genes. The primary objective of cancer therapy is to impede the growth and progression of tumors by targeting and rectifying specific mutations while reinstating the expression of dysregulated genes. The immunotherapeutic technique known as adoptive cell therapy (ACT) involves harnessing immune cells, particularly T cells, for combating tumor cells (Jensen 2015). Currently, there are two main approaches being studied in the field of ACT: transgenic T cell receptor (TCR)-T cell therapy and chimeric antigen receptor (CAR)-T cell therapy (Fan 2016).

1.2 *Source of CRISPR-Cas*

The Clustered Regularly Interspaced Short Palindromic Repeats (CRISPR) system, an instrument for virus defense, emerged from bacteria (Hu *et al.* 2023). The repetitive sequence within the CRISPR sequence is extensively conserved, and when the virus invades bacteria, the Cas protein in the bacteria will cut out a part of the viral DNA and put it into the spacer of the repeat sequence, thus forming clusters, regularly spaced, short palindromic repeats. Bacteria collect viral DNA and then archive their identities. Once the Cas protein finds the

DOI: 10.1201/9781003587590-2

same sequence, that is, a virus, the Cas protein will cut off the virus and protect the bacteria from being infected by the virus, so this is an efficient bacterial defense mechanism (Figure 1), and the simulation of this defense mechanism is to carry out the basis of gene editing. First, use the principle of complementary base pairing of DNA at the gene editing site to design a guide RNA. After the guide RNA binds to the Cas protein, it will find the corresponding DNA fragment site that needs gene editing, and cut the DNA at this site. At the same time, if a correct gene is delivered as a template, then the cell has the opportunity to use the correct template to repair the gap in DNA and complete gene editing.

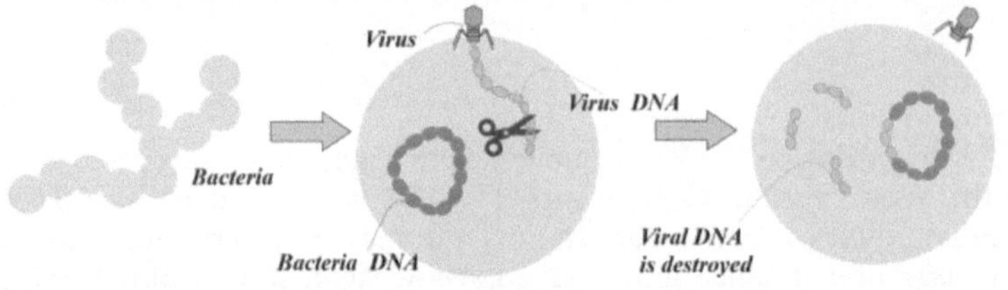

Figure 1. Origin of the CRISPR/Cas system. (Photo/Picture credit: Original).

1.3 *The CRISPR-Cas development process*

One of the most significant technological advancements of the last 30 years is gene editing technology. In 1996, the preliminary generation of gene editing technology genetically engineered zinc finger nucleases (ZFNs) was developed and made public. A process for changing biological things in an artificial way. 2009 saw the development of transcription-like activator effector nucleases (TALENs), a second-generation gene editing technique (Moscou and Bogdanove 2009). Both ZFNs and TALENs technologies need to design, synthesize and assemble complex protein modules with specific DNA recognition functions. The construction period is long and the steps are cumbersome, making it difficult to perform high-throughput gene editing, which greatly limits their popularization and application.

Until 2012, CRISPR technology appeared, which only needs to follow the principle of DNA-RNA base pairing, and uses RNA-mediated nuclease to combine with DNA target sequence to achieve the purpose of gene editing. Its appearance makes up for the shortcomings of various editing technologies. This system is simple, precise with high editing efficiency, which greatly reduces the technical threshold and enables gene editing to enter various research fields such as plants, animals, and microorganisms on a large scale, triggering a new round of upsurge of gene editing research (Zhu *et al.* 2009). In 2014, CRISPR Therapeutics, Editas Medicine, and Intellia Therapeutics the three world-renowned gene editing therapy companies, were founded by three leaders in the field of CRISPR (Emmanuelle Charpentier, Feng Zhang, Jennifer A. Doudna) and started CRIPSR A new chapter in gene therapy. In view of the risk of uncontrollable DNA repair caused by double-strand breaks, David Liu invented the base editor in 2016 and the lead editor in 2019 (Anzalone *et al.* 2019), which made up for the defects of CRISPR itself, and gene editing officially Enter the era of precision (Figure 2).

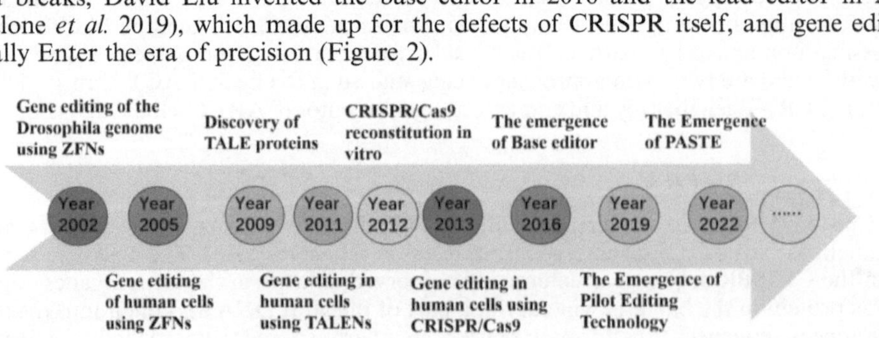

Figure 2. The progression of gene editing techniques. (Photo/Picture credit: Original).

2 CRISPR-CAS9 SYSTEM'S COMPONENTS

2.1 *Varieties of CRISPR-Cas*

CRISPR-Cas, the prokaryotic immune system, functions as a natural safeguard. In the process of constantly fighting against viruses, the diversity of Cas genes has also been greatly enriched. The CRISPR-Cas system has been split into two primary categories, each with six types and 33 subtypes, because of the function of Cas proteins in bacterial immune defense. The effectors of the first category (class I) that cleave exogenous nucleic acids are multi-protein complexes consisting of different Cas proteins, which include types I, III, and IV, comprising 16 distinct subtypes, and the second category (class II) includes Types II, V, VI and 17 subtypes require only one Cas nuclease with a large multifunctional binding domain, among which Cas9 exists in all type II systems (Figure 3). Among the different CRISPR-Cas systems, the class II CRISPR-Cas system known as CRISPR-Cas9 is extensively employed (Gao *et al.* 2022).

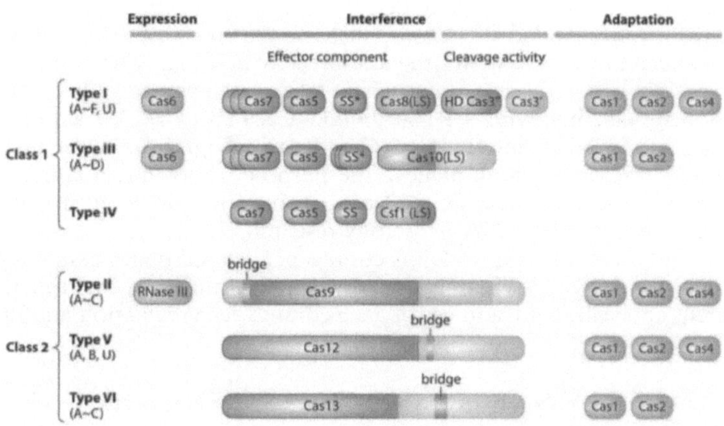

Figure 3. Classes and proteins are present in CRISPR/Cas systems (Yoshizumi *et al.* 2018).

2.2 *The similarities and differences of Cas9, Cas12 and Cas13*

Cas9, Cas12, and Cas13 are different types of proteins in the CRISPR system that have some similarities and differences in the way they function in gene editing and gene regulation.

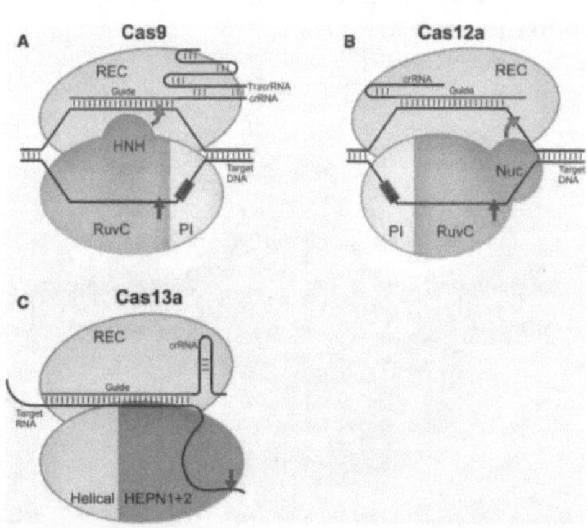

Figure 4. Cas9, Cas12, and Cas13 of Class II (Schindele *et al.* 2018).

Cas9 (Figure 4A) is the earliest widely used CRISPR protein. It can combine with CRISPR RNA (crRNA) and transcription unit type RNA (tracrRNA) to form a complex, and realize DNA double-strand cutting by recognizing a specific sequence of target DNA. In gene editing, after Cas9 cuts the target DNA, it can guide repair through non-homologous end-joining repair mechanism (NHEJ) or homologous recombination (HDR), and realize genetic modification.

Cas12 (also known as Cpf1) (Figure 4B) is another class of CRISPR proteins. Cas12 can recognize the target double-stranded DNA (dsDNA) only under the guidance of crRNA, and target the thymine-rich PAM site, and specifically cut the target sequence. Single-stranded DNA (ssDNA) in a heterosexual cleavage reaction. Different from Cas9, Cas12 has its own RNA processing enzyme activity, which can cut DNA and RNA, so it has more potential applications in gene editing and gene regulation. Compared with Cas9, Cas12 requires a shorter crRNA for target recognition, which helps to simplify the design of CRISPR systems. In addition, the cut-end structure produced by Cas12 is also different from that of Cas9, so it may have different effects on different types of gene editing and repair mechanisms.

Cas13 (Figure 4C) is a class of RNA-guided RNA-cutting enzymes in the CRISPR system (Ye 2019). Cas13 is an R-guided RNA endonuclease that possesses the ability to precisely cleave single-stranded target RNA with the assistance of crRNA. Moreover, Cas13 exhibits trans-cleavage activity when triggered by specific targets and can be utilized in non-specific cleavage reaction systems involving ssRNA. Unlike Cas9 and Cas12, Cas13 is mainly used for gene regulation and RNA interference. Cas13 can recognize and cut target RNA by binding to specific crRNA, so as to achieve the purpose of down-regulating or degrading specific RNA molecules. This makes Cas13 have application potential in gene expression regulation, virus resistance and RNA pathology research.

In summary, Cas9 is mainly used for DNA cutting and gene editing, Cas12 has the ability to cut DNA and RNA, and Cas13 is mainly used for RNA cutting and gene regulation. Each of them has different application advantages in gene editing, gene regulation and research.

3 THE FUNDAMENTALS OF THE CRISPR-CAS9 GENE EDITING TECHNIQUE

3.1 *System composition*

The natural CRISPR-Cas9 system is comprised of three elements (Figure 5): the Cas9 protein, crRNA, and tracrRNA. Within this assemblage, the crRNA and tracrRNA combine through local base pairing to create a gRNA (guide RNA). Following the attachment of the gRNA to Cas9, the gRNA serves as a guide, instructing this protein to recognize and cleave the object's DNA sequence. To simplify experimental design and enhance the stability of the gRNA, researchers have fused the crRNA and tracrRNA into a single RNA molecule called sgRNA (single-guide RNA) (Liu and Xu 2021).

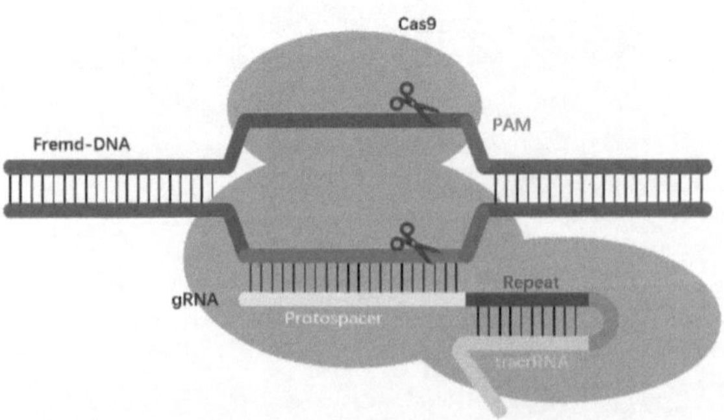

Figure 5. The CRISPR-Cas9 system's constituents. (Photo/Picture credit: Original).

3.2 *Basic principles*

The fundamental components of CRISPR-Cas9 technology consist of the Cas9 protein responsible for DNA double-strand cleavage and a guiding gRNA that facilitates target recognition. The technical principle of CRISPR-Cas9 includes two basic processes of gRNA-guided Cas9 targeting DNA cleavage and DNA repair (Figure 6).

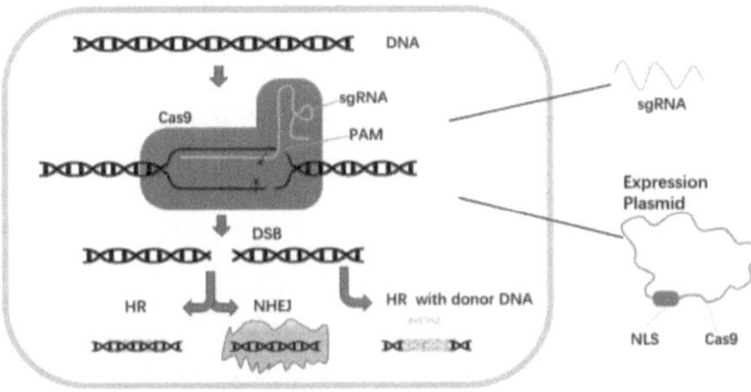

Figure 6. Working model of CRISPR/Cas9. (Photo/Picture credit: Original).

Initially, the Cas9 protein precisely severs the designated DNA sequence, resulting in a breakage of the DNA strands. The Cas9 protein comprises two nuclease domains, each capable of cleaving single strands of DNA independently. In order to effectively identify the target sequence, the Cas9 protein must fulfill two requirements: (1) a nucleotide pairing contact involving the target DNA and the gRNA's 20 nucleotides at the 5' end; (2) the 3' end of the target DNA has a suitable PAM sequence (PAM is cas9 specific recognition site, cas9 will cut at the third base upstream of PAM). Once CRISPR/Cas9 has cleaved the target DNA, a double-strand break (DSB) is created. This DSB serves as the foundation for all endonuclease-based gene editing. The DNA repair mechanism in the cell then engages to correct the DSB, altering the DNA sequence in the process. There are two primary mechanisms responsible for repairing DNA: non-homologous end joining (NHEJ) and homology -directed repair (HDR) (Josef 2006). NHEJ and HDR are both commonly employed mechanisms for DNA repair.

3.3 *Two DNA repair mechanisms*

Non-homologous end joining (NHEJ) (Figure 7) is a rapid and common DNA repair mechanism for repairing DNA double-strand breaks (DSBs). In NHEJ, when a DNA break occurs, the repair mechanism directly joins the broken DNA ends to each other without requiring the search for a homologous DNA template. NHEJ, which often takes place in the G1 and G2 stages of the organism's life cycle, is quick and independent of homologous DNA sequences, making it crucial in circumstances where cells urgently require DNA repair. Nevertheless, due to its independence from homologous sequences, the NHEJ repair process has the potential to introduce insertion, deletion mutations, or incorrect junctions, which in turn may result in gene mutations and functional abnormalities.

Homology-mediated repair (HDR) (Figure 7) is another DNA repair mechanism that repairs the break by finding a homologous DNA sequence around the site of a DNA break and using this sequence as a template. In the S and G2 phases of DNA double-strand fracture fix, HDR typically takes place. During this time, sequences of identical DNA can come from different regions of the same chromosome or from paired chromosomes. The HDR mechanism generally maintains the accuracy of the DNA sequence because it uses homologous DNA as a template for repair, avoiding insertion or deletion mutations. Due to its precision, HDR is commonly used for precise gene editing in genetic engineering and gene repair (Jansen 2002).

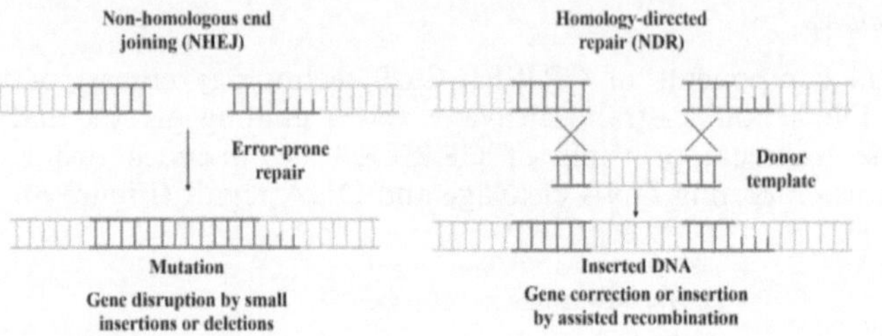

Figure 7. Two DNA repair mechanisms (NHEJ and HRD). (Photo/Picture credit: Original).

4 UTILIZING CRISPR/CAS9-BASED GENE EDITING TECHNOLOGY FOR ANTI-TUMOR THERAPY

4.1 *CAR-T cell immunotherapy*

Chimeric antigen cell therapy (CAR)-T is an immune therapy based on CAR (Corrales and Matson 2017). CAR-T cell therapy shows great potential as an effective treatment for diverse cancer types. It involves using a signaling molecule called CAR (chimeric antigen receptor) that binds to a specific antibody. This makes it possible for Tlymphocytes to identify and target tumor cells. Most clinical trials now being conducted use homologous the CAR-T cells, which are obtained from individuals, engineered to express the CAR, then multiplied in the lab before being reintroduced into the patients (Fesnak *et al.* 2016). Indeed, there are concerns regarding the cost and variability of T cells in patients, which can impact the effectiveness of the universal CAR-T cell approach.

Large-scale production of universal CAR-T (UCAR-T) cells, which are created from T cells taken from healthy donors and offer greater product consistency, has significantly broadened the application potential of CAR-T cell treatment (Dimitri *et al.* 2022). Currently, the development of UCAR-T cells predominantly involves the knockout or silencing of the T cell receptor (TCR) and β2-microglobulin (β2M) genes (Wang *et al.* 2023). The leading technology for the development and implementation of UCAR-T cells is CRISPR/Cas9 gene knockout (Figure 8). Eyquem *et al.* employed CRISPR-Cas9 technology to disrupt the constant region of TCRα, targeting the 5' end of its first exon with a specific guide RNA (sgRNA). The CD19 CAR gene sequence and symmetry arms were then inserted into the cells using an Adeno-associated virus (AAV). The CD19 CAR gene was introduced into the TCR locus by homologous recombination.

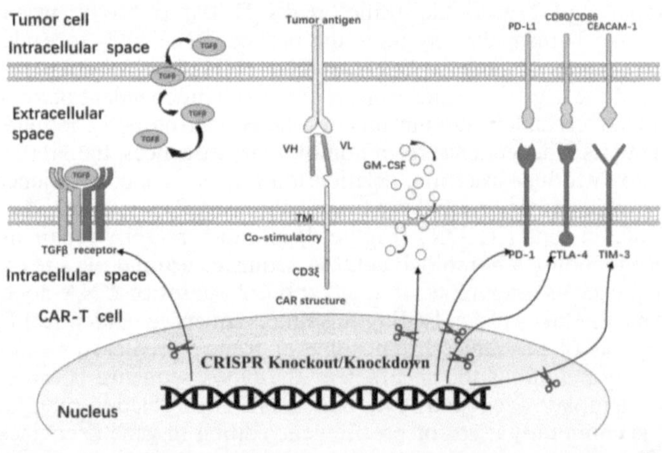

Figure 8. Utilizing CRISPR/Cas9-based gene editing technology for anti-tumor therapy. (Photo/Picture credit: Original).

4.2 *TCR-T cell therapy*

TCR-T cell treatment also belongs to ACT. By identifying the tumor antigen of the patient as the therapeutic target, the TCRα/β heterodimer that specifically recognizes the tumor antigen is used for gene transduction into T cells, and the interaction between TCR and antigenic peptide-the main tissue is improved. The affinity of the major histocompatibility complex (MHC) molecular complex enables T lymphocytes to efficiently recognize target cells (Quan *et al.* 2021). A promising method of immunotherapy is TCR-T cell treatment, as it enables T cells to be engineered with specific TCRs that can recognize and respond to tumor antigens presented by MHC molecules. Contrarily, CAR-T cell therapy is limited to targeting proteins on the cell's exterior. TCR-T cells have a distinct edge over other immune cells for treating solid cancers because they can identify intracellular tumor-specific antigens. This expanding field holds significant potential for improving the effectiveness of immunotherapy in cancer treatment (Xu *et al.* 2022).

TCR-T treatment, however, has a limited range of target antigens since it needs MHC molecules to function effectively for adequate antibody presentation.

Cancer cells can achieve immune escape by down-regulating the expression level of MHC molecules, which is a major shortcoming of TCR-T cell therapy. Gene editing of TCR-T cells using CRISPR-Cas9 technology enables them to recognize a wider range of tumor antigens and reduce dependence on MHC (Figure 9).

The fact that there are instances of recipient T cells that still have their original TCRs is a crucial factor to take into account with TCR-T cell treatment. These endogenous TCRs serve as competitors to transgenic TCRs for binding to CD3. Additionally, the mismatch between native TCRs and transgenic TCRs can potentially lead to the formation of hybrid TCR dimers (Ghaffari and Khalili 2021). In order to solve these difficulties, the native TCR and genes were switched out for genes that include artificial tumor-specific TCR elements created using the CRISPR/Cas9 technique (Ghaffari and Khalili 2021). When compared to regular TRC-T cells, the transgenic TCR's expression and functionality were improved by TCR knockdown. To mitigate the risk of mispairing, an alternative approach is the utilization of a stable Vα/Vβ single-chain TCR (sc TCR) replacement.

In 2020, a groundbreaking human clinical trial (Wei *et al.* 2022) reported the use of multiplex CRISPR/Cas9 editing to target TRAC, TRBC, and PDCD1 in T cells. This process aims to reduce TCR incompatibilities and improve immunity against tumors. To allow the identification of tumor cells, an artificial cancer-specific TCR transgene was additionally inserted. The modified T cells were administered into the patients and remained there for a period of up to nine months. These findings imply that the simultaneous use of genome modification and TCR transmission holds great promise for enhancing the creation of safer and more effective tumor immunotherapy.

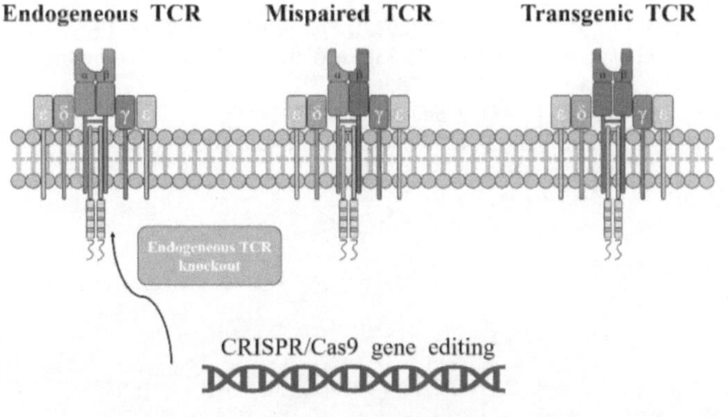

Figure 9. The structure of TCR dimers and the utilization of CRISPR/Cas9 in TCR-T cell therapy. (Photo/Picture credit: Original).

5 CONCLUSION

The precise transformation of CAR-T cells and TCR-T cells can be achieved through CRISPR/Cas9 gene editing technology. In CAR-T cells, CRISPR/Cas9 can realize gene knockout and modification against tumor immune escape and improve the specific recognition of target antigens by CAR-T cells. These topics include overcoming the problem of autologous therapeutic rejection, improving T cell depletion, fighting tumor microenvironment suppression, and minimizing the toxicities and adverse reactions of CAR-T treatments in the future. CRISPR/Cas9 technology is capable of being applied to alter TCR transcription and functionality, MHC antigen generation and presentation levels, and both. These changes can improve TCR-T cells' capacity for immunological assault against tumor cells.

Great strides will be made in comprehension of the signal transduction networks involved in tumor start and development if the gene-editing method CRISPR/Cas9 is used to investigate the development of malignancies. Moreover, it offers novel perspectives in the development of tumor treatment strategies.

REFERENCES

Anzalone A.V., Randolph P.B., Davis J.R., Sousa A.A., Koblan L.W., Levy J.M., Chen P.J., Wilson C., Newby G.A., Raguram A. and Liu D.R. (2019). *Nature*. 576, 149 .

Corrales L., Matson V., Flood B., Spranger S. and Gajewski T.F. (2017). *Cell Res.* 27, 96–108.

Dimitri A., Herbst F. and Fraietta J.A. (2022). *Mol Cancer.* 21, 78.

Eyquem J., Mansilla-Soto J., Giavridis T., Van Der Stegen S.J.C., Hamieh M., Cunanan K.M., Odak A., Gonen M. and Sadelain M. (2017). *Nature*. **543**, 113–117.

Fan X.H. (2016). *In vitro and in vivo anti-tumor activity of chimeric antigen receptor T cells targeting lung cancer marker Mesothelin.* Phd Thesis. Shanghai.

Fesnak A.D., June C.H. and Levine B.L. (2016). *Nat. Rev. Cancer*. 16, 566–81.

Gao W.S., Dou J.P., Wei S., Liu X.J., Zhang Z.F. and Li Y.N. (2022). *Curr Biotech.* 12, 532–538.

Ghaffari S., Khalili N. and Rezaei N. (2021). *J Exp Clin Canc Res.* 40, 1.

Hu Y.C., Cao C.H., Zheng L.G., Shen J.T., Zhao W. and Dai L. (2023). *Chem J Chinese U.* 44, 65–77.

Jansen R., Van Embden J.D.A., Gaastra W., Schouls L.M. (2002). *Omics*. 6, 23–33.

Jensen MC. (2015). *Science*. 350, 6260.

Josef J. (2006). *Nat. Rev. Mol. Cell biol.* 7, 335–46.

Liu H.J. and Xu Y.W. (2021). *Adv Cardiovascular Dis.* 42, 1117–1119.

Moscou MJ. and Bogdanove AJ. (2009). *Science*. 326, 5959.

Quan J.L., Kang Y.L., Zhang W.L., Tian H. and Gao X.D. (2021). *Prog Pharm Sci.* 45, 725–734.

Schindele P., Wolter F. and Puchta H. (2018). *Febs Lett.* 592, 12.

Wang C., Zhang Z.P. and Li Y.C. (2023). *J Chin Pharm Univ.* 54, 141–149.

Wei S.W., Chao G., Min Y.Z., Li Y., Lu J.C., Huang X.Y., Cai J.B., Zhang P.F., Cui Y.H. and Ke A.W. (2022). *Mol Cancer*. 21, 1

Xu D.J., Zhou Q., He Z.Y., Li M.L. and Si J.B. (2022). *Pharm Biotechnol.* 29, 192–200.

Ye W.W. (2019). Structural biology research on Cas13b-mediated CRISPR RNA maturation and recognition, MD, Fujian.

Yoshizumi I., Mart K. and Mart F. (2018). *J Bacteriol.* 200,7.

Zhu P.H., Zhu Q., Wang Y.F. and Feng B. (2009). *J LIFE SC.* 30, 1003–1009.

Biological Sciences and Environmental Health – Gao (Ed.)
© 2025 the Author(s), ISBN: 978-1-032-96016-6

β2-adrenergic receptors: Structure, distribution, and treatment of heart failure

Yunru Wang
School of Biochemical Engineering, Beijing Union, Beijing, China

ABSTRACT: Heart failure refers to the inability of the heart to produce sufficient venous return and blood supply required for tissue metabolism. It is often caused by various diseases that weaken the contractile capacity of the heart muscle, leading to a decrease in cardiac output, and resulting in a series of symptoms and signs. The incidence of heart failure is about 0.3%~2.0% in the general population, while it exceeds 10.0% in the elderly over 65 years old. The β2-adrenergic receptor is widely distributed throughout the body in different organs and tissues, with higher levels of expression in vascular and bronchial smooth muscle cells. It plays an important role in the regulation of cardiac activity. In recent years, many studies have shown significant differences in signal transduction between different subtypes of β2-adrenergic receptors and their mediated cardiac responses. Although the β2-adrenergic receptor-mediated catecholamine effect is not very important under physiological conditions (except in the frog heart), it plays an important role in heart failure and post-infarction heart disease. This review briefly introduces the structure of cardiac β2-adrenergic receptors, their distribution in the human body, and their signal transduction under the pathological conditions of heart failure. It further discusses the characteristics of β2-adrenergic receptor signal transduction and the latest research progress in its relationship with congestive heart failure.

1 INTRODUCTION

Adrenergic receptor-mediated catecholamine effects play an important role in the regulation of cardiovascular function. In 1948, Ahlquist first divided adrenergic receptors into two subtypes – α2- and β2-adrenergic receptors – based on the different reactions of sympathetic drugs in blood vessels. In 1967, Lands *et al.* further divided β2-adrenergic receptors into β1 and β2 subtypes according to their different pharmacological properties. The rapid development of molecular biology theory and technology has provided a broader field for studying the biological characteristics of receptors. In 1986, Dixon first deduced the primary structure and corresponding gene of the β2-adrenergic receptor by cloning the cDNA of the human β2-adrenergic receptor and found that the β2-adrenergic receptor is a member of the G protein-coupled receptor superfamily. The human β2-adrenergic receptor is a polypeptide chain composed of 413 amino acids, which is divided into three functional domains: extracellular domain, transmembrane domain, and intracellular domain. The extracellular domain and intracellular domain include three loops, and the transmembrane domain penetrates the membrane seven times (7TM). The classical theory holds that, as a member of the G protein-coupled receptor superfamily, the signal transduction process of the β2-adrenergic receptor begins with specific agonists binding to the receptors to promote the activation of Gs protein adenylate cyclase (AC). AC then catalyzes cyclic adenosine monophosphate (cAMP) production, which activates cAMP-dependent protein kinase A (PKA). The activation of PKA phosphorylates intracellular effector proteins exerts a series

DOI: 10.1201/9781003587590-3

of biological effects, including myocardial contraction and energy metabolism. In addition to these rapid effects, the activation of β2-adrenergic receptors can also cause effects such as gene transcription, cell growth, and apoptosis. This indicates that β2-adrenergic receptor signal transduction is a cascade reaction (phosphorylation cascade reaction), so its regulation also occurs at multiple levels, such as G protein-coupled receptor kinase, cAMP phosphodiesterase, and protein phosphatase. It was previously believed that only the β1-adrenergic receptor could regulate myocardial systolic function. Recently, it has been found that β1-adrenergic receptors and β2-adrenergic receptors jointly regulate myocardial systolic function. Cardiovascular disease is one of the most significant threats to human health. In 2011, the World Health Organization reported that 173 million people died of cardiovascular disease worldwide, accounting for 30% of global deaths (Chesley *et al.* 2000; Liu *et al.* 2010).

2 STRUCTURE AND DISTRIBUTION OF β2 ADRENOCEPTORS

2.1 *Structure of β2-adrenergic receptors*

The structure of the β2-adrenergic receptor is composed of seven transmembrane α-helix regions in the core, with the N-terminus located outside the membrane. The N-terminus is the external part of the receptor, containing the adhesion sequence and glycosylation site, which are involved in the localization and recognition of the receptor (Figure 1). Intramembrane C-terminus: The C-terminus, located inside the cell, is involved in the internalization of receptors and downstream signal transduction following receptor activation. There are three outer loops and three inner loops; the third inner loop connects TM5 and TM6, a key region for interaction with the G protein. Most ECL2 amino acids form an α-helix structure, while a small portion forms a random coil structure. Among them, ECL2 has an important physiological function, which forms a lid-like structure that covers the ligand binding site, which may impede the entry and exit of ligands. The conserved cysteine residues, Cys184 and Cys190, interact with some residues and ligands on TM3, while Cys190 also interacts with Cys191 to form a disulfide bond. This bond is of great significance for stabilizing the crystal structure of the receptor and binding ligands (Konstam and Remme 1998).

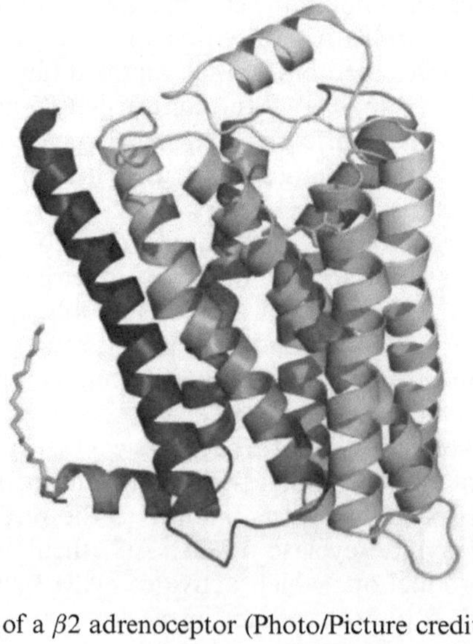

Figure 1. Structure diagram of a β2 adrenoceptor (Photo/Picture credit: Original).

2.2 *Distribution of β2-adrenergic receptors in the human body*

The β2-adrenergic receptor is mainly distributed in the heart, bronchus, blood vessels, and other areas of the human body, with notable concentrations in the sinus node, coronary artery, and other places. Abnormal expression of β2-adrenergic receptors can lead to conditions such as heart failure, bronchitis, hypertension, and other diseases (Table 1).

Table 1. Distribution of β2-adrenergic receptors in the human body.

Organ	Distribution	Effect
Heart	Sino-auricular node	β1, β2 – Acceleration
	Ectopic pacemaker	β1, β2 – Acceleration
	Myocardial contraction	β1, β2 – Reinforcement
	Coronary artery	β2 – Relaxation
Bronchus	Bronchial smooth muscle	β2 – Relaxation
	Bronchial mucosal blood vessels	A – Contraction (eliminates edema)
Blood vessel	Skin, mucosal blood vessels	A – Contraction
	Renal vascular	A – Contraction (decreased renal blood flow)
	Skeletal muscle blood vessels	β2 – Relaxation

3 β2-ADRENERGIC RECEPTOR AND HEART FAILURE

3.1 *β-adrenergic receptor signal transduction pathway*

3.1.1 *β1-adrenergic receptor signaling pathway*

Under various pathological conditions, such as heart failure, the continuous activation of β1-adrenergic receptors causes an increase in intracellular Ca^{2+} concentration, resulting in the conversion of the signaling pathway from the β1-AR-Gs-AC-cAMP-PKA pathway to the β1-AR-Gs-intracellular Ca^{2+} and calmodulin-dependent protein kinase (CaMK) II (β1-AR-Gs-Ca^{2+}-CaMKII) pathway. This promotes processes such as myocardial hypertrophy and myocardial cell apoptosis, contributing to the myocardial remodeling process and further aggravating heart failure (Zhu *et al.* 2003).

3.1.2 *β2-adrenergic receptor signaling pathway*

In contrast to β1-adrenergic receptors, which primarily couples with Gs proteins, β2-adrenergic receptors can promiscuously couple with both Gs (stimulatory G protein) and Gi (inhibitory G protein). The promiscuous coupling of β2-adrenergic receptors with Gs and Gi forms the structural and functional basis of its unique biological effects. The β2-adrenergic receptor/Gi coupling inhibits the positive inotropic and positive effects mediated by β2-adrenergic receptor/Gs (James and Robbins 2011). The coupling of β2-adrenergic receptors with Gs protein and Gi protein is one of the important mechanisms for regulating cardiac function.

The positive inotropic effect refers to the coupling of β2-adrenergic receptors with Gs protein, which enhances the contractility of cardiomyocytes by activating adenylyl cyclase and increasing intracellular cAMP levels. This is crucial for enhancing cardiac pumping function.

On the other hand, positive relaxation refers to the coupling of β2-adrenergic receptors and Gs protein, which promotes the rapid relaxation of cardiomyocytes by activating adenylate cyclase and increasing cAMP levels. This allows the heart to fill efficiently during diastole and prepares it for the next contraction.

However, when the β2-adrenergic receptor couples with Gi protein, the activation of Gi protein inhibits the activity of adenylate cyclase, resulting in decreased cAMP levels (Chesley *et al.* 2000). This inhibits the positive inotropic effect and positive relaxation effect, thereby weakening the contractility and diastolic capacity of cardiomyocytes. In general, activation of these receptors can increase both cardiac contractility and heart rate.

3.2 *Drugs for heart failure*

3.2.1 *β receptor antagonist*

The cardiovascular protective effect of adrenaline receptor antagonists was proposed around 1970. Historically, the development of these antagonists has gone through three different stages, resulting in three generations of treatments for chronic heart failure (Asano *et al.* 2001). While all adrenaline receptor antagonists can block adrenaline receptor signaling, their clinical effects vary.

Propranolol, a first-generation adrenergic receptor antagonist, targets both $\beta1$- and $\beta2$-adrenergic receptors with high affinity but has no effect on α-adrenergic receptors. More than 20% of patients with chronic heart failure are affected by first-generation treatments. The resistance to adrenergic receptor antagonists in some patients is due to cardiac contractile function and increased afterload.

Metoprolol, a second-generation drug, is a selective $\beta1$-adrenergic receptor antagonist. This selectivity helps avoid side effects on the peripheral vasculature and lungs. The third generation of β-adrenergic receptor antagonists, also known as vasodilator β-adrenergic receptor antagonists, includes drugs such as carvedilol and bucindolol. These are primarily used to treat hypertension. At clinically effective doses, carvedilol is not highly selective between $\beta1$ and $\beta2$ adrenoceptors; the drug also has an affinity for α1-adrenergic receptors. As a result, carvedilol acts as an antagonist of the $\alpha1/\beta1/\beta2$ adrenoceptors. The vasodilatory effect of third-generation drugs is mainly attributed to their antagonism of α1-adrenergic receptors. By binding and blocking the postsynaptic membrane, the α1-adrenergic receptor signaling pathway dilates blood vessels and reduces peripheral vascular resistance. By blocking β-adrenergic receptors, they inhibit renin secretion in the kidneys, thereby suppressing the renin-angiotensin-aldosterone system and producing an antihypertensive effect. Therefore, in patients with congestive heart failure, third-generation adrenergic receptor antagonists show better efficacy compared to first-generation and second-generation drugs (Malik *et al.* 2015).

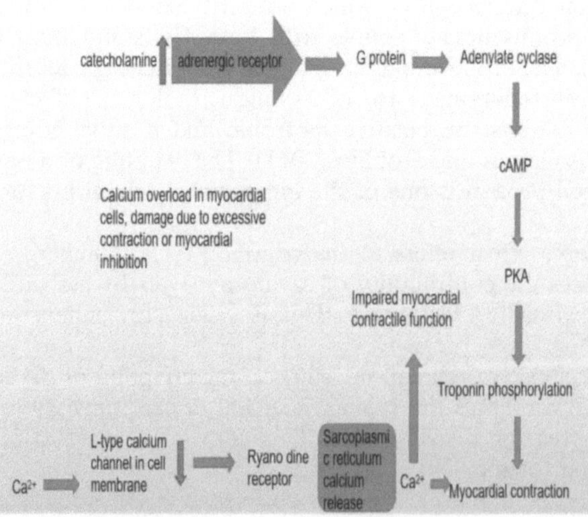

Figure 2. Continuous activation of β-adrenergic receptors inducing intracellular Ca^{2+} signaling pathways.

3.2.2 *β2-adrenergic receptor agonist combined with β1-adrenergic receptor antagonist*

In patients with chronic heart failure, the expression of β1-adrenergic receptors is downregulated by about 50%, reducing the ratio of β1- to β2-adrenergic receptors from the normal 8:2 to 6:4 (Gauthier *et al.* 2007). At this stage, targeting the β2-adrenergic receptor becomes more critical. When fecosterol and metoprolol are combined, the expression of the β2-adrenergic receptor does not decrease. Considering the cardiotoxicity of β1-adrenoceptors and the cardioprotective effects of β2-adrenoceptors, the combination of β2-adrenoceptor agonists and β1-adrenoceptor antagonists can be explored as a new strategy for the treatment of heart failure (Jessup *et al.* 2009).

3.2.3 *β2-adrenergic receptor function-biased agonist*

Based on the studies of the mechanism of the β-adrenergic receptor signaling pathway, it has been proposed that combining β1-adrenergic receptor antagonists with β2-adrenergic receptor-Gs signaling pathway-biased agonists could be a new strategy for the treatment of heart failure.

Carvedilol activates the cardioprotective pathway so that the drug has a better clinical effect compared to other drugs that can only exert β-adrenergic receptor inhibitory function. The clinical effect of carvedilol is thought to be primarily mediated by β-arrestin pathway bias (Hunt *et al.* 2009). Given the constant expression of β2-adrenergic receptors in heart failure, biased activation of the β2-adrenergic receptor β-arrestin signaling pathway can reduce apoptosis and enhance myocardial contraction, which is a new strategy for the treatment of heart failure.

The combination of β2-adrenergic receptor Gs signaling pathway agonists and β-adrenergic receptor blockers in the treatment of heart failure is clear, and the effect is significant. Furthermore, due to cavedilol's activation of the β-arrestin signaling pathway, the pathway compared to β-adrenergic receptor blockers has more advantages in the treatment of heart failure.

As research on β-adrenergic receptors, especially on the signaling pathway of β2 adrenergic receptors and their physiological effects (including the eutectic structure of β2 adrenergic receptors and various functionally biased ligands), deepens, we can expect advancements in understanding the polymorphisms of β2-adrenergic receptor genes and molecular configurations. This progress will likely lead to the development of a new generation of β2-adrenergic receptor function-biased drugs and combined treatment strategies with other heart failure drugs, heralding a new era for personalized and precise medical practices in heart failure patients.

4 CONCLUSION

During heart failure, the expression of β-adrenergic receptors is significantly downregulated, while the activity of circulating adrenergic receptors increases. The rise in plasma adrenaline levels may compensate for the decrease in adrenergic receptor expression, maintaining the activity of intracellular pathways. Future research will primarily focus on the effects of different drugs on myocardial cell surface β-adrenergic receptors. Clarifying the roles of receptors and systemic levels of adrenaline will effectively guide the treatment of heart failure.

At the same time, we look forward to the emergence of new drugs that can not only lower the level of adrenaline in the blood circulation and reduce damage to target organs but also restore the sensitivity of myocardial cell surface β-adrenergic receptors to maintain the normal function of myocardial cells.

Due to the complex pathological mechanisms of cardiovascular diseases, combined drug therapies targeting different mechanisms (or targets) may achieve better results. Two examples illustrate this approach: First, the combination of angiotensin receptor II blockers and enkephalin inhibitors, which has been shown to have better therapeutic effects than standard therapy, significantly reducing the incidence of cardiovascular endpoint events (cardiovascular death, hospitalization for heart failure, etc.). Second, the use of enalapril folic acid tablets (Yiye) that target high homocysteine levels, which damage vascular endothelium and contribute to the formation of atherosclerosis. High homocysteine levels also increase the risk of stroke, and combining antihypertensive drugs, such as Enalapril, with folic acid has been proven to reduce this risk in large evidence-based medicine studies.

In summary, exploring disease pathophysiological mechanisms and discovering new pathogenic factors, as well as designing combined treatments targeting different pathways, will remain key areas of research for new drugs. The role of β-adrenergic receptors in the pathogenesis of heart failure has been extensively studied, evolving from an initial understanding of the cardiotoxicity of positive inotropic drugs to the current β-adrenergic receptor antagonists. Given the complexity of the adrenaline signaling pathway and the different disease conditions, it is necessary to balance the cardiotoxicity and cardioprotective effects of different receptors. Appropriate β2-adrenergic receptor signaling pathway-biased agonists can be screened from existing β2-adrenergic receptor agonists and their derivatives. At the same time, considering the polymorphism of the patient's β-adrenergic receptor gene, the most effective treatment plan can be selected. More clinical evidence is needed to validate the feasibility of combining β2-adrenergic receptor agonists with β1-adrenergic receptor antagonists in the treatment of heart failure.

REFERENCES

Asano, K., Zisman, L. S., Yoshikawa, T., Headley, V., Bristow, M. R. and Port, D. J. (2001). Bucindolol, a nonselective β1-and β2-adrenergic receptor antagonist, decreases β-adrenergic receptor density in cultured embryonic chick cardiac myocyte membranes. *Journal of Cardiovascular Pharmacology*, 37(6), 678–691.

Chesley A., Lundberg M. S., Toshinobu A., Xiao R. P., Ohtani S., Lakatta E. G. and Michael T. C., (2000). The β2-adrenergic receptor delivers an antiapoptotic signal to cardiac myocytes through Gi-dependent coupling to phosphatidylinositol 3′-kinase. *Circulation Research*, 87(12), 1172–1179.

Chesley, A., Lundberg, M. S., Asai, T., Xiao, R. P., Ohtani, S., Lakatta, E. G. and Crow, M. T. (2000). The beta(2)-adrenergic receptor delivers an antiapoptotic signal to cardiac myocytes through G(i)-dependent coupling to phosphatidylinositol 3'-kinase. *Circulation Research*, 87(12), 1172–1179.

Gauthier C., Seze-Goismier C., Rozec B., (2007). Beta 3-adrenoceptors in the cardiovascular system. *Clinical Hemorheology and Microcirculation*, 37, 193–204.

Hunt S.A., Abraham W.T. and Chin M.H. (2009). American heart association task force on practice guidelines: developed in collaboration with the international society for heart and lung transplantation. *Circulation* 119, 14.

James, J., and Robbins, J. (2011). At the source: treating heart failure by altering muscle motor function. *Circulation Research*, 109(1), 5–7.

Jessup M., Abraham W. T., Casey D. E., Feldman A. M., Francis G. S., Ganiats T. G., Konstam M. A., Mancini D. M., Rahko P. S., Silver M. A., Stevenson L. W., Yancy C. W. (2009). 2009 Writing Group to Review New Evidence and Update the 2005 Guideline for the Management of Patients with Chronic Heart Failure Writing on Behalf of the 2005 Heart Failure Writing Committee, Jessup M, Abraham W T, *et al.* 2009 focused update: ACCF/AHA guidelines for the diagnosis and management of heart failure in adults: a report of the American College of Cardiology Foundation/American Heart Association Task Force on Practice Guidelines: developed in collaboration with the *International Society for Heart and Lung Transplantation Circulation*, 119, 1977–2016.

Konstam, MA and Remme, WJ. (1998). Treatment guidelines in heart failure. *Prog. Cardiovasc. Dis*,41,65–72.

Liu H., Xu Y., Zhang Y.J., Zhang Z.Y. and Ni S.S., (2010). Construction of down-regulated cell model of β2 adrenergic receptor, *Chinese Medical Association*, 7,112–113.

Lowes, B. D., Minobe, W., Abraham, W. T., Rizeq, M. N., Bohlmeyer, T. J., Quaife, R. A., and Bristow, M. R. (1997). Changes in gene expression in the intact human heart. Downregulation of alpha-myosin heavy chain in hypertrophied, failing ventricular myocardium. *The Journal of Clinical Investigation*, 100(9), 2315–2324.

Malík, I., Muselík, J., Stanzel, L., Csöllei, J. and Maruniak, M. (2015). In vitro antioxidant potential of para-alkoxy-phenylcarbamic acid esters containing 4-(4-fluoro-/3-trifluoromethylphenyl) Piperazin-1-Yl Moiety. *Fresenius Environmental Bulletin*, 24(7), 2310–2318.

Zhu, W. Z., Wang, S. Q., Chakir, K., Yang, D., Zhang, T. and Brown. (2003). Linkage of β1-adrenergic stimulation to apoptotic heart cell death through protein kinase A–independent activation of Ca 2+/calmodulin kinase II. *The Journal of Clinical Investigation*,111,617–625.

Biological Sciences and Environmental Health – Gao (Ed.)
© 2025 the Author(s), ISBN: 978-1-032-96016-6

Induced pluripotent stem cells and CRISPR/Cas9 gene editing combined treatment of genetic disorder: Mechanisms, applications, and future

Hantao Wang
The School of Medicine, Imperial College London, London, UK

ABSTRACT: The treatment of genetic disorder is a severe health issue worldwide and has garnered significant attention from the medical and biological fields. While previously, most treatments focus on alleviating the specific complications of genetic diseases instead of effective therapy that can completely eradicate them. However, the emerging iPSCs and CRISPR/Cas9 gene editing combined treatment shows promise in providing complete treatment for patients with genetic diseases. This paper discusses the basic principles and practical application case analysis of this therapy, as well as its advantages, disadvantages, and future possibilities. It shows that CRISPR/Cas9 gene editing can be effectively combined with iPSCs technology in multiple degrees. The CRISPR/Cas9 system can improve the success rate of reprogramming somatic cells and promote the successful generation of iPSCs. It is also used to modify or remove disease-causing genes before iPSCs proliferation. This paper also includes two real life examples of treatment: β-thalassaemia and Huntington's disease. Therapy and modelling based on the iPSCs and CRISPR/Cas9 system are highly patient-specific and can provide valuable experimental data for medical treatment. While there are potential threats in the research process, the treatment still offers unimaginable potential benefits for human society.

1 INTRODUCTION

Throughout human history, small changes in genetic sequences had led to the emergence of a wide variety of genetic diseases. From aplasia, the first genetic disease discovered, to various genetic diseases such as beta thalassemia, Huntington's disease, cystic fibrosis, and others, a large portion of the population is now affected. For newborns, the percentage of live births affected by genetic disorders already exceeded 5%, and genetic disorders caused miscarriages accounted for more than two-thirds of all (Roth and Marson 2021). People of different regions and age groups suffer from genetic diseases. Unfortunately, there are few direct curative therapies available, with most treatments only able to relieve symptoms. In the case of β-thalassemia, the most reliable therapy is hematopoietic stem cell transplantation (or bone marrow transplantation) but restricts by the limitation of human leukocyte antigen (HLA)-matched stem cell donors and patients with other genetic diseases also face a similar challenge too (Trakarnsanga *et al.* 2022).

However, new solutions have emerged in recent years with the continuous advancement of biotechnology, one spotlight is the Induced Pluripotent Stem Cells (iPSCs) therapy. This provides patients with genetic diseases with a sustainable and patient- or disease-specific cell resource that also allows external gene editing (Trakarnsanga *et al.* 2022; Wattanapanitch 2021). By applying convenient CRISPR gene editing to iPSCs cells, it is possible to

DOI: 10.1201/9781003587590-4

effectively relieve the scarcity of HLA-matched stem cell donors and treat more patients. This combined treatment offers both researchers and patients hope to completely eradicate these diseases. Nevertheless, there are still many potential problems in growing usable gene-edited iPSCs, with the three main issues being tumorigenicity, heterogeneity, and genetic instability (Poetsch *et al.* 2022; Yamanaka 2020). Furthermore, the utilization of iPSCs and gene editing therapy in society encounters a variety of ethical criticisms and challenges.

This paper provides a summary of the combination of iPSCs and CRISPR therapy, with the hope of providing help and reference for the faster adoption of this therapy in clinics for different types of genetic diseases. To achieve this, the paper begins by explaining the fundamental principles of iPSCs and CRISPR combination therapy before delving into two well-known genetic disorders that have been treated with this therapy: β-thalassemia and Huntington's disease. And finally concludes by assessing potential future advancements and challenges associated with this therapy.

2 IPSC REPROGRAMMING AND CRISPR/CAS9 EDITING MECHANISMS

2.1 *iPSC reprogramming mechanism*

The iPSCs reprogramming was found by Yamanaka in 2026, the process involves using four key transcription factors (TFs) OCT4, SOX2, KLF4, and cMYC (OSKM) to reprogram terminally differentiated somatic cells (usually human fibroblasts) (Deng *et al.* 2021; Zhang *et al.* 2020). There are two ways to utilize these TFs. The traditional way uses retroviral vectors (RVs) or lentiviral vectors (LVs) to deliver the human genes for these TFs into target somatic cells. However, this method carries a risk of off-target gene activation and heterogeneous reprogramming (Sokka *et al.* 2022), which can produce aberrant iPSCs. Another way involves using the CRISPR/Cas9 system to directly activate endogenous loci, which in turn activates the promoters of OSKM and causes their transcription. Although the two methods use different mechanisms, they both prompt the activation of OSKM and other assisting TFs to initiate the reprogramming process. The key reprogramming process typically starts with the activation of Oct4, which binds to many Oct4 target genes, including mainly miRNAs promoter regions, along with Sox2 (Shi and Jin 2010; Teshigawara *et al.* 2017). These target genes are highly involved in maintaining pluripotency. In humans, this step occurs almost simultaneously with the mesenchymal-to-epithelial transition (MET), as Oct4 and Sox2 can bind to the promoter region of epithelial-associated miRNA and help epithelial genes up-regulation. Therefore, MET can be seen as a crucial and symbolic event in the deviation of iPSCs. Klf4 and c-Myc also cooperate in inducing a pluripotent competent state at a slightly later stage. While the comprehensive reprogramming process is not yet fully understood, these observed steps allow for the reactivation of cells' pluripotency, establishing iPSCs lines with the same pluripotent state as natural embryonic stem cells (ESCs) (Doss and Sachinidis 2019). During this process, some cells acquire a similar pluripotent gene network and epigenetic profile as ESCs, enabling them to differentiate into any type of somatic cell (Doss and Sachinidis 2019).

2.2 *CRISPR/Cas 9 gene editing mechanism*

For the CRISPR/Cas9 system, it was discovered by Ishino in 1987, is a part of the bacterial immune system. Its primary function is to prevent the insertion of viral genetic information during infection. The CRISPR/Cas9 system consists of two components: the Cas9 enzyme and single-guide RNA (sgRNA). The nucleotide sequence of sgRNA is complementary to target DNA, allowing the Cas9 protein to locate the target genes on the genome. Once the Cas9 protein has found the target gene, it acts as a molecular scissor to cut it. The cell then repairs the "damaged" DNA sequence through non-homologous end joining (NHEJ) or homology-directed repair (HDR). The NHEJ pathway involves insertion and deletion, which results in premature stop codons and DNA frameshift, causing target gene inactivation. The HDR pathway replaces the mutated DNA sequence with another homologous chromosome, inserting the correct DNA sequence in the cutting site during the repair process. While the HDR pathway is less efficient since it only occurs in the G or S phase of the cell cycle, it is more reliable and stable than NHEJ as its repair mechanism is more accurate (Bhardwaj *et al.* 2022). CRISPR-Cas9 gene editing can be combined with iPSCs in various stages of genetic disease therapy. As previously mentioned, it can facilitate the reprogramming process of iPSCs since the CRISPR/Cas9 system is highly specific. Its DNA sequence binding specificity is only determined by the sgRNA it carries, allowing for precise control of the activation and expression of OSKM without the need for complex DNA binding protein design (Hockemeyer and Jaenisch 2016). Compared to traditional OSKM activation methods, the CRISPR/Cas9 system is faster, more efficient, and easier to operate and design. Apart from promoting iPSCs reprogramming, the CRISPR/Cas9 system can also directly modify disease-causing genes. Many known genetic diseases are caused by single gene mutation, such as CAG repeats in Huntington's disease or mutation of beta globulin gene in beta-thalassemia. When the sequence of the disease-causing gene is known, scientists can modify or remove genes that cause diseases by editing the sequence of the sgRNA.

3 IPSCS AND CRISPR/CAS9 COMBINED TREATMENT IN β-THALASSEMIA

Thalassemia is one of the most widespread inherited autosomal recessive disorders on Earth and causes a severe public health issue. It is caused by mutations in the alpha and beta-globin genes, which prevent the production of usable global. This results in red blood cells that do not mature properly or transport oxygen effectively, leading to persistently lower haemoglobin concentrations than normal. Long-term blood transfusion is the most common treatment, but it can only maintain basic survival and does not fully cure the disease. Patients may experience complications such as iron overload, high fever, and cardiovascular disease after transfusion. Those patients who receive multiple blood transfusions that in areas with low sanitation may also face the risk of infections such as viral hepatitis, gram-positive cocci infection, or fungal infection (Ebrahimi *et al.* 2021). β-thalassemia is a particularly serious form of thalassemia. Nevertheless, the new treatment that combines iPSCs and CRISPR/Cas9 gene editing has brought hope for patients with β-thalassemia. iPSCs that are reprogrammed from patients' somatic cells can provide a sustained and gene-editable source of cells that are homologous to the patient. The CRISPR/Cas9 gene editing system can effectively modify the beta globulin gene mutation in these iPSCs with homozygous β-thalassemia through the HDR pathway (Wattanapanitch 2021). After the gene editing, the iPSCs become heterozygous for β-thalassemia and then undergo hematopoietic and erythroid differentiation. The final differentiated iPSCs restore the expression of the HBB gene and β-globulin, offering a potential pathway to recovery for patients (Wattanapanitch *et al.* 2018).

4 IPSCS AND CRISPR/CAS9 COMBINED TREATMENT IN HUNTINGTIN'S DISEASE

Huntington's Disease is a dominant and neurodegenerative disorder that primarily affects middle-aged individuals. In patients, many CAG repeats occur in the DNA sequence that encodes the Huntingtin (HTT) protein, causing misfolding of the HTT protein, which leads to the degeneration of the stratal gray matter and cerebral cortex atrophy (Ferrari Bardile *et al.* 2023). Early-stage patients may experience mild cognitive impairment and ineffective coordination of limb movements, which progressively worsen with age, ultimately resulting in movement disorders, cognitive disorders, and neuronal dysfunction. Currently, available treatments can only alleviate individual symptoms of Huntington's Disease and cannot directly eradicate it. Like the treatment of β-thalassemia, in iPSCs lines derived from patients, the CRISPR/Cas9 complex can recognize and cut the repeated CAG fragments by altering the sgDNA sequence. This will cause a reduction in mutated HTT expression and partial recovery of the patient's motor and speech function. Multiple sgRNAs are combined in actual treatment to target different target genes and achieve multiplex gene changes (Alkanli *et al.* 2023). In new experiments, modified Cas9 nucleases are used, which can alter the energy of the Cas9/sgRNA complex and effectively reduce off-target binding and off-target effects (Sokka et al. 2022).

In addition to therapies that have already been applied to actual treatments, iPSCs are widely used to establish neurodegenerative disease models, providing opportunities for in vitro experiments and the cultivation of patient-specific therapies. The CRISPR/Cas9 system itself can also be utilized to produce animals with genetically mutated genomes that are responsible for human diseases, which can be used to study the pathology of diseases.

The occurrence of iPSCs and CRISPR/Cas9 combined therapy is a significant breakthrough in the fields of medicine and biology. This advancement has brought renewed hope for the complete cure of many diseases that were previously deemed incurable. Besides Beta-thalassemia and Huntington's disease, there are many other diseases that can be treated. iPSCs can serve as a cellular source for degenerative diseases like Alzheimer's disease, Friedreich ataxia, and Parkinson's disease. Moreover, numerous prevalent genetic diseases have the potential to be cured, and there is even the possibility of completely eradicating inherited genetic diseases in the human population.

5 ADVANTAGES OF THE COMBINED TREATMENT

The unique ability of induced pluripotent stem cells (iPSCs) to self-renew and differentiate into diverse cell types makes them an unparalleled and sustainable source for medical treatment. By reprogramming patient-derived cells, ethical concerns around using ESCs can be effectively avoided. Patient-specific iPSCs can perfectly meet the needs of patients and are more easily accepted by their bodies, effectively avoiding many complications of immune rejection after transplantation. The use of the CRISPR/Cas9 system can effectively solve the low efficiency and randomness of reprogramming, as it can target the promoter region of OSKM to control the opening and closing of its factors to guide somatic cell reprogramming. Compared to traditional transfer methods through RVs or LVs, the CRISPR/Cas9 complex is more stable and efficient. The forced expression of transcription factors in traditional gene editing may cause off-target gene activation and heterogeneous reprogramming, making the output iPSCs more like the original cells rather than true pluripotent stem cells.

The combination treatment can be taken to another level by creating disease models (Doss and Sachinidis 2019). The foundation of human pathology is mainly based on experimental observation, but it is still difficult to obtain usable cell sources from patients or establish unique human disease models due to a lack of effective clinical trial opportunities. This greatly delays and limits the development of treatment methods. Common non-clinical efficacy models that can be used to investigate, such as animal models, face a high risk of failure during the transition to humans. The virtually limitless proliferation potential of iPSCs makes them ideal for use in thousands of experiments, and they are also more cost-effective than obtaining cells directly from patients. Furthermore, iPSCs derived from the patient's own cells can be used to develop personalized therapies, establishing special case models for individual patients. One significant advantage is that these models can reduce the drug wastage. The common dosage of drugs can only be roughly given based on the patient's performance, but such judgments are often not accurate enough and not specific to each patient. Overdoses may cause serious side effects while underdosing can be ineffective and wasteful. Patients' specific model can help to find suitable dosage more accurately. In addition, iPSCs are easy to obtain and have high differentiation abilities, which can expedite the elucidation of pathological physiological mechanisms of diseases in basic research and safety pharmacology. Several countries, including the United States, Mexico, and Panama, are establishing relevant laws and systems for iPSCs disease treatment, and putting them into practical clinical use.

6 DISADVANTAGES AND CHALLENGES OF THE COMBINED TREATMENT

While iPSCs and CRISPR/Cas9 technology combined treatment offers numerous advantages, it is still important to acknowledge the potential risks and defects that come with its development. One of the most concerning risks is the possibility of tumorigenicity in iPSC therapy. The high proliferation ability of iPSCs is its most attractive feature but it is also a double-edged sword. Undifferentiated iPSCs during proliferation period have a high risk of developing into teratomas or malignant tumours due to the possible gene mutation. The inappropriate regulation of the reprogramming factors, such as c-Myc, a mutated gene that often occurs in human cancer, inside the cell can also cause the iPSCs carcinogenesis. Additionally, heterogeneity, reprogrammed iPSCs may retain certain epigenetic memories of the original cells, which can result in differentiation into specific types of cells during differentiation rather than complete reset programming. This will be an obstacle for these cells to be applied to the downstream circumstances. Although more precise gene editing controls and improved in vitro directed differentiation pathways are commonly used to reduce these possibilities, it has not been eliminated. Moreover, in vitro culture of iPSCs may still have genetic instability such as chromosomal abnormalities and loss of the original gene sequence, which currently has no effective resolution (Yamanaka 2020).

In addition to the technical level, the iPSCs and CRISPR/Cas9 technology combined treatment technology still faces certain ethical issues at the social level. Unlike the problems arising from the use of ESCs, the combination treatment itself does not have a high ethical rejection, but some potential downstream uses of iPSC cell derivatives may be very sensitive. For example, large-scale genetic sequencing of patients and the use of patient-derived cells as iPSC sources may trigger a stalemate similar to the famous HeLa cell lawsuit, not only touching on the patient's right to know and the attribution of cell usage rights but also easily arousing public concerns about privacy and confidentiality in medical care. In addition, some iPSC cell derivatives are injected into non-human animals after the establishment of disease models. The impact of these derivatives on organisms is unknown, but they may cause animal protectionists' vigilance and protests to a great extent (Takashima *et al.* 2023).

7 CONCLUSION

This paper highlights the potential of combining iPSCs and CRISPR/Cas9 gene editing in genetic disease and disease modelling. Reprogramming somatic cells using the CRISPR/Cas9 system can avoid off-target gene activation and heterogeneous reprogramming and generate iPSCs sources needed by patients more efficiently and accurately. Moreover, CRISPR/Cas9 gene editing is fast, convenient, and easy to design. Medical staff can quickly learn and utilize this technique without requiring extensive training and practice. This benefit makes it highly advantageous for developing countries, as it is cost-effective and does not require significant resources to cultivate skilled personnel. For genotypic diseases caused by known mutation sequences, precise cutting can be performed by changing the sgRNA sequence in CRISPR/Cas9 complex, and disease-causing genes can be modified and processed by NHEJ or HDR pathway. Furthermore, the use of iPSCs as a cell source can also avoid ethical issues and immune rejection associated with the use of ESCs. This technology is currently in the clinical stage with patients suffering from β-thalassaemia and Huntington's Disease receiving treatment. Research is also being conducted to explore treatment options for other genetic and degenerative diseases such as Alzheimer's, Down's syndrome, and haemophilia. Combining iPSCs and CRISPR/Cas9 gene editing technology can also be used to establish human-specific disease models for research and discovery of more possible therapies. Although problems such as carcinogenesis and iPSCs heterogeneity may be encountered during research and experimentation, as the specific pathway of iPSCs reprogramming and CRISPR/Cas9 gene editing becomes clearer, these dangers may be gradually resolved. The combination of gene editing and iPSCs therapy can cover more than just the simple treatment of genetic diseases. Disease models based on these technologies can be applied to a range of diseases such as cardiovascular diseases, cancer, and leukaemia. Additionally, these two technologies can also be applied to in vitro organ cultivation to reduce the plight of human organs being in short supply. The application prospects of the interaction and combination of these two technologies are difficult to estimate. In the coming future, perhaps iPSCs and CRISPR/Cas9 combination therapy will become one of the treatment options accessible to all patients around the world.

REFERENCES

Alkanli S.S., Alkanli N., Ay A. and Albeniz I., (2023). *Mol Neurobiol.* **60** (3), 1486

Bhardwaj S., Kesari K.K., Rachamalla M., Mani S., Ashraf G.M., Jha S.K., Kumar P., Ambasta R.K., Dureja H., Devkota H.P., Gupta G., Chellappan D.K., Singh S.K., Dua K., Ruokolainen J., Kamal M.A., Ojha S. and Jha N.K., (2022). *J Adv Res.* **40**, 207

Deng W., Jacobson E.C., Collier A.J. and Plath K., (2021). *Curr Opin Genet Dev.* **70**, 89

Doss M.X. and Sachinidis A., (2019). *Cells.* **8** (5)

Ebrahimi M., Mohammadi-Asl J., Rahim F., (2021). *Ann Hum Biol.* **48** (4), 307

Ferrari Bardile C., Radulescu C.I. and Pouladi M.A., (2023). *Trends Mol Med.*

Hockemeyer D. and Jaenisch R., (2016). *Cell Stem Cell.* **18** (5), 573

Poetsch M.S., Strano A., Guan K., (2022). *Stem Cells.* **40** (6), 546

Roth T.L. and Marson A., (2021). *Annu Rev Pathol.* **16**, 145

Shi G. and Jin Y., (2010). *Stem Cell Res Ther.* **1** (5), 39

Sokka J., Yoshihara M., Kvist J., Laiho L., Warren A., Stadelmann C., Jouhilahti E.M., Kilpinen H., Balboa D., Katayama S., Kyttala A., Kere J., Otonkoski T., Weltner J. and Trokovic R., (2022). *Stem Cell Reports.* **17** (2), 413

Takashima K., Minari J., Chan S. and Muto K., (2023). *Regen Ther.* **24**, 294

Teshigawara R., Cho J., Kameda M. and Tada T., (2017). *Lab Invest.* **97** (10), 1152

Trakarnsanga K., Thongsin N., Metheetrairut C., Tipgomut C., Poldee S. and Wattanapanitch M., (2022). *Sci Rep.* **12** (1), 15551

Wattanapanitch M., (2021). *Methods Mol Biol.* 2211, **193**

Wattanapanitch M., (2021). *Methods Mol Biol.* **2211**, 193

Wattanapanitch M., Damkham N., Potirat P., Trakarnsanga K., Janan M., U.P.Y, Kheolamai P., Klincumhom N. and Issaragrisil S., (2018). *Stem Cell Res Ther.* **9** (1), 46

Yamanaka S., (2020). *Cell Stem Cell* **27** (4), 523.

Zhang L., Wang Y., Zhang Y., Wang L. and Huang H., (2020). *Cell Reprogram.* **22** (2), 99

Biological Sciences and Environmental Health – Gao (Ed.)
© 2025 the Author(s), ISBN: 978-1-032-96016-6

Model construction of human knee joint based on organ chips

Hanyu Tian
Department of Biomedical Engineering, The Hong Kong Polytechnic University (PolyU), Hong Kong, China

ABSTRACT: As people's lifestyle requirements become higher, knee joint diseases are becoming more and more common, and seriously affect the quality of life of patients. Knee arthritis is a common disease and causes cartilage to age and changes in the cells within the joint. However, traditional disease models can only restore or replace the real in vivo environment of humans to a certain extent. The organ-on-a-chip technology uses a microfluidic-based physiological system to fully simulate the human environment. This technology has been applied to osteoarthritis by many people, simulating human blood vessel modeling and human bone tissue. Organ chips can accurately represent the tissue structure and cell response of the human body under the environment of simulating the natural tissue environment of the human body. And more precise control of cell types and experimental results. Although there are still major challenges, the development of organ-on-a-chip can completely change the process of drug research and provide more efficient and diversified treatment methods for disease treatment. Advances in organ-on-a-chip technology mark a critical step in the connection between theoretical medicine and clinical trials, enabling the rapid development of future medical care.

1 INTRODUCTION

As people's lives become more and more tiring, knee joint diseases are emerging in an endless stream, which is related to the high incidence of such diseases, the serious decline in people's quality of life, and some people's own disabilities or genetic problems. And osteoarthritis is the 11th disease affecting humans and one of the most common diseases in the elderly (Kim and Keating 2019). Osteoarthritis is a very deformable disease that causes cartilage aging and rapid aging of chondrocytes and dedifferentiation of chondrocytes, and this disease usually affects the entire joint. Since this disease will affect many joint tissues, and the current traditional disease model research is often limited by the limitations of animal experiments and in vitro cell culture, it is difficult to accurately simulate the pathogenesis of human joint diseases. In recent years, chip technology based on organ chips has been increasingly prominent. This review starts from the organ-on-a-chip technology, discuss its application in the construction of human joint disease models, summarize the existing research results, and look forward to the future development.

2 DIFFERENT ORGAN CHIP APPLICATION SCENARIOS

2.1 *The principle of organ chip technology*

Organ-on-a-chip is the most advanced technology in the field of 3D culture technology. Organ-on-a-chip and micro-physiological systems can more effectively reproduce natural

DOI: 10.1201/9781003587590-5

tissue environment samples, human tissue structure, and cell-specific responses (Tian *et al.* 2015). And on human bone-like tissue and human fat, microfluidic technology can still create a good environment for experiments (Loskill *et al.* 2017; Mansoorifar *et al.* 2020). As shown in Figure 1, Organ chips can have various sizes and shapes, but they all contain hollow channels, which can cultivate various living cells and tissues of the human body under the flowing artificial liquid. In some designs, for example, the Figure 1d shown that the organ chip can also realize the simulation of the whole body of the human body by coupling two or more organ chips. The application of induced pluripotent stem cells in this respect is of great significance. The most basic organ-on-a-chip is an organ-on-a-chip that is optically transparent and has two channels driven mechanically. It is usually made by soft lithography using PDMS. Different cell tissues are cultured on the bottom as well as on top of the matrix-coated membrane. For example, when performing alveolar simulation, the bottom of the cells is usually liquid, and the top can be air, which simulates the actual situation of human alveolar cells through air.

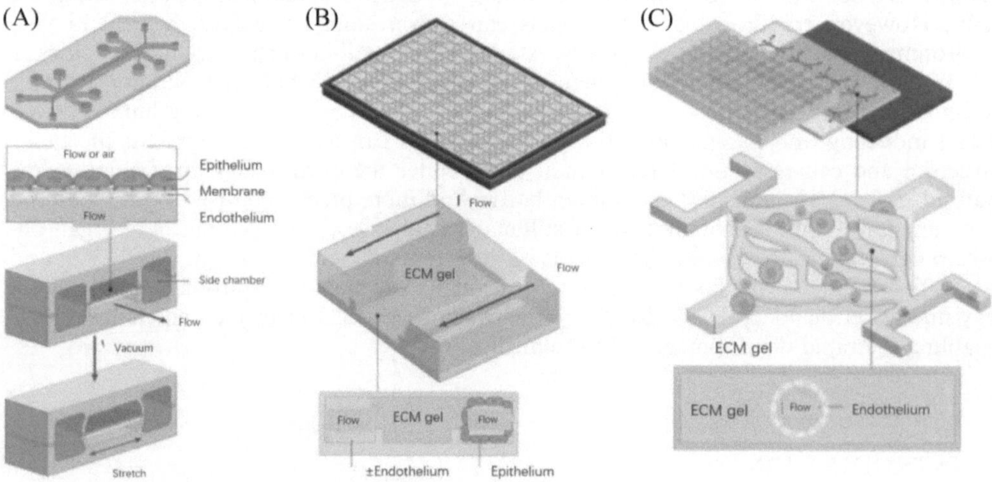

Figure 1. Different organ-on-chips models A) The organ chips' classic model; B) Three-channel chip; C) Communication of multiple organ chips (Loskill *et al.* 2017).

2.2 *Pyramid concentration gradient*

Microfluidics now use pyramidal concentration gradient generators and downstream cell culture modules. Due to the Raynaud effect, the liquid presents a laminar flow when it passes through the serpentine channel of the microfluidic chip. Under the pyramidal concentration gradient generator, the laminar flow can combine with the adjacent flow and diffusely mix through the serpentine channel. The result is a dilution of the solution and a series of concentration gradients at the outlet.

2.3 *Microphysiology WAT chip*

When simulating the physiological environment of adipose tissue in the human body, there is another microphysiological system, which is mainly composed of medium channels, circular cell chambers and microporous membranes. This is similar to the blood circulation in the body. The medium channel serves as the connector of each channel, constantly delivering fresh nutrients and other drugs or artificially added factors into this microphysiological environment, and transporting some metabolic waste and many biological Factors are transported from the microphysiological environment. And in microfluidics, the volume and flow of nanoliter fluid can be compared and controlled in time and laterally. Compared to standard cell cultures, the use of very small liquids prevents non-physiological explanations for autocrine production of cells. And independent culture medium and tissue chambers make the whole system more flexible in structure and operation (Loskill *et al.* 2017).

2.4 *Organ chips applied in bone*

Bone tissue tends to be arranged in a more complex structure due to its mineralized matrix. The dense matrix layer around the bone tissue contains blood vessels and nerve fibres, so it can be said that the nerves innervate the bone tissue and define the bone tissue from a biological point of view. Compared with traditional 2D culture, microfluidic technology has an in vivo environment that is closer to the human body itself. This can be achieved by inventing some more novel microdevices, such as this microdevices, which can monitor and control the exchange between cells and oxygen and nutrients in real time (Mansoorifar *et al.* 2020).

3 EVALUATING THERAPIES USING ORGAN CHIPS AS MODELS

3.1 *Prediction of knee osteoarthritis using organ chips*

Osteoarthritis of the knee is a chronic all-joint disease characterized by degeneration or loss of cartilage and inflammation of the synovial membrane. The current non-surgical treatment for knee osteoarthritis includes physical and drug methods as treatment methods. Drug treatment includes injection of class IA drugs, or corticosteroids and mesenchymal stromal cells (Caldwell *et al.* 2006). However, these methods still have large side effects in treating patients. For example, in an analysis by Jevsevar *et al.*, it showed that patients who were injected with drugs such as acetaminophen still suffered from severe knee pain compared with those injected with placebo. patients (Jevsevar *et al.* 2018). And if these drugs fail, the patient faces a much riskier total knee replacement. Although total knee replacement surgery is the best treatment for OA, it is also very risky. Most patients indicated that there would still be more sequelae after surgery, and a long recovery time was required (Goodman *et al.* 2014). However, the cycle of developing new drugs is very long, so the use of organ chips, that is, microphysiological systems, has become more advantageous in this regard.

Organ chips can enable each organ to perform independently in vitro, and then through artificial connections, a relatively intact human simulation system can be established for in vitro experiments. For example, Meagan J once established a joint system composed of osteocartilage, fat, and fiber analogues, and, like the Figure 2, organ chips are used to explore the relationship between osteoarthritis and biomechanics. The joint system was cultivated for one month before the osteoarthritis was stimulated by chemical methods. And the genotype and phenotype changes of the samples obtained by the system were compared with the samples of osteoarthritis, and it was proved that the simulation of this system can fully indicate the disease characteristics of osteoarthritis. It better simulates the human knee cartilage (Li *et al.* 2022). In the experiment, hBMSC (human bone marrow-derived stem cells) were used to generate the micro-joint physiological system. All microarticular systems were generated from human bone marrow-derived stem cells that were cultured for 28 days in osteogenic medium (10% FBS, 1x antibiotics, 10-7M dexamethasone) to generate OC tissue. But the whole system needs three parts, and the remaining two parts are AT and SFT. AT is a medium for adipogenesis, and SFT is cultured for 21 days after human bone marrow-derived stem cells are expanded by 80-90% in a T300 flask and then GM is switched to a cellulose-producing medium.

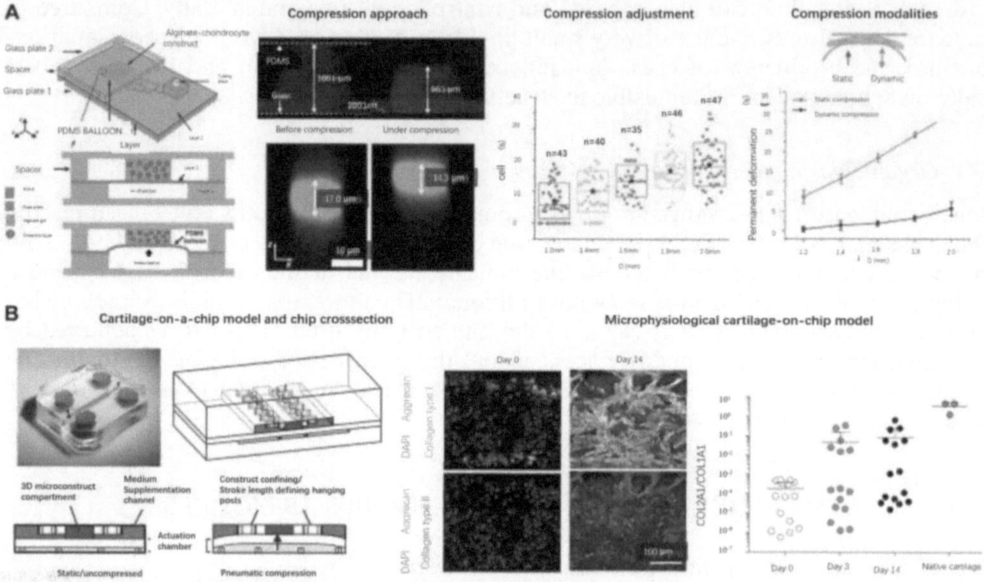

Figure 2. Exploring the impact of biomechanics on osteoarthritis through organ-on-a-chip A) Conditions showing that microfluidic gases can transfer mechanical stress to study bone derivation mechanisms. B) Development of a cartilage-on-a-chip with 3D Cartilage Structure (Rothbauer *et al.* 2022).

Finally, more and more evidence showed that the organ-on-a-chip and microphysiological system can be used as a new tool for studying human knee osteoarthritis. Various models and methods can replicate one or more components of the knee joint for simulation. And hBMSC can allow people to further design the fat group and fibre group, so as to facilitate the further engineering design of analogues.

Occhetta *et al.* developed a cartilage-on-a-chip model of the relationship between osteoarthritis and mechanical loading (Occhetta *et al.* 2019). Nuclear factor-κB is an important factor related to chondrocyte development, and this factor plays an important role in the process of osteoarthritis. Many of them are associated with signaling (Feng *et al.* 2017; Xu *et al.* 2021). Due to the importance of this factor, further experiments on it have been carried out by Jevsevar *et al.* And it has performance in mouse model and organ-on-a-chip model.

3.2 *Model prediction of knee joint bones and blood vessels using organ chips*

Organ chips can not only predict human cartilage, but also model blood vessels and bone tissue. Compared with the traditional in vitro culture model, the microfluidic model, especially the organ-on-a-chip platform, provides more release tissue culture conditions and improves clinical analysis capabilities. Since human bone tissue is a highly mineralized tissue, it only performs basic human functions, such as movement and support. Due to the complex structure of bone cells, as well as the tight junctions between bone cells and neighboring cells, this will affect the results during the experiment. The microfluidic device can promote cell culture and development. Compared with traditional 2D cell culture, it can more easily simulate the living environment of cells and improve the tight junction of cells. Because we can artificially control the proliferation of cells. For example, Amin Mansoorifar's group controlled the flow rate of bone cells and showed the growth of cells under different flow rates. It also proved that bone cells can grow smoothly and carry out experiments under microfluidic conditions. In Figure 3, people apply organ chips to human bone tissue.

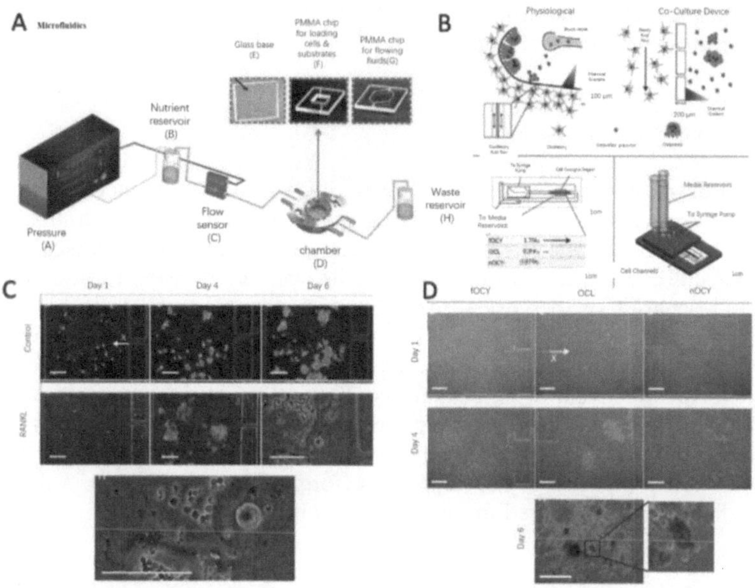

Figure 3. Application of Organ Chips on Bones. A) The entire microfluidic system is displayed, which is composed of a high-precision pressure pump, nutrient solution, waste storage, flow sensor, and microfluidic chamber. B) This figure shows how the two physiological environments are simulated using microfluidic devices and compared with the devices installed on the manifold. C) This graph shows osteoclasts cultured in RANKL-supplemented medium on days 1, 4, and 6 and the control group. D) This figure shows images of fOCY, OCL and nOCY cells on days 1 and 4 of culture. and shows TRAP+ staining of osteoclasts on day six. (Mansoorifar *et al.* 2020).

4 FUTURE CHALLENGES AND OPPORTUNITIES

In the past few decades, only animal models have made great achievements in biology and medicine. However, with the development of the times, people are increasingly aware of the limitations of existing animal models, especially in the simulation of some human bodies that cannot achieve most of the synchronization with the human body. Products after various mouse experiments still need a lot of time for human clinical trials. But organ-on-a-chip is still in its infancy, but the ability to use organ-on-a-chip can overcome the old animal experimental models and the methods we have been using for decades.

Although organ-on-a-chip is developing very rapidly, it still needs a lot of development, and it cannot be applied in clinical medicine at the current level, especially for the development of drugs. One of the key challenges is that the organ chip cannot fully simulate the internal environment of a whole human body, and currently only a small part of the simulator tubes are connected. Most of the organs have not yet been connected, and real organ chips have not been achieved, which can be used to replace human experiments.

At present, the most important construction method of organ chips is to use PDMS to construct, because PDMS requires low cost, and has good optical permeability and gas permeability. However, PDMS has a natural defect, that is, it can absorb some small molecule hydrophobic substances (Meer *et al.* 2017). In order to prevent this problem, it is still necessary to use other carriers, such as the use of nanomaterials. Modifying the nanomaterials to be hydrophilic or making the nanomaterials unable to further combine with PDMS prevents the drug in them from being absorbed by PDMS, resulting in the failure of the experiment. In order to improve this shortcoming, we still need to continue to pay attention to the alternative materials of PDMS, thinking that in the future, better materials can be provided for the model of organ chips.

5 CONCLUSION

With the rapid development of science and technology and the advancement of organ chip technology, more novel materials and methods can be used to simulate human organs in a deeper level. Organ chips can provide a more accurate human physiological model and a more physiologically relevant and predictive in vitro platform in the future, and realize the integration and progress of theoretical medicine and clinical medicine in a way that traditional technologies cannot match. As emphasized in this review, the advancement of organ-on-a-chip can provide more reliable clinical trial evaluation in the future, and can effectively and greatly shorten the cycle of clinical trials. This move can provide a more convenient method for the future development of the pharmaceutical industry. We can artificially speed up or slow down the reaction process, and strictly control the dose to shorten the cycle. It is conceivable that after the further development of organ chip technology in the future, people's various diseases will be cured in more diverse and efficient ways.

REFERENCES

Caldwell B., Aldington S., Weatherall M., Shirtcliffe P., and Beasley R., (2006). *Journal of the Royal Society of Medicine* **99**, 132.

Feng S., Bowden N., Fragiadaki M., Souilhol C., Hsiao S., Mahmoud M., Allen S. T., Pirric D., Blanca Tardajos Ayllon, Akhtar S., Thompson A. S., Jo H., Weber C., Ridger V., Schober A. and Evans P. G., (2017). *Arteriosclerosis, Thrombosis, and Vascular Biology* **37**, 2087.

Goodman S. B., Konttinen Y. T. and Takagi M., (2014). *Journal of Long-Term Effects of Medical Implants* **24**, 253.

Jevsevar D. S., Shores P. B., Mullen K., Schulte D. M., Brown G. A., and Cummins D. S., (2018). *Journal of the American Academy of Orthopaedic Surgeons* **26**, 325.

Kim C. and Keating A., (2019). *Gerontology* **65**, 294.

Li Z., Lin Z., Liu S., Yagi H., Zhang X., Yocum L., Romero-Lopez M., Rhee C., Makarcyzk M. J., Yu I., Li E. N., Fritch M. R., Gao Q., Goh K. B., O'Donnell B. T., Hao T., Alexander P. G., Bhushan Mahadik, J. P. Fisher, and Goodman S. B., (2022). *Advanced Science* **9**, 2105909.

Loskill P., Sezhian T., Tharp K. M., Lee-Montiel F. T., Jeeawoody S., Reese W. M., Zushin P.-J. H., Stahl A., and Healy K. E., (2017). *Lab on a Chip* **17**, 1645.

Mansoorifar A., Gordon R., Bergan R. C., and Bertassoni L. E., (2020). *Advanced Functional Materials* **31**, 2006796.

Occhetta P., Mainardi A., Votta E., Vallmajo-Martin Q., Ehrbar M., Martin I., Barbero A. and Rasponi M., (2019). *Nature Biomedical Engineering* **3**, 545.

Rothbauer M., Reihs E. I., Fischer A., Windhager R., Jenner F., and Toegel S., (2022). *Frontiers in Bioengineering and Biotechnology* **10**, 886360.

Tian K., Zhong W., Zhang Y., Yin B., Zhang W., and Liu H., (2015). *Molecular Medicine Reports* **13**, 67.

van Meer B. J., de Vries H., Firth K. S. A., van Weerd J., Tertoolen L. G. J., Karperien H. B. J., Jonkheijm P., Denning C., IJzerman A. P., and Mummery C. L., (2017). *Biochemical and Biophysical Research Communications* **482**, 323.

Xu Z., Ke T., Zhang Y., Guo L., Chen F., and He W., (2021). *Molecular Medicine* **27**, 80.

Biological Sciences and Environmental Health – Gao (Ed.)

Research progress and prospects of mesenchymal stem cells for neurodegenerative disease treatment

Ziyan He
College of Basic Medical Sciences, Shanghai Jiao Tong University, Shanghai, China

ABSTRACT: As the global population continues to age, there is a mounting emphasis on addressing a myriad of aging-related ailments, with a particular spotlight on neurodegenerative diseases. These neurological conditions are often marked by their irreversible nature, a characteristic that becomes even more daunting when considering the limited therapeutic options currently available to mitigate the progression of these disorders. Amidst this challenging landscape, mesenchymal stem cells (MSCs) have emerged as a beacon of hope and have swiftly become a central subject of extensive scientific research. One of the primary reasons for the burgeoning interest in MSCs is their accessibility. Furthermore, they exhibit a plethora of therapeutic potentials. Their innate qualities include capabilities for neuroregeneration, providing neuroprotection, and modulating immune responses, making them a promising candidate for therapeutic interventions. This comprehensive paper delves into the potential of MSCs-based treatments specifically tailored for neurodegenerative ailments. It elucidates the underlying mechanisms of various therapeutic approaches, such as transplantation therapy, exosome therapy, and gene-modification therapy. By analyzing their therapeutic outcomes in diverse animal models, this review offers a holistic understanding of their efficacy. Moreover, in light of the challenges and gaps identified in existing research, the paper also charts out potential avenues for future investigations, aiming to further refine and optimize MSCs-based interventions for neurological disorders.

1 INTRODUCTION

The global population is undergoing a significant transformation as it ages at an unprecedented pace. Ageing is intricately interlinked with physical degeneration, leading to heightened susceptibility to disease and mortality. Notably, neurodegenerative disorders have received considerable attention among the ailments associated with the ageing process. The significance of neurodegeneration and its subsequent cognitive decline holds particular prominence, exerting a substantial influence on health span and overall quality of life.

The complex mechanisms beneath neuronal impairments present a significant barrier to an in-depth comprehension of the pathogenic events involved, impeding the creation of efficient remedies. Additionally, the central nervous system (CNS) has a limited ability for regeneration, rendering it arduous to target extensive neuronal cell death. Furthermore, the majority of drugs encounter formidable challenges in traversing the blood-brain barrier (BBB), exacerbating the difficulties in controlling these conditions.

Numerous therapeutic strategies have undergone extensive exploration over the course of several decades. However, a definitive cure remains elusive, necessitating a steadfast focus on preventive approaches. Particular groups of neurons, like dopaminergic and cholinergic neurons, as well as motor neurons, experience increasing degeneration in neurodegenerative illnesses, resulting in particular types of neurologic impairment. Since stem cell transplantation

DOI: 10.1201/9781003587590-6

has the potential to have a variety of reparative responses within the CNS, it seems to be a viable therapeutic alternative. Neuronal stem cells (NSCs) represent the primary physiological niche in neurodegenerative disorders, for its capability of self-renewing and differentiating into neurons and glia cells. Promising evidence of functional advantages following NSC transplantation has been found in animal models of diverse neurodegenerative disorders (Forotti *et al.* 2019). In many studies, transplanted human neural stem cells (hNSCs) have been observed to form cell clusters near the injection site in the grownup brain, demonstrating restricted migration capabilities that may restrict their therapeutic efficacy (Öz *et al.* 2023).

While NSCs demonstrate some therapeutic potential, their ability to replace damaged or lost neurons in the affected regions may be limited. NSCs that have been transplanted can induce an immune response, leading to rejection or damage to the transplanted cells. What is more, the source of neural stem cells raises ethical concerns. Obtaining them from fetal tissue or embryos raises ethical dilemmas and limits their widespread use. Meanwhile, the majority of studies identify nutritional and immunomodulatory benefits as the key treatment method, rather than neuronal replacement. Previous researches on NSCs indicate that their therapeutic benefits may be linked to paracrine action (Dause *et al.* 2022).

By contrast, mesenchymal stem cells (MSCs) are derived from a variety of tissues, including bone marrow, umbilical cord and adipose tissue, rendering them more readily obtainable and prepared for various stem cell applications. The high proliferation and differentiation potential of MSCs makes it possible to expand them through in vitro culture, which results in a sufficient number of cells for transplantation. Furthermore, MSCs possess the capacity to transform into a range of cell types, including neurons, glial cells, and vascular cells, which entails improved functional recovery. MSCs have a low level of surface antigen expression, which may reduce the risk of immune rejection (Yoshida *et al.* 2020). The stimulation of neurogenesis, synaptogenesis, neuronal differentiation, and amyloidogenesis and/or microglia activation by MSCs has been reported in studies, which mutually results in a reduction in Aβ accumulation and cognitive recovery (Moreno-Jiménez *et al.* 2019).

In vivo injection of MSCs inhibits neuroinflammation and secretes growth factors in neurodegenerative disease models. A growing amount of data from preclinical studies support the multispectral differentiation and immunomodulatory properties of MSC (Li *et al.* 2023). However, only a few studies have received regulatory approval and marketing authorization for MSC-based therapeutic product (Krampera and Blanc 2021).

This review elucidates the current state of therapeutic strategies involving mesenchymal stem cells (MSCs) for neurodegenerative disease treatment. Besides, intricate mechanisms underlying MSC-mediated therapeutic effects were expounded (Figure 1). Furthermore, a critical assessment of the obstacles encountered among MSC-based therapies is presented, along with the identification of essential pathways for future research endeavours.

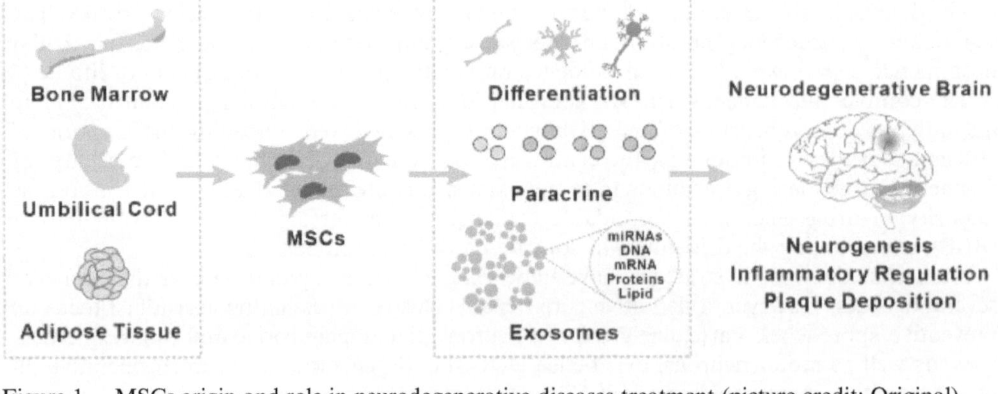

Figure 1. MSCs origin and role in neurodegenerative diseases treatment (picture credit: Original).

2 MECHANISM AND APPLICATION OF MSCS TRANSPLANTATION FOR NEURODEGENERATIVE DISEASES

MSCs are defined as cells that can self-renew and develop mesenchymal tissue characteristics. MSCs produce therapeutic effects mainly through differentiation, immunomodulation and secretion of neurotrophic factors.

MSCs have the potential for multidirectional differentiation, with capability to transform into cells not only within the mesodermal lineage but also encompassing endodermal and neural ectodermal cells, notably neurons and glial cells. Stereotactic injection delivers MSCs directly to the lesion area. Behavioural abnormalities in neurotoxin 6-hydroxydopamine-induced Parkinson's disease (PD) rat model were ameliorated by intracerebroventricularly injected bone marrow-derived mesenchymal stem cells (BM-MSCs), for they partially differentiated into nestin and GFAP expressing cells (Chen *et al.* 2017). Intravenously infused MSCs are able to cross the blood-brain barrier (BBB) to migrate towards the focal area through chemotaxis, secreting various neurotrophic factors, finally differentiate into neuron-like cells. After being injected, BM-MSCs were able to home in the damaged brain and exerted a therapeutic effect on PD rat model through a multi-methodic effect (Ahmed *et al.* 2016).

Neuroimmune cells (namely microglia and astrocytes), when stimulated into a pro-inflammatory state, are widely implicated as pathological agents in numerous neurodegenerative disorders. These cells assume a pivotal role in the advancement of said neurodegenerative conditions (Lampe *et al.* 2019; Schain and Kreisl 2017). MSCs exert immunomodulatory effects that intricately regulate inflammatory responses within the context of neurodegenerative diseases, ultimately culminating in the mitigation of cerebral tissue damage. By releasing an array of soluble mediators such as tumour necrosis factor, interleukin, ciliary neurotrophic factor and neurotrophic factor, MSCs hold potent anti-inflammatory capabilities (Sobacchi *et al.* 2017). Study shows that MSCs exert immunosuppressive effects, dampening immune responses and restraining microglial activation through the induction of tumour necrosis factor-stimulated gene-6 expression (Liu *et al.* 2019). Na *et al.* demonstrated that the transplantation of MSCs elicits a dual impact on inflammation: it promotes microglial activation while concurrently attenuating the NLRP3 inflammasome, thereby instigating an anti-inflammatory milieu (Na *et al.* 2020).

Moreover, MSCs have the capacity to secrete neurotrophic factors, thereby fostering neuronal growth, enhancing regenerative processes. Jia *et al.* applied human umbilical cord MSCs to an Alzheimer's disease (AD) mouse model, demonstrating its ability to promote synaptic plasticity and mediate cognitive enhancement by secreting hepatocyte growth factor through activation of cMet-AKT-GSK3β signalling pathway (Jia *et al.* 2020). Park *et al.* proved intravenous injection of human adipose-derived MSCs to have therapeutic effects on PD mice by restoring BDNF and GDNF expression to protect dopaminergic neurons (Park and Chang 2020).

3 APPLICATION OF MSCS-DERIVED EXOSOMES IN NEURODEGENERATIVE DISEASES

Further research has revealed that the therapeutic functions of MSCs primarily occur through paracrine signalling pathways, with exosomes emerging as a key component of their paracrine effects. Exosomes are small extracellular vesicles (EVs) secreted by cells with a lipid bilayer membrane (Cocozza *et al.* 2020). MSC-Derived Exosomes (MSC-Exo) encompass a diverse array of components, ranging from small molecules, lipids, nucleic acids to proteins. These constituents have the potential to exert profound effects on a series of cellular processes, specifically cell migration, proliferation, apoptosis and immune regulation. This capability holds substantial promise for mitigating deficits associated with neurodegenerative diseases. A study using APP/PS1 mice shows that MSC-Exo exhibits targeting of the cortex and hippocampus via intravesical administration and is able to improve cognitive function (Cui *et al.* 2019). It was demonstrated that there was a reduction in Aβ levels and plaque deposition in the brain, as well as a decrease in astrocyte and microglia activation, expression of synaptic protein 1 and PSD95 was enhanced and cognitive deficits was rescued (Cui *et al.* 2019). Chen *et al.* proved PD rats model exhibited no trouble with MSC-Exos getting through the BBB and into the substantia nigra for dopaminergic neurons, which reduced apoptotic cell death and the asymmetric rotation caused by apomorphine (Chen *et al.* 2020).

Exosomes derived from MSCs not only replicate the functions of MSCs but also offer distinct advantages, including immunomodulatory properties and a reduced risk of tumorigenicity. Studies have shown that MSC-derived exosomes have broad immunomodulatory capacity (Xie *et al.* 2020). Exosomes are smaller and have low/no expression of membrane surface tissue antigens compared to MSCs and are demonstrated to inhibit immune rejection (Qian *et al.* 2020). Clinical safety of MSCs is highly challenged due to its tumorgenicity (Jeong *et al.* 2011). Exosome therapy is a cell-free therapy that largely solves this problem. Moreover, due to its nano-scale volume and stability, the production and preservation of MSC-Exo demonstrates great value in clinical use. MSCs can generate a large number of exosomes of the same composition, which is suitable for large-scale production. Particularly, engineered exosomes with enhanced targeting and therapeutic efficacy have demonstrated tremendous potential in clinical applications and drug delivery (Guo *et al.* 2020). The surface of MSC-Exos can also be modified and utilized as engineered exosomes for targeted delivery (Gandham *et al.* 2020).

4 CHALLENGES AND FUTURE PERSPECTIVES FOR MSC-BASED THERAPIES

However, there are still challenges associated with MSC-based therapies, including unclear mechanisms and heterogeneity. The mechanisms through which MSCs exert their effects can vary in different experimental and pathological contexts (Moll *et al.* 2019). The lack of standardized evaluation criteria further hinders the assessment of treatment efficacy. Moreover, MSCs derived from different tissue sources exhibit significant heterogeneity that cannot be overlooked. Certain inconsistencies have been observed between results obtained in in vitro settings and those in animal models, as well as disparities between preclinical data and clinical outcomes in ongoing trials. Single-cell multi-omics analysis provides effective information to further explain MSC therapeutic mechanisms and elucidate the issue of MSC heterogeneity. In MSC produced from different origins, single-cell transcriptome studies reconstruct progressive cellular senescence. Gao *et al.* points out that perinatal MSCs have fewer senescent cells when contrasted with adult MSCs, and altered multispectral differentiation capacity and impaired immunosuppression were observed when BM-MSCs were isolated from aged donors (Gao *et al.* 2023). On the other hand, the culture conditions of MSC have an important influence on their growth status and pluripotency. Studies have been conducted to optimize MSC culture from monolayer culture to microcarrier culture and different culture medium (Koh *et al.* 2023; Pilgrim *et al.* 2022). The optimization and standardization of MSC culture conditions will contribute to homogeneity and quality in mass production.

Genetic modification proves to be an efficient method for enhancing the therapeutic outcomes of MSCs. Hu *et al.* have illustrated that the introduction of brain-derived neurotrophic factor to cholinergic-like neuronal grafts derived from human umbilical cord MSCs leads to heightened acetylcholine release and increased ChAT levels in the hippocampus (Hu *et al.* 2019). This intervention also intensifies astrocyte and microglia activation and fosters neurogenesis, resulting in a substantial enhancement of spatial learning and memory in AD rats. Another study has provided evidence that the overexpression of neurotrophin-3 facilitates the differentiation of BM-MSCs into neurons, leading to an improvement in cognitive function in experimental AD rats (Yan *et al.* 2021). In summary, genetically modified MSCs exhibit enhanced therapeutic potential by overexpressing neurotrophic factors that promote directed differentiation, increase survival, and reduce immune rejection (Zhou *et al.* 2023).

MSCs can undergo genetic engineering to introduce various genes, and in addition to that, exosomes can also undergo functional modification with specific genes or miRNAs. Li *et al.* has effectively inhibited autophagy and pyroptosis using miR-188-3p-modified exosomes in MPTP-induced PD mice and proved modified exosomes to be restorative to neuronal damage in the substantia nigra (Li *et al.* 2021). An increasing body of research has started to explore MSC-derived exosomes as a potent nanocarrier for augmenting their neurotherapeutic potential. These exosomes can encapsulate diverse payloads, encompassing growth factors, small molecule drugs and nucleic acids like mRNAs, miRNAs, and siRNAs. Gene modified exosomes by expressing organ targeted protein linked with Lamp2b on the exosomal membrane enhanced exosome target delivery, which shed lights on various and broad engineering therapy (Kim *et al.* 2018). What is more, selective sorting of RNA targets can be achieved by designing exosome surface functionalization to generate therapeutic exosomes (Salunkhe *et al.* 2020). Accordingly, the development of more standardized, safer, and efficient therapeutic approaches based on MSCs holds great promise for the treatment of neurodegenerative diseases. These advancements will offer valuable support for addressing neurodegenerative conditions and furthering human health.

5 CONCLUSION

MSCs offer distinctive benefits in the clinical treatment of neurodegenerative disorders. Apart from their capacity to differentiate into both glial cells and neurons, offering promising avenues for cell replacement therapy, MSCs hold significant clinical potential in areas such as nutrition, immunomodulation, and neuroprotection. These attributes effectively mitigate the risk of immune rejection and enhance the quality of life for patients. MSCs-derived exosomes preserve several therapeutic attributes of their parent MSCs, such as the capacity to regulate neural synapse development, stimulate angiogenesis, and facilitate tissue repair. The therapeutic potential of MSC and their exosomal therapy in neurodegenerative diseases has been evaluated in various clinical trials over the past decade, but the safety and efficacy in humans have not yet been demonstrated (Ghasemi *et al.* 2023). An imperative mandate exists for the continued exploration of safer, more efficacious, and feasible therapeutic modalities. The optimization of the preparation procedure, delivery methodology, and determination of the ideal dosage for both MSCs and their derived exosomes assumes an essential role in the quest to furnish enhanced therapeutic interventions for patients. The pursuit of a more profound comprehension of these underlying mechanisms stands poised to significantly bolster the therapeutic advancement of MSCs, thereby augmenting their latent therapeutic efficacy.

REFERENCES

Ahmed H. H., Salem A. M., Atta H. M., Eskandar E. F., Farrag A. R. H., Ghazy M. A., Salem N. A., and Aglan H. A., (2016). *World. J. Stem. Cells.* **8**, 106.

Chen D. D., Fu W., Zhuang W., Cui L., Li F., and Wang X., (2017). *J. Neurosci. Res.* **95**, 907.

Chen H. X., Liang F. C., Gu P., Xu B. L., Xu H. J., Wang W. T., Hou J. Y., Xie D. X., Chai X. Q., and An S. J., (2020). *Cell Death Dis.* **11**, 1.

Cocozza F., Grisard E., Martin-Jaular L., Mathieu M., and Théry C., (2020). *Cell.* **182**, 262.

Cui G., Guo H., Li H., Zhai Y., Gong Z., Wu J., Liu J., Dong Y., Hou S., and Liu J., (2019) *Immun. Ageing.* **16,** 10.

Dause T. J., Denninger J. K., Smith B. M., and Kirby E. D., (2022). *Exp. Neurol.* **355**, 114142.
Forotti G., Nizzardo M., Bucchia M., Ramirez A., Trombetta E., Gatti S., Nereo Bresolin, Giacomo Pietro Comi, and Corti S., (2019). *Exp. Neurol.* **321**, 113041.
Gandham S., Su X., Wood J., Nocera A. L., Alli S. C., Milane L., Zimmerman A., Amiji M., and Ivanov A. R., (2020). *Trends Biotechnol.* **38**, 1066.
Gao Y., Cheng Y., Chen Y., Wang W., Li H., Zheng W., Zhu P., An J., Duan Y., Sun T., Liu X., Xue F., Liu W., Fu R., Han Z., Zhang Y., Yang R., Cheng T., Wei J., and Zhang L., (2023). *Nat. Commun.* **14**, 4373.
Ghasemi M., Roshandel E., Mohammadian M., Farhadihosseinabadi B., Akbarzadehlaleh P., and Shamsasenjan K., (2023). *Stem Cell Res Ther.* **14**, 122.
Guo M., Yin Z., Chen F., and Lei P., (2020). *Alzheimers. Res. Ther.* **12**, 109.
Hu W., Feng Z., Xu J., Jiang Z., Feng M., (2019). *Brain Res.* **1710**, 61–73
Jeong J. O., Han J. W., Kim J. M., Cho H. J., Park C., Lee N., Kim D. W., and Yoon Y., (2011). *Circ. Res.* **108**, 1340.
Jia Y., Cao N., Zhai J., Zeng Q., Zheng P., Su R., Liao T., Liu J., Pei H., Fan Z., Zhou J., Xi J., He L., Chen L. X., Nan X., Yue W. and Pei X., (2020). *Adv. Sci.* **7**, 1903809.
Kim H., Yun N., Mun D., Kang J.-Y., Lee S.-H., Park H., Park H., and Joung B., (2018). *Biochem. Biophys. Res. Commun.* **499**, 803.
Koh B., Sulaiman N., Fauzi M. B., Law J. X., Ng M. H., Yuan T. L., Azurah A. G. N., Mohd Yunus M. H., Idrus R. B. H. and Yazid M. D., (2023). *Int. J. Mol. Sci.* **24**, 3745.
Krampera M. and Le Blanc K., (2021). *Cell Stem Cell.* **28**, 1708.
Lampe L., Zhang R., Beyer F., Huhn S., Kharabian Masouleh S., Preusser S., Bazin P., Schroeter M. L., Villringer A., and Witte A. V., (2019). *Ann. Neurol.* **85**, 194.
Li H., Dai H., and Li J., (2023). *J. Adv. Res.* **45**, 15.
Li Q., Wang Z., Xing H., Wang Y. and Guo Y., (2021). *Mol. Ther. Nucleic Acids.* **23**, 1334.
Liu Y., Zeng R., Wang Y., Huang W., Hu B., Zhu G., Zhang R., Li F., Han J., and Li Y., (2019). *Brain Res.* **1724**, 146422.
Moll G., Ankrum J. A., Kamhieh-Milz J., Bieback K., Ringdén O., Volk H.-D., Geissler S., and Reinke P., (2019). *Trends Mol. Med.* **25**, 149.
Moreno-Jiménez E. P., Flor-García M., Terreros-Roncal J., Rábano A., Cafini F., Pallas-Bazarra N., Ávila J. and Llorens-Martín M., (2019). *Nat. Med.* **25**, 554.
Na L., Wang S., Liu T., and Zhang L., (2020). *Biomed Res Int.* **2020**, 1.
Öz T., Kaushik A., and Kujawska M., (2023). *World J. Stem Cells* **15**, 687.
Park H. and Chang K.A., (2020). *Int. J. Mol. Sci.* **21**, 8129.
Pilgrim C. R., McCahill K. A., Rops J. G., Dufour J. M., Russell K. A., and Koch T. G., (2022). *Front. Vet. Sci.* **9**, 859025.
Qian X., An N., Ren Y., Yang C., Zhang X. and Li L., (2020). *Stem Cell Rev. Rep.* **17**, 411.
Salunkhe S., Dheeraj, Basak M., Chitkara D., and Mittal A., (2020). *J. Control Release.* **326**, 599.
Schain M. and Kreisl W. C., (2017). *Curr. Neurol. Neurosci. Rep.* **17**, 25.
Sobacchi C., Palagano E., Villa A., and Menale C., (2017). *Front. Bioeng. Biotechnol.* **5**, 32.
Xie M., Xiong W., She Z., Wen Z., Abdirahman A. S., Wan W., and Wen C., (2020). *Front. Immunol.* **11**, 13.
Yan Z., Shi X., Wang H., Si C., Liu Q., Du Y., (2021). *Front. Cell Neurosci.* **15**, 629356.
Yoshida S., Miyagawa S., Toyofuku T., Fukushima S., Kawamura T., Kawamura A., Kashiyama N., Nakamura Y., Toda K., and Sawa Y., (2020). *Sci. Rep.* **10**, 4593.
Zhou H., He Y., Xiong W., Jing S., Duan X., Huang Z., Nahal G. S., Peng Y., Li M., Zhu Y. and Ye Q., (2023). *Bioact. Mater.* **23**, 409.

Biological Sciences and Environmental Health – Gao (Ed.)
© 2025 the Author(s), ISBN: 978-1-032-96016-6

Targeting microglia and its relationship with TREM-2 in Alzheimer's disease

Shunjie Lin
International School, Clinical Medicine, Jinan University, Guangzhou, China

ABSTRACT: Patients with Alzheimer's disease (AD) experience cognitive decline, memory lapses, and impairments in novel object recognition, none of which have been robustly ameliorated by contemporary mainstream treatments based on amyloid beta (Aβ)-protein hypothesis. The potential involvement of microglial phagocytosis and the correlation between triggering receptors expressed on myeloid cell-2 (TREM2) and microglia in the pathologically excessive accumulation of Aβ in the hippocampus and cortex is noteworthy. This study investigates the role of TREM2 and its downstream signaling-mediated microglia biological functions, explores the time-dependent features of the TREM2 effect on Aβ deposition, and analyzes a novel monoclonal antibody (mAb) that promotes the TREM2 expression (4D9, Ab18, and CGX101). Specifically, the study examines recent evidence suggesting TREM2 is a key regulator of microglial function and that loss of TREM2 function increases the risk of Alzheimer's disease. Studies showing TREM2 deficiency results in reduced microglial phagocytosis and lipid transport, leading to amyloid plaque accumulation have been discussed. The study also highlights new mAbs like 4D9 that enhance TREM2 signaling and microglial survival, resulting in reduced amyloid levels in mouse models. Overall, modulating TREM2 presents a promising therapeutic approach to enhancing microglial function and clearance of amyloid aggregates that drive Alzheimer's progression. Further research into the timing and dosing of TREM2-targeting therapies will provide essential insights into their clinical potential and safety.

1 INTRODUCTION

The global prevalence of dementia, including Alzheimer's disease (AD), is projected to rise significantly, exceeding 152.8 million by the year 2050, a substantial increase from the 50 million reported in the Global Burden of Disease Study in 2019 (Dementia Forecasting Collaborators 2022). Particularly noteworthy is the growing body of evidence, especially in the aftermath of the coronavirus disease 2019 (COVID-19) pandemic, which elucidates the COVID-19-induced alterations in immune function and the exacerbation of neuropsychiatric symptoms in AD. These findings underscore a close correlation between higher mortality rates in AD and COVID-19 (Eikelboom *et al.* 2021).

Clinically, non-amnestic AD presentations, as defined by the 2011 National Institute on Aging and Alzheimer's Association (NIA-AA) criteria for AD (McKhann *et al.* 2011), are characterized by impairments in language, visuospatial abilities, and executive dysfunction. In the first three to ten years after diagnosis, patients experience a gradual decline in mental capacity and social abilities, including forgetfulness and emotional apathy. Subsequently, patients more severely develop cognitive deficits, which may encompass communication challenges, disorientation, confusion, and memory loss, leading to dementia and, in some cases, even death (Qiu *et al.* 2023).

While the amyloid beta (Aβ) cascade hypothesis remains the predominant theory explaining the pathophysiology of AD, other possible mechanisms, such as inflammatory

DOI: 10.1201/9781003587590-7

response, oxidative stress, and cholinergic circuit disruption, have been put forth. Unfortunately, the precise etiology of AD is still poorly understood due to the complexity of its pathology mechanism (Qiu *et al.* 2023).

For decades, scientists have focused on developing anti-amyloid treatments, but with limited success in significantly improving cognitive impairment in AD patients, leading to discouragement among pharmaceutical companies from developing drugs targeting amyloid. However, recent research has emphasized TREM2's role as a regulator of microglial survival, chemotaxis, clustering, and the phagocytosis of Aβ via TREM2/DAP12 and downstream signaling pathways. Over the past five years, this discovery has gained significant attention, prompting Denali Therapeutics to develop a novel AD therapeutic candidate, 4D9, which has undergone initial clinical trials. This progress has reignited interest in Aβ clearance through TREM2-mediated phagocytosis (Schlepckow *et al.* 2020).

On the other hand, the surge in research on TREM2 has prompted critical thinking about whether TREM2 overexpression is beneficial at all stages of Aβ deposition, as well as other pathological models, such as tauopathies, neuronal loss, and plaque-associated apolipoprotein. Consequently, to address these concerns comprehensively, the pharmacological effects of TREM2 agonists should be established in phase 2 clinical trials.

2 MICROGLIAL PHAGOCYTOSIS OF ABETA IN ALZHEIMER'S DISEASE

In the domain of neurodegenerative disease, microglia play a dual role akin to a double-edged sword. On one hand, they contribute to memory loss through synaptic clearance via the complement mechanism; on the other hand, they promote the health of the central nervous system (CNS) via the phagocytosing Aβ, thereby influencing the pathological progression of AD (Li *et al.* 2023). In recent research, authors have aimed to use different models of AD, including APP/PS1, 5XFAD mouse model, and *Caenorhabditis elegans*, to investigate whether stimulating microglial pathophysiology, morphology, and function can reduce cognitive impairment by enhancing the efficiency of phagocytosing Aβ1-40 and Aβ1-42 accumulation (Schocha *et al.* 2021).

Although the effectiveness of enhancing the phagocytic process has been demonstrated, it remains unclear whether TREM2-mediated phagocytosis is beneficial for clearing Aβ clearance. To solve this problem, a comprehensive examination of how TREM2 signaling regulates microglial biological function and how altered TREM2 expression affects Aβ burden is required. Most studies using TREM2 knockout-induced pluripotent stem cells (hiPSC) co-cultured with microphages suggest that TREM2 deletion impairs microglial survival, clustering, and Aβ phagocytosis, both in vivo and in vitro (Ulland and Marco 2018).

Moreover, researchers are committed to uncovering the mechanisms that govern the transformation of homeostatic microglia into different pathological microglial states in AD and normal aging. These distinct microglial states, such as white matter-associated microglia (WAM) and disease-associated microglia (DAM), have shown neuroprotective potential in AD and are dependent on the TREM2 signaling pathway. Consequently, current pharmacological approaches aim to enhance their conversion by augmenting TREM2 signaling (Li *et al.* 2023).

2.1 *TREM2/DAP12 regulates microglial chemotaxis*

To validate the regulatory role of TREM2 in physiological and pathological microglia states, previous research has already highlighted that TREM2/DAP12 is involved in and supports microglial survival, proliferation, chemotaxis, aggregation, and phagocytic capacity.

In vitro studies have provided valuable insights into the impact of TREM2 deficiency on microglial function. When TREM2 is deficient, the migration distance of microglia is reduced, which is strongly inhibited further when N9 microglia are pre-incubated with Genistein (a general tyrosine kinase inhibitor) and Piceatannol (a selective SYK inhibitor).

These inhibitors effectively block the activation and phosphorylation of SYK 38, subsequently impeding TREM2/DAP12 activation. However, treating TREM2 deficient microglia with the chemotactic stimuli CCL2 and C5a can significantly enhance their migration toward chemokines. Consistent with these in vivo experiments, apoptotic neurons in the absence of TREM2 are surrounded by a reduced number of clustered macroglia compared to wild-type, and this aggregation occurs at a slower rate (Mazaheri *et al.* 2017).

Taken together, these findings underscore the critical role of TREM2 in facilitating the attraction of microglia toward sites of injured neurons. Furthermore, CCK7 and ERK signaling, downstream of spleen tyrosine kinase (SYK) activation, also contribute to microglial chemotaxis. Previous studies have revealed that ERK activation stimulates CCK7, which further triggers the phosphorylation of CXCR4, while its downstream signaling via SDF-1α enhances microglial chemotactic migration. Especially in the Aβ phagocytic process, mRNA and membrane-bound protein levels of CXCR4 are significantly reduced in the TREM2 knockout (KO) group. This reduction in CXCR4 expression impairs microglial movement toward Aβ, as the downstream induction of SDF-1α, which typically enhances microglial chemotaxis, is blocked in the absence of TREM2 (McQuade *et al.* 2020).

2.2 *TREM2/DAP12 regulates microglial survival*

Trem2/DAP12 not only regulates microglial migration but also plays a crucial role in promoting microglial survival and proliferation. Studies using TREM2 KO mice brains and microglia have revealed significant increases in pro-caspase 3, Bcl-2, and cleaved-caspase, indicating an accelerated apoptosis process and disruption of normal microgliosis. These findings support the hypothesis that TREM2 is essential for cell-cycle regulation. Mechanistically, the activation of the Wnt/β-catenin pathway downstream of TREM2/DAP12 is involved in mediating microglial survival. Also, β-catenin can be modulated by the SYK/PI3K/Akt pathway. Thus, promoting Wnt/β-catenin signaling via the PI3K/AKt pathway can restore the impaired microglia proliferation in the TREM2 KO/KD group (Zheng *et al.* 2017).

As a downstream component of the PI3K/AKT pathway, mTOR contributes to physiological fitness in response to Aβ and stressful environments. It has been emphasized that mTOR stimulation by Cyclocreatine and Dectin-1 treatment, which increases energetic capacity, can rescue TREM2-deficient microglia from autophagy and apoptosis, thereby enhancing their survival and proliferation (Ulland and Marco 2018).

Recent research has also focused on improving the shifting from the M1 to M2 microglial phenotype. It has been found that the C57BL/6 mice model, exposed to a high-dose lipopolysaccharide (LPS) injection for 7 days exhibited an increase in the M2 microglia phenotype, which has enhanced anti-inflammatory function in the CNS and is accompanied by a higher TREM2 expression level compared to the 4-day group (Li *et al.* 2023). Interestingly, *Alpinia oxyphylla*, a traditional Chinese medicine, promotes M2 polarization, protects neurons from oxidative stress, and preserves cognitive function. Moreover, TREM2 is essential for mediating the effects of Chrysin treatment on increasing the M2 level through the PI3K/AKT/GSK3β and BDNF/TrkB/TLR4 pathways (Li *et al.* 2023).

2.3 *TREM2/DAP12 regulates microglial phagocytosis*

Canonically, shedding of the TREM2 N-terminal domain inhibits phagocytic function without affecting the anti-inflammatory action, demonstrating that the full-length TREM2 molecule is necessary for efficient phagocytic function of microglia. This function relies on the downstream SYK/PI3K/AKT/PLCγ2 activation pathway (Yao *et al.* 2019). In addition, PLCγ2 is responsible for cholesterol metabolism and functions downstream of Toll-like receptors (TLRs) to independently regulate the inflammatory environment of microglia, separate from its interaction with TREM2. Interestingly, deletion of PLCγ2 induces various changes, affecting not only phagocytosis but also the microglial association around the Aβ plaques and even microglial survival itself Another important signaling pathway, PI3L/AKT/C/EBPα, has been found to upregulate the transcription of downstream CD36 and its expression in microglia, further improving TREM2-mediated phagocytosis (Li *et al.* 2023).

3 DISTINCT ROLES OF TREM2 IN DIFFERENT STAGES OF Aβ DEPOSITION

Most researchers agree that TREM2 positively regulates microglial biological function, promotes M2 phenotype polarization, and ameliorates cognitive impairment in AD pathology (McQuade *et al.* 2020). However, in vitro studies suggest that Aβ accumulation is strongly related to TREM2 levels, which contradicts the findings of in vivo research (Ulland and Marco 2018). The inconsistency in these findings can be summarized as follows: TREM2 appears to exacerbate Aβ deposition in the early stage but promotes Aβ clearance in later stages, indicating a time- and/or age-dependent role for TREM2 in regulating Aβ phagocytosis (Schocha *et al.* 2021). These conclusions are based on experiments using different mice models and examining different aspects of Aβ accumulation, including the microglia-plaque association and phagocytosis, macroglial exosome expression, and R47H mutation of TREM2.

For instance, in the APP/PS1 mouse model, 2-month-old Trem2-deficient mice showed a significant reduction in Aβ plaque number and area in the cortex and hippocampus. At 4 months, no obvious differences were observed, while at 8 months, the Aβ area increased, although there was no significant change in the number of Aβ plaques. This suggests that the absence of TREM2 may lead to the diffusion of plaques and an extension of fibrils. However, both early and late stages showed a reduction in CD45, a biomarker of myeloid cells, especially those surrounding amyloid plaques (Jay *et al.* 2017).

Similar results have been observed in the 5XFAD mouse model, where TREM2 knockout did not affect Aβ levels in the hippocampus in the 4-month stage, but a rocketing accumulation of Aβ was noted by 8 months (Wang *et al.* 2016). Another PS2APP TREM2 knockout mice model, spanning from a 4-month to 22-month period, which is the longest duration experiment, provided an amazing result that 6–7-month female groups show more severe Aβ deposition than that of male concomitant reduction in microglial cluster and phagocytosis. However, plaque burden reduction was observed surprisingly in 12-month-old females and 19–22-month-old males (Meilandt *et al.* 2020). These results are also consistent with the 2019 study, indicating that TREM2 knockout exacerbates Aβ plaque in the early stage but that this trend diminishes in later stages (Parhizkar *et al.* 2019). Moreover, TREM2-knockout led to Aβ plaques having a more diffuse and less dense morphology compared to TREM2 wildtype mice (Meilandt *et al.* 2020; Wang *et al.* 2016). Notably, the ratio of Aβ 42 to Aβ 40, along with an increase in fibril Aβ oligomers in the hippocampus, indicated that the absence of TREM2 will increase the accumulation of fibrillar Aβ rather than soluble forms (Meilandt *et al.* 2020).

In another study utilizing APP/PS1 mice of different ages (4, 7, and 10 months) and subjecting them to oligonucleotide (ASOs) treatment, it was found that at 10 months, post-plaque stages showed a significant decrease in TREM2 mRNA levels and a concurrent reduction in plaque accumulation, with microglial activation remaining lower even one month after ASO treatment (Schocha *et al.* 2021). A recent study also revealed that TREM2 expression and its positive regulators, miR-146a, increased while the negative regulator, miR-34a-5p, decreased in the AD group compared with aged-matched healthy controls. However, TREM2-expressing monocytes significantly reduced when treated with LPS-induced neuroinflammation and Aβ 42, indicating a down-regulation effect of the inflammatory milieu while also enhancing TREM2 expression. Undeniably, cooperative anti-inflammatory treatments not only alleviate the inflammatory milieu but also enhance the TREM2 expression and modulate microglial phenotypes. It has been reported that Curcumin and Hydroxysafflor Yellow A inhibit LPS-induced and Aβ-induced neuroinflammation, respectively, by promoting the TREM2 /TLR4/NF-$_{\kappa}$B pathway in BV2 cells (Rosa *et al.* 2023).

Research has focused not only on TREM2-dependent phagocytosis but also on microglial exosomes, which express unique membrane proteins that promote microglial binding to Aβ and facilitate phagocytosis (Huang *et al.* 2022). Additionally, the TREM2 R47H variant, acting as the influential risk factor, has garnered significant attention from researchers. To investigate the TREM2^{R47H} mutation effect on amyloid plaque, previous data have revealed that TREM2-heterozygous and homozygous human stem cell-derived monocytes and microglia-like cells showed impaired Aβ phagocytosis, though this impairment was not observed in the TREM2 R47H variant group. Recent research established the FXFAD/TREM2^{R47HNSS} (normal splice site) mouse model aimed to prevent cryptic splicing events, revealing that soluble Aβ 40 increased in the hippocampus and decreased in the cortex, while insoluble Aβ 40 did not show any differences at 4-month age. However, by 12 months, Aβ plaque size increased in both brain regions, and soluble Aβ 42 and insoluble Aβ 40 and Aβ 42 increased in the hippocampus and cortex, respectively. Furthermore, impaired microglial association with plaques and a reduction in microglial size and number were observed in this model at 4 months of age, but these changes were no longer evident at the later 12-month disease stage (Tran *et al.* 2023).

Both the PS2APP TREM2-deleted model and the R47H TREM2-expressing BV-2 microglia model emphasized that microglia exposed to phosphatidylserine induced more neuronal loss and axonal atrophy, dependent on the exposure of phosphatidylserine, than the wild-type group. This further proved the notion that TREM2-dependent microgliosis helps maintain the compacted, condensed form of Aβ, which prevents neurotoxicity (Meilandt *et al.* 2020). In light of these findings, it is crucial to consider not only the quantity of Aβ but also the effects of TREM2 on its various forms when studying amyloid pathology.

4 WILL AGONIZING TREM2 BECOME A PROMISING THERAPY FOR ALZHEIMER'S DISEASE?

Since Denali Therapeutics introduced the novel therapeutic candidate 4D9 antibody for AD patients in 2020, several other antibodies with similar mechanisms aimed at enhancing the positive effects of TREM2 have been reported. Numerous research studies have analyzed the impact of those antibodies on different aspects of AD-associated pathology and have sought to identify and resolve their limitations and disadvantages.

4.1 *mAb 4D9, Ab18, and CGX101*

Monoclonal antibody (mAb) 4D9, an IgG2a antibody, is designed to prevent the shedding of TREM2 through metalloproteinase- and disintegrin-mediated mechanisms, especially α-secretase. Another antibody, AD9, selectively agonizes TREM2 through a dual mechanism by specifically binding to the stalk region epitope near the ADAM cleavage site and activating downstream SYK signaling. Research has shown that 4D9 binds to cell surface TREM2 in bone marrow-derived macrophages (BMDMs), enhancing full-length TREM2 expression, which is crucial for microglial biological function and survival. Additionally, 4D9 reduces the formation of soluble TREM2 (sTREM2) and promotes the survival of BMDMs after withdrawal of macrophage colony-stimulating factor (M-CSF), a condition that partially reduces TREM2. This survival-promoting effect was not observed in the control group. In vivo, AD9 demonstrated target engagement by binding to and significantly reducing sTREM2 levels in cerebrospinal fluid in a dose-dependent manner. Furthermore, AD9 promotes the transformation of microglial states from homeostatic to DAM, accompanied by a selective reduction in soluble Aβ42 (Schlepckow *et al.* 2020).

Although AD9 research has demonstrated its beneficial effects in both in vivo and in vitro assays, previous data have raised concerns about whether TREM2 agonists, which are primarily standard IgG antibodies, can effectively penetrate the brain through the blood-brain barrier (BBB) (Kathryn M. 2022). To address this, Denali Therapeutics introduced "transport vehicles," such as the transferrin receptor (TfR), to facilitate the penetration of monoclonal antibody transport through the BBB via receptor-mediated transcytosis (RM), with these approaches currently undergoing initial clinical trials (Jacob 2023).

Following the AD9 topical issue, the design of Ab18 aimed to enhance brain uptake through the BBB by converting the traditional bivalent immunoglobulin G1 (IgG1) to a tetravalent immunoglobulin (TVD-Ig), which showed over a tenfold increase in distribution. The authors emphasized that the agonist effect of Ab18 did not interfere with the natural ligands such as phosphatidylcholine (PC), phosphatidylserine (PS), or oligomeric amyloid-beta (o$A\beta$) binding to TREM2, which are crucial for promoting microglial clustering, phagocytic function, and metabolism. Furthermore, by enhancing the valency from Ab18 to Ab18 TVD-lg through antibody engineering, the EC50 was successfully reduced to 0.42 nM, significantly improving penetration efficiency. Interestingly, a substantial increase in downstream pSYK activation was observed at a 10nM concentration of Ab18 TVD-Ig but not at 100nM. The authors further elucidated the efficacy of the novel Ab18 TVD-Ig/αTfR treatment, which specifically targeted both TREM2 and TfR. Inspired by Denali Therapeutics' approach, this treatment was administered to 5XFAD AD mice, leading to improved outcomes such as reduced $A\beta$ deposition, ameliorated cognitive deficits, and preserved synaptic integrity, attributed to its enhanced brain delivery (Zhao *et al.* 2022).

It is undeniable that TfR facilitates the transportation of protein into the CNS, drawing significant attention and serving as a noteworthy example for others to follow (Kariolis *et al.* 2020). A recent study has demonstrated the potential of an activating antibody targeting TREM2 with a BBB transport vehicle (ATV: TRM2), which elicits a broader impact on microglial states. This effect was evidenced by a significant upregulation of DAM states and four distinct clusters around the plaques, which exhibited more convex solid forms and shorter branches in terms of morphological changes. Furthermore, the ATV:TREM2 treatment reversed survival defects observed under conditions of low macrophage colony-stimulating factor (M-CSF) in vitro, while surprisingly enhancing microglial phagocytosis in vivo and upregulating the expression of phagocytosis-associated genes, including AXL, Itgax, and Lgals3. To elucidate the mechanisms behind the accelerated uptake of ATV: TREM2 in the brain, DOAT labeling was employed, demonstrating a persistent increase in signal intensity after 96 hours (Lengerich *et al.* 2023).

The promising monoclonal antibody AL002a has led to the chronic activation of TREM2, amelioration of elevated Abata-related genes, and the recruitment of microglial cells around plaques. Additionally, it has demonstrated improved performance in AD mouse model assays, particularly in novel object recognition. Notably, AL002a has shown target engagement in Phase 1 clinical trials (Jacob 2023).

4.2 *Current concern about mAb*

The development of mAb aimed at enhancing TREM2 activation has become a mainstream approach for novel AD therapeutic candidates. The advantage of their specific binding to TREM2 epitopes further prevents unpredictable side effects, such as gastrointestinal overstimulation induced by non-CNS selective acetylcholinesterase inhibitors, which often limits the administration of the effective dose (Jacob 2023). However, chronic activation of TREM2 is associated with an exacerbation of neuritic plaques and the promotion of tau spreading in the 5XFAD AD mouse model, raising concerns about whether TREM2 overexpression is beneficial in all AD-associated pathology (Jacob 2023). TREM2 plays a complex role in tau-targeted experimental models that generate conflicting hypotheses.

Regrettably, there is a paucity of research investigating the impact of the mAbs on tauopathies (Aleksandra and Weiner 2020). Additionally, the stimulation of boosting homeostatic microglia toward DAM states may lead to the induction of APOE expression, consequently increasing plaque-associated APOE and driving amyloid aggregation. Previous studies have also shown inconsistent results regarding synaptic pruning pathology (Lewcock *et al.* 2020). In summary, the effects of TREM2 overactivation induced by mAbs on various pathologies, including amyloid plaques, appear to be dose- and time-dependent and remain an area of ongoing investigation.

5 DISCUSSION

Besides AD, other conditions such as atherosclerosis, liver cirrhosis, and cancer exhibit similar pathological features, such as chronic inflammation, protein aggregation, and elevated levels of cell apoptosis (Aleksandra and Weiner 2020). To break this pathological vicious cycle, targeting TREM2-regulated phagocytosis has emerged as a promising therapeutic approach. However, overexpression of TREM2 may not always yield benign outcomes. For example, in gastric cancer research, significant increases in TREM2 mRNA and protein levels compared to healthy gastric tissue have been observed. Additionally, the authors emphasized a substantial adverse relationship between TREM2 levels and prognosis in a cohort of 317 patients. Similar findings regarding the role of TREM2 in patient prognosis have been reported in studies involving glioma and hepatocellular carcinoma (Aleksandra and Weiner 2020).

6 CONCLUSION

TREM2/DAP12 signaling plays a crucial role in maintaining microglial functions, such as survival, chemotaxis, recruitment around amyloid plaques, and phagocytosis of these plaques. TREM2 also exhibits a time-dependent role in plaque accumulation in various diseases. While TREM2-targeted therapeutics hold promise for the future, the dual-edged effect of TREM2 on specific diseases and at different stages must be carefully considered in therapeutic development.

REFERENCES

Aleksandra D., Weiner A. and Amit I. (2020). *Cell* **181**,6: 1207–1217

Eikelboom, W.S., Esther van den B., E. H. Singleton, MSc, S. J. Baart, M. Coesmans, A. E. Leeuwis, C. E. Teunissen, Bart N.M. van B., Yolande A.L. P., P. Scheltens, W. M. van der Flier, Rik Ossenkoppele and J. M. Papma. (2021). *Neurology* **97**,13: e1276–e1287

GBD 2019 Dementia Forecasting Collaborators. (2022). Estimation of the Global Prevalence of Dementia in 2019 and Forecasted Prevalence in 2050: An Analysis for the Global Burden of Disease Study 2019'. *The Lancet. Public Health* 7,2: e105–e125

Huang S., Liao X., Wu J., Zhang X., Li Y., Xiang D. and Luo S. (2022). *FEBS Letters* **596**, 8: 1059–1071

Jacob G. (2023). *Neural Regeneration Research* **18**, 12: 2680–2681.

Jay T. R., Hirsch A. M., Broihier M. L., Miller C. M., Neilson L. E., Ransohoff R. M., Lamb B. T. and Landreth G. E. (2017). *The Journal of Neuroscience* **37**,3: 637–647

Kariolis M. S., Wells R. C., Getz J. A., Kwan W., Mahon C. S., Tong R., Kim D., Srivastava A., Bedard C., Henne K. R., Giese T., Assimon V. A., Chen X., Zhang Y., Solanoy H., Jenkins K., Sanchez P. E., Kane L., Miyamoto T., Chew K. S., Pizzo M. E., Liang N, Calvert M. E. K., DeVos S. L., Baskaran S., Hall S., Sweeney Z. K., Thorne R. G., Watts R. J., Dennis M. S., Silverman A. P. and Yu Y. J. Z. (2020). *Sci. Transl. Med.* **12**, 545: e1359

Lewcock J. W., Schlepckow K., Paolo G. D., Tahirovic S., Monroe K. M. and Haass C. (2020). *Neuron* **108**, 5: 801–821

Li Y., Xu H., Wang H., Yang K., Luan J. and Wang S. (2023). *Biomedicine & Pharmacotherapy* **165**: 115218

Mazaheri F., Snaidero N., Kleinberger G., Madore C., Daria A., Werner G., Krasemann S., Capell A., Trümbach D., Wurst W., Brunner B., Bultmann S., Tahirovic S., Kerschensteiner M., Misgeld T., Butovsky O. and Haass C. (2017). *EMBO Reports* **18**, 7: 1186–1198

McKhann G. M., Knopman D. S., Chertkow H., Hyman B.T., Jack Jr. C. R., Kawas C. H., Klunk W. E., Koroshetz W. J., Manly J. J., Mayeux R., Mohs R. C., Morris J. C., Rossor M. N., Scheltens P., Carrillo M. C., Thiest B., Weintraub S., and Phelps C. H. (2011). *Alzheimers Dement.* **7**, 3: 263–269

McQuade A., Kang Y. J., Hasselmann J., Jairaman A., Sotelo A., Coburn M., Shabestari S. K., Chadarevian J. P., Fote G., Tu C. H., Danhash E., Silva J., Martinez E., Cotman C., Prieto G. A., Thompson L. M., Steffan J. S., Smith I., Davtyan H., Cahalan M., Cho H. and Blurton-Jone M. (2020). *Nature Communications* **11**: 5370

Meilandt W. J, Ngu H., Gogineni A., Lalehzadeh G., Lee S., Srinivasan K., Imperio J., Wu T., Weber M., Kruse A. J, Stark K. L, Chan P., Kwong M., Modrusan Z., Friedman B. A., Elstrott J., Foreman O., Easton A., Sheng M. and Hansen D. V. (2020). *Journal of Neuroscience* **40**, 9: 1956–1974

Parhizkar S., Arzberger T., Brendel M., Kleinberger G., Deussing M., Focke C., Nuscher B., Xiong M., Ghasemigharagoz A., Katzmarski N., Krasemann S., Lichtenthaler S. F., Müller S. A., Colombo A., Monasor L. S., Tahirovic S., Herms J., Willem M., Pettkus N., Butovsky O., Bartenstein P., Edbauer D., Rominger A., Ertürk A., Grathwohl S. A., Neher J. J., Holtzman D. M., Luehmann M. M. and Haass C. (2019). *Nature Neuroscience* **22**: 191–204.

Qiu W., Liu H., Liu Y., Lu X., Wang L., Hu Y., Feng F., Li Q. and Sun H. (2023). *Med. Res. Rev.* **43**,4: 1091–1140

Rosa F. L., Agostini S., Piancone F., Marventano I., Hernis A., Fenoglio C., Galimberti D., Scarpini E., Saresella M. and Clerici M. (2023). *International Journal of Molecular Sciences* **24**, 10: 8626.

Schlepckow K., Monroe K. M., Kleinberger G., Cantuti-Castelvetril L., Parhizkar S., Xia D., Willem M., Werner G., Pettkus N., Brunner B., Sülzen A., B. N., Hampel H., Xiang X., Feederle R., Tahirovic S., Park J. I., Prorok R., Mahon C., Liang C., Shi J., Kim D, J., Sabelström H., Huang F., Di Paolo G., Simons M., Lewcock J. W. and Haass C. (2020). *EMBO Molecular Medicine* **12**,4: e11227

Schocha K. M., Ezerskiy L. A., Morhausa M. M., Bannona R. N., Sauerbecka A. D., Shabsovicha M., Jafarnejadb P., Rigob F., and Millera T. M. (2021). *PNAS.* **118**, 27: e2100356118

Tran K. M., Kawauchi S., Kramár E. A., Rezaie N., Liang H. Y., Sakr J. S., Gomez-Arboledas AN., Arreola M. A., da Cunha C., Phan J., Wang S., Collins S., Walker A., Shi K., Neumann J., Filimban G., Shi Z., Milinkeviciute G., Javonillo D. I., Tran K., Gantuz M., Forner S., Swarup V., Tenner A. J., LaFerla F. M., Wood M. A., Mortazavi A., MacGregor G. R. and Green K. N. (2023). *Molecular Neurodegeneration* **18,** 1: 12

Ulland, T. K. and Marco C. (2018). *Nature Reviews Neurology* **14**: 667–675

van Lengerich B., Zhan L., Xia D., Chan D., Joy D., Park J. I., Tatarakis D., Calvert M., Hummel S., Lianoglou S., Pizzo M. E., Prorok R., Thomsen E., Bartos L. M., Beumers P., Capell A., Davis S. S., de Weerd L., Dugas J. C., Duque J., Earr T., Gadkar K., Giese T., Gill A., Gnörich J., Ha C., Kannuswamy M., Kim D., Kunte S. T., Kunze L. H., Lac D., Lechtenberg K., Leung A. W, Liang C., Lopez I., McQuade P., Modi A., Torres V. O., Nguyen H. N., Pesämaa I., Propson N., Reich M., Robles-Colmenares Y., Schlepckow K. I., Slemann L., Solanoy H., Suh J. H., Thorne R. G., Vieira C., Wind-Mark K., Xiong K., Yu Z. Y. J., Diaz D., Dennis M. S., Huang F., Scearce-Levie K., Watts R. J., Haass C., Lewcock J. W., Paolo G. D., Brendel M., P. E. S. and Monroe K. M. (2023). *Nature Neuroscience.* **26**, 3: 416–429

Wang Y., Ulland T. K., Ulrich J. D., Song W., Tzaferis J. A., Hole J. T., Yuan P., Mahan T. E., Shi Y., Gilfillan S., Cella M., Grutzendler J., DeMattos R. B., Cirrito J. R., Holtzman D. M. and Colonna M. (2016). *Journal of Experimental Medicine* **213**, 5: 667–675.

Yao H., Coppola K., Schweig J. E., Crawford F., Mullan M. and Paris D. (2019). *Frontiers in Cellular Neuroscience* **13**: 457.

Zhao P., Xu Y., Fan X., Li L., Li X., Arase H., Tong Q., Zhang N. and An Z. (2022). *MAbs* **14**, 1: 2107971

Zheng H., Jia L., Liu C., Rong X., Zhong L., Yang L., Chen X., Fryer J. D., Wang X., Zhang Y., Xu H. and Bu G. (2017). *The Journal of Neuroscience* **37**, 7: 1772–1784

Biological Sciences and Environmental Health – Gao (Ed.)

Mechanisms of melanocyte death in vitiligo: Oxidative stress and autoimmunity

Ruiming Ye
Biology Department, College of Arts & Sciences, Georgia State University, Atlanta, USA

ABSTRACT: Vitiligo is a common pigmentary disorder characterized by localized or generalized depigmentation of the skin and mucous membranes. The pathogenic mechanism of vitiligo is closely linked to oxidative stress and immune responses involving CD8 T cell activity. Elaborating on the characteristics and specific modes of action of these mechanisms can offer deeper insights into vitiligo. Oxidative stress can lead to cell death regulation, including autophagy and ferroptosis, while disrupted immunological modulation on cell survival may lead to cell apoptosis and necrosis. These death mechanisms could largely contribute to the pathogenesis of vitiligo. Evidence suggests that the death of melanocytes in vitiligo may not be solely caused by oxidative stress or immune system dysfunction alone, but by a combination of both. This review explores the two primary pathogenic mechanisms of vitiligo – oxidative stress and autoimmunity– and their contribution to melanocyte death, as well as potential interaction between the two.

1 INTRODUCTION

Vitiligo is a chronic dermatological condition characterized by blotches on various parts of the skin due to depigmentation. The prevalence rate is approximately 0.5%, with an incidence rate of about 0.54% in China. The affected areas often display creamy white spots with irregular edges. The skin in this area can also turn white, and the inside of the nose and mouth can also be affected, usually occurring symmetrically on both sides of the body. Vitiligo usually begins to appear after exposure to the sun. While vitiligo is not associated with disturbing sensations such as itching or pain, it can have a negative impact on an individual's self-esteem and even lead to mental health issues such as anxiety or depression due to the disfiguring nature of the spots, which can interfere with their social interactions.

To make matters worse, the efficacy of existing vitiligo treatments remains suboptimal. More advanced therapies, such as phototherapy (psoralen combined with ultraviolet-A and narrow-band ultraviolet-B), topical treatments (corticosteroids, calcineurin inhibitors), and systemic treatments (corticosteroids), continue to be both practically and economically burdensome. The widespread prevalence of this chronic disease, coupled with unsatisfactory treatment outcomes, highlights the need for further research into the pathogenesis of vitiligo. In recent years, studies on the etiology and mechanism of vitiligo have become increasingly in-depth, leading to the proposal of various theories, but the etiology of vitiligo is still uncertain.

2 OXIDATIVE STRESS

Oxidative stress arises from an imbalance of oxidants and antioxidants, occurring when there is an excess of oxidants and insufficient antioxidants. Although several theories exist

DOI: 10.1201/9781003587590-8

about the etiology of vitiligo, oxidative stress is widely considered a key factor. Excessive reactive oxygen species (ROS) play a major role in triggering oxidative stress within cells in the human body. ROS are natural by-products of cellular metabolism and include peroxides (PXs), superoxides, and hydrogen radicals. The excessive accumulation of ROS, combined with a reduced cellular ability to scavenge ROS, is a hallmark of cellular oxidative stress and is strongly linked to the pathogenesis of vitiligo (Dalmazi *et al.* 2016). High concentrations of ROS contribute to the destruction of melanocytes (MCs) by causing structural and functional damage to DNA, lipids, proteins, and metabolites (Sastry *et al.* 2019). In addition, ROS-induced oxidative stress triggers widespread organelle dysfunction, disrupts cellular metabolic pathways, and weakens cellular defense against attack from oxidative agents. With the deepening of research, increasing evidence shows that there is a close correlation between oxidative stress and keratinocytes, mitochondrial damage, and endoplasmic reticulum (ER) stress.

2.1 *Main factor causing oxidative stress: Reactive oxygen species*

ROS are oxygen-containing chemically reactive chemicals. They are highly reactive and easily interact with other molecules in the body, causing damage to cells and tissues when they are present in excess. The excess part of ROS is mainly generated from three parts. First, ROS comes from the production of melanin. Tyrosinase (Tyr) is an enzyme that limits the rate of melanin synthesis. It can convert tyrosine into dihydroxyindole through a series of reactions. Dihydroxyindole is oxidized into indole quinone, and the redox cycle from indole to quinone generates ROS (Denat *et al.* 2014). Second, the generation of ROS also comes from the energy metabolism of mitochondria (Figure 1) (Dell *et al.* 2007). The production of melanin is an energy-consuming process, while the biosynthesis of ATP produces ROS. Third, external environmental stimuli can lead to excessive production of ROS, and ultraviolet light is a more common way to stimulate excessive production of ROS. When ultraviolet rays irradiate cells, an immediate reaction occurs in the cells to produce ROS (Hofer *et al.* 2019). Phenols can combine with Tyr to generate ROS. These factors predispose MCs to the accumulation of ROS, leading to oxidative stress.

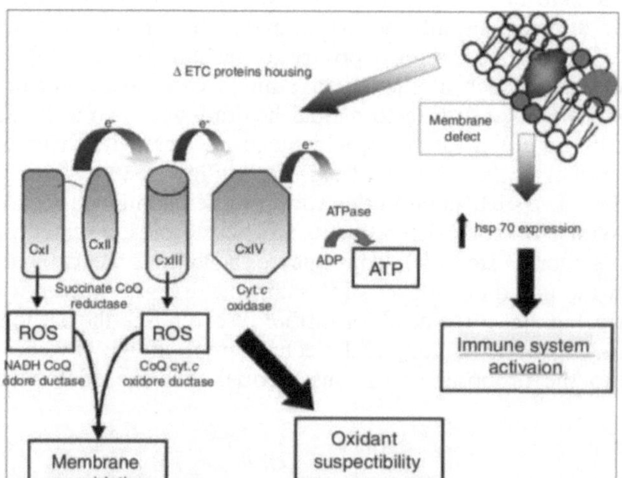

Figure 1. ROS production in mitochondrial energy metabolism (Dell *et al.* 2007).

In addition to excessive ROS production, the weakened ability of cells to scavenge ROS is the direct cause of ROS accumulation in epidermal cells. There are three main defense mechanisms in cells against oxidants. The first is to rely on molecules with antioxidant effects, such as pycnogenol, glutathione (GSH), thioredoxin (TRX) (Karlenius and Tonissen 2010), and vitamin C, among others. Their molecular weight is small, so they can reach places where antioxidant enzymes cannot reach, react with ROS, and eliminate or delay the accumulation of ROS. The second is antioxidant enzymes, including catalase, TRX reductase, GSH reductase, and other antioxidant enzymes. They can quickly break down the ROS produced by cells, but they can't reach everywhere, and they can't remove all ROS. The third is the function of damage repair enzymes, which repair biomolecules damaged by oxidative damage. Cellular oxidative stress caused by ROS overproduction weakens cellular defense mechanisms against oxidants.

Studies have shown that in vitiligo patients, highly concentrated ROS induce oxidative stress in epidermal cells. In their skin lesions, ROS content is significantly increased, and antioxidant enzyme activity is dramatically reduced. One plausible hypothesis regarding the effect that oxidative stress puts on epidermal cells in vitiligo patients is that it causes damage to biomolecules in MCs, leading to progressive loss of MC function.

2.2 *Sites of ROS generation and victims of oxidative stress: Mitochondria*

Mitochondria are double-membrane organelles that meet the energy and metabolic needs of aerobic cells. Mitochondria control many unique mechanisms, such as mitochondrial dynamics, mitochondrial biogenesis, and mitophagy. At the same time, mitochondria are also the main target of many stimuli, including ROS. Although ROS are generated from many different sources, the vast majority of ROS in cells originate from mitochondria. ROS generated by exogenous stimuli attack mitochondria, destroy their function, and damage mitochondria. Damaged mitochondria are the primary endogenous source of ROS generation, which leads to increased ROS levels and creates a vicious circle.

Excessive ROS damages mitochondrial DNA (mtDNA), and the damaged mtDNA becomes a new antigen, triggering the production of corresponding antibodies. Another way in which oxidative stress damages mitochondria is by disrupting the integrity of the cytochrome c (Cytc) complex. The principal route for safeguarding mitochondria, upholding their equilibrium, and ensuring proper cellular functioning is through the mitochondrial unfolded protein response (UPRmt). This process, which can be triggered by excess ROS, protects and restores damaged mitochondria. However, prolonged UPRmt can affect the normal functioning of mitochondria, resulting in mitochondrial damage.

Oxidative stress induced by ROS damages MCs by affecting ATP and mtDNA production within mitochondria. Vesicular exocytosis and pore-forming channels are the two primary mechanisms involved in the extracellular release of ATP, with the pore-forming channel mechanism capable of functioning under conditions of oxidative stress. Studies have shown that the ATP levels in the lesional and perilesional skin of vitiligo patients are higher compared to that in normal skin (Ahn *et al.* 2020). When ATP is released from the cell through the pore-forming channel, the expression of CXC motif chemokine ligands 9 (CXCL9) in keratinocytes is increased, accelerating the transformation of MC-specific CD8 T cells into cells associated with vitiligo skin lesions. Normally, mitochondria have unique mechanisms to keep mtDNA intact. However, oxidative stress can induce mtDNA damage, leading to impaired release of mtDNA into the cytoplasm or circulation. The amount of circulating mtDNA in the peripheral blood of patients with vitiligo is increased, and its change is closely related to the severity of mtDNA oxidative damage. In addition, mtDNA modifications caused by ROS and reactive nitrogen accumulation can lead to the formation of neoantigens, which may trigger autoimmune responses in vitiligo.

In summary, mitochondria are the primary producers of ROS in MCs. Excessive ROS can disrupt various balance mechanisms within mitochondria, leading to mitochondrial damage, triggering cellular immune responses, and promoting mitochondria-mediated MC death.

3 MELANOCYTE DEATH ASSOCIATED WITH OXIDATIVE STRESS

A prominent feature of vitiligo is the breakdown of the epidermis caused by the destruction of MCs, with oxidative stress identified as one of the primary causes. Therefore, it is important to elucidate the death-regulation pathway of MCs in vitiligo.

3.1 *Autophagy regulation*

Autophagy is a form of cell death regulation in vitiligo. It can be activated by many intracellular stress conditions, such as oxidative and ER stress, among others. Under these conditions, it initiates autophagosome formation via the unc-51-like autophagy-activating kinase 1 (ULK1) complex for phagocyte assembly and the class III phosphatidylinositol 3-Kinase (PI3KC3)-Beclinl complex for nucleation. Subsequently, the Atg12/Atg5/Atg16 complex kicks in to boost the conversion of microtubule-associated protein 1 light chain 3 (LC3) to the LC3II complex.

Many studies have suggested autophagy as an important factor in the cell death of vitiligo patients. Cells regulate autophagy through the energy sensor AMPK activation and subsequent mTORC1 inhibition. AMPK-mTORC1 signaling contributes to the autophagy activation in MCs (Bastonini *et al.* 2021). The study found that the LC3II/LC3I ratio and the level of Atg5 were elevated compared with healthy control MCs. In contrast, P62, the mammalian target of rapamycin, and Tyr activity levels in vitiligo MCs were obviously decreased (Cui *et al.* 2019). LC3II/LC3I and Beclin I protein levels were significantly reduced in N-acetyl-L-cysteine (NAC) treated vitiligo MCs, demonstrating that autophagy induction may be associated with redox related to imbalance (Bastonini *et al.* 2021). In vitiligo patients, ROS damages the structure and function of cells, particularly mitochondria, which may lead to impaired autophagy. This is consistent with a study that found reduced mitophagy in MCs in patients with vitiligo.

In summary, autophagy not only has the ability to maintain cell homeostasis but also participates in the pathogenesis of vitiligo. However, whether autophagy plays a dominant role in regulating MC death in vitiligo requires further investigation.

3.2 *Ferroptosis*

Ferroptosis is primarily driven by the function of ferrous ions or ester oxygenase, which catalyze the oxidation of the highly expressed unsaturated fatty acids on the cell surface, leading to peroxidation of liposomes and ultimately cell death. In addition, it is characterized by a decrease in the expression of the antioxidant system GSH and GSH peroxidase 4 (GPX4), a selenium-dependent enzyme that catalyzes lipid PXs, thereby preventing the process of ferroptosis. Unlike other forms of cell death, ferroptosis involves smaller mitochondria with denser mitochondrial membrane structures, reduced or absent mitochondrial cristae, and ruptured outer membranes. At the same time, ferroptosis also manifests as increased lipid peroxidation and increased ROS.

MCs express relatively high levels of bioavailable iron compared to other vitiligo-associated cells. Under external stimuli, the ferrous iron level and unsaturated fatty acid oxidation in MCs increase at the same time. An increase in oxidation levels can lead to an imbalance between oxidation and anti-oxidation, leading to an increase in ROS. It is widely recognized that nuclear factor E2-related factor 2 (Nrf2) plays a crucial role in the antioxidant response and in regulating cell proliferation and survival signaling. Most of the genes involved in the regulation of ferroptosis are regulated by transcriptional signaling of Nrf2, which include heme oxygenase-1 (HO-1) and GPX4. These lines of evidence demonstrate that Nrf2 is a crucial regulator. In fact, the activation and impairment of Nrf2 and those downstream genes are considered to be part of the pathological process of vitiligo. HO-1 can lead to ferroptosis, which is manifested by the excessive formation of Fe2+ to promote oxidation in reverse.

In summary, ferroptosis is suggested to be linked to MC death in vitiligo, and the specific regulatory role of GPX4 in the condition warrants further investigation.

4 IMMUNOLOGICAL MODULATIONS OF MELANOCYTES

4.1 *Innate immunity in melanocytes*

The innate immune system is non-specific and lacks memory in its pathogenic defense, which serves as the frontline defense against invading pathogens, consisting of multiple layers of physical barriers, innate immune cells, and relevant molecules. Cells or molecules in the innate immune system recognize and act on pathogens non-specifically. However, they can also mistakenly identify self-antigens, leading to the destruction of target cells and the development of autoimmune diseases.

Multiple damage-associated molecular patterns (DAMPs) have been demonstrated to be present in the perilesional skin of vitiligo patients. In fact, DAMPs containing MC-specific neoantigens, such as inducible heat shock protein 70 (HSP70i) and high-mobility group-box-1 (HMGB1), are induced and transported out of the intracellular environment. This group of signal-carrying DAMPs then stimulates the activation of innate immunity. Researchers have proved that MCs can release the chromatin-associated nuclear protein HMGB1 upon oxidative stress, and it can further affect the survival of MCs (Mou *et al.* 2018). In addition, HMGB1 can bind free DNA and HMGB1-DNA complexes, enhance the maturation of dendritic cells (DCs) in vitiligo patients, and promote the production of cytokines and chemokines, such as CXC motif chemokine ligand 16 (CXCL16) and interleukin-8 by keratinocytes (Cui *et al.* 2019). Heat shock proteins (HSPs) may be important candidates for bridging skin stress through innate immune responses. Essentially, HSP70i, a ubiquitous cytoprotectant against apoptosis, may enhance the delivery of MC antigens to major histocompatibility complex class II expressed on MCs, thereby enhancing the immunogenicity of stressed MCs. Both HSP70i and HMGB1 bind to PRRs on DCs, triggering their maturation and antigen presentation processes (Cui *et al.* 2019). DCs activated by DAMPs release a series of cytokines into the extracellular environment, while stimulated keratinocytes produce interleukin-1β, interleukin-18, CXCL9, CXC motif chemokine ligand 10 (CXCL10), and CXCL16 (Cui *et al.* 2019). Under endogenous and exogenous stress, natural killer (NK) cells and innate lymphocyte-1 (ILC1) secrete interferon-γ (IFN-γ), which induces the expression of CXC motif chemokines on the surface of MCs, including the CXC chemokine receptor 3 (CXCR3B), and triggers the release of CXCL9, CXCL10, and CXCL11 from keratinocytes and MCs. CXCL10 then activates CXCR3B, triggering MC apoptosis (Tulic, Cavazza, and Cheli 2019).

4.2 *Adaptive immunity in melanocytes*

Unlike the innate immune system, the adaptive immune system responds specifically to antigens. The adaptive immune system can create immunological memory upon an initial stimulation and generate a stronger response while stimulated with the same antigen the next time. In vitiligo, adaptive immunity contributes to the specific killing of MCs, leaving nearby cells unaffected. It is also a major player in the destruction of MCs in vitiligo. In this section, we primarily discuss T cells rather than B cells, as the role of B cell-dominated humoral immunity in the pathogenesis of vitiligo remains an unresolved puzzle.

After pro-inflammatory signals are triggered in the skin, DCs within draining lymph nodes can process and present MC antigens. This leads to the creation of MC-specific antibodies by CD8 cytotoxic T lymphocytes (CD8 CTLs). In autoimmune diseases, such as multiple sclerosis, rheumatoid arthritis, and vitiligo, CD8 CTLs play a pivotal role (Sabatino *et al.* 2019). Within the sequence of events leading to extensive MC destruction, CD8 CTLs execute the final stage, launching a definitive and lethal assault on MCs during the pathogenesis of vitiligo. Research reveals the presence of lymphocytic infiltrates predominantly composed of CD8 CTLs at the edges of depigmented lesions. These cells induce apoptosis in MCs through diverse pathways. Notably, two widely discussed pathways involve the secretion of perforin and granzyme, as well as the activation of the Fas-FasL mechanism (Deng *et al.* 2019). Nonetheless, there exists a divergence of opinions regarding the relative impact of these mechanisms on MC destruction in vitiligo. Studies utilizing a mouse model, where autoimmunity against normal MCs was prompted by DNA immunization against xenoforms of dopachrome isomerase, demonstrated that perforin is necessary for autoimmune MC destruction, with Fas-FasL's role being less critical (Bowne *et al.* 1999).

5 IMMUNOLOGICAL MODULATION OF MELANOCYTE DEATH

5.1 *Apoptosis*

Apoptosis is typically prompted by physiological or pathological factors that initiate a complex network of regulations governed by the activation of caspases and molecules, such as Bcl-2/Bax. Excessive apoptosis can contribute to conditions such as autoimmune diseases, neurodegenerative disorders, and ailments such as vitiligo. As apoptosis is initiated when signals favoring cell death surpass those supporting survival, the ratio of Bcl-2/Bax assumes significance in deciding the susceptibility of cells to induced apoptosis. Research indicates that the Bcl-2/Bax ratio in perilesional MCs is lower compared to control MCs. Consequently, Bcl-2 and Bax expression could potentially make MCs more prone to undergoing apoptosis.

The initiation of apoptosis through the extrinsic apoptotic signaling pathway relies on interactions mediated by transmembrane receptors. T lymphocyte-mediated mechanisms have been proposed as significant contributors to the loss of MC. Research indicates that levels of IFN-γ, secreted by CTL, type 1 helper T cells, NK, and ILC1, are increased in vitiligo patients. Similarly, as previously mentioned, the immune system induces apoptosis through IFN-γ-triggered expression of CXC-motif chemokine receptor CXCR3B on MC surfaces, coupled with the release of CXCL10 from both keratinocytes and MCs. This leads to the activation of CXCR3B by CXCL10, subsequently prompting MC apoptosis. Notably, heightened levels of CXCL10 in the serum and the infiltrated IFN-γ-producing cells, including CD8 TCL, have also been observed in those undergoing anti-programmed cell death-1 therapy (Larsabal *et al.* 2017). This observation lends support to the disrupted role of apoptosis in vitiligo MCs.

To summarize, apoptosis has been firmly established as a pivotal process in the demise of vitiligo MCs. Nonetheless, various studies have highlighted distinctions between MC death and conventional apoptosis, indicating the potential involvement of alternate cell death regulation for the pathogenesis of vitiligo.

5.2 *Necrosis*

Necrosis denotes an irreversible cell or organismal demise caused by external or internal physical factors (e.g., heat, stress, and radiation), chemical agents, (e.g., strong alkalis, acids, and toxins), and biological triggers (e.g., endotoxins and pathogens). Once tissue death occurs, it cannot be reversed. This contrasts with apoptosis, a natural and regulated form of cell death, whereas necrosis generally refers to pathological or abnormal cell death triggered by external agents. A key distinction between necrosis and apoptosis lies in the associated inflammation, with necrosis often leading to inflammatory responses, whereas apoptosis typically does not.

Research indicates that MCs can experience necrosis when subjected to stimulation in controlled settings. The percentage of cells undergoing necrosis rises with increasing hydrogen peroxide concentrations. Surface levels of cell surface calreticulin (CRT) increase with increased apoptosis. Under oxidative stress, elevated CRT expression promotes the apoptosis of MCs. The exposure to CRT also boosts the apoptotic process of H2O2-induced MCs, causing the activation of proinflammatory factors (Zhang *et al.* 2014). Consequently, necrosis could be linked to specific stimuli in certain types of vitiligo. However, it might not be the primary mode of MC death, especially given that most vitiligo patients do not experience intense (chemical stimuli, mechanical stimuli, etc.) irritation, and visible macroscopic signs of inflammation are absent on the skin of vitiligo lesions.

6 INTERACTION OF OXIDATIVE STRESS AND IMMUNITY

The two main theories for the pathogenesis of vitiligo involve MC death due to the autoimmune system and oxidative stress-mediated destruction of MCs. While both autoimmune system and oxidative stress may contribute to vitiligo pathogenesis, their effects can vary among patients, despite their mutually exclusive nature. The synergistic interaction between oxidative stress and autoimmune mechanisms could lead to the loss of MCs, as previously proposed. For example, in addition to direct MC toxicity, ROS can also induce autoimmune attacks against MCs in a variety of ways. Excessive accumulation of ROS leads to oxidative stress and destroys MCs, especially the mitochondria of MCs. After the MCs are destroyed, final clearance is completed by CD8 CTLs, which indicates that both oxidative stress and the autoimmune system are involved in the process from destruction to clearance of MCs. In addition, oxidative stress can induce MCs to produce HMGB1, and HMGB1 is involved in DC maturation and antigen presentation in the autoimmune system. In fact, in addition to the evidence mentioned above, phagocytosis can also prove the close connection between oxidative stress and the autoimmune system.

7 PHAGOPTOSIS: SUPPORTING OXIDATIVE STRESS THEORY AND IMMUNITY HYPOTHESIS

Previously, phagocytosis was considered a secondary process that followed apoptosis or necrosis, with the prevailing belief that phagocytes primarily engulfed dead cells or those nearing death. However, current understanding reveals that phagocytosis can actively lead to the death of living cells. This phenomenon, known as primary phagocytosis or phagoptosis, occurs when "eat me" signals become transiently exposed and/or "don't eat me" signals diminish on the membranes of living cells, triggering the process of phagocytosis.

The most typical "eat me" signal is the exposure of phosphatidylserine (PS) on the cell surface. In healthy unactivated cells, PS is exclusively expressed in the inner layer of the cellular membrane. However, under oxidative stress, PS is exposed and activated in MCs. Another major "eat me" signal is CRT, which stimulates lipoprotein receptor-related protein in phagocytes to further promote the phagocytosis process. In the context of vitiligo, an experiment demonstrated a significant increase in CRT mRNA levels induced by H2O2 treatment. Specifically, PIG1 and PIG3V cells showed increases of more than 2- to 4-fold at

2 hours post-treatment. Additionally, CRT levels were found to be higher during the active phase of the condition compared to the stable phase (Zhang *et al.* 2014).

The role of phagocytic processes in the loss of MCs within vitiligo remains uncertain due to the lack of in vivo evidence demonstrating the presence of phagocytes alongside cellular remnants and the fact that investigations in vitro are often done without phagocytes. Phagocytosis is clearly regulated by both oxidative stress and the autoimmune system. Nonetheless, it is apparent that MCs hold the potential to modulate "eat me" and "don't eat me" signaling, necessitating a more comprehensive investigation.

8 CONCLUSION

In fact, the pathogenic mechanism of vitiligo is still complex and mysterious. The death of MCs is associated with a variety of cell death mechanisms, and no clear conclusion can be drawn. The ignorance of pathogenesis limits the development of related therapies, and so far, there is still no effective cure for all of the different types of vitiligo. However, the scientific approach advanced in recent years has yielded some interesting results confirming the potential clinical implications of oxidative stress and the immune system. Oxidative stress induced by ROS plays a crucial role in the MCs of patients with vitiligo. The immune system is the last resort to kill MCs. Although MC loss may result from a variety of etiologies, the interaction between oxidative stress and the immune system is clearly one of the key pathways. Further research into the correlation between oxidative stress and immunity responses could enhance our understanding of MC loss in vitiligo patients and identify the triggers for immune system activation.

REFERENCES

Ahn Y., Seo J., Lee E. J., Kim J. Y., Park M. Y., Hwang S., Almurayshid A., Lim B. J., Yu J. W. and Oh S. H., (2020). *J. Invest. Dermatol.* **140**,9.

Bastonini E., Kovacs D., Raffa S., delle Macchie M., Pacifico A., Iacovelli P., Torrisi M. R. and Picardo M., (2021). *Cell Death Dis.* **12**,318.

Bowne W. B., Srinivasan R., Wolchok J. D., Hawkins W. G., Blachere N. E., Dyall R., Lewis J. J. and Houghton A. N., (1999). *J. Exp. Med.* **190**,11.

Cui T., Zhang W., Li S., X. et al. (2019). *J. Invest. Dermatol.* **139**, 10.

Denat L., Kadekaro A. L., Marrot L., Leachman S. A. and Abdel-Malek Z. A., (2014). *J. Invest. Dermatol.* **134**,6.

Deng Q., Luo Y., Chang C., Wu H., Ding Y. and Xiao R., (2019). *Front. Immunol.* **10**.

Di Dalmazi G., Hirshberg J., Lyle D., Freij J. B. and Caturegli P., (2016). *Immun. Highlights.* **7**, 11

Dell'Anna M. L., Ottaviani M., Albanesi V., Vidolin A. P., Leone G., Ferraro C., Cossarizza A., Rossi L. and Picardo M., (2007). *J. Invest. Dermatol.* **127**,5.

Hofer S., Stonig M., Wally V., Hartmann A., Fuchs D., Hermann M., Paparella M., Ganzera M. and Gostner J. M., (2019). *ALTEX.* **36**,2.

Karlenius T. C. and Tonissen K. F., (2010). *Cancers.* **2**,209.

Larsabal M., Marti A., Jacquemin C., Rambert J., Thiolat D., Dousset L., Taieb A., Dutriaux C., Prey S., Boniface K. and Seneschal J., (2017). *J. Am. Acad. Dermatol.* **76**,5.

Mou K., Liu W., Miao Y., Cao F., Li P., (2018). *J. Cell. Mol. Med.* **22**,61

Sabatino J. J., Wilson M. R., Calabresi P. A., Hauser S. L., Schneck J. P. and Zamvil S. S., (2019). *Proc. Natl. Acad. Sci. U. S. A.* **116**, 51.

Sastry K. S., Naeem H., Mokrab Y. and Chouchane A. I., (2019). *Oxid. Med. Cell.* Longev. **2019**.

Tulic M. K., Cavazza E., Cheli Y., Jacquel A., et al. (2019). *Nat. Commun.* **10**,1.

Zhang Y., Liu L., Jin L., Yi X., Dang E., Yang Y., Li C. and Gao T., (2014). *J. Invest. Dermatol.* **134**,1

Biological Sciences and Environmental Health – Gao (Ed.)

Acute myeloid leukemia with mutated TP53

Jie Xu
Letters and Science Department, University of California Berkeley, USA

ABSTRACT: Acute myeloid leukemia (AML) is a serious and prevalent malignant disease of the blood system. During its onset, abnormal original cells and immature cells in the bone marrow are generated in large quantities, which gather in the bone marrow, disrupting normal hematopoiesis. Various factors affect its onset, such as ionizing radiation, chemical influence, and genetic inheritance. TP53 is an important tumor suppressor gene, with mutations found in more than 50% of human tumors; such mutations may be key contributors to the main pathogenesis factors of human tumors. Studies have shown that TP53 gene abnormality is associated with the onset of AML. By exploring the specific mechanism of the TP53 mutation in AML, observing the general rule and characteristics of its mutation, and focusing on the target therapy, the role of TP53 mutation in other cancers is also described.

1 INTRODUCTION

Within the intricate landscape of blood cancers, myelodysplastic syndromes (MDS) and acute myeloid leukemia (AML) emerge as distinctive entities closely connected to the TP53 gene—a pivotal player in maintaining genomic stability. In contrast to patients with functional, wildtype p53-producing TP53, those with MDS and AML complicated by TP53 mutations respond poorly to induction chemotherapy, hypomethylating agents (HMA), and venetoclax-based treatment, resulting in poor prognosis.

AML represents a diverse spectrum of hematological malignancies characterized by unrestrained immature myeloid cell proliferation in the bone marrow and blood circulation. A prominent genetic anomaly closely linked to AML is the mutation of the TP53 gene, a pivotal guardian of cellular integrity responsible for overseeing cell cycle checkpoints and facilitating DNA repair mechanisms.

This article digs into the intricate landscape of AML, with a particular emphasis on the significance of TP53 mutations in the development and progression of this disease, the common mutation pattern in this gene, and its role in AML development. It will also explore some of the most effective treatment strategies for AML patients with TP53 mutations. Moreover, it will also discuss the importance of TP53 in other types of cancer.

2 NORMAL FUNCTIONS OF TP53 GENE

Originally identified as an oncogene, research in the past decades has shown that TP53 is, in fact, a critical tumor suppressor, playing a cytogenetically significant role (Ozaki 2011). The TP53 gene, located on chromosome 17p13.1, encodes the p53 protein, often referred to as "the guardian of the genome." As a transcription factor, the p53 protein is involved in many signal transduction pathways, including DNA damage response, oncogene activation, and

DOI: 10.1201/9781003587590-9

cellular stress, by binding directly to DNA in all cells (Daver *et al.* 2022). This positions TP53, along with its subunits located on chromosome 17p13.1, as regulators for many functions, including cell cycle arrest, DNA repair, translation, metabolism and proliferation, apoptosis, and cellular senescence (Daver *et al.* 2022). Under normal conditions, p53 levels are kept low through ubiquitin-mediated proteasomal degradation, ensuring a controlled response to cellular stress. Upon encountering stress signals such as DNA damage or oncogene activation, p53 is stabilized and activated, leading to the transcriptional upregulation of its target genes. As p53 activates, cells enter a cell cycle arrest state, allowing DNA repair processes to address the damage and maintain genomic integrity. If the damage is severe and irreparable, p53 induces apoptosis to eliminate the damaged cells, preventing the propagation of potentially harmful mutations.

Consequently, TP53 mutations in AML disrupt the normal functions of the TP53 gene, which is involved in cell cycle regulation, DNA repair, and apoptosis. These mutations impede the capacity of p53 to bind to DNA and properly regulate target genes. Leukemic cells with TP53 mutations exhibit uncontrolled cell proliferation, impaired DNA repair mechanisms, resistance to apoptosis, and increased genomic instability.

Understanding the detailed nuances of TP53 functionalities is an ongoing research focus in the p53 field. While decades of research have revealed the basic functions of TP53, much remains to be learned about this important gene, especially its correlation to immunology. For example, the research report by Sabapathy and Lane (2019) presented a novel angle of understanding the functionality by studying the antibodies associated with TP53. Recent research by Mendez *et al.* (2019) indicates that TP53's functions not only extend beyond guarding genomic integrity, but it also acts as a guardian of tumor immunosurveillance. Mendez's article went in-depth on the immunological functions of TP53, investigating antiviral immunity and suppression of virus-associated cancer, activation of NK cell ligands, restriction on tumor progression, and regulation of metabolism due to its correlation with OXPHOS (Mendez *et al.* 2019).

3 COMMON MUTATION PATTERNS IN TP53

Within the realm of cancer genetics, the mutation pattern of TP53 stands out prominently. It is, in fact, one of the most frequently mutated genes across various cancer types. Baugh *et al.* (2018) underscore that TP53 mutations are pervasive, occurring in approximately 50%–60% of human cancers. This statistic is particularly striking, as it highlights the gene's central role in tumorigenesis. Furthermore, an astounding 90% of these TP53 mutations are categorized as missense mutations, with the majority of them occurring in the gene's DNA-binding domain.

To delve deeper into the specifics of TP53 mutations, it is crucial to understand that these mutations encompass both missense point mutations and small deletions. These genetic changes are typically followed by the loss of alleles on chromosome 17p13.1's short arm, collectively leading to a malfunction in the TP53 gene. The review published on *Frontier Oncology* by Mendez *et al.* (2019) elucidates that while these mutations may not exhibit the extensive codon range changes seen in chromosomal aneuploidy, their impact can be astonishingly lethal.

These seemingly subtle missense mutations and small deletions have far-reaching consequences because they result in mutational inactivation of TP53. Mutational inactivation refers to the process whereby mutations in the TP53 gene result in the loss or impairment of its normal function. This loss of function is far from a solitary event; rather, it sets off a series of downstream effects that vary depending on the specific karyotype of the cancer. According to Mendez *et al.* (2019), they can precipitate a cascade of detrimental effects, such as the elevation of inflammatory cytokine levels and a substantial increase in tumor initiation. This underscores the critical role TP53 plays in regulating inflammatory responses and tumor suppression. This intricate interplay between TP53 mutations and the broader genomic landscape further emphasizes the gene's paramount significance in the context of cancer biology.

4 ROLE OF TP53 MUTATION IN ACUTE MYELOID LEUKEMIA

The role of TP53 mutations in AML is significant and has been extensively studied. TP53 mutation is responsible for 6% of AML, and it is grouped with chromosomal aneuploidy into a subgroup responsible for 13% of AML for their correlation (Mendez *et al.* 2019). TP53 mutations in AML are often associated with complex karyotypes, characterized by numerous chromosomal abnormalities. These complex karyotypes indicate higher genomic instability and increased genetic complexity within leukemic cells. TP53 mutations contribute to the acquisition of additional mutations and chromosomal abnormalities, leading to disease progression and therapy resistance.

TP53 mutations also confer resistance to standard chemotherapeutic agents used in AML treatment, such as anthracyclines and cytarabine (Döhner *et al.* 2009). The loss of p53 function disrupts the apoptotic response and impairs DNA repair mechanisms, enabling leukemic cells to survive and proliferate in the presence of DNA damage induced by chemotherapy. Consequently, patients with AML complicated by TP53 mutations frequently have a poorer response to standard therapies like chemotherapy and are at a higher risk of relapse after the administration of the treatment. Studies have associated TP53 mutated AML with higher relapse rates and inferior overall survival compared to NON-muted cases (Döhner *et al.* 2009; Rücker *et al.* 2011). TP53-mutated AML is considered a high-risk subgroup, and the presence of TP53 mutations is an independent adverse prognostic factor. These patients often exhibit more aggressive disease features, including higher white blood cell counts and more frequent extramedullary involvement. They are generally considered high-risk and may require alternative or intensified treatment approaches. Allogeneic hematopoietic stem cell transplantation (allo-HSCT) is often considered in eligible patients with TP53-mutated AML, as it provides a chance for cure by eradicating leukemic cells and replacing them with healthy donor cells. However, even with allo-HSCT, this disease subgroup remains challenging to treat due to its high relapse rate and transplant-related complications (Döhner *et al.* 2009; Rücker *et al.* 2011). The impact of TP53 mutation on patients choosing allo-HSCT has been discussed in the following section.

Understanding the foundational mutation landscape of TP53 may explain the poor prognosis and treatment resistance. TP53 mutations in AML often co-occur with other genetic alterations, further influencing disease outcomes. FLT3-ITD, NPM1, and DNMT3A mutations are common co-occurring mutations (Mendez *et al.* 2019). The presence of these mutations alongside TP53 mutations may confer additional adverse prognostic implications and impact treatment responses.

Large-scale sequencing efforts have yielded valuable insights into the genetic landscape of AML, shedding light on the complexity of this hematologic malignancy. In a large study undertaken by the Cancer Genome Atlas Network, whole exome and whole genome sequencing were employed to analyze 200 de novo AML samples. This thorough genomic investigation uncovered a list of recurrently altered genes in AML, providing crucial information for understanding the disease's pathogenesis (Cancer Genome Atlas Research Network 2013).

One striking finding from this research is the relatively low number of mutations observed in coding genes within AML patients, averaging approximately 13 mutations per individual (Cancer Genome Atlas Research Network 2013). Despite the relatively low mutation burden, these genetic alterations play pivotal roles in the disease's development and progression. Among these mutations, five stood out as recurrent, highlighting their significance in AML.

The concept of mutual exclusivity observed across diverse combinations of mutations is particularly noteworthy. This linkage pattern suggests that different genetic mutations may converge on common pathways or mechanisms, leading to the emergence of AML. Among the recurrently mutated genes, mutual exclusivity was notably observed between mutations in NPM1, RUNX1, CEBPA, TP53, and transcription factor-fusion genes (Cancer Genome Atlas Research Network 2013). These findings imply that these specific genetic alterations may independently drive AML through different biological processes, and when one occurs, the likelihood of the others diminishes significantly.

However, the complexity of AML genetics extends beyond mutual exclusivity, as co-occurrence of mutations was also noted. For instance, FLT3-ITD, DNMT3A, and NPM1 mutations were found to co-occur in some AML patients (Cancer Genome Atlas Research Network 2013). This co-occurrence suggests potential interactions or synergistic effects between these genetic changes, further highlighting the intricate interplay of genetic alterations in AML pathogenesis.

The extensive genomic analysis conducted by the Cancer Genome Atlas Network has unraveled critical insights into the genetic underpinnings of AML. While AML is characterized by a relatively low number of coding gene mutations per patient, recurrent mutations, mutual exclusivity, and co-occurrence patterns have illuminated the intricate genetic landscape of the disease. These findings offer valuable avenues for further research and therapeutic exploration, ultimately aiming to improve the understanding of AML and the development of targeted treatments for this complex malignancy.

5 TREATMENT METHODS FOR TP53-MUT ACUTE MYELOID LEUKEMIA

The presence of TP53 mutations in AML poses significant challenges to treatment decision-making. Patients with TP53-mutated AML have demonstrated resistance to standard chemotherapeutic regimens as well as lower response rates to traditional induction therapies.

5.1 *Allogeneic hematopoietic stem cell transplantation*

The medical procedure known as allogeneic hematopoietic stem cell transplantation (allo-HSCT) is used to treat certain hematological cancers, such as AML with TP53 mutations. In allo-HSCT, healthy donor stem cells, normally from a genetically matched relative or unrelated donor, are transplanted into the patient after their own diseased bone marrow and immune system have been suppressed or eliminated through chemotherapy and/or radiation treatment. By replacing cancerous cells with healthy ones, these donor stem cells can create a new, healthy immune system and restore blood cell production in the recipient. In the case of TP53-mutated AML, allo-HSCT is considered a potential curative approach, as it offers the opportunity to replace the compromised bone marrow with genetically normal stem cells, potentially leading to disease remission and long-term survival in eligible patients. However, outcomes remain suboptimal due to the high risk of relapse and transplant-related complications. Numerous studies have consistently revealed that individuals afflicted with TP53-mutated AML or MDS face a daunting 80% to 90% escalated risk of relapse and mortality after receiving allogeneic stem cell transplantation (allo-SCT), as opposed to their TP53 wildtype counterparts (Lindsley *et al.* 2017; Medeiros *et al.* 2016; Yoshizato *et al.* 2017). The majority of these post-allo-SCT relapses and fatalities tend to occur among patients who exhibit concurrent chromosome 17 abnormalities or complex karyotypes, which signify a multifaceted disease state (Loke *et al.* 2022). Nevertheless, among TP53-mutated AML patients, the detection of allo-SCT during their first remission (CR1) has demonstrated the potential to significantly diminish the risk of relapse by as much as 80% and reduce the risk of death by up to 70% (Short *et al.* 2020). Unfortunately, regardless of age or physical condition, only a small proportion of TP53-mutated AML patients manage to progress to have the option of allo-SCT in CR1. This percentage ranges from 0% to 33% in various published series, with reduced response rates, insufficient blood cell recovery, elevated early mortality rates, and premature relapse emerging as the main barriers to choosing allo-SCT for a full recovery in this particular patient population (Kim *et al.* 2021; Short *et al.* 2020; Welch *et al.* 2016).

Given that the prognosis for patients who do not achieve morphologic remission before receiving allo-SCT is often poor and that this situation is made considerably worse in the case of TP53-mutated AML, this strategy seems prudent. It is significant to note that the removal of TP53 mutations prior to allo-SCT has been established as a positive prognostic factor. Therefore, patients who successfully achieve TP53 mutation clearance or demonstrate a mutation burden of less than 5% as measured by next-generation sequencing should be considered for transition to allo-SCT despite the possible risk of relapse (Hunter *et al.* 2016).

5.2 *Combination therapy*

Elderly patients and individuals with comorbidities often face daunting challenges when it comes to treating AML. For these groups, the conventional intensive chemotherapy or allogeneic cell transplantation regimens can be prohibitively risky. Fortunately, a beacon of hope emerges in the form of combination therapy involving venetoclax, a BCL-2 inhibitor, and hypomethylating agents (HMA). As highlighted in *Blood*, a comprehensive study published by DiNardo *et al.* (2018), this innovative treatment approach has garnered significant attention for its potential to offer safer and more effective options. In their phase 1b study, DiNardo and colleagues reported that patients treated with venetoclax combined with decitabine or azacitidine showed a higher rate of complete remission (CR) + CR with incomplete count recovery (CRi), prolonged median duration of CR + CRi, and a longer median overall survival compared to those not receiving the combination therapy: 67% versus 47%, 11.3 months versus 5.6 months, and 17.5 months versus 7.2 months, respectively (DiNardo *et al.* 2018).

Building upon this promising foundation, a more recent review by Daver *et al.* (2022) shed further light on the significant impact of this combination therapy, indicating that it can lead to enhanced rates of achieving complete remission or complete remission with incomplete hematologic recovery (CR+CRi) in TP53-mutated AML patients. These approaches not only hold promise in achieving higher rates of remission and prolonged survival but also offer hope to patients who may not be eligible for more aggressive treatments, thereby reshaping the therapeutic paradigm for this challenging hematologic malignancy.

Furthermore, the Food and Drug Administration's approval of venetoclax in 2020 for use in combination with azacitidine, decitabine, or low-dose cytarabine specifically for elderly patients and those with comorbidities underscores the clinical significance and relevance of these findings. This regulatory approval not only validates the efficacy and safety of this treatment but also paves the way for more accessible and tailored therapeutic options in the future.

5.3 *Other treatment*

In recent years, novel therapeutic approaches targeting specific vulnerabilities associated with TP53-mutated AML have emerged. One promising strategy involves the use of small molecules that reactivate mutant p53, such as PRIMA-1 (PRIMA-1Met) and APR-246, which have shown promising preclinical and early clinical activity in restoring p53 function and inducing leukemic cell death (Zatloukalová *et al* 2018). Furthermore, novel agents targeting specific genetic alterations co-occurring with TP53 mutations, such as IDH1/2 inhibitors, may also have a role in the management of TP53-mutated AML (Medeiros *et al.* 2017).

6 TP53 IN OTHER TYPES OF CANCER

In addition to its involvement in AML, TP53 mutations are observed in various other types of cancer, both hematological and solid tumors. The TP53 gene is known as a tumor suppressor gene, and its mutation or inactivation contributes to tumor development and progression. Some examples of cancer types in which TP53 mutations are frequently found are discussed as follows:

Colorectal cancer: TP53 mutations are commonly detected in about 50% of colorectal cancer patients, particularly in the advanced stages of the disease (Iacopetta 2003). These mutations often correlate with poor prognosis and resistance to chemotherapy.

Breast cancer: Approximately 30% of TP53 mutations are found in a subset of breast cancer cases, particularly those associated with hereditary breast and ovarian cancer syndrome (BRCA1/2 mutations) (Shahbandi *et al.* 2020). TP53 mutations in breast cancer are associated with aggressive tumor behavior and resistance to treatment.

Lung cancer: TP53 mutations occur in about 50% of non-small cell lung cancer (NSCLC), a subgroup that makes up 80% of all lung cancer cases (Sun *et al.* 2023). TP53 mutations in NSCLC are associated with increased tumor aggressiveness, resistance to chemotherapy, and poor patient outcomes.

Ovarian cancer: TP53 mutations of about 96% are frequently observed in high-grade serous ovarian cancer, the most common and aggressive subtype within this category (Oien and Chien 2016). TP53 mutations are associated with early tumor initiation and progression, as well as resistance to chemotherapy.

Pancreatic cancer: TP53 mutations are common in pancreatic ductal adenocarcinoma (PDAC), with about 50% to 75% of patients having TP53 mutations (Morton *et al.* 2022), a highly lethal malignancy. TP53 mutations in PDAC are associated with tumor progression, metastasis, and resistance to therapy.

The main takeaway from these data is that the frequency and impact of TP53 mutations can vary among different cancer types and patient populations. The specific type and location of TP53 mutations can also influence their functional consequences and clinical implications.

7 CONCLUSION

This paper explores the characteristics of TP53 mutations in AML and other cancers. The association between TP53 and AML involves multiple mechanisms, and the mutated genes are correlated with clinical features and prognosis. However, the existing clinical evidence is not strong, and further clinical research is needed to identify potential targets for treatment and better guide the formulation of individualized treatment plans to improve the long-term survival outcomes for cancer patients.

REFERENCES

Baugh E.H., Ke H., Levine A.J., Bonneau R.A. and Chan C.S. (2018 Jan). Why are there hotspot mutations in the TP53 gene in human cancers? Cell Death Differ. **25**(1):154-160. DOI: 10.1038/cdd.2017.180. Epub 2017 Nov 3. PMID: 29099487; PMCID: PMC5729536.

Cancer Genome Atlas Research Network. 2013. *New England Journal of Medicine*. **368**(22):2059–74.

Daver N.G., Maiti A., Kadia T.M., Vyas P., Majeti R., Wei A.H., Garcia-Manero G., Craddock C., Sallman D.A. and Kantarjian H.M. (2022). TP53-Mutated myelodysplastic syndrome and acute myeloid leukemia: Biology, current therapy, and future directions. *Cancer Discov.* 12(11):2516–2529, 10.1158/2159-8290.CD-22-0332. *Erratum in: Cancer Discov.* 2022 Dec;**12**(12):2954. PMID: 36218325; PMCID: PMC9627130.

DiNardo C.D., Pratz K., Pullarkat V., Jonas B.A., Arellano M., Becker P.S., Frankfurt O., Konopleva M., Wei A.H., Kantarjian H.M., Xu T., Hong W.J., Chyla B., Potluri J., Pollyea D.A., Letai A. (2019 Jan 3). Venetoclax combined with decitabine or azacitidine in treatment-naive, elderly patients with acute myeloid leukemia. *Blood.* **133**(1):7–17. DOI: 10.1182/blood-2018-08-868752. Epub 2018 Oct 25. PMID: 30361262; PMCID: PMC6318429.

Döhner H., Estey E.H., Amadori S., Appelbaum F.R., Büchner T., Burnett A.K., Dombret H., Fenaux P., Grimwade D., Larson R.A., Lo-Coco F., Naoe T., Niederwieser D., Ossenkoppele G.J., Sanz M.A., Sierra J., Tallman M.S. and Löwenberg B., C.D. (2010 Jan 21). Bloomfield; European LeukemiaNet. Diagnosis and management of acute myeloid leukemia in adults: recommendations from an international expert panel, on behalf of the *European LeukemiaNet. Blood.* **115**(3):453–74. DOI: 10.1182/blood-2009-07-235358. Epub 2009 Oct 30. PMID: 19880497.

Hunter A.M., Komrokji R.S., Yun S., Al Ali N., Chan O., Song J., Hussaini M., Talati C., Sweet K.L., Lancet J.E., Padron E., List A.F. and Sallman D.A. (2021 Feb 23). Baseline and serial molecular profiling predicts outcomes with hypomethylating agents in myelodysplastic syndromes. *Blood Adv.*;**5**(4):1017–1028. DOI: 10.1182/bloodadvances.2020003508. PMID: 33591325; PMCID: PMC7903224.

Iacopetta B. (2003 Mar). TP53 mutation in colorectal cancer. *Hum Mutat.* **21**(3):271–6. DOI: 10.1002/humu.10175. PMID: 12619112.

Kim K., Maiti A., Loghavi S., Pourebrahim R., Kadia T.M., Rausch C.R., Furudate K., Daver N.G., Alvarado Y., Ohanian M., Sasaki K., Short N.J., Takahashi K., Yilmaz M., Tang G., Ravandi F., Kantarjian H.M., DiNardo C.D. and Konopleva M.Y. (2021 Oct 15). Outcomes of TP53-mutant acute myeloid leukemia with decitabine and venetoclax. *Cancer.*;**127**(20):3772–3781. DOI: 10.1002/cncr.33689. Epub 2021 Jul 13. PMID: 34255353; PMCID: PMC10462434.

Lindsley R.C., et al. (2017). *The New England Journal of Medicine*. **376**(6):536–47.

Loke J., Labopin M., Craddock C., Cornelissen J.J., Labussière-Wallet H., Wagner-Drouet E.M., Van Gorkom G., Schaap N.P.M., Kröger N.M., Veelken J.H., Rovira M., Menard A.L., Bug G., Bazarbachi A., Giebel S., Brissot E., Nagler A., Esteve J. and Mohty M. (2022 Aug 1). Additional cytogenetic features determine outcome in patients allografted for TP53 mutant acute myeloid leukemia. *Cancer.* **128** (15):2922–2931. DOI: 10.1002/cncr.34268. Epub 2022 May 25. PMID: 35612815; PMCID: PMC9545190.

Medeiros B.C., Fathi A.T., DiNardo C.D., Pollyea D.A., Chan S.M. and Swords R. (2017 Feb). Isocitrate dehydrogenase mutations in myeloid malignancies. *Leukemia.* **31**(2):272–281. DOI: 10.1038/leu.2016.275. Epub 2016 Oct 10. PMID: 27721426; PMCID: PMC5292675.

Mendez L.M., Posey R.R. and Pandolfi P.P. (2019 Nov). The Interplay Between the Genetic and Immune Landscapes of AML: Mechanisms and Implications for Risk Stratification and Therapy. *Front Oncol.* **7**;9:1162. 10.3389/fonc.2019.01162. PMID: 31781488; PMCID: PMC6856667.

Morton J.P., Timpson P., Karim S.A., Ridgway R.A., Athineos D., Doyle B., Jamieson N.B., Oien K.A., Lowy A.M., Brunton V.G., Frame M.C., Evans T.R. and Sansom O.J. (2010 Jan 5). Mutant p53 drives metastasis and overcomes growth arrest/senescence in pancreatic cancer. *Proc Natl Acad Sci U S A.* 107 (1):246–51. DOI: 10.1073/pnas.0908428107. Epub 2009 Dec 14. Erratum in: *Proc Natl Acad Sci U S A.* 2022 Apr 26;**119**(17):e2204610119. PMID: 20018721; PMCID: PMC2806749.

Oien D.B. and Chien J. (2016). TP53 mutations as a biomarker for high-grade serous ovarian cancer: are we there yet? *Transl Cancer Res*;**5**(Suppl 2):S264–S268. DOI: 10.21037/tcr.2016.07.45.

Ozaki T. and Nakagawara A. (2011). *Cancers (Basel)*. **3**(1):994–1013.

Rücker F.G., Schlenk R.F., Bullinger L., Kayser S., Teleanu V., Kett H., Habdank M., Kugler C.M., Holzmann K., Gaidzik V.I., Paschka P., Held G., von Lilienfeld-Toal M., Lübbert M., Fröhling S., Zenz T., Krauter J., Schlegelberger B., Ganser A., Lichter P., Döhner K. and Döhner H. (2012 Mar 1). TP53 alterations in acute myeloid leukemia with complex karyotype correlate with specific copy number alterations, monosomal karyotype, and dismal outcome. *Blood.***119**(9):2114–21. DOI: 10.1182/blood-2011-08-375758. Epub 2011 Dec 20. PMID: 22186996.

Sabapathy K. and Lane D.P. (2019). Understanding p53 functions through p53 antibodies. *J Mol Cell Biol.* 11 (4):317–329, 10.1093/jmcb/mjz010. Erratum in: *J Mol Cell Biol.* 2019 Dec;**11**(12):1105. PMID: 30907951; PMCID: PMC6487784.

Shahbandi A., Nguyen H.D., Jackson J.G. (2020 Feb). TP53 Mutations and Outcomes in Breast Cancer: Reading beyond the Headlines. *Trends Cancer.* **6**(2):98–110. doi: 10.1016/j.trecan.2020.01.007. Epub 2020 Feb 5. PMID: 32061310; PMCID: PMC7931175.

Short N.J., Montalban-Bravo G., Hwang H., Ning J., Franquiz M.J., Kanagal-Shamanna R., Patel K.P., DiNardo C.D., Ravandi F., Garcia-Manero G., Takahashi K., Konopleva M., Daver N., Issa G.C., Andreeff M., Kantarjian H. and Kadia T.M. (2020 Nov 24). Prognostic and therapeutic impacts of mutant

TP53 variant allelic frequency in newly diagnosed acute myeloid leukemia. *Blood Adv.* **4**(22):5681–5689. DOI: 10.1182/bloodadvances.2020003120. PMID: 33211826; PMCID: PMC7686900.

Sun H., Ren P., Chen Y., et al. (2023). Optimal therapy for concomitant EGFR and TP53 mutated non-small cell lung cancer: a real-world study. *BMC Cancer.* **23**, 198. https://doi.org/10.1186/s12885-023-10637-4.

Welch J.S., Petti A.A., Miller C.A., Fronick C.C., O'Laughlin M., Wilson R.S., Baty J.D., Duncavage E.J., Tandon B., Lee Y.S., Wartman L.D., Uy G.L., Ghobadi A., Tomasson M.H., Pusic I., Romee R., Fehniger T.A., Stockerl-Goldstein K.E., Vij R., Oh S.T., Abboud C.N. , Cashen A.F., Schroeder M.A., Jacoby M.A., Heath S.E., Luber K., Janke M.R., Hantel A., Khan N., Sukhanova M.J., Knoebel R.W., Stock W., Graubert T.A., Walter M.J., Westervelt P., Link D.C., DiPersio J.F. and Ley T.J. (2016 Nov 24). TP53 and Decitabine in Acute Myeloid Leukemia and Myelodysplastic Syndromes. *N Engl J Med.* **375** (21):2023–2036. DOI: 10.1056/NEJMoa1605949. PMID: 27959731; PMCID: PMC5217532.

Yoshizato T., Nannya Y., Atsuta Y., Shiozawa Y., Iijima-Yamashita Y., Yoshida K., Shiraishi Y., Suzuki H., Nagata Y., Sato Y., Kakiuchi N., Matsuo K., Onizuka M., Kataoka K., Chiba K., Tanaka H., Ueno H., Nakagawa M.M., Przychodzen B., Haferlach C., Kern W., Aoki K., Itonaga H., Kanda Y., Sekeres M.A., Maciejewski J.P., Haferlach T., Miyazaki Y., Horibe K., Sanada M., Miyano S., Makishima H. and Ogawa S. (2017 Apr 27). Genetic abnormalities in myelodysplasia and secondary acute myeloid leukemia: impact on outcome of stem cell transplantation. *Blood.*;**129**(17):2347–2358. DOI: 10.1182/blood-2016-12-754796. Epub 2017 Feb 21. PMID: 28223278; PMCID: PMC5409449.

Zatloukalová P., Galoczová M. and Vojt⊠šek B. (2018 Winter). Prima-1 and APR-246 in Cancer Therapy. Klin Onkol. **31**(Suppl 2):71–76. English. DOI: 10.14735/amko20182S71. PMID: 31023027.

Biological Sciences and Environmental Health – Gao (Ed.)

Role of MYCN gene in high-risk neuroblastoma

He Liang
Nanchang Institute of Technology, HangZhou, China

ABSTRACT: Neuroblastoma is a prevalent solid tumor affecting young children, arising from developing neural crest cells. Neuroblastoma exhibits genetic, morphological, and clinical heterogeneity, manifesting in different areas such as the abdomen, neck, adrenal glands, and pelvis. The MYC protein serves as a primary regulatory factor for cellular fate and is a short-lived transcription factor strictly controlled by the ubiquitin proteasome system. MYCN promotes tumorigenesis in Neuroblastoma. Abnormal amplification of MYCN is strongly linked to an unfavorable prognosis in patients. This review focusing on MYCN involve in various biological processes such as metastasis, self-renewal, proliferation and angiogenesis. In non-amplification neuroblastoma cases, downregulation of MYCN promotes tumor progression. To our knowledge, the essentiality of the MYCN signaling pathway in the biology of neuroblastoma is so far underscored. This article reviews the various targeted therapies that regulate the protein stability and transcriptional level of MYCN, emphasizing its feasibility as a therapeutic target for high-risk neuroblastoma.

1 INTRODUCTION

Neuroblastoma (NB) is the most common extracranial solid tumor in children. It predominantly affects children under the age of 5 and accounts for approximately 7% of all childhood cancers, with a mortality rate of around 15% (Matthay *et al.* 2016). NB can present as localized disease or widespread metastasis, with rare instances of spontaneous regression. While low to intermediate-risk NB can be managed by surgical resection alone, High-risk NB often proves fatal. Aggressive multimodal therapies, including chemotherapy, radiation therapy, and surgery, have improved the 5-year survival rate from less than 20% to over 50%. Thus, understanding the underlying molecular mechanisms of NB is crucial in developing safer and more effective treatment strategies.

MYCN is a member of the MYC gene family. In primary NB tissues, *MYCN* amplification has a strong statistical correlation with the 17q21-ter alteration, the most common genetic aberration in NB, with an incidence rate of 38-65%. *MYCN* amplification is recognized as a significant biological marker associated with a negative prognosis in NB. During early development, it is highly expressed in migrating neural crest cells. In normal mouse sympathetic adrenal gland development, it plays a key role in the regulation of cell proliferation and ventral migration within the neural crest (Figure 1) (Hatton *et al.* 2006).

2 RISK STRATIFICATION IN NEUROBLASTOMA

Risk stratification is very helpful in determining the likelihood of cure and determining the appropriate level of treatment in NB children. Low-risk NB cases can typically be effectively

DOI: 10.1201/9781003587590-10

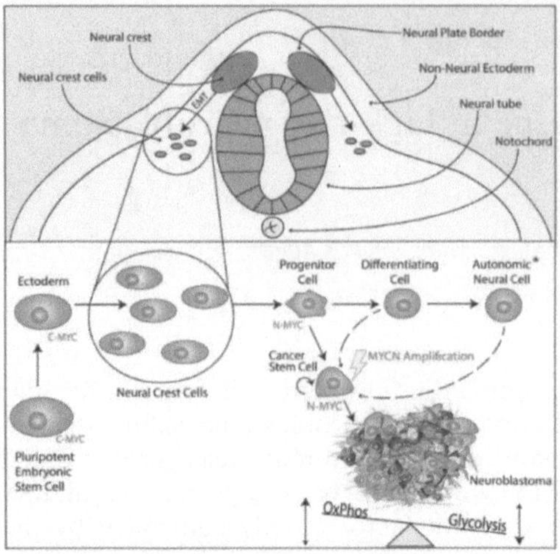

Figure 1. MYCN promotes tumorigenesis in Neuroblastoma (Hatton *et al.* 2006).

managed through surgical intervention alone, whereas high-risk NB cases require intensified treatment to maximize the chances of cure. Initially, the Children's Oncology Group (COG) relied on the International Neuroblastoma Staging System (INSS) to categorize patients into three risk groups: low, intermediate, and high-risk. However, the field is presently transitioning towards the adoption of the International Neuroblastoma Risk Group Staging System (INRGSS). The INRG classification assigns children to one of 16 pretreatment groups labeled A through R, based on several factors, and subsequently divides them into four overall risk groups: very low-risk, low-risk, intermediate-risk, and high-risk.

3 MYCN AMPLIFICATION IN HIGH-RISK NEUROBLASTOMA

Research on NB has demonstrated that targeted expression of *MYCN* in peripheral neuroblasts of mice using the rat tyrosine hydroxylase (TH) promoter led to NB development, confirming that aberrant *MYCN* expression can initiate this disease within migratory neural crest cells. *MYCN* amplification plays multifaceted roles in the pathogenesis of NB tumors.

3.1 *Metastasis*

Approximately 50% of patients with NB tumors experience metastasis, which involves the spread of tumors to various locations including the bone marrow, bone, lymph nodes, liver, and brain. The level of *MYCN* expression has been associated with invasive and metastatic behavior. Notably, previous research has indicated that *GAS7*, as an evolutionarily conserved gene, is involved in multiple developmental pathways as a suppressor of tumor metastasis. In cases where *MYCN* amplification is present, the expression level of *GAS7* is significantly lower compared to cases without *MYCN* amplification. Studies using animal model systems have shown that reducing *GAS7* expression can promote the metastasis of *MYCN* amplification NB cells (Dong *et al.* 2021). Overexpression and genetic alterations of *LIN28B* has been found repress let-7 family genes in mature tumors (Balzeau *et al.* 2017). This inhibitory effect increased *MYCN* expression. *FAK* are upregulated in *MYCN* amplification NB cell lines and tumor specimens by bioinformatics analysis. Further analysis revealed that MYCN could bind to the *FAK* promoter region. Also was confirmed in vitro and in vivo experiments. In addition, the application of RNA interference and/or small molecule inhibitors against *FAK* reduced the invasion and migration ability of NB cell lines (Megison *et al.* 2013). Together, these studies demonstrate that *MYCN* and its regulatory proteins promote NB genesis (Table 1).

Table 1. Genes regulated by MYCN in Neuroblastoma.

Model System	Regulated by *MYCN*	Functions	References
Cell lines, Mouse Zebrafish	*GAS7*	Migration, Invasion, Metastasis	Dong *et al.* 2021
Cell lines, Mouse	*LIN28B*	Migration, Invasion, Metastasis	Balzeau *et al.* 2017
Cell lines, Mouse	*FAK*	Migration, Invasion, Metastasis	Megison *et al.* 2013

3.2 *Proliferation*

Research has shown that *MYCN* can increase the proliferation of NB cells through multiple mechanisms. Specifically, *TRPM6* and *TRPM7* have been identified as transcriptional targets of *MYCN* in NB. The proteins TRPM6 and TRPM7 can promote the uptake of calcium and magnesium in cells and enhance cell proliferation. *HMGA1* is an important regulator of cell growth, and *MYCN* increases cell proliferation by upregulating the expression of *HMGA1*. *E2F2* can activate transcription behind *MYCN*, promoting cell proliferation through the activation and progression of cell cycle-induced transcription. Research has found that *SHMT2* is highly expressed in NB with *MYCN* amplification. This enzyme breaks down serine and the resulting glycine can be used in methyl biosynthesis to promote cell proliferation.

3.3 *Angiogenesis*

Angiogenesis is a biological process through which preexisting vessels give rise to new capillary blood vessels. The *MYCN* oncogene is capable of stimulating tumor angiogenesis, thereby facilitating the progression of NB. Biopsy samples from NB patients with and without *MYCN* amplification were compared, as well as samples derived from NB cell line xenografts, using the chick chorioallantoic membrane (CAM) assay to measure angiogenic ability, demonstrated that the angiogenic velocity of all *MYCN* amplification samples was significantly higher than that of non- amplification samples. Notably, *MYCN* knockout mice either perish in utero or manifest severe cardiovascular abnormalities, underscoring the fundamental role of *MYCN* in normal cardiovascular development. Increasing evidence suggests that drugs that interfere with angiogenesis can impede the progression of NB. Consequently, employing anti-angiogenic strategies may represent an efficacious approach to treating NB.

3.4 *Apoptosis*

MYCN can bind to the promoter of the p53 gene and stimulate its expression. *MDM2*, an E3 ligase, is the major antagonist of p53, promoting its ubiquitination and inhibition. *MDM2* can be directly induced by *N-MYC* but is also regulated by feedback mechanisms. *MDM2* is intriguingly known as a transcriptional target of *p53*, while MYCN can concurrently enhance the transcription of *MDM2* and *p53*. The activation of *MYCN* in *MDM2* and *p53* explains the potential of MYCN amplification in NB to exhibit chemotherapy resistance and relapse (Maerken *et al.* 2009).

Loss of Caspase-8 function in NB is considered as a mechanism by which *MYCN* amplification enables evasion of apoptosis. The loss of Caspase-8 enhances the production of tumor necrosis factor-related apoptosis-inducing ligands and induces apoptosis resistance in NB tumors.

3.5 *Differentiation*

MYCN plays an important role in the process of embryonic development. Mutations in human *MYCN* have been linked to birth defects. Mouse embryos that lack *MYCN* perish around E11.5 and display severe developmental deficiencies in multiple organs and tissues. The presence of endogenous *C-MYC* or *N-MYC* is vital for the pluripotency and self-renewal of mouse embryonic stem cells (ESCs) and induced pluripotent stem cells (iPSCs). The simultaneous loss of these two genes is incompatible with the maintenance of pluripotency and leads to spontaneous differentiation. Furthermore, the overexpression of *MYCN* during neural crest cell differentiation can lead to an increase in neurons.

3.6 *Immune surveillance*

Immunotherapy combined with chemotherapy has emerged as a new treatment strategy. Multiple omics analyses of NB cells have identified a multitude of tumor-related genes and antigens. Notably, the *MYCN* and the ganglioside surface antigen GD2 have been found to be particularly important. n clinical trials, Daratumumab has been shown to improve patient survival rates (Ladenstein *et al.* 2013). It is worth noting that, in high-risk NB cohorts, T cell and cytotoxic cell markers and CD8+ infiltration are lower in *MYCN* amplification tumors compared to *MYCN* non- amplification tumors, suggesting that the low infiltration of tumor-infiltrating lymphocytes (TILs) is at least partly associated with *MYCN* amplification. The possible reasons for reduced TIL infiltration in *MYCN* amplification tumors may include reduced attraction and activation of lymphocytes by *MYCN* amplification cells, as well as diminished immunogenicity.

4 HIGH-RISK NEUROBLASTOMA WITHOUT MYCN AMPLIFICATION

In NB, once amplification of the *MYCN* is detected, it is classified as high-risk and treated according to the therapeutic protocols for high-risk NB. However, for *MYCN* non-amplification NB, there is currently a lack of better clinical or prognostic indicators. The summarization and analysis of its genetic characteristics and pathogenesis have expanded the genetic diagnostic strategies for NB.

4.1 *Chromosomal gains and losses*

Nearly all high-risk NB patients exhibit periodic changes in chromosomal copy number, and the specific alterations have been identified to have prognostic relevance. In approximately one-third of high-risk patients, 11q deletion is inversely associated with *MYCN*-driven high-risk NB. In *MYCN* non-amplification NB, gain or loss of whole chromosomes can result in hyperdiploidy (defined as a DNA index >1), which is a prognostic variable that is particularly meaningful in infants with *MYCN* non-amplification NB, with better outcomes observed in patients with hyperdiploidy compared to patients with normal diploidy (DI of 1).

4.2 *CircRNAs regulation*

CircRNA is an important non-coding RNA that has been extensively studied in the pathogenesis of NB. Increasing evidence suggests its involvement in tumor cell proliferation, invasion, and migration. For high-risk NB without *MYCN* amplification, it has been suggested that non-coding RNAs (ncRNAs) may play a crucial role. In a study analyzing transcriptome data from 104 NB patients across all risk groups, Comparing the tumor samples of high-risk NB patients with MYCN amplification or non-amplification, it was found that the abundance and expression of CircRNAs were negatively correlated with

MYCN expression. *MYCN* comprehensively inhibited CircRNAs expression by upregulating the expression of *DHX9* RNA helicase (Fuchs *et al.* 2023). Moreover, CircRNAs have been found to have dual functions in promoting tumor progression and inhibiting tumor initiation. Both upregulation and downregulation of CircRNA expression have the potential to inhibit tumor growth, highlighting its potential as a therapeutic target.

5 THERAPEUTIC STRATEGIES FOR HIGH-RISK NEUROBLASTOMA

In *MYCN* amplification NB, inhibiting the transcription or expression of *MYCN* through RNA interference and CRISPR knockout led to increased apoptosis and differentiation, as well as reduced cell viability. These findings provide a potential therapeutic approach for treating *MYCN*-driven NB by blocking *MYCN* expression. However, MYCN, as a transcription factor, does not have binding sites for small molecules and cannot be directly targeted by drugs. Strategies for the treatment of *MYCN*-driven NB encompass several approaches. Firstly, targeting proteins that are either upstream or downstream of the cellular pathways involving MYCN, such as the acetyl-lysine binding domain (bromodomain), can be an effective strategy. Secondly, directing therapeutic interventions towards genes involved in regulating MYCN mRNA or protein stability holds promise. Furthermore, activating p53-induced apoptosis is another avenue to pursue in combating this disease. Lastly, inducing NB differentiation has been identified as a potential strategy (Huang and Weiss 2013).

5.1 *BET bromodomain inhibitors*

One strategy to suppress MYCN gene expression is to use the inhibitors that specifically target the bromodomain and the extra-terminal domain (BET) family. BET proteins function as transcriptional regulators, JQ1 (a BET inhibitor) can block the growth of *MYCN* targets and MYCN. In xenograft models derived from patients with NB and the TH-MYCN mouse model, JQ1 inhibits the growth of *MYCN* amplification NB, significantly increases overall survival in treated mice, promotes tumor cell apoptosis, and reduces proliferation. GSK1324726A (I-BET726), similarly, inhibits BET and MYCN expression, induces cytotoxicity, and suppresses cell growth.

5.2 *HDAC inhibitors*

Targeting histone deacetylases (HDACs) has been demonstrated as an effective therapeutic strategy for *MYCN*-driven NB. Several preclinical studies have shown the efficacy of HDAC inhibitors (HDACis) in *MYCN*-driven cancers. For instance, the SIRT1 inhibitor Cambinol reduced tumor incidence in a Th-MYCN driven NB mouse model. Vorinostat (SAHA), a histone deacetylase (HDAC) inhibitor, significantly enhanced cytotoxic effects in a panel of NB cell lines and completely blocked tumor growth in *MYCN* transgenic mice and zebrafish. Therefore, HDAC inhibitors offer a promising targeted therapeutic approach for *MYCN* amplification NB.

5.3 *Antagonists of MDM2*

Unlike many other malignant tumors, NB rarely exhibits p53 mutations. Specifically targeting the p53/MDM2 pathway in NB using inhibitors can be a promising therapeutic strategy. Several studies have demonstrated the efficacy of various MDM2 inhibitors in the treatment of NB. For instance, Nutlin-3, an antagonist, specifically targets p53 in the p53-MDM2 pathway and induces cell apoptosis, showing anti-tumor effects in both chemo-sensitive and resistant NB cell lines. The second-generation Nutlin, RG7388 showed better antitumor efficacy and lower toxicity in experiments.

5.4 *Regulators of MYCN protein stability*

Aurora A kinase (AURKA) has the capability to stabilize MYCN through protein-protein interactions, thereby safeguarding MYCN from proteasomal degradation. Consequently, inhibiting AURKA serves as a secondary approach for targeting MYCN in cases of NB. Research has shown that the application of MLN8237 (alisertib), an AURKA inhibitor, to NB cells induces cellular senescence, inhibits cell proliferation, and hampers tumor growth in mouse models (Yang *et al.* 2020).

5.5 *Inducers of differentiation*

Some studies have reported that promoting the differentiation of developing neural crest cells can reduce the occurrence of NB. It is known that *MYCN* can inhibit the differentiation pathway, Therefore, various strategies have been proposed to disrupt the expression of *MYCN* and reduce the development, growth, and dissemination of NB. One strategy targets the Max protein, a MYCN/MYC associated factor. 10058-F4 and 10074-G5, by disruption of the association between MYCN and transcription factor Max, inhibit MYCN-MAX heterodimer transactivation of gene expression and induce differentiation and apoptosis in *MYCN* amplification NB (Müller *et al.* 2014). WNT3A/RSPO2 signaling regulates the phosphorylation of cyclin D1, BMP4, and RB proteins and plays a role in the differentiation or progression of NB, suggesting its potential as a therapeutic target for NB.

6 CONCLUSION

Neuroblastoma is known as the "king of pediatric tumors" and is a major malignant tumor that threatens the lives of children. *MYCN* amplification plays various roles in High-risk NB and acts as transcriptional factor, promoting tumor metastasis, proliferation, self-renewal, inhibiting differentiation and cell cycle arrest. Unfortunately, *MYCN* cannot be directly targeted by drugs, and targeted therapies against *MYCN* primarily focus on its transcriptional level and protein stability. Currently, there are several inhibitors targeting the upstream and downstream proteins involved in *MYCN*-mediated pathways. Preclinical studies using bromodomain inhibitors to specifically disrupt *MYCN* expression levels have shown promising results and have been tested in children with advanced-stage NB. Additionally, there is literature suggesting that MYCN inhibited the expression of CircRNAs by upregulating the expression of DHX9, indicating that CircRNAs may play an important role in tumorigenesis of high-risk NB without *MYCN* amplification. Therefore, identifying new driving factors and therapeutic targets is of utmost importance in the treatment of NB.

REFERENCES

Balzeau, J. et al. (2017). *Frontiers in Genetics*, 8, 31.
Dong, Z. et al. (2021). *Cancer Research*, 81(11), 2995–3007.
Fuchs, S., et al. (2023). *Nature Communications,* 14(1), 3936.
Hatton, B. A. et al. (2006). *Cancer Research,* 66, 8655–8661.
Huang M. and Weiss W.A. (2013). *Cold Spring Harb Perspect Med.* 3(10): a014415.
Ladenstein, R. et al. (2013). *mAbs*, 5, 801–809.
Matthay, K. K. et al. (2016). *Nature Reviews Disease Primers*, 2, 16078.
Megison, M. L. et al. (2013). *Clinical & Experimental Metastasis*, 30(5), 555–568.
Müller, I., Larsson, K., Frenzel, A., et al. (2014). *PLOS One*, 2019(5), e97285.
Van Maerken, T. et al. (2009). *Journal of the National Cancer Institute,* 101(22), 1562–1574.
Yang, Y., Ding, L., Zhou, Q., et al. (2020). *Cancer Cell International*, 20, 9.

Chapter 2
Nutrition, health, and disease prevention

Biological Sciences and Environmental Health – Gao (Ed.)
© 2025 the Author(s), ISBN: 978-1-032-96016-6

The impact of high-fiber diet on diabetes and obesity in middle-aged adults

Yang Zhao
Faculty of Medicine, Macau University of Science and Technology, Macau, China

ABSTRACT: Middle-aged people are at high risk for both diabetes and obesity, so preventing and improving obesity and diabetes in middle-aged people has become an important issue. Numerous studies have shown that dietary fiber has a direct or indirect effect on diabetes and obesity. This study aims to explore the potential of a high-fiber diet as an intervention for individuals with diabetes and obesity. The paper delves into the definition of a high-fiber diet, the prevalent causes of type 2 diabetes and obesity among middle-aged adults, the effects of a high-fiber diet on managing diabetes and obesity in this population, and the practicality of implementing a high-fiber diet on a larger scale. Recent studies are examined to reveal that a high-fiber diet exhibits promising potential for effectively controlling diabetes and obesity in middle-aged adults, suggesting its feasibility for widespread adoption. This study contributes to addressing the challenges of obesity and diabetes in the middle-aged population.

1 INTRODUCTION

Diabetes and obesity stand out as two of the most perilous diseases frequently discussed in the 21st century. These afflictions exert a profoundly adverse influence on human well-being. Individuals in middle age find themselves particularly susceptible to both diabetes and obesity, underscoring the urgency of addressing and ameliorating these health challenges in this demographic. Furthermore, the demands of work and other pressures often leave middle-aged individuals with limited time for physical exercise, rendering dietary enhancement a viable avenue for intervention. A wealth of studies has underscored the direct and indirect impact of dietary fiber on diabetes and obesity. High-fiber diets have garnered considerable attention due to their rich fiber content. Moreover, dietary fiber is readily accessible, primarily sourced from whole grains, fruits, and vegetables. Consequently, embracing a high-fiber diet holds promise as a strategy to preempt and alleviate diabetes and obesity within the middle-aged populace.

A high-fiber diet is characterized by an elevated intake of dietary fiber, which constitutes the seventh major nutrient crucial for human health. Dietary fiber serves six primary physiological functions, encompassing the promotion of intestinal well-being, regulation of blood sugar levels to prevent type 2 diabetes, facilitation of satiety and weight management, prevention of disorders in lipid metabolism and cardiovascular ailments, impact on mineral absorption, and deterrence of specific tumor formations (Rong 2015). Generally, a diet exceeding 30g of daily dietary fiber intake is classified as high in fiber, with an upper threshold around 75-80g per day. The achievement of a high-fiber diet predominantly involves the augmentation of fiber-rich food sources such as vegetables, fruits, whole grains, legumes, nuts, and seeds (Weickert and Pfeiffer 2018). In terms of staple foods, research suggests that prioritize the consumption of whole grain foods over refined grains. This approach enhances dietary fiber content while curtailing sugar intake. This strategy serves to

DOI: 10.1201/9781003587590-11

uphold healthy body weight in middle-aged individuals, mitigating the risk of overweight and obesity, while concurrently staving off prediabetes and type 2 diabetes.

2 THE MAIN CAUSES OF DIABETES AND OBESITY IN MIDDLE-AGED PEOPLE

2.1 *Obesity*

Obesity is a chronic disease characterized by excess adiposity, which impairs health (Abdul *et al.* 2023). It is a global health problem that increases the risk of type II diabetes mellitus (T2DM), cardiovascular disease and dyslipidemia (Heppner and Tilve 2015). Obesity stands as one of the prevalent afflictions in contemporary society, with a notable incidence among adults, particularly within the middle-aged demographic. Within this age group, several contributing factors underlie the propensity for obesity, with three primary factors coming to the fore: medication side effects, hormonal imbalances, and reduced physical activity.

Middle-aged individuals are characterized by an increased susceptibility to multiple health issues. Consequently, patients often resort to medication for treatment or preventive measures. Some medications contain hormones that can influence appetite regulation, potentially intensifying cravings and leading to overeating. Certain hormones can also disrupt metabolic processes, culminating in weight gain and even obesity.

Being the primary caregivers and breadwinners within family dynamics, middle-aged individuals shoulder substantial life pressures from both work and home responsibilities. This chronic stress can disrupt hormonal balance, frequently manifesting in an increased appetite. Consequently, hormonal imbalances often precipitate weight gain in these individuals.

The demanding responsibilities of work and personal life can render middle-aged individuals time-strapped, impeding regular exercise routines. Irregular, insufficient physical activity coupled with heightened caloric intake results in a positive energy balance, fostering weight gain and eventually obesity.

2.2 *Diabetes*

Type 2 diabetes stands as one of the most prevalent maladies in contemporary society, posing grave threats to nerve function and cardiovascular health. It is a multifactorial disorder, characterized by an ominous octet with predominant components being insulin resistance and β-cell dysfunction (Bhansali *et al.* 2020). By impinging on the body's utilization of insulin, this disease disrupts sugar metabolism. It holds the dubious distinction of being a primary catalyst for debilitating conditions such as blindness, kidney failure, heart attacks, strokes, and lower limb amputations. Notably, the middle-aged population bears a significant burden of type 2 diabetes, with its origins rooted in metabolic factors, genetic predisposition, obesity, and unhealthy lifestyle practices. The hereditary aspect of type 2 diabetes is well-established, such that individuals with diabetic parents face an elevated risk of developing the condition themselves.

Obesity looms as a pivotal risk factor for type 2 diabetes. The excess adiposity prompts cellular insensitivity to insulin, resulting in diminished sugar uptake by cells and impaired insulin secretion. This, in turn, culminates in elevated blood sugar levels due to a combination of insulin resistance and inadequate insulin secretion, ultimately paving the way for type 2 diabetes. Unfavorable lifestyle habits and conditions like hypertension serve as critical precursors to prediabetes, which is often a harbinger of type 2 diabetes. Elements such as disrupted sleep patterns and erratic eating schedules play a role. Prolonged physical inactivity contributes to insulin resistance, whereby cells become less responsive to insulin's prompts. Consequently, blood sugar levels rise, ultimately fostering the onset of type 2 diabetes.

3 THE EFFECT OF HIGH-FIBER DIET ON DIABETES

Type 2 diabetes mellitus (T2DM) is distinguished by a triad of insulin resistance, impaired β-cell function, and perturbed glucose and lipid metabolism. In light of this, it becomes imperative to address insulin resistance, expedite the restoration of glucose and lipid metabolism to normalcy, and modulate the composition of intestinal flora to ameliorate the manifestations of type 2 diabetes .

Dietary fiber assumes a pivotal role in this endeavor. Research results indicated that higher dietary fiber intake was significantly associated with reduced risk of newly-diagnosed T2DM (Jin *et al.* 2021). It can augment insulin secretion and enhance insulin sensitivity within the body. Interference of grain fiber with dietary protein absorption could also explain the improved IR in participants consuming high-fiber diets (Weickert and Pfeiffer 2018). Additionally, it facilitates heightened glucose uptake, curbs lipid accumulation, and mitigates hepatic glucose production. The reduction in oxidative stress also reflects, in part, the advantages of a diet high in dietary fiber for diabetes treatment. Therefore, high-fiber diets have a significant positive effect on the cure of diabetes.

3.1 *Positive effect of dietary fiber on insulin resistance*

At the current stage, research has demonstrated that dietary fiber yields a notable positive impact on insulin resistance within various organ tissues including the liver, skeletal muscle, and adipose tissue.

Diets that produce a hyperglycemic response lead to overproduction of insulin, which induces hepatic lipogenesis, leading to the development of insulin resistance and fatty liver (Brockman *et al.* 2012). The liver, functioning as a critical target for insulin action, significantly influences glycogen synthesis and breakdown along with gluconeogenesis. Thus, enhancing liver insulin resistance constitutes a vital mechanism in the context of dietary fiber-induced hypoglycemic effects. Within the liver, dietary fiber principally ameliorates insulin resistance by regulating both glucose production and lipid accumulation.

Skeletal muscle, being the foremost consumer of glucose in the body, plays a pivotal role in systemic insulin resistance. Consequently, enhancing insulin sensitivity within skeletal muscle becomes a pivotal strategy in reducing blood glucose levels. Dietary fiber reduces insulin resistance primarily by promoting glucose uptake by skeletal muscle cells. Skeletal muscle consumes large amounts of glucose, making its insulin resistance a key factor in the worsening of type 2 diabetes mellitus (T2DM). Dietary fiber intake has been shown to have a positive trend in correlation with skeletal muscle strength (Frampton *et al.* 2021). However, dietary fiber effectively promotes the uptake and utilization of glucose by skeletal muscle, thereby greatly reducing insulin resistance in skeletal muscle (Wang *et al.* 2020).

Adipose tissue represents another significant insulin target and is a key focus in insulin resistance intervention. The principal means by which dietary fiber improves insulin resistance within adipose tissue is by heightening lipolysis. Research reveals that cereal-based dietary fiber can elevate serum adiponectin levels in mice subjected to a high-sugar and high-fat diet. This, in turn, increases the expression of proteins involved in the processes of lipolysis and browning. This cascade activates the cAMP-PKA-HSL metabolic pathway, consequently fostering fat cell lipolysis and contributing to the amelioration of insulin resistance (Wang *et al.* 2020). It has been shown that grain dietary fiber leads to a significant reduction in the relative size and volume of adipocytes in HFD-induced obesity (Han *et al.* 2017). A study involving an 8-week intervention with corn insoluble dietary fiber (HAM-RS2) in individuals with Type 2 diabetes and insulin resistance indicated that HAM-RS2 augmented the expression of genes such as triglyceride lipase, perilipin, adiponectin, and hormone-sensitive lipase in patients. This increase in gene expression translated to enhanced fat decomposition, augmented glucose uptake by muscle tissue, and ultimately an improvement in insulin resistance within both fat and muscle tissue (Wang *et al.* 2020).

3.2 *The effect of dietary fiber on improving glucose and lipid metabolism disorders*

Glucose metabolism disorders encompass irregular enzyme activity in relation to glucose and fructose within the body, along with abnormal blood sugar levels resulting from tissue and organ impairments. Manifestations include hyperglycemia, insulin resistance, disrupted lipid metabolism, weight gain, obesity, pancreatic islet dysfunction, and tissue damage. These characteristics, notably prevalent in Type 2 Diabetes Mellitus (T2DM), underscore the severe implications of glucose metabolism disorders. Dietary fiber assumes a pivotal role in ameliorating these disorders, exerting influence on specific enzymes involved in glucose metabolism. By modulating glycogen synthesis and breakdown, dietary fiber interventions contribute to addressing glucose metabolism disruptions. Additionally, short-chain fatty acids, generated through this process, can be assimilated into circulation, impacting host metabolic regulation or serving as substrates for other microorganisms. Research indicates enhanced insulin sensitivity, regulated weight, reduced inflammation, and potentially lower metabolic disease risk through augmented levels of gut-derived short-chain fatty acids (Myhrstad *et al.* 2020).

Intestinal flora, a dynamic ecosystem of microorganisms in the digestive process, significantly contributes to digestion. Imbalanced intestinal flora commonly characterizes patients with T2DM. Enhancing the intestinal flora holds paramount importance in alleviating T2DM symptoms (Xie *et al.* 2021). A central principle lies in the microbial degradation of dietary fiber through carbohydrate enzymes encoded within the gut. This breakdown influences the composition of intestinal bacteria, thereby impacting the balance of species and strains in the colon (Xie *et al.* 2021). Alterations in the intestinal flora consequently induce changes in short-chain fatty acids, which, in turn, contribute to the enhancement of glucose and lipid metabolism. This intricate interplay also holds significance in addressing obesity-related concerns.

4 THE EFFECT OF HIGH-FIBER DIET ON OBESITY

Obesity has emerged as a critical health concern, linked to elevated risks of chronic ailments such as cardiovascular disease, type 2 diabetes, and specific cancers. The middle-aged population is particularly vulnerable to obesity, often hindered by time constraints for effective exercise due to work and daily pressures. Thus, identifying practical approaches to address obesity in this demographic becomes imperative, and enhancing the diet of middle-aged individuals with obesity has become a pivotal avenue for intervention. Evidence from around the globe suggests that dietary fiber, especially when consumed in fiber-rich diets, may have beneficial effects on all parameters of weight management as well as metabolic disorders associated with obesity (Bozzetto *et al.* 2018). The incorporation of dietary fiber holds promise as a potent strategy.

At the macro level, dietary fiber exhibits the capacity to stimulate intestinal peristalsis, optimizing digestive processes. With its high water-absorption and intestinal retention attributes, dietary fiber slows down gastrointestinal transit, promoting satiety while hindering rapid sugar and fat release and absorption. This mechanism reduces energy storage. Additionally, dietary fiber prolongs chewing time during food consumption, thereby enhancing the sensation of satiety in individuals (Morell *et al.* 2014). Soluble fiber extends the duration of satiety signal release (Fiszman and Varela 2013). Consequently, elevating the proportion of dietary fiber within the diet structure effectively diminishes the ratio of sugary to fatty foods, thus curtailing daily calorie intake while upholding satiety levels. Furthermore, dietary fiber stabilizes blood glucose levels, augments insulin secretion, and bolsters insulin sensitivity, mitigating insulin resistance and curtailing fat accumulation. Research suggests that insoluble dietary fiber from flaxseed cake (FIDF) and soluble dietary fiber from flaxseed cake (FSDF) could potentially counter obesity by boosting basal metabolism, regulating gut flora, and promoting short-chain fatty acid (SCFA) production.

FIDF and FSDF each play distinct roles in modulating obesity development, with FSDF showcasing greater efficacy in weight reduction, serum lipid metabolism regulation, and energy equilibrium enhancement. This underscores the ability of certain dietary fibers to effectively combat obesity (Zhao *et al.* 2023).

At the micro level, dietary fiber exerts its influence on obesity through multifaceted mechanisms. Primarily, specific fiber types, such as soluble fiber, can bind to cholesterol in the intestines, curbing its absorption into the bloodstream. This culminates in reduced blood cholesterol levels, subsequently lowering the risk of obesity-related complications like heart disease. Additionally, dietary fiber wields the capacity to modulate gut microbiota composition. By providing nutrients to beneficial gut bacteria, dietary fiber fosters an environment conducive to their growth. Research demonstrates that soybean insoluble dietary fiber (SIDF) intervention enhances short-chain fatty acid (SCFA) content and prompts satiety hormone secretion via the fermentation of beneficial bacteria (Wang *et al.* 2021). The intervention of SIDF could potentially prevent obesity in mice on a high-fat diet (HFD) by regulating gut microbiota composition, thereby marking SIDF as a possible ingredient in functional foods.

Dietary fiber's significance in managing obesity among middle-aged adults transcends both macro and micro perspectives. On the macro level, it fosters satiety, curtails energy intake, and deters excessive fat accumulation. At the micro level, it influences cholesterol metabolism, governs gut microbiota composition, and modulates hormonal regulation. research showed that though viscous fiber as a monotherapy did not provide clinically meaningful weight loss, co-administration of viscous fiber with an energy-restricted diet might alternatively offer a more effective approach (Jovanovski *et al.* 2020). In totality, incorporating fiber-rich foods in the diet emerges as an efficacious strategy to manage weight and diminish the health risks associated with obesity in middle-aged adults.

5 FEASIBILITY OF SCALING UP A HIGH FIBER DIET ON A LARGE SCALE

The widespread implementation of high-fiber diets faces a crucial issue: the availability of foods that meet the requirements of such diets for local populations. Therefore, it is essential to ascertain the accessibility of suitable foods across different regions globally. While crop varieties differ among regions, it's evident that foods aligning with the high-fiber dietary criteria are present in all studied areas. Prices for grains, vegetables, and fruits adhering to high-fiber standards naturally fluctuate based on the region, making price feasibility evaluation challenging. Additionally, diverse cooking methods across regions may impact nutrient absorption. Consequently, when promoting high-fiber diets in various areas, the influence of cooking practices on nutrient content must be considered, adjusting food quantities accordingly. Furthermore, the acquisition of high-fiber foods supports their large-scale utilization.

The pivotal determinant of the viability of broad high-fiber diet adoption lies in public acceptance. The advent of the global information age has empowered people to access extensive health-related information, heightening their awareness of health's significance. This trend is particularly pronounced among middle-aged individuals. In regions susceptible to modern society's prevalent diseases, middle-aged individuals attach significant importance to healthy diets, driven by health concerns and a desire for longevity. Consequently, this age group exhibits substantial receptiveness to high-fiber diets, aiding in disease prevention. A mounting body of scientific research validating the impact of high-fiber diets on averting and managing various conditions has positively influenced the public's perception and acceptance of these diets. Furthermore, the growing availability and variety of high-fiber food products, including whole grain breads, soy items, and oatmeal, indicate their popularity among consumers. This suggests that a diverse array of high-fiber foods resonates well with consumers, thereby affirming the feasibility of promoting high-fiber diets in terms of public acceptance.

6 CONCLUSION

The comprehensive exploration of dietary fiber's impact on obesity and diabetes within the middle-aged population, as detailed throughout this paper, substantiates the positive effects of a high-fiber diet structure on mitigating these conditions. Drawing from the section elucidating the influence of dietary fiber on obesity in middle-aged individuals, it is evident that the high-fiber diet structure holds considerable relevance for addressing obesity. As a regular meal, high-fiber diet with its low-calorie characteristics can reduce the calories in food; as a substitute meal, high-fiber diet in the water-saturated state of the dietary fiber satiety and its ability to reduce the appetite can reduce people's intake of food. Therefore, for middle-aged people, high-fiber diet, whether it is to prevent obesity or treatment of obesity, presents a positive impact. Adding fiber to low-calorie/low-fat foods may enhance satiety, but the feeling of fullness may be short-lived due to the low energy and fat content of diet meals.

For middle-aged diabetes, dietary fiber in the high-fiber diet has excellent glycemic control, which has a positive effect on diabetes prevention and diabetes treatment. Research supports that consumption of at least 25 g/day total dietary fiber may prevent type 2 diabetes. In addition, the high-fiber diet has excellent universality, the food that meets the requirements is relatively easy to obtain, and high-fiber food has a certain degree of public acceptance in the middle-aged population, so the promotion of the high-fiber diet in the middle-aged population should be relatively feasible and easy to implement.

In conclusion, high-fiber diets exhibit substantial efficacy in controlling obesity and type 2 diabetes within the middle-aged demographic, warranting recognition and emphasis. It is plausible that the widespread adoption of high-fiber diets could make a positive impact on the global challenges posed by diabetes and obesity.

REFERENCES

Abdul W. R., Cohen R. and C. Le Roux C.W., (2023). *Ann. Med*, **55**, 2203517.

Bhansali S., Bhansali A., Dutta P., Walia R. and Dhawan V., (2020). *J Cell Mol Med*, **24**, 2832.

Bozzetto L., Costabile G., Della Pepa G., Ciciola Q., Vetrani C., Vitale M., Rivellese A.A. and Annuzzi G., (2018). *Nutrients*, **10**, 943.

Brockman D. A., Chen X. and Gallaher D. D., (2012). *Nutr Metab*, **9**, 100.

Fiszman S. and Varela P., (2013). *Food Hydrocoll*, **32**, 147.

Frampton J., Murphy K.G., Frost G. and Chambers E., (2021). *J Cachexia Sarcopenia Muscle*, **12**, 2134.

Han S.F., Jiao J., Zhang W., Xu J. Y., Zhang W. B., Fu C. L. and Qin L. Q., (2017). *Nutrition*, **33**, 118.

Heppner P. and Tilve D., (2015). *FRONT NEUROSCI-SWITZ*, **9**, 92.

Jin F., Zhang J. and Shu L., (2021). *J NUTR*, **20**, 1.

Jovanovski E., Mazhar N., Komishon A., Khayyat R., Li D., Sonia B.M., Khan T., Jenkins A. L., Smircic-Duvnjak L., Sievenpiper J.L., Vuksan V., (2020). *AM J CLIN NUTR*, **111**, 471. Morell P., Fiszman S. M., Varela P. and Hernando I., (2014). *Food Hydrocoll*, **41**, 343.

Myhrstad M. C. W., Tunsjø H., Charnock C. and Telle-Hansen V.H., (2020). *Nutrients*, **12**, 859.

Rong Y. *The relationship between cereal fiber intake and risk of gestational diabetes mellitus* (Huazhong University of Science and Technology, 2015).

Wang B., Yu H., He Y., Wen L., Gu J., Wang X., Miao X., Qiu G. and Wang H., (2021). *Food Funct*, **12**, 7923.

Wang Y. F., Yang X. H., Cao J. H., Qu C. F., Zhang L. P., Miao J. L. and Xie W. C., (2020). *Food & Machinery*, **36**,6.

Weickert M. O. and Pfeiffer A. F. H., (2018). *J NUTR*, **148**, 7.

Xie J., Ma M. T., Chen X. J., Xu Z. K., Li Z. J. and Sui Z. Q., (2021). *Farm Product Processing*, **2**, 67.

Zhao M., Wang B., Li L. and Zhao W., (2023). *Nutrients*, **15**, 1718.

Biological Sciences and Environmental Health – Gao (Ed.)

The association between gut microbiome and hypertension in China based on current Chinese nutrients

Ziqi Chen
College of Public Health, Chongqing Medical University, Chongqing, China

ABSTRACT: In China, Cardiovascular disease (CVD) is the top cause of death. Hypertension, which is an important risk factor for CVD, could be prevented by following a healthy diet. A healthy diet can not only provide sufficient and balanced nutrients but also benefit the maintenance of normal gut microbiome. The gut microbiome affects the risk of hypertension by involving the regulation of the gut barrier and producing various microbiota. Hence, by preventing intestinal barrier dysfunction and intestinal microbiome imbalance, a healthy diet could reduce inflammation and decrease the risk of hypertension. The current Chinese diet provides insufficient and imbalanced nutrients, which could lead to gut microbiome imbalance and increase the risk of hypertension. Several dietary patterns such as the Mediterranean diet (MD) and the Dietary Approaches to Stop Hypertension (the DASH diet) could decrease blood pressure. Among healthy dietary patterns, the Jiangnan diet, which is a conventional Chinese diet pattern, could be a possible solution for those who are with or at risk of hypertension in China.

1 INTRODUCTION

It is proved that the food people's daily intake greatly affects their health. A healthy diet, which consists of sufficient, balanced, and safe food could prevent people from many noncommunicable diseases (NCDs) (WHO 2003). From 1997 to 2006, a nutrition transition happened in China. The shift in Chinese diet in the past 10 years, represents an increase in red meat and processed meat consumption, a moderate increase in the consumption of fruits, nuts and seeds, fish, and dairy products, and a decrease in the intake of whole grain. The study also points out that most of the Chinese daily diet did not provide enough nutrients to meet their daily needs (Liu *et al.* 2021). Such poor nutrition status is a risk factor for many NCDs. CVD is one of the NCDs and it is one of the leading causes of global mortality (G.B. o. 2020). Among several factors that affect the risk of CVD, one of the main factors is hypertension which is associated with daily nutrient intake (Arnett *et al.* 2019; Naqvi *et al.* 2021; Yang *et al.* 2020; Yu *et al.* 2018). In China, the top leading cause of death from 2009 to 2019 is CVD. Hypertension, which is a risk factor for CVD, became the top risk factor of mortality in 2019 (G.B.o. 2020). However, hypertension can be prevented by cultivating healthy eating behaviors (Arnett *et al.* 2019; Yu *et al.* 2018).

There are many studies on the association between food and blood pressure. The DASH diet and the MD are two famous solutions that benefit people to control their blood pressure in a safe range (Arnett *et al.* 2019; Yu *et al.* 2018). In addition, the Jiangnan diet is a traditional Chinese diet that could benefit people with hypertension as well (Wang *et al.* 2020). Apart from nutrients in food that benefit the patient with hypertension, the food benefits the growth and colonization of the gut microbiome as well and the gut microbiome plays an important role in blood pressure management (Naqvi *et al.* 2021). The bacterial

DOI: 10.1201/9781003587590-12

genome is much bigger than the human genome (about 150 times greater). In the human gut, there are more than 2900 commensal and opportunistic species and most of the gut bacteria reside in the colon (about 1011 per gram content). The colon provides the gut microbiome with an ideal environment that is rich in nutrients and lacks oxygen. The Firmicutes and Bacteroidetes are two main phyla that contribute more than 90% of intestinal bacteria (Naqvi *et al.* 2021).

The microbiome exists largely different among people and dietary factor plays an important role in the composition of the gut microbiome. Besides the dietary factor, many factors which include age, disease, medication, and lifestyle can affect the intestinal microbiome as well (Campaniello *et al.* 2022). Determined by these factors, the diversity, richness, and composition of the microbiota, and products of gut microbiome have great individual differences. The metabolites of the microbiome can be absorbed and cause a change in the receptor sensitivity, immunomodulatory, and signaling function of the host. Thus, in different diseases or different stages of the disease, the gut microbiome can present variations (Campaniello *et al.* 2022). In patients with cardiovascular diseases, the change in particular species is observed compared to the normal and the shift could change the metabolites of the gut microbiome (Campaniello *et al.* 2022; Naqvi *et al.* 2021). Among the metabolites, short fatty acids (SCFAs), bile acids (BAs), lipopolysaccharide (LPS), and trimethylamine N-oxide (TMAO) have different effects on blood pressure (Yang *et al.* 2023).

There are few articles about the association between these microbiota products and their effect on blood pressure in China. Thus, to better understand how diet affects hypertension by the gut microbiome, this article aims to discuss the association between microbiome and hypertension and dietary factors that can affect the gut microbiome. This article will also discuss the current diet and some possible dietary advice for patients with hypertension in China.

2 GUT MICROBIOME AND HYPERTENSION

Through gut barrier dysfunction and gut metabolites, the gut microbiome is involved in the regulation of blood pressure (Verhaar *et al.* 2020; Witkowski *et al.* 2020; Yang *et al.* 2023).

2.1 *Gut barrier dysfunction and hypertension*

Among people with imbalanced gut microbiome, decreased probiotics and promoted number of harmful bacteria are two characteristics of the gut microbiome. Such imbalance could increase blood pressure by generating inflammation (Witkowski *et al.* 2020). The imbalanced gut microbiota could elevate the blood pressure levels by eroding the normal function of the intestinal barrier as well. An animal experiment observed an enhanced permeability caused by the decline of the tight junction proteins, goblet cells, and shorter villi and the increment of the gut tissue's stiffness in rat models of hypertension (Santisteban *et al.* 2017). The normal gut barrier could prevent the host from systemic inflammation caused by exotoxin and endotoxin, while the increased intestinal permeability and impaired gut structure could lead to systemic inflammation among patients with gut barrier dysfunction. The systemic inflammation can lead to endothelial cell dysfunction which is a risk factor of hypertension (Santisteban *et al.* 2017; Verhaar *et al.* 2020; Witkowski *et al.* 2020; Yang *et al.* 2023).

2.2 *Gut metabolites and hypertension*

The other important way the gut microbiome affects blood pressure is through metabolites of the intestinal microbiome. The blood level of SCFAs, TMAO, and LPS have a deep relationship with hypertension. In patients with hypertension, the decline of SCFAs and increase of TMAO and LPS are observed and these changes could raise the blood pressure level of the patient (Verhaar *et al.* 2020; Yang *et al.* 2023).

The SCFAs, which mainly consist of acetate, propionate, and butyrate, are protective factors against hypertension (Yang *et al.* 2020). The intake of dietary fiber and SCFA-producing gut microbiome are two main factors that affect the levels of SCFAs in fecal and plasma. The SCFAs can be produced by the human body, while most of the SCFAs (about 90%) come from the gut microbiome. The indigestible dietary fiber is the main resource for the gut microbiome to produce SCFAs, while protein and peptides can also be utilized in SCFAs production. Most of the SCFAs (about 90-95%) can be absorbed by the colonic epithelial cells rapidly and efficiently. Ruminococcaceae and Lachnospiraceae are two main gut microbiota that produce butyrate and propionate and acetate are primarily produced by Bifidobacterium spp and mucin-degrading bacteria. The plasma SCFAs are mainly comprised of acetate and propionate, while most butyrate is used by colonocytes as a primary energy source (Verhaar *et al.* 2020; Yang *et al.* 2020, 2023). By regulating the immune response and inflammation, which include inhibiting histone deacetylase (HDACs) and activating G-protein-coupled receptors (GPCRs), The SCFAs could affect blood pressure (Yang *et al.* 2023). GPR4, GPR43, and GPR109A are GPCRs that are located on the cell surface and the SCFAs can activate the GPCRs, which is one of the major approaches for SCFAs to regulate the function of different systems. Through GPCRs, SCFAs could prevent inflammation and benefit the integrity of the gut structure. The activation of GPCRs could reduce the risk of hypertension by increasing the regulatory T cells (Treg) and decreasing inflammatory mediators. On the other hand, the SCFAs can affect hypertension by involving the neuromodulation mechanism of blood pressure. Via activating the GPCRs which are located on the sympathetic ganglia and the vagus nerve, the SCFAs participate in the neurofeedback of the gut and the regulation of the sympathetic nervous directly (Verhaar *et al.* 2020; Yang *et al.* 2023). The restraining of HDACs is another important method that SCFAs involve in blood pressure modulation. By suppressing HDACs, the SCFAs could decrease the risk of hypertension. The HDACs, which affect the epigenetic DNA modification by regulating the acetylation of histone protein, are mainly expressed by the endothelial, immune, and vascular smooth muscle cells. The activity of HDACs could be inhibited by SCFAs to either forbid or enable the expression of specific genes, which allows SCFAs to involve vascular inflammation by affecting pro-inflammatory cytokines. By inhibiting the HDACs, the SCFAs prevent vascular inflammation by regulating the function of macrophages and dendritic cells and alleviating the inflammation induced by TNFα- or LPS. The SCFAs could affect the recruitment and migration of immune cells to participate in the envelopment of vascular inflammation as well. Hence, the SCFAs contribute to the modulation of inflammatory expression, vascular integrity, and the prevention of cardiovascular diseases, by impeding the normal function of HDACs (Li *et al.* 2018; Yang *et al.* 2023). Besides, as one of the major energy sources of colonocytes, SCFAs are involved in the maintenance of normal gut barrier by promoting the proliferation and growth of colonocytes, which could protect the host from hypertension by inhibiting inflammation (Verhaar *et al.* 2020).

The nutrients such as carnitine, choline, and lecithin, which can be found in animal products, especially in egg yolks and meat, can enable the gut microbiome to produce trimethylamine (TMA). Among intestinal microbiome, bacterium from the families Clostridia and Enterobacteriaceae are the major producers of TMA. TMA can be absorbed into blood plasma and be oxidized into TMAO by flavin monooxygenase 3 (FMO3) in the liver (Witkowski *et al.* 2020; Yang *et al.* 2023). The plasma level of TMAO is a risk factor for atherosclerosis and the TMAO could raise blood pressure by causing atherosclerosis. Although the exact mechanisms remain to be explored, several mechanisms of how TMAO affects the risk of atherosclerosis have been proposed (Verhaar *et al.* 2020; Witkowski *et al.* 2020).

TMAO could be involved in cholesterol metabolism. TMAO disrupts cholesterol clearance by inhibiting the bile acids pool size (Witkowski *et al.* 2020). Besides, in FMO3 knockdown mice, which have low TMAO level, the absorption of lipid and cholesterol production is limited. In addition, the FMO3 knockdown also leads to the acceleration of reverse cholesterol transport, which decreases the risk of atherosclerosis in mice (Warrier *et al.* 2015). The microbiome participates in the modulation of platelet function through TMAO production. By causing platelet hyperreactivity and thrombotic events, TMAO contributes to the increment of atherosclerosis risk. In addition, dose-dependently association between TMAO concentration and responsiveness of platelet aggregation has been observed. Via such mechanism, the dietary choline can be utilized by the gut microbiome for TMA production and increase the risk of hypertension (Zhu *et al.* 2016). TMAO could also participate in inflammation generation by affecting the expression of inflammatory cytokines. By boosting the productivity of the pro-inflammation cytokines and inhibiting the production of the anti-inflammatory cytokine, the TMAO could lead to atherosclerosis (Verhaar *et al.* 2020).

However, the plasma level of TMAO expresses high variability whether within-individual or inter-individual, which disrupts the comparison of different studies. The composition of food intake, kidney function, and intestinal microbiome can affect the plasma level of TMAO (Verhaar *et al.* 2020; Witkowski *et al.* 2020; Yang *et al.* 2023). The consumption of meat, especially red meat consumption is an important dietary factor that can raise circulating TMAO levels. A three 4-week isocaloric diets study, which divided volunteers into three groups by dietary protein type (non-meat, white meat, red meat), observed an increment among the red meat groups' plasma level of TMAO. Red meat provides abundant carnitine for the gut microbiome in TMA production. Red meat consumption could reshape the gut microbiome to benefit TMA production by utilizing carnitine as well. However, the intake of red meat does not influence TMA production by utilizing choline. Besides, by reducing fractional renal excretion, the red meat diet can increase the plasma concentration of TMAO (Wang *et al.* 2019). Although TMAO can affect the risk of hypertension, the exact mechanism of how TMAO is involved in hypertension is still unproven (Verhaar *et al.* 2020; Yang *et al.* 2023).

As the major component of bile, Bas decreases the risk of hypertension by modulating lipid metabolism, increasing energy utilization, regulating intestinal microbiome, and maintaining normal function of the gut barrier. Besides, the Bas also affects hypertension by participating in TMAO metabolism. The Bas can affect FMO3 to regulate the plasma level of TMAO by activating the farnesoid X receptor (FXR) (Verhaar *et al.* 2020).

The increment in the blood level of LPS is a risk factor for hypertension. The LPS is a bacterial endotoxin that originates from Gram-negative bacteria. The disorder of the gut microbiome and dysfunction of the gut barrier can increase the plasma level of LPS. An abnormal gut microbiome provides more LPS than the normal one and can be absorbed by the gut more easily in patients with gut leakiness. On the other hand, as an antigen, the LPS could lead to dysfunction of intestinal mucosal and increment of gut barrier permeability by generating intestinal inflammation. The LPS generates inflammation by activating the toll-like receptors on the surface of immune cells in host circulation, which could promote the risk of hypertension (Yang *et al.* 2023).

3 GUT MICROBIOME AND DIET

3.1 *Some diet patterns decrease the risk of hypertension*

A healthy diet pattern benefits the maintenance of normal gut microbiome and decreases the risk of hypertension. The MD and the DASH diet are two well-known diet patterns that could decrease the risk of hypertension. Apart from these diets, the Jiangnan diet is a Chinese traditional healthy diet pattern that could affect the risk of hypertension as well.

By following the MD, the risk of hypertension could be decreased. According to a study, by following the MD, the mortality and the incidence of cardio and cerebro-vascular disease could be decreased (Sofi *et al.* 2010). The MD emphasizes the intake of olive oil, whole grains, vegetables, fruits, legumes, and nuts. The MD also recommends moderate consumption of dairy products, seafood or fish, eggs, wine, and poultry. The MD suggests that the intake of red meat and sweets should be less often. Although people mainly benefit from the combined effects of the MD, olive oil, which is one of the features of the MD, might be more effective in decreasing blood pressure than other components of the MD. Olive oil not only provides unsaturated fat but also provides polyphenols which could decrease blood pressure by protecting vascular. Apart from olive oil, the MD also recommends a plenty consumption of nuts, vegetables, fruits, and whole grains, which benefit the patient with hypertension as well. The MD is also known for its taste. Thus, it is easier for people to change their diet pattern to the MD and adhere to it (Davis *et al.* 2015; De Pergola & D'Alessandro 2018).

The DASH diet was shown the ability to decrease blood pressure whether in normal people or people with hypertension. Among people with younger age or high sodium intake, the DASH diet is more effective in blood pressure lowering. The DASH diet encourages people to consume more whole grains, vegetables, fruits, low or free-fat dairy products, legumes, and nuts but limits the intake of sugar-sweetened beverages, red meat, and processed meat. Thus, compared to other dietary patterns, the DASH diet emphasizes low consumption of sodium and fat especially the dietary cholesterol and saturated fat but a vast intake of dietary fiber, potassium, magnesium, and calcium. The DASH diet is also tasty and easy for people to follow (Castro-Barquero *et al.* 2020; Filippou *et al.* 2020).

Compared to North China, the burden of NCDs including hypertension is lower in Southern China. In Jiangsu, Anhui, and Zhejiang, especially around the downstream reaches of the Yangtze River, residents share some features of diet and cooking style. Such a local diet emphasizes high consumption of vegetables, fruits, fish and shrimp, and legumes and moderate intake of whole-grain rice, plant oils (mainly rapeseed oil), and red meat. The Jiangnan diet suggests people should limit the consumption of salt, or millet wine. The Jiangnan diet also emphasizes all the ingredients should be fresh and in season. The Jiangnan diet recommends people prepare their food by steaming or boiling in water or frying in a lukewarm-fire. The consumption of vegetables and fruits in season, fish, and squeezed rapeseed oils which are rich in polyunsaturated and Omega-6 fatty acids could be the feature to explain the lower burden of hypertension in Southern China. Although convincing evidence is insufficient to illustrate the benefit of the Jiangnan diet, the Jiangnan diet might appear more adherence for its taste and cost in China compared to the MD and the Dash diet (Wang *et al.* 2020).

3.2 *The current Chinese diet*

The current Chinese diet cannot maintain a healthy gut microbiome which could increase the risk of NCDs.

The Chinese dietary pattern is shifting to the Western dietary pattern. Chinese tend to consume refined grains rather than whole grains. Chinese also consume more red meat, processed meat, sugar-sweetened beverages, fried food, and saturated fat. Although the consumption of fruits, nuts, eggs, dairy products, and fish increases moderately, the consumption of these foods is still insufficient and cannot benefit the prevention of CVD (Wang *et al.* 2020). Such diet pattern shifting is the most important risk factor for CVD in recent years (Wang *et al.* 2022).

In 2019, among patients with CVD in China, the top six leading dietary risk factors are a diet high in sodium, the diet low in whole grains, the overconsumption of red meat, low fruits consumption, low legumes consumption, and low fiber intake. The high sodium intake is the most serious dietary risk in China from 2009 to 2019. The death number contributed by it is more than the sum of the 2nd and 3rd dietary risk factors and it is the most rapidly increasing dietary risk factor. The issue of low legumes consumption keeps deteriorating rapidly. Its contribution to mortality in patients with CVD exceeds the low fruits consumption and becomes the 4th dietary risk factor in 2019. From 2009 to 2019, the three dietary risk factors that the patient with CVD managed to improve are diet low in vegetables, fruits, and fiber. However, the issue of low fruits consumption is still serious for its contribution to mortality in patients with CVD.

4 CONCLUSION

The gut barrier dysfunction and gut microbiota are two ways that gut microbiome is involved in hypertension. An imbalanced gut microbiome could cause gut barrier dysfunction. In people with gut barrier dysfunction, the bacteria and some microbiota that could generate inflammation are more likely to appear in blood and may lead to hypertension eventually. The diet could affect the microbiota. For instance, the dietary fiber intake benefits the production of SCFA which could decrease the risk of hypertension but the consumption of red meat can increase the plasma level of TMAO which is a risk factor for hypertension. Hence, a healthy diet could decrease the risk of hypertension by maintaining a normal barrier dysfunction and a normal intestinal microbiome.

The diet can affect the composition of the gut microbiome. A healthy diet pattern could decrease the risk of hypertension and also benefit a normal gut microbiome. However, the current Chinese diet pattern is high in red meat, sugar-sweetened beverages, processed meat, fried food, and sodium. Meanwhile, the intake of legumes, nuts, vegetables, fruits, and dairy products is insufficient. Although the blood pressure-lowering effect of the DASH diet and the MD is well-proved, serval foods recommended by the two dietary pattern is hard to obtain or too expensive and the taste of the two diets might not fit the Chinese. The Jiangnan diet, which emphasizes the food groups similar to those diet patterns, could be a practical diet pattern because it is a traditional diet pattern widely accessed by the residents around the downstream reaches of the Yangtze River. Thus, the Jiangnan diet might be a dietary pattern for the Chinese to maintain a normal gut microbiome, decrease blood pressure, and reduce the risk of hypertension. Due to lack of relative article, this article does not discuss the direct association between diet and gut microbiome. More studies are needed to validate the role of the current Chinese diet in hypertension to meet the serious burden of hypertension in China.

REFERENCES

Arnett D.K., Blumenthal R.S., Albert M.A., Buroker A.B., Goldberger Z.D., Hahn E.J., Himmelfarb C.D., Khera A., Lloyd-Jones D., McEvoy J.W., Michos E.D., Miedema M.D., Muñoz D., Smith S.C., Jr., Virani S.S., Williams K.A., Sr., Yeboah J., and Ziaeian B. (2019). *Circulation*, **140**, e596–e646

Campaniello D., Corbo M.R., Sinigaglia M., Speranza B., Racioppo A., Altieri C., and Bevilacqua A. (2022). *Nutrients*, **14**

Castro-Barquero S., Ruiz-León A.M., Sierra-Pérez M., Estruch R., and Casas R. (2020). *Nutrients*, **12**

Davis C., Bryan J., Hodgson J., and Murphy K. (2015). *Nutrients*, **7**, 9139–53

De Pergola G. and D'Alessandro A. (2018). *Nutrients*, **10**

Filippou C.D., Tsioufis C.P., Thomopoulos C.G., Mihas C.C., Dimitriadis K.S., Sotiropoulou L.I., Chrysochoou C.A., Nihoyannopoulos P.I., and Tousoulis D.M. (2020). *Adv Nutr*, **11**, 1150–1160

G.B.o. Disease, "GBD Compare". November 11, 2020.

Li M., van Esch B., Wagenaar G.T.M., Garssen J., Folkerts G., and Henricks P.A.J. (2018). *Eur J Pharmacol*, **831**, 52–59

Liu M.-w., McNaughton S.A., He Q.-q., and Leech R. (2021). *International Journal of Behavioral Nutrition and Physical Activity*, **18**, 1–11

Naqvi S., Asar T.O., Kumar V., Al-Abbasi F.A., Alhayyani S., Kamal M.A., and Anwar F. (2021). *Biomedicine & Pharmacotherapy*, **134**, 111156

Santisteban M.M., Qi Y., Zubcevic J., Kim S., Yang T., Shenoy V., Cole-Jeffrey C.T., Lobaton G.O., Stewart D.C., Rubiano A., Simmons C.S., Garcia-Pereira F., Johnson R.D., Pepine C.J., and Raizada M.K. (2017). *Circ Res*, **120**, 312–323

Sofi F., Abbate R., Gensini G.F., and Casini A. (2010). *Am J Clin Nutr*, **92**, 1189–96

Verhaar B.J.H., Prodan A., Nieuwdorp M., and Muller M. (2020). *Nutrients*, **12**

W.H. Organization, (2003). Diet, nutrition, and the prevention of chronic diseases: report of a joint WHO/FAO expert consultation. Vol. **916**. World Health Organization.

Wang J., Lin X., Bloomgarden Z.T., and Ning G. (2020). *Journal of Diabetes*, **12**, 365–371

Wang Y., Feng L., Zeng G., Zhu H., Sun J., Gao P., Yuan J., Lan X., Li S., Zhao Y., Chen X., Dong H., Chen S., Li Z., Zhu Y., Li M., Li X., Yang Z., Li H., Fang H., Xie G., Lin P.H., Chen J., and Wu Y. (2022). *Circulation*, **146**, 303–315

Wang Z., Bergeron N., Levison B.S., Li X.S., Chiu S., Jia X., Koeth R.A., Li L., Wu Y., Tang W.H.W., Krauss R.M., and Hazen S.L. (2019). *Eur Heart J*, **40**, 583–594

Warrier M., Shih D.M., Burrows A.C., Ferguson D., Gromovsky A.D., Brown A.L., Marshall S., McDaniel A., Schugar R.C., Wang Z., Sacks J., Rong X., Vallim T.A., Chou J., Ivanova P.T., Myers D.S., Brown H. A., Lee R.G., Crooke R.M., Graham M.J., Liu X., Parini P., Tontonoz P., Lusis A.J., Hazen S.L., Temel R.E., and Brown J.M. (2015). *Cell Rep*, **10**, 326–338

Witkowski M., Weeks T.L., and Hazen S.L. (2020). *Circ Res*, **127**, 553–570

Yang F., Chen H., Gao Y., An N., Li X., Pan X., Yang X., Tian L., Sun J., Xiong X., and Xing Y. (2020). *Biomed Pharmacother*, **130**, 110503

Yang Z., Wang Q., Liu Y., Wang L., Ge Z., Li Z., Feng S., and Wu C. (2023). *Clin Exp Hypertens*, **45**, 2195135

Yu E., Malik V.S., and Hu F.B. (2018). *J Am Coll Cardiol*, **72**, 914–926

Zhu W., Gregory J.C., Org E., Buffa J.A., Gupta N., Wang Z., Li L., Fu X., Wu Y., Mehrabian M., Sartor R. B., McIntyre T.M., Silverstein R.L., Tang W.H.W., DiDonato J.A., Brown J.M., Lusis A.J., and Hazen S. L. (2016). *Cell*, **165**, 111–124

Biological Sciences and Environmental Health – Gao (Ed.)
© 2025 the Author(s), ISBN: 978-1-032-96016-6

Serotonin regulation by gut microbiota and eating disorders

Chongdi Fan
SPCS, Queen Mary University of London, London, UK

ABSTRACT: Investigation into how gut microbiota may affect human health is a burgeoning area in neuroscience and microbiology. Increasing evidence supports the existence of the gut-brain axis, in which the gut microbiome affects the central nervous system (CNS) through neurogenic, immune, and endocrine pathways. Human diseases concerning eating disorders are thought to result from intestinal serotonin dysbiosis, leading to impaired serotonin production. The mechanisms by which metabolites produced by gut microbiota regulate neurotransmitters have been investigated thoroughly. Short chain fatty acids (SCFAs) bind to G-protein coupled receptors on enterochromaffin cells, hence triggering it to secrete tryptophan hydroxylase, the enzyme that is responsible for catalyzing the 5-HT (serotonin) synthesis. This review discusses the concept of the gut-brain axis, the function of SCFA as a microbial metabolite in serotonin production, treatment methods for eating disorders (EDs), and various clinical trials related to ED treatment methods.

1 INTRODUCTION

Eating disorders (EDs) are becoming increasingly prevalent, with binge eating disorder (BED) being the most common, accounting for one-third of the population (Thursby and Juge 2017). Recent studies have highlighted a strong connection between EDs and the gastrointestinal (GI) tract. The human GI tract hosts a diverse range of microbiotas, with approximately 2000 species and around 10^14 bacteria colonizing the GI tract (Chen *et al.* 2021).

Gut microbiotas have different roles in maintaining a balanced physiological system inside the human body, and microbiomes are involved in the immune system, metabolism, endocrine system, and manipulating the brain function through the bidirectional gut-brain axis connection, which operates via the vagus nerve and blood circulation (Silva *et al.* 2020). Dysbiosis, or imbalance of gut microbiota, is greatly associated with pathogenesis and psychopathology (Thursby and Juge 2017), largely due to the imbalance of serotonin levels and other neurotransmitters. Serotonin is produced through the interaction of microbiota metabolites, particularly short-chain fatty acids (SCFAs) and enterochromaffin (EC) cells (Guzel and Mirowska-Guzel 2022).

This review summarizes how the regulation of serotonin levels can help with treating EDs by interacting with the central nervous system (CNS). It explores the mechanism through which gut microbiota influences the CNS through the gut-brain axis, the production of serotonin, and the role of dysbiosis leading to EDs. The relevant treatment methods are also discussed.

 DOI: 10.1201/9781003587590-13

2 GUT-BRAIN AXIS

2.1 *Evidence for gut-brain axis*

The gut-brain axis refers to the interactive network between gastrointestinal activities and the CNS. The hypothetic views on the new concept of the gut-brain axis did not disappear until research was carried out in 1998 by Sudo *et al.* (Appleton 2018). According to their clinical study, three groups of mice – germ-free (GF), specific pathogen-free (SPF), and gnotobiotic – were compared to test the hypothalamic-pituitary-adrenocortical (HPA) axis response to stress (Appleton 2018; Sudo *et al.* 2004). The HPA axis allows the adjustment of hormone levels in response to stress, connecting the endocrine system to the CNS (James *et al.* 2020).

In the cortex of GF mice, a fall in brain-derived neurotrophic factor (BDNF) level was monitored, whereas the SPF mice were not affected; in addition, neither group showed different sensitivity to ether stress (Appleton 2018; Sudo *et al.* 2004). The reason may be that the commensal microbiota in the enteric system of the mice was an essential environmental determinant in regulating the stress response by affecting the limbic system (Appleton 2018). Further studies also proved that the GI tract and CNS were connected through the vagus nerves, constructing the bidirectional network between them. Since the HPA axis and GI tract allow the brain to influence intestinal activities, various physiological functions can be affected. The most significant ones are the production of neurotransmitters, functioning immune responses, emotional processes, and cognitive functioning (Appleton 2018; Sjostedt *et al.* 2021; Terry *et al.* 2022), all of which can affect the gut microbiota directly.

2.2 *Short-chain fatty acids*

SCFAs produced in the GI tract are crucial when regulating brain functioning through metabolic pathways. SCFAs originate from metabolites of specialized gut microbiota, particularly *Firmicutes*, including species such as *Lactobacillaceae*, *Ruminococcaceae*, and *Lachnospiraceae* (Fusco *et al.* 2023). These microbiotas can produce hydrolytic enzymes to hydrolyze complex polysaccharides such as dietary fibers and resistant starch (Fusco *et al.* 2023; Silva *et al.* 2020). The hydrolyzed substances are then converted to form SCFAs through anaerobic fermentation in the large intestine (Tomás-Pejó *et al.* 2023). Its chemical features are characterized by short carbon chains with no more than six carbon atoms. In most cases, acetate (2C) is the primary product of anaerobic fermentation, comprising 60% of the total SCFAs, followed by propionate (3C) and butyrate (4C) (Silva *et al.* 2020). In addition, a small proportion (less than 1%) of SCFAs is synthesized through amino acid fermentation (Fusco *et al.* 2023; Silva *et al.* 2020).

SCFAs exert local effects to ensure the physiological health of the human body. For example, a vast majority of related research on butyrate has shown anti-tumor properties: it can trigger apoptosis in replicating cancer cells by inhibiting histone deacetylase (Siddiqui and Cresci 2021). SCFAs also play a pivotal role within the gut-brain axis. They can improve the integrity and permeability of the blood-brain barrier by crossing it through monocarboxylate transporters and inhibiting the expression of tight junction proteins (Cryan *et al.* 2019; Silva *et al.* 2020). Consequently, SCFAs can further influence neuroinflammation in the CNS by increasing neurogenesis, leading to improved cognitive function and memory (Fusco *et al.* 2023; Silva *et al.* 2020; Valdes *et al.* 2018).

3 MICROBIOTA AND SEROTONIN PRODUCTION

3.1 *Role of serotonin*

Neurotransmitters play a crucial role in transmitting signals between synapses of neurons and glial cells. Various neurotransmitters, such as aminobutyric acid, glucagon-like peptide

1, glycine, and serotonin, can be synthesized in the intestine through microbiota metabolism (Chen *et al.* 2021; Silva *et al.* 2020). The discovery of serotonin (5-HT) can be traced back to 1937, when Vittorio Espramer found it in the intestine lumen, initially naming it enteramine (Guzel 2022). Serotonin exerts its effect on both the GI tract and CNS. In the GI tract, serotonin increases muscle motility by binding onto the serotonin receptors, such as 5-HT1A, 5-HT1P, and 5-HT2A (Guzel 2022), promoting the contraction and relaxation of the intestinal muscles. It also plays a role in regulating sleep by influencing the CNS through the various neurons in the varus nerve and contributes to maintaining excellent cognitive function, mood regulation, sleep, and eating behavior (Guzel and Mirowska-Guzel 2022; Silva *et al.* 2020).

3.2 *Serotonin production*

Trillions of microbiota in the gut are involved in the intestinal serotonergic system, with serotonin being generated in three main ways:

(1) Certain types of bacteria secrete serotonin precursors and directly release them into the gut lumen.
(2) Metabolites of microbiota, such as SCFAs, interact with epithelial cells, stimulating them to release luminal serotonin.
(3) Secretion of metabolites can affect the level of serotonin synthesis enzymes, thereby regulating the rate of serotonin release.

Serotonin levels in the human body can be raised either by taking probiotics or through production by gut microbiota (Blake *et al.* 2022). SCFAs and other microbial metabolites are essential in producing luminal serotonin by binding to specific receptors on enteroendocrine cells, such as G-protein coupled receptors (GPCRs) (Silva *et al.* 2020) and olfactory receptor 78 (OLF78) (Guzel 2022). SCFAs and other secondary bile acids can further trigger 5-HT secretion by activating enterochromaffin (EC) cells, a type of enteroendocrine cell known as the 'on' mechanism (Guzel 2022).

The serotonergic enzyme tryptophan hydroxylase (TPH1) is secreted from EC cells and catalyzes the synthesis of 5-hydroxytryptophan (5-HTP) from amino acid L-tryptophan (Layunta *et al.* 2021), which eventually leads to the production of serotonin 5-HT. It is noticeable that TPH1 acts as a rate-limiting enzyme in serotonin production. Sufficient evidence has indicated that acetate and butyrate can increase the mRNA of TPH1 (Blake *et al.* 2022).

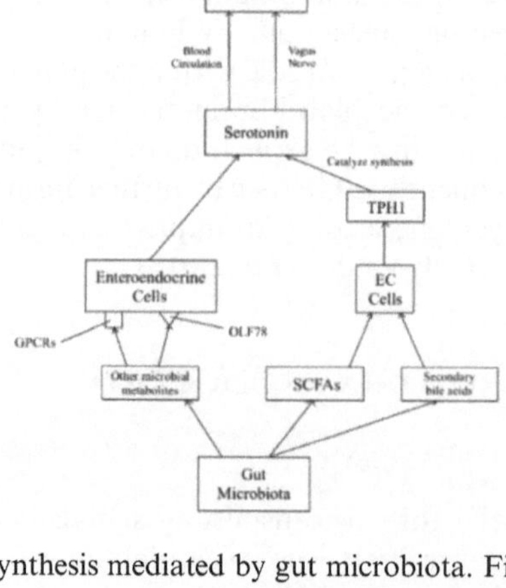

Figure 1. Neurotransmitter synthesis mediated by gut microbiota. Figure credit: Original.

3.3 *Mechanism of serotonin signaling*

Serotonin signaling is a bidirectional process within the human body. Serotonin synthesized by EC cells can enter the bloodstream directly to reach the CNS, as well as their precursors (Figure 1). In addition, serotonin is involved in signal transmission within the neurons of the vagus nerve. Scientific research on serotonin receptors has classified the known 18 receptors into seven families, from 5HT-1 to 5HT-7 (Layunta *et al.* 2021), each playing a distinct role in regulating normal physiological functions. For example, the 5HT-5 receptor is involved in intestinal secretion and regulates the neuroendocrine function of the CNS (Guzel 2022; Layunta *et al.* 2021).

4 SEROTONIN DYSBIOSIS LEADING TO EATING DISORDERS

Alterations in microbiota composition have been linked to potential mental health disorders. A microbiota profile made by Castellini *et al.* explored the relationship between the concentration of bacterial fecal microbiota and EDs, using different alpha diversity estimators to quantify the bacterial richness in each controlled group with anorexia nervosa (AN), bulimia nervosa (BN), and healthy control (HC) groups (Table 1). The results demonstrated a significant difference between the HC and ED groups, with the ED groups showing lower bacterial diversity in their fecal samples (Castellini *et al.* 2023).

Table 1. Clinical trials in eating disorder treatment methods.

Authors	ED type	Samples	Treatment	Results	References
Fitzsimmons-Craft *et al.*	AN, BN	N = 690 females	CBT-ED	No significant difference in abstinence; significant reduction in binge eating	Fitzsimmons-Craft *et al.* 2020
Fitzsimmons-Craft *et al.*	Not specified	N = 700 females	Chatbot based on the student bodies program	Significant reduction in weight concern in the intervention group; reduction in ED psychopathology in the intervention group	Fitzsimmons-Craft *et al.* 2022
Lock *et al.*	AN, BN	N = 30 adolescents	FBT+CRT or FBT+AT	Greater cognitive improvement in FBT+AT group; similar outcomes between groups	Lock *et al.* 2018; Nandini *et al.* 2023
Le Grange *et al.*	AN, BN, BED	N = 97 adolescents	FBT, CBT-E	Greater rate of weight gain in FBT than CBT-E at EOT	Le Grange *et al.* 2022
Melisse *et al.*	BED	N = 180	CBT -E	Reduction in binges in the intervention group; 40% showed full recovery	Melisse *et al.* 2023
Glashouwer *et al.*	AN, BN, EDNOS	N = 51 females	Placebo control	No difference between groups in primary outcome measure	Glashouwer *et al.* 2018
Wye *et al.*		N = 100 adolescents	FBT	Not yet recruiting	Eliza *et al.* 2023

Abbreviations: ED, Eating disorder; AN, Anorexia nervosa; BN, Bulimia nervosa; BED, Binge eating disorder; EDNOS, Eating disorders not otherwise specified; ARFID, Avoidant restrictive food intake disorder; CBT, Cognitive behavioral therapy; FBT, Family-based treatment; CRT, Cognitive remediation therapy.

4.1 *Eating disorders*

There is ongoing debate about whether EDs can be categorized as psychopathology due to their multifactorial etiopathogenesis. The causes of EDs range from biological factors to social pressures and emotional triggers, such as traumatic experiences. EDs are often linked to psychiatric disorders, as they usually occur with mood and anxiety disorders (Steiger and Psychiatry 2004). Therefore, a comprehensive approach is required to recognize and diagnose these clinical syndromes. EDs are primarily classified into two main syndromes, as discussed.

4.1.1 *Anorexia nervosa*

This condition involves self-imposed starvation behavior due to an intense fear of gaining weight, resulting in anxiety and severe malnutrition. There are two subtypes of AN: BED is characterized as long-term overeating episodes without purging. BED is the most common eating disorder, especially in the female population. More than 80% of the BED patients also suffer from other psychiatric syndromes (Duan *et al.* 2022). PED (purge eating disorder) involves self-induced vomiting or other methods to avoid gaining weight.

4.1.2 *Bulimia nervosa*

In contrast to AN, BN involves binge eating followed by purging, which can occur through vomiting or excessive exercise. These behaviors are often triggered by dietary dyscontrol or compulsive exercises (Steiger and Psychiatry 2004).

The emotional impact of ED is significant, with patients often experiencing intense negative emotions after binging or purging, such as guilt, embarrassment, and anxiety. There is no denying that intestinal microbiomes are closely related to EDs, particularly through their impact on the level of serotonin expression, which controls eating behavior. When EC cells are stimulated, resulting in a high level of serotonin, the CNS receives signals that reduce the desire to eat, potentially leading to AN syndrome. Conversely, low serotonin levels can promote binge eating, making BN more likely to occur (Steiger and Psychiatry 2004).

5 TREATMENT METHODS AND CLINICAL TRIALS FOR EATING DISORDERS

Treatment methods for EDs are limited due to the complexity and evolving understanding of these conditions. However, several approaches have demonstrated effectiveness, including cognitive behavioral therapy (CBT), psychotherapy, and pharmacological treatments (Duan *et al.* 2022). Additional measures, such as family-based treatment methods and cognitive behavioral therapy, are also being explored to alleviate symptoms. Ongoing clinical trials continue to investigate the efficacy of various physiological treatment methods, including family-based and cognitive behavioral therapies (Nandini *et al.* 2023).

5.1 *Selective serotonin reuptake inhibitors*

Selective serotonin reuptake inhibitors are widely used as anti-depressants. They work by blocking the serotonin transporter (5-HT transporter) on presynaptic neurons, inhibiting the reuptake of serotonin, thus promoting neuronal signaling by raising the serotonin levels of 5-HT in the synaptic cleft (Blake *et al.* 2022; Duan *et al.* 2022). Fluoxetine has been validated to be used in treating BN, while lisdexamfetamine has been used to cure BED (Panda *et al.* 2023). So far these two anti-depressants represent the primary pharmacological treatments available for EDs.

5.2 *Probiotics*

Probiotics promote the growth and proliferation of beneficial gut microbiota, such as those that synthesize SCFAs through anaerobic fermentation of their metabolites. Additionally, probiotics can inhibit the neuroendocrine stress response (Fattorusso *et al.* 2019), which may reduce the risk of anxiety and other mental health issues.

5.3 *Nutrient supplements*

Supplementing with vitamins and other essential nutrients can potentially improve symptoms of EDs. Patients with EDs often show deficiencies in vitamin and trace elements, with zinc being the most common deficiency, accounting for 60% of the population, followed by vitamin D (Panda *et al.* 2023). Taking nutrient supplements in appropriate amounts is suggested to improve the intestinal environment and overall health.

5.4 *Clinical trials*

Numerous clinical trials are exploring the hypothesis on the effectiveness of CBT on reducing ED psychopathology. One such study by Ellen E. Fitzsimmons-Craft tested the hypothesis that a digital CBT guided program would reduce ED psychopathology in female students. The online platform, SB-ED, incorporates components of CBT tailored for EDs, screens students with EDs, and addresses stress, body image and mood, and relapse prevention. The results showed a significant difference in the eating disorder examination questionnaire global score in the intervention group: a reduction from 3.62 to 2.70, demonstrating the effectiveness of CBT as an EDs treatment method. This clinical trial provides strong evidence for the efficacy and acceptability of digital CBT in standard care (Fitzsimmons-Craft *et al.* 2020).

6 CONCLUSION

The gut microbiota plays a significant role in regulating eating behaviors and emotions through its interaction with the gut-brain axis and neurotransmitter production, particularly serotonin. Interestingly, the full internal activity of the microbiome hasn't been completely discovered. While recent studies in the mechanism of 5-HT production have illuminated how SCFAs bind to GPCRs and OLF78 to promote serotonin secretion into the bloodstream, the complete mechanisms remain partially understood. Further, the discovery of the 'on' mechanism indicates serotonin is also secreted by EC cells under the stimulation of SCFAs and other secondary bile acids. Nonetheless, the 'on' mechanism by which EC cells exert their effect in treating EDs is not clearly identified, necessitating further research in EC cells with 5-HT secretion. The vast majority of the population has realized the severity of the impact of EDs on humans. However, treating EDs, especially through the pharmacological pathways, is a relatively new field to neuroscience and microbiology. Although there are approved antidepressants for treating BN and BED, there is no validated medication for AN. Given the fast development of technology, the future of ED pharmaceutics would mainly depend on further study and evidence on the gut microbiota and neurotransmitter activities.

REFERENCES

Blake A.E., Peter T. and Arthur P. (2022). *Current Opinion in Biotechnology*. **78**, 958–1669

Castellini G., Cassioli E., Vitali F., Rossi E., Dani C., Melani G., Flaccomio D., D'Andria M., Monroy M. M., Galli A., Cavalieri D., Ricca V., Bartolucci G.L. and De Filippo C. (2023). *Sci. Rep.* **13**, 11753

Chen Y., Xu J. and Chen Y. (2021). Nutrients. **13**, 2099
Cryan J.F., O'Riordan K.J., Cowan C., Kiran S., Bastiaanssen T. and Boehme M. (2019). **99**, 1877–2013
Duan H., Zhu L., Li M., Zhang B. and Fang S. (2022). *Front. Pharmacol.* **13**, 949823
Eliza V.W., Brittany M., Kyra C., Hyun-Joon Y., Nandini D., Cara B. and James D. L. (2023). *Contemporary Clinical Trials.* **124**, 107036
Fattorusso A., Di G.L., Dell'Isola G.B., Mencaroni E. and Esposito S. (2019). *Nutrients.* **11**, 521
Fitzsimmons-Craft E.E., Chan W.W., Smith A.C., Firebaugh M., Fowler L.A., Topooco N., DePietro B., Wilfley D.E., Taylor C.B. and Jacobson N.C. (2022). *Int. J. Eat. Disord.* **55**, 343–353
Fitzsimmons-Craft E.E., Taylor C.B., Graham A.K., Sadeh-Sharvit S. and Balantekin K.N. (2020). *JAMA. Netw. Open.* **3**, 2015633
Fusco W., Lorenzo M.B. and Cintoni M., Porcari S., Rinninella E., Kaitsas F., Lener E., Mele M.C., Gasbarrini A., Collado M.C., Cammarota G. and Ianiro G. (2023). *Nutrients.* **15**, 2211
Glashouwer K. A., Neimeijer R. A. M., de Koning M. L., Vestjens M. and Martijn C. (2018). *Journal of Consulting and Clinical Psychology.* **86**, 1046–1055
Guzel T. and Mirowska-Guzel D. (2022). *Molecules.* **27**, 1680
J. Appleton. Inter Med (Encinitas). **17**, 28–32. (2018)
James P.H., Nawshaba N., Marissa A.S. and Evelin M.C. (2020). *Stress.* **23**, 617–632
Layunta E., Buey B., Mesonero J.E. and Latorre E. (2021). *Front. Endocrinol.* **12**, 748254
Le Grange D., Eckhardt S., Dalle Grave R., Crosby R., Peterson C., Keery H. and Martell C. (2022). *Psychological Medicine.* **52**, 2520–2530
Lock J., Fitzpatrick K. K., Agras W. S., Weinbach N. and Jo B. (2018). *European Eating Disorders Review.* **26**, 62–68
Melisse B., Evd. Berg, Jonge M., Blankers M., Furth E., Dekker J. and Beurs E. (2023). *J. Med. Internet. Res.* **25**, 40472
Nandini D., Brittany E. M., Kyra C., Eliza Margaret Van Wye and James D. (2023). *Lock Journal of Clinical Child & Adolescent Psychology.* **52**, 159–170
Panda, Swati S., Akankshya N., Srishti S., and Palok A. (2023). *Metabolites.* **13**, 488
Siddiqui M.T. and Cresci G.A.M. (2021). *J. Inflamm. Res.* **14**, 6025–6041
Silva YP., Bernardi A. and Frozza RL. (2020). *Front. Endocrinol.* **11**, 25
Sjostedt P., Enander J. and Isung J. (2021). *Front. Psychiatry* **12**, 682–868
Steiger H. (2004). *J. Psychiatry. Neurosci.* **20**, 20–9.
Sudo N., Chida Y., Aiba Y., Sonoda J., Oyama N., Yu X., Kubo C. and Koga Y. (2004). *J. Physiol.* **558**, 263–275
Terry S.M., Barnett J.A., and Gibson D.L. (2022). *J. Eat Disord.* **10**, 154
Thursby E. and Juge N. (2017). *Biochem. J.* **474**, 1823–1836
Tomás-Pejó E., González-Fernández C., Greses S., Kennes C., Otero-Logilde N., Veiga M.C., Bolzonella D., Müller B. and Passoth V. (2023). *Biotechnol. Biofuels.* **16**, 96
Valdes A.M., Walter J., Segal E. and Spector T.D. (2018). *BMJ.* **361**, 2179

Biological Sciences and Environmental Health – Gao (Ed.)

Role of trimethylamine oxide (TMAO) produced by gut microbiota in heart failure

Yingqi Hong
Biology, College of Mount Saint Vincent, USA

ABSTRACT: Heart failure (HF) is a pressing worldwide health issue that calls for creative preventive and treatment methods. The gut microbiota has a role in more than just digestion; dysbiosis that results in an increase in toxic metabolites might hasten the onset of HF. Trimethylamine N-oxide (TMAO), a molecule produced by gut microbes digesting food precursors, has gained attention as a connection between the gastrointestinal tract and the cardiovascular system. Elevated TMAO levels consistently correlate with a higher HF risk and poorer outcomes, strongly suggesting its involvement in HF development and progression. Clinical studies and animal models have revealed a mechanistic role for TMAO in inflammation, oxidative stress, and endothelial dysfunction. Dietary interventions targeting oxidized TMAO precursors and microbial composition offer promising avenues for alleviating HF. Challenges include the individualized nature of the gut microbiota and the need for long-term safety assessments. This review explores the emerging links between the gut microbiota, TMAO, and HF and highlights the complexities and opportunities in this evolving field. The intricate interrelationships between the gut microbiota, TMAO, and HF provide important insights into the pathomechanisms of HF, as well as directions for future clinical therapeutic strategies. The insights presented highlight the multifaceted nature of the etiology of HF and the interconnectedness of different physiologic processes. The gut microbiota and TMAO are expected to become dynamic therapeutic targets in the complex treatment to HF, bringing new perspectives for heart failure prevention and management.

1 INTRODUCTION

Heart failure (HF) is a complicated and widespread illness that poses a serious worldwide public health risk. A series of unpleasant symptoms, as well as greater mortality and morbidity rates, are caused by the heart's diminished ability to pump blood effectively (Savarese *et al.* 2023). The 8.9 million heart failure cases in China in 2020 alone serve as a stark reminder of the disease's widespread prevalence (Ma *et al.* 2023). Additionally, the prevalence of HF is highest in Central Europe, North Africa, and the Middle East, where there are between 1133 and 1196 cases per 100,000 people, while rates are lowest in Eastern Europe and Southeast Asia, where there are between 498 and 595 cases per 100,000 people (Savarese *et al.* 2023). This stark geographical variation underscores the multifaceted nature of HF's determinants and its complex interplay with a multitude of factors.

Traditionally, heart failure has been attributed to a combination of genetic predisposition, lifestyle choices, and comorbidities (Kaviarasan *et al.* 2022). However, as research advances, an increasingly intricate and holistic picture of heart failure etiology is emerging. Beyond the conventional factors, attention is shifting towards the intricate microbial ecosystem residing within the gastrointestinal tract, known as the intestinal flora.

DOI: 10.1201/9781003587590-14

The intestinal flora constitutes a rich and diverse consortium of microorganisms that inhabit the gastrointestinal tract. Recent breakthroughs in scientific understanding have revealed their profound impact on immune regulation, which extends far beyond the gut, encompassing distant organs, including the heart. The key to understanding the complex interplay between gut microorganisms and HF is the idea of a bidirectional communication channel between the gut and the circulatory system.

The understanding of TMAO's mechanistic contribution to HF pathophysiology has expanded significantly. Oxidized trimethylamine has also been connected to the increase of inflammation, oxidative stress, and endothelial dysfunction in addition to its negative effects on cardiovascular health (Oria *et al.* 2020). These mechanisms are recognized as pivotal drivers of HF development and progression.

This comprehensive review aims to unravel the intricate web of connections between gut flora, heart failure, and TMAO. The multifaceted factors and their potential as therapeutic targets for HF management are discussed. Key aspects to be explored include the modulation of gut microbes through dietary interventions aimed at TMAO reduction and the analysis of clinical findings. By shedding light on the multifaceted roles of gut flora and TMAO in HF's development and progression, this review strives to contribute to a deeper understanding of this complex interplay, with the ultimate goal of advancing innovative strategies for HF prevention and treatment.

2 EFFECTS OF GUT MICROBIOTA ON HEART FAILURE VIA TMAO

2.1 *The link between gut microbes and heart failure*

Increasing research is pointing to the significance of gut flora in cardiovascular disease. Gut flora produces biometabolites that act in a variety of ways to influence the body. At the initiation of heart failure, the small and large intestinal walls undergo a thickening and heightened permeability. Dysbiosis is brought on concurrently by changes in the quantity and make-up of gut flora. Increased quantities of pathogenic bacteria, including Candida, and decreased amounts of anti-inflammatory microorganisms define this dysbiosis. These shifts contribute to an upsurge in detrimental metabolites, thereby intensifying systemic inflammatory reactions. Consequently, this cascade of events inflicts damage upon the myocardium, subsequently hastening the advancement of heart failure (Pasini *et al.* 2016). This is increasingly recognized as a driver of heart failure progression. Inflammation due to dysbiosis can trigger a systemic immune response and affect the myocardial remodeling process, thus contributing to the development and progression of HF (Jia *et al.* 2019). Whereas, TMAO has been identified as a metabolite closely associated with cardiovascular disease and can be used as a risk factor indicator to monitor the heart failure process. The complex relationship between gut microbes and HF is also mediated through their role in shaping the host immune response. Perturbation of this relationship can promote immune dysfunction and inflammatory cascades as one of the factors contributing to the development of HF (Szabo *et al.* 2021).

2.2 *Influencing factors of intestinal flora on TMAO production*

Synthesis of trimethylamine TMAO through the metabolism of dietary precursors by intestinal microorganisms involves complex interactions that are influenced by a range of factors. The production of oxidized trimethylamine depends not only on the availability of its precursors, but is also regulated by the composition and activity of the intestinal microbiota. Dietary composition, as a significant influencing factor, plays a crucial role in regulating the production of oxidized trimethylamine. Oxidized trimethylamine is produced by microbial conversion of dietary components rich in choline, phosphatidylcholine and carnitine (Jia *et al.* 2022). These precursors are notably abundant in foods like beef and pork, eggs, and some shellfish, which encourages the production of oxidized trimethylamine during gut microbial metabolism (Romano *et al.* 2015). In contrast, diets rich in plant foods provide less substrate for the production of oxidized trimethylamine. The complex link between dietary intake and trimethylamine oxide levels emphasizes the potential of dietary interventions as a strategy to modulate trimethylamine oxide-mediated cardiovascular risk. In addition, changes in intestinal flora species and their relative abundance significantly affected TMAO levels. As effective makers of TMA from dietary precursors, some bacterial taxa have been found (Tang and Chen 2022). The balance between these TMA-producing bacteria and other gut microbes that metabolize TMA or produce competing metabolites contributes to the overall TMA production rate.

2.3 *Effects of dietary intervention on gut microbiota and TMAO*

A key approach to altering the production of TMAO involves manipulating the intake of choline, carnitine and phosphatidylcholine. Gut microorganisms break down these nutritional precursors to create TMA, which can then be oxidized to create TMAO. It has been shown that TMAO concentrations are significantly correlated with fish and egg intake (Hamaya *et al.* 2020). Consumption of fish and eggs in SFFQ apples was significantly correlated with higher TMAO concentrations after controlling for demographic factors and adjusting for food groups in concert. The 7DDR evaluation confirmed the relationship between TMAO concentrations and fish consumption as being favourable (Hamaya *et al.* 2020). Prebiotics and probiotics are another avenue of dietary intervention targeting the gut flora; Prebiotics are indigestible dietary fibers that favorably influence the development of healthy gut microbes, potentially preventing the spread of harmful bacteria like Clostridium difficile (Moludi *et al.* 2021). This holds some promise for reducing TMA output.

3 EFFECT OF TMAO ON HEART FAILURE

3.1 *Biosynthesis pathways and regulatory factors of TMAO*

In the complex interaction between the dietary elements, gut microbiota, and heart failure, TMAO is an essential player. Its formation is a complex process that begins with the metabolism of food precursors, primarily trimethylamine (TMA), by gut microbes. TMA is a precursor to TMAO and is produced through the metabolic breakdown of certain food components. Foods rich in the amino acid choline, as well as compounds such as creatine and creatinine in muscle tissue, are the main sources of these precursors. Red meat, chicken, fish, and eggs are just a few of the common foods that contain a lot of choline. (Romano *et al.* 2015). In the intricate ecosystem of the human gut, specific microorganisms play a key role in converting these precursor substances into TMA. During digestion, these food precursors are subjected to microbial enzymes in the gut. Certain microorganisms possess the enzymatic mechanisms required to convert choline, creatine, and creatinine into TMA (Romano *et al.* 2015). The absorption of TMA into the bloodstream and transport to the liver occurs once it is produced in the gut. Here, a key role is played by hepatic flavin monooxygenase 3 (FMO3), which oxidizes TMA, thereby converting it to TMAO, a compound of interest for its role in cardiovascular health and HF.

The factors that regulate TMAO levels are multifactorial and encompass a range of variables, including the composition of the gut flora, the number of choline-rich foods consumed, and a variety of other factors (Romano *et al.* 2015). The composition and diversity of the gut bacteria have a significant impact on the pace at which dietary precursors are converted to TMA. In addition, an individual's dietary choices play a crucial role, as consuming more choline-rich foods can lead to elevated levels of TMAO. Finally, the enzymatic activity of FMO3 in the liver is a key determinant of the conversion of TMA to TMAO.

3.2 *TMAO's part in the onset of heart failure*

A key mechanism by which TMAO affects the development of HF is its pro-inflammatory properties (Figure 1). The presence of elevated levels of TMAO is linked to an increase in inflammatory markers. Nuclear factor-B (NF-B) pathway activation and increased production of pro-inflammatory genes are brought about by elevated levels of TMAO (Yang *et al.* 2019). This chronic low-grade inflammation is considered a hallmark of HF progression and can lead to decreased myocardial contractility and exacerbate cardiac dysfunction (Tang and Chen 2022). TMAO-mediated inflammation may further perpetuate the vicious cycle, and the inflamed tissue may provide a favorable environment for the proliferation of TMAO-producing bacteria, which in turn amplifies TMAO levels. The effect of oxidized trimethylamine on endothelial function is another way in which it contributes to the development of HF. TMAO activates endothelial dysfunction and cardiometabolic complications via a number of mechanisms, including decreased endothelial cell viability, excessive reactive oxygen species (ROS) production, increased vascular inflammation, and vascular calcification leading to atherosclerotic plaques and decreased vascular tone. (Shanmugham *et al.* 2023). Oxidized trimethylamine has been shown to impair endothelial nitric oxide synthesis, a key mediator of vascular relaxation and homeostasis. Endothelial dysfunction may lead to impaired vasodilatory function, increased oxidative stress, and an unfavourable vascular environment. In addition, TMAO-induced endothelial dysfunction may impede nutrient and oxygen delivery to cardiac tissue and exacerbate myocardial injury (Shanmugham *et al.* 2023). The thioredoxin interacting proteins-NOD, LRR, and pyrin structural domain-containing protein 3 (TXNIP-NLRP3), which have been demonstrated to create ROS when TMAO is present, are regulated by oxidative stress, which is a significant factor in cardiac remodelling in HF (Figure 1) (Shanmugham *et al.* 2023). Elevated levels of oxidized trimethylamine are associated with increased reactive oxygen species production and diminished antioxidant defences. This oxidative imbalance can lead to cellular damage, apoptosis, and fibrosis, resulting in detrimental cardiac remodelling (Oria *et al.* 2020). Furthermore, TMAO-induced oxidative stress can exacerbate mitochondrial dysfunction, impair energy production, and compromise overall cardiac function.

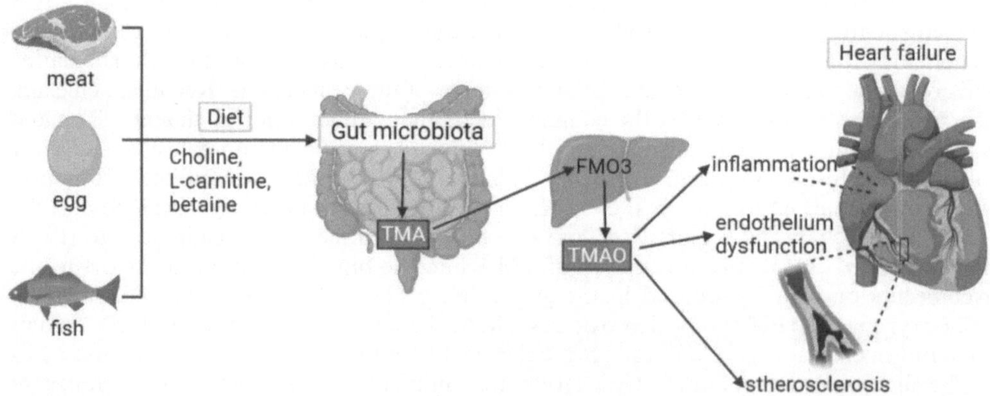

Figure 1. The formation of trimethylamine N-oxide (TMAO) and how it affects the heart are shown in this schematic. By metabolizing dietary precursors present in meals like meat, eggs, and fish that include choline, L-carnitine, and betaine, intestinal microbes produce trimethylamine (TMA). After that, FMO3 in the liver oxidizes TMA to create TMAO. High TMAO levels have been linked to heart issues, affecting blood vessels, inflammation, etc., and speeding the development of heart disease, which in turn affects heart failure. Figure created using Biorender.com.

3.3 *Associations between TMAO and heart failure in clinical studies*

Numerous clinical research has looked into the connection between TMAO concentrations and HF in the general population (Table 1). High TMAO concentrations have repeatedly been linked to an increased risk of severe cardiovascular events, including the onset and progression of HF. One notable study found that, even after adjusting for conventional risk variables, greater TMAO concentrations were still independently linked to a higher risk of incident HF. This outcome was likewise attained with additional carnitine modification (Wei *et al.* 2022). In addition, TMAO levels showed a dose-response relationship with the risk of HF, reinforcing the potential clinical significance of TMAO as a predictive biomarker. Elevated levels of TMAO are linked to a worse prognosis for individuals with heart failure, including an increase in mortality and hospitalization owing to heart failure exacerbation. TMAO has a predictive value for heart failure prognosis (Jia *et al.* 2022). These findings emphasize the potential of TMAO as a prognostic indicator for heart failure treatment.

Table 1. Clinical trials of how diet affects TMAO and the effect of TMAO on prognosis in heart failure.

Author	Subjects	Results	Reference
Yiming Dai *et al.* 2022	Relationship between diet and urinary TMAO and its precursors in children.	The presence of fish, meat, or eggs in school-age children's urine can affect TMAO and its precursors. TMAO concentrations are positively linked to high levels of dietary diversity.	Dai *et al.* 2022
Rikuta Hamaya *et al.* 2020	Association of diet with circulating TMAO concentration.	Fish intake had a significant impact on TMAO concentrations, but not red meat consumption. TMAO concentrations were negatively linked to uPDI, an unhealthy dietary pattern.	Hamaya *et al.* 2020
Toru Suzuki *et al.*	The relationship between TMAO and the prognosis of acute heart failure.	Age, blood urea, and eGFR were the primary predictors of TMAO, with diabetes, smoking status, atrial fibrillation, and NYHA classification playing a minor role.	Suzuki *et al.* 2016
Qiu Weida *et al.* 2022	Plasma TMAO and NT-proBNP combined have a predictive value for the likelihood of recovery and length of hospitalization for IHF patients.	The risk of all-cause death was highest in the group with high TMAO+high NT-proBNP in the study of 189 patients with ischemic heart failure, and IHF patients with increased levels of both. biomarkers were more likely to be hospitalized. Patients stayed in hospitals longer.	Qiu *et al.* 2022
Nan Li *et al.* 2022	Acute myocardial infarction and heart failure patients' prognoses are associated to TMAO.	In patients with AMI and HF, high TMAO levels before to PCI were independently connected to a higher risk of MACE, especially in people with high hsCRP levels.	Li *et al.* 2022

Abbreviations: TMAO, Trimethylamine N-oxide; uPDI, Unhealthy Dietary Pattern Index; eGFR, Estimated Glomerular Filtration Rate; NYHA, New York Heart Association; NT-proBNP, N-terminal pro-B-type natriuretic peptide; IHF, Ischemic Heart Failure; HF, Heart failure; AMI, Anterior Myocardial Infarction; PCI, Percutaneous Coronary Intervention; MACE, Major Adverse Cardiovascular Events; hsCRP, high-sensitivity C-reactive protein.

3.4 *The potential of TMAO and gut microbiota as heart failure treatment targets*

The intricate relationships between the gut microbiota and TMAO have come to light as a promising avenue in the search for novel treatment approaches for HF. The complicated link between gut microorganisms and TMAO formation, as well as their effect on cardiovascular health, brings up new opportunities for targeted therapies in the treatment of HF. The potential to modulate gut microbial composition to mitigate cardiovascular risk, including HF, has attracted considerable attention. Emerging evidence suggests that interventions targeting the gut microbiota, such as dietary changes, have the potential to alter microbial homeostasis in ways that are beneficial in reducing oxidized trimethylamine production. TMAO, a metabolite derived from the processing of dietary precursor microorganisms, has emerged as a biomarker linking gut microbial activity to cardiovascular health. The risk of HF onset and development has repeatedly been linked to elevated levels of TMAO. The role of trimethylamine oxide as a potential contririsbutor to adverse cardiac remodeling, inflammation, and oxidative stress further emphasizes its importance in the pathophysiology of HF.

Utilizing TMAO as a therapeutic target requires a multifaceted approach. Dietary interventions that limit the intake of trimethylamine oxide precursors and promote the growth of beneficial gut microbes can serve as the cornerstone of such strategies. By modulating gut microbial composition, these interventions may be effective in reducing trimethylamine oxide production and its deleterious cardiovascular effects.

4 CONCLUSION

The intricate relationship between the gut microbiota, TMAO, and HF has been elucidated. Once viewed as an unassuming digestive companion, the gut microbiota has evolved into a complex coordinator of myriad physiological processes that extend far beyond digestion. The gut microbiome has a major impact on inflammation, metabolism, and immunity, and its critical role in cardiovascular health is being newly recognized. Heart failure's complicated development has been connected to abnormalities in the composition and operation of the gut microbiota. Chronic inflammation, oxidative stress, and immune dysfunction induced by the gut microbiota are potential catalytic mechanisms of heart failure. The profound impact of the gut microbiota on immune regulation and systemic inflammation creates a dynamic environment that escalates heart failure risk. In addition, microbial TMAO plays a critical role as a sentinel biomarker that effectively monitors the trajectory of heart failure. Elevated levels of TMAO signal adverse cardiovascular outcomes, including increased risk of heart failure and prognostic implications. The far-reaching effects of TMAO also include the promotion of inflammation, endothelial dysfunction, and adverse cardiac remodeling, all of which are key factors in the intricate pathophysiology of heart failure.

Although existing studies have yielded valuable insights, there is still uncharted territory in the intricate field of gut microbiota, TMAO, and heart failure, which underscores the urgency of continued research. Delving into the subtle interactions between these factors is critical to unraveling the intricate mechanisms behind them and refining targeted interventions. The challenges posed by significant individual differences in gut microbial composition, genetic susceptibility, and environmental influences must be squarely addressed in order to bridge the gap between research findings and effective clinical strategies. Future research efforts are expected to make progress in several key areas. Further elucidation of the molecular and cellular mechanisms of the gut microbiota-TMAO-heart failure axis is critical for a more comprehensive understanding of the axis. With this knowledge, specific therapies that are based on the individual microbial profiles and genetic predispositions of patients might be developed. To ascertain the long-term security, effectiveness, and sustainability of initiatives focusing on this axis, longitudinal studies must also be carried out. Modulation of gut microbial composition through dietary interventions aimed at reducing TMAO precursors offers a potential avenue for heart failure prevention and treatment. The ability to develop personalized therapeutic strategies based on an individual's gut microbiota profile heralds a paradigm shift in heart failure treatment. In addition to dietary interventions, direct targeting of TMAO biosynthetic pathways or innovative microbial manipulation to reduce TMAO production is a promising avenue for future research and clinical translation.

REFERENCES

Dai Y., Zhang J., Wang Z., Xu S., Zhang Q., Duan Z., Tan R., Qi X., Guo J., Chang X., Wu C. and Zhou Z., (2022). *Nutrients*, **14**, 3419

D'Oria R., Schipani R., Leonardini A., Natalicchio A., Perrini S., Cignarelli A., Laviola L. and Giorgino F., (2020). *Oxidative Medicine and Cellular Longevity*, **2020**, 5732956

Hamaya R., Ivey K. L., Lee D. H., Wang M., Li J., Franke A., Sun Q. and Rimm E. B., (2020). *The American Journal of Clinical Nutrition*, **112**, 1448–1455

Jia Q., Li H., Zhou H., Zhang X., Zhang A., Xie Y., Li Y., Lv S. and Zhang J., (2019). *Cardiovascular Therapeutics*, **2019**, 5164298

Jia Q., Li H., Zhou H., Zhang X., Zhang A., Xie Y., Li Y., Lv S. and Zhang J., (2022). *Chinese Journal of Heart Failure and Cardiomyopathy*, **27**, 242–246

Kaviarasan V., Mohammed V. and Veerabathiran R., (2022). *Egypt Heart Journal*, **74**, 5

Li N., Zhou J., Wang Y., Chen R., Li J., Zhao X., Zhou P., Liu C., Song L., Liao Z., Wang X., Yan S., Zhao H. and Yan H., (2022). *ESC Heart Failure*, **9**, 3846–3857

Ma M., Wang Z., Fan J. and Hu S., (2023). *Chinese Journal of General Medicine*, **26**, 3975–3994

Moludi J., Saiedi S., Ebrahimi B., Alizadeh M., Khajebishak Y. and Ghadimi S. S., (2021). *Journal of Cardiovascular Translational Research*, **14**, 299–307

Pasini E., Aquilani R., Testa C., Baiardi P., Angioletti S., Boschi F., Verri M. and Dioguardi F., (2016). *JACC. Heart Failure*, **4**, 220–227

Qiu W. D., Xiao X. J., Xia S., Gao Z. P. and Li L. W., (2022). **50**, 684–689

Romano K. A., Vivas E. I., Amador-Noguez D. and Rey F. E., (2015). *mBio*, **6**, e02481

Savarese G., Becher P. M., Lund L. H., Seferovic P., Rosano G. M. C., and Coats A. J. S., (2023). *Cardiovascular Research*, **118**, 3272–3287

Shanmugham M., Bellanger S. and Leo C. H., (2023). *Pharmaceuticals* (Basel, Switzerland), **16**(4), 504

Suzuki T., Heaney L. M., Bhandari S. S., Jones D. J. and Ng L. L., (2016). *Heart (British Cardiac Society)*, **102**, 841–848

Szabo T. M., Frigy A. and Nagy E. E., (2021). *International Journal of Molecular Sciences*, **22**, 13053

Tang H. Y. and Chen M., (2022). *Chinese Journal of Cardiovascular Medicine*, **27**, 196–199

Wei H., Zhao M., Huang M., Li C., Gao J., Yu T., Zhang Q., Shen X., Liang J., Li N., Zhao C., Wang Z., Dong E., Zheng L. and Wang D., (2022). *Frontiers in Medicine*, **16**, 295–305

Yang S., Li X., Yang F., Zhao R., Pan X., Liang J., Tian L., Li X., Liu L., Xing Y. and Wu M., (2019). *Frontiers in Pharmacology*, **10**, 1360

Biological Sciences and Environmental Health – Gao (Ed.)

The therapeutic effect of BDNF on Alzheimer's disease

Yizhen Shi
Oversea Education College, Nanjing Tech University, Nanjing, JiangSu Province, China

ABSTRACT: Alzheimer's Disease (AD) is one of the focus objects of today's research. It is a neurological disease that influence cognition, function, and behavior and is gradual and irreversible. At present, speech loss, memory blockage, cognitive impairment, and mobility difficulties are the primary symptoms of Alzheimer's disease in elderly people. Researchers have found progress in the treatment of AD, but there is still a research gap and adequate understanding of the problem of AD. Brain-derived neurotrophic factor (BDNF) is closely associated with AD, with a decrease in BDNF, adverse symptoms such as schizophrenia and obsessive-compulsive disorder may develop. Therefore, by collecting data about AD and analyzing BDNF, this paper explores the effect of BDNF in treating AD. Neuronal function in key memory circuits of the brain (the entorhinal cortex and hippocampus) is regulated by BDNF, a nervous system growth factor. In animal models, BDNF inhibits cell loss, facilitates cell functions, and builds new connections between neuronal cells. According to previous biological studies, BDNF, which is activated by the tyrosine receptor B, can be identified as a reasonable candidate for AD.

1 INTRODUCTION

Brain-derived neurotrophic factor (BDNF), a critical factor affecting memory and learning, is found throughout the human nervous system. People with Alzheimer's disease (AD) have reduced levels of this protein. Whether a person has AD or not, acute physical exercise of a moderate to high intensity would raise plasma BDNF levels. Even still, when at rest, healthy people have higher levels of BDNF than AD sufferers. There are no studies on how continuous exercise affects BDNF levels in AD patients when they are at rest (Rosliza *et al.* 2018). People with AD would experience an increase in BDNF levels during a hypothetical endurance training program, whether it was interval training or continuous training. Their neuropsychological and physiological capabilities. There is a progressive process of the change of the symptoms of AD, the beginning is not aware of the changes in the body, showing a state of asymptomatic; To mild cognitive (mild cognitive impairment [MCI]) and/or neurobehavioral (mild behavioral impairment [MBI]) changes, and eventually to the most severe form of AD, showing slow movement and memory loss. Researchers and medical professionals have developed a number of ways to distinguish the stages of AD, and these methods are different and have their own shortcomings, but they can detect the cause of AD. By diagnosing the severity of the disease, the researchers named each stage of AD differently.

Most older people develop AD because of persistent nerve blockage in the brain. In today's world, the drugs developed can only improve the course of the disease to a certain extent, but they cannot completely cure it. The course of AD lasts for a long period, which can last 20 years or more.The symptoms of Alzheimer's disease can be roughly divided into three stages. In the first three years, the symptoms are mild, and patients may experience extreme or diminished mood, blurred vision, and memory loss. Patients in the second stage, which is the longest, gradually lose their ability to act independently and display non-self-conscious behavior.In the third stage, the patient will essentially be unconscious and frequently feel lethargic.

DOI: 10.1201/9781003587590-15

After many investigations and studies, it is concluded that the expression level of BDNF is indeed related to Alzheimer's disease. Therefore, regulating BDNF expression in the body has become an effective treatment for improving AD (Laura *et al.* 2018).

Two potential pathologic markers of AD are extracellular amyloid beta (A) plaques and intracellular neurofibrillary tangles (nft). The brain of AD patients contains A large amount of aggregate A plaque deposits, and too much or too little beta protein will produce adverse reactions; Plaque deposits usually occur decades before the disease is apparent, and the changes in the brain begin during the asymptomatic period. nft is formed when an abnormal accumulation of hyperphosphorylated tau protein is observed 10-15 years before the onset of symptoms, so early diagnosis is particularly important in cases of AD.

2 BASIC INFORMATION ABOUT BDNF

2.1 *Structure and function of BDNF*

The symptoms of Alzheimer's disease can be roughly divided into three stages. In the first three years, the symptoms are mild, and patients may experience extreme or diminished mood, blurred vision, and memory loss. Patients in the second stage, which is the longest, gradually lose their ability to act independently and display non-self-conscious behavior.In the third stage, the patient will essentially be unconscious and frequently feel lethargic. Studies have found that the BDNF expression is associated with AD, and it can be further used as a drug to treat Alzheimer's disease by adjusting the level (Harikesh *et al.* 2022).

The severity of extracellular amyloid beta (A) plaques and intracellular neurofibrillary tangles (nft) are the two factors that best translate the extent to which the symptoms of AD reach. AD can lead to neurodegeneration, brain cells will shrink, even simple household activities can not be completed, and there will be temporary memory loss. Beta deposits in the brains of AD patients are either due to reduced clearance of A or excessive production of A; Plaque deposits typically occur 20 years or more before the onset of cognitive impairment. nft is caused by the unusual state of the hyperphosphorylated tau protein, but they may be predicted and prevented in advance.

BDNF is a secretable polypeptide composed of 119 amino acid residues. Studies have shown that BDNF is widely distributed in brain, and those with AD have lower levels of BDNF than the general population. It is vital for the maintenance of the development of the central nervous system (CNS). It is widely present in the hippocampus, cortex, nerve tissue, and other areas in the body, and has a significant impact on the expression of nerves in the body (Sanjay *et al.* 2022).

BDNF is a neurotrophic factor widely expressed in the brain, especially in the hypothalamus, limbic system and hippocampus, and is mainly produced by glutamergic neurons and glial cells. Skeletal muscle cells, smooth muscle cells, endothelial cells, and activated immune cells are all capable of expression of BDNF in the periphery. BDNF can be found in platelets, which are the most important peripheral reservoirs, and the level of BDNF is 100-1000 times higher than that in neurons.

2.2 *Source of BDNF*

BDNF was first detected in the pig brain in 1982 and has since been investigated by many researchers. Because pig, human, mouse, and human BDNF have exactly the same amino acid coding sequence, and have striking similarities with nerve growth factor (NGF) sequence, At the heart of the nerve growth factor family is BDNF. It has been confirmed that BDNF exists in the CNS of higher animals and becomes an indispensable nerve growth factor for development and homeostasis regulation. BDNF can activate downstream signals by binding with the receptor tyrosine-protein kinase B (TrkB) on the surface of neuron membranes through target origin, secretory and paracrine ways, and is vital for the development, differentiation, function maintenance and synaptic plasticity of neurons (Jianming *et al.* 2021).

It is widely present in the human body and is the most abundant neurotrophic factor found in the human body so far. It can be found in the heart, kidneys, lungs, T cells, and cerebellum. BDNF usually increase during development and aging in the entorhinal cortex, a key memory center in the brain as well as the most important place where AD often affects short-term memory loss. BDNF is found to be decreased in AD patients.

3 THE MECHANISM OF BDNF FUNCTION

3.1 *Protective effect of BDNF to AD*

This basic protein not only participates in the repair and regulation of neurons, but also prevents neuronal apoptosis, interfering with the development of dendrites, axons and synapses (Ting *et al.* 2021).

There are two forms of BDNF, namely, BDNF precursor BDNF (proBDNF) and mature BDNF (mBDNF). proBDNF and mBDNF jointly maintain nerve homeostasis mBDNF/proBDNF imbalance can damage neuronal plasticity, lead to neuronal death, and participate in the occurrence of neuropsychiatric diseases, including anxiety, depression, schizophrenia, and AD, PD and other neurodegenerative diseases pathophysiological mechanism. The more biologically active proBDNF in the cerebrospinal fluid of AD patients can induce apoptosis. The level of proBDNF and BDNF in the cerebrospinal fluid of AD patients was largely more than that of the healthy people, while the proBDNF/BDNF ratio is significantly increased, thus inducing neuron death and synaptic plasticity (Jie *et al.* 2019).

3.2 *Inhibition of β-amyloid production by BDNF*

β-amyloid protein formed by APP hydrolysis is a part of neuroinflammatory plaques, its presence would cause nerve inflammation and other damage, and then threaten the prominent growth and development, resulting in serious neurological damage (Eremenko *et al.* 2019). It is also recognized as a major cause of Alzheimer's disease. Cutting the APP with ADAM-10 releases beta-amyloid, resulting in sAPP alpha, which has a neuroprotective effect on the human body. The redistribution of BDNF to ADAM-10 on the cell surface can enhance ADAM-10 cutting processing of APP, which can reduce the concentration of *β*-amyloid protein to achieve the purpose of protecting nerve tissue. These results indicated that BDNF can indirectly regulate the pathway of amyloid production (Eremenko *et al.* 2019).

Table 1. Clinical trials of drugs that affect BDNF to treat AD.

Subjects	Treatment	Results	References
Male 5xFAD mice	The nerve can be protected by adding glial cells in a motion-induced manner	reversed cognitive impairment-without affecting neurogenesis, neuronal loss	Irina *et al.* 2020
225 subjects	Irisin expressed in the brain and activated expression of BDNF in the mouse hippocampus	CSF levels of Aβ42, but not Aβ40	Mychael *et al.* 2020

(*continued*)

Table 1. Continued

Subjects	Treatment	Results	References
a mouse model	ADTC5 is used to deliver BDNF into the brain	BDNF can be transported to the brain by ADTC5	Brain *et al.* 2020
Forty AD patients	Myokines were measured by ELISA	The patient showed positive results in this test	Elisa *et al.* 2019
3xTg-AD mice	Exenatide	The weight and glucose metabolism of mice were not affected by exenatide treatment	Manuela *et al.* 2019
Tg-APP/PS1 mice	Hyperoxygenation treatment changes	HT22 Treating Hippocampal cells with Aβ42 increased the expression of hypoxia-related genes	Juli *et al.* 2019
Adult male TSs	Behaviour and MRI tests	Donepezil significantly improved the spatial cognitive deficits induced by aβ1-40, and reversed the temporal Angle	Hong *et al.* 2018
AD rats	MWM test	CX691 (0.3 mg/kg) can improve the memory ability and spatial learning function of AD rats	Nazanin *et al.* 2018
5xFAD mice	7,8-dihydroxyflavone	Cortical beta plaque deposition can be reduced by treatment with 7, 8-DHF	Aytan *et al.* 2018
175 healthy subjects and 222 with prodromal	Magnetic resonance imaging	Within the normal and pathological aging, Met carriers and APOE E4 carriers lack compensatory mechanisms	Gomar *et al.* 2019

3.3 *BDNF-TrkB pathway*

The basis of AD neurodegeneration has been approved to be related to the loss of BDNF/TrkB activity, especially the decreased BDNF mRNA and protein transcription in the hippocampus and frontal cortex, which are closely related to cognitive impairment. The BDNF gene expression in the prefrontal cortex is associated with the neuropathology of AD amyloid plaques, neuroinflammatory plaques, and neuronal tangles. Compared to the normal group, the proBDNF transcription in the hippocampus of AD patients was increased. In addition, the study found that compared with normal people, the expression level of proBDNF in the cerebrospinal fluid of AD and the proBDNF/BDNF ratio were higher, which speculated that the progression of AD disease could be detected by the changes of BDNF (Wanbing *et al.* 2023).

After transcription and translation of BDNF gene, the proBDNF is formed. pro-BDNF can not only exist as the precursor of mBDNF, but also play a biological function different from mBDNF. pro-BDNF and mBDNF play opposite roles in regulating apoptosis. Pro-BDNF is hydrolyzed by the tissue plasminogen activator (tPA) plasminase system to produce mBDNF. tyrosine kinase receptor B (TrkB) is a high-affinity receptor for BDNF. After the two binding, the intracellular region of TrkB is activated, and the phosphorylation level of TrkB itself is increased. Thus, activating downstream phosphatidylinositol 3-kinase (PI3K)/ protein kinase B (PI3K) (PKB), Ras/mitogen-activated protein kinase (MAPK) and phospholipase C-γ1 (Phospholipase C-γ1) (PLC-γ1)/ protein kinase C (PKC) and other signaling pathways (Figure 1).

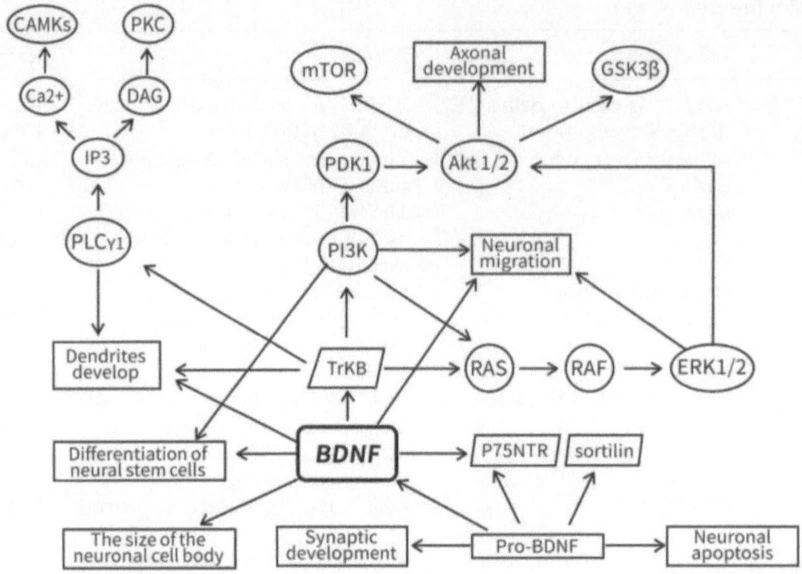

Figure 1. Mechanism of TrkB and BDNF functions. Figure credit: Original.

The condition of AD is closely related to the expression of the hippocampus, and the BDNF/TrkB signaling pathway is related to the learning and memory ability of the hippocampus, which is another way that BDNF acts on AD. BDNF binds to activated tyrosine kinase receptor B to stabilize synaptic development and prevent nerve cell apoptosis. When trkB is selectively spliced with mRNA, three forms of BDNF trkB are produced, which include the full-length catalytic receptor (TRKb.fl) and the two truncated forms (TrkB). T1 was highly expressed in non-neuronal cells. FL in the adult brain. In neuroblastoma cells or hippocampal primary neurons, BDNF rapidly enhanced the TrkB on the membrane surface in a short period of time. However, longer treatments (minutes to hours) can result in reduced TrkB levels on the membrane surface. To improve synaptic plasticity, BDNF modifies presynaptic transmitter release or increases postsynaptic transmitter sensitivity to regulate synaptic efficacy. The neurotransmitter acetylcholine, which regulates cognitive function, was reduced in the hippocampus of AD patients, and the expression of BDNF protein was positively associated with ACh content.

The expression levels of BDNF and TrkB were decreased in AD. A remarkable decrease in BDNF and TrkB mRNA levels was also found in non-AD Tau disease. It has also been reported that polymorphism in BDNF is associated with the risk of developing AD. Therefore, BDNF may be a protective factor in the pathogenesis of AD. BDNF can protect neurons from Aβ toxicity in vitro or in vivo. When living brain sections of the entorhinal cortex or hippocampus were incubated with BDNF, long-term enhanced (LTP) damage caused by Aβ was prevented (Lievyn *et al.* 2020).

4 CONCLUSION

An early diagnosis of AD can become critical as treatments that change the associated disease pathology become useful—especially such treatments may be more effective in facilitating cognitive function, as well as prolonging independence, when given during early stage of AD. For the sake of early treatment, more people are seeking help at the earliest signs of AD.

Patients will be able to manage their symptoms in the present, seek different treatment options, and plan their sleep and diet, which may affect the deterioration of their symptoms, improve their physical fitness, and ultimately form a benign outcome. By targeting and improving the underlying biological mechanisms, coupled with good living habits to improve psychological status, AD can be treated to the greatest extent possible. This approach Outlines common ways for clinicians to diagnose AD early in the treatment process, determine the best outcomes for AD, and how to effectively and cost-effectively incorporate them into current clinical practice.

REFERENCES

Aytan N., Choi J., Carreras I., Crabtree L., Nguyen B., Lehar M., Kraysztof Blusztajin J., B. G, J and Dedeoglu A. (2018). *Eur. J. Pharmacol.* **828**

Brain M. K., Liqin Z., Molinar Eduardo R. and Teruna S. (2020). *J. Med. res. Arch.***8**

Elisa C., Denise G., Giovanni S., Alberto C., Margherita B., Paolo M., Angelo A., Cheristian L., Ildebrando A., Carlo F. and Lucio T. (2019). *SIN.* **40**, 793–810

Eremenko E., Mittal O., Berner K., Kamenetsky N., Nemirovsky A., Elyahu Y. and Monsonego A. (2019). *EBioMedicine.* **43**, 424–434

Gomar J., Conejero-Goldberg C., Huey E., Davies P., T. E, Idberg G. (2019). *Neurobiol. Aging.* **39**

Harikesh D., Anamika D., Kavita G. and Arunabha Y. (2022). *Int. J. Neurosci.*

Hong Z., Shiwei N., Hongbin Z., Shude L. and Jianlin J. (2018). *Metab Brain Dis.* **33**, 1961–1974

Irina B., Mariia I., Annika S., Marina I., Sanna L., Hennariik K., Alessandra V., Heikki T., Frederick W., Mustafa A., Tarja M., Alexandra G., Heikki T. and Katja M. K. (2020). *J. Neuroinflammation.* **17**

Jianming L., Chun C., Hee E. A., Xia L. Shan-Ping Y., Fredric M., Ivette S., Gong J., Shengxi W. and Keqiang Y. (2021). *Neuropharmacology.***197** 108737

Jie W., Zhi-Hao, Hee E., Xia L., Shan-Ping Y., Fredric M., Ivette S., Gong J., Shengxi W. and Keqiang Y. (2019). *PNAS.***116**

Juli C., Hye-Jin K., Jung-Eun L., Yunjin L., Ju-young S. and Pyung-Lim H. (2019). *Aging cell.***18**, e12888

Laura M. G., Agata C. and Enrico R. (2018). Aging. **10**, 1791–1792

Lievyn E., Thomas V., Sylvie M., Anna-Gaelle V., Nathalie O., Remi N., Claudia L., Jean Luc F. and Pierre Olivier L. (2020). *EURAPA.* **17**, 2

Manuela B., Alberto G., Vanessa C., Marco O., Roosano L., Annamaria C. and Stefano S. (2019). *J. Alzheimer's Dis.***70**, 3

Mir Z., Rosliza, Naeem B., Muhammad Nadeem I., Bin Simbak N., ALA Z., Mohammad Ariff T., Khalili M., Amjad Kamal M. and Amin Baig A. (2018). *Res. J. Pharm. Technol.* **11,** 4317

Mychael L., Felipe C. R., Felipe K. S., Claudia D., Naima A., Bart V., Fernanda T., Paulo M., Felice Fernanda D. and Sergio F. (2020). *Amst.***12**, e12034

Nazanin M., Ali S., Iman F., Mohammad A., Amir M., Elham K. and Ayat K. (2018). *Iran J Basic Med Sci.* **21**, 7

Sanjay A., Takahisa K. and Jagdish S. (2022). *Int. J. Biol. Macromol.* **208**, 901–911

Ting W., Shengnan G., Kun Z., Shaoru C. and Ting L. (2021). *Int J Pharmacol.* **17**

Wanbing W., Yanzhong L., Fangling M., Xuan S., Kai C., Rengong Z., Chen W., Honghua Z., YunWu Z., GuoJun B., XiaoFen C. and Li Z. (2023). *Brain Behav. Immun.* **113**, 275–288

Biological Sciences and Environmental Health – Gao (Ed.)
© 2025 the Author(s), ISBN: 978-1-032-96016-6

Effect of Mediterranean diet on overweight and obesity in adults

Jiayi Shi
College of Food Science and Technology, Yunnan Agricultural University, Kunming, China

ABSTRACT: Overweight and obesity are widespread global health issues that present significant risks to health and have received growing attention. The treatment of these conditions has been widely researched by scholars. At present, the Mediterranean diet (MD) is widely promoted as one of the healthiest dietary patterns by experts in many countries. It offers a rich array of nutrients while emphasizing low-sugar, low-fat, light, and simple meals. A number of studies have shown that MD has a significant effect on weight loss in adults with overweight and obesity. This paper aims to analyze the mechanisms behind the weight loss effects of MD on overweight and obese patients, as well as the therapeutic benefits of combining MD with exercise therapy for health issues in women. This research seeks to provide a basis for future treatments of overweight, obesity, and other chronic diseases.

1 INTRODUCTION

With the advancement of society and the alteration of people's habits, the proportion of overweight and obese people has reached unprecedented levels. However, these conditions often go unnoticed in their early stages, gradually becoming a hidden threat to public health. The 2020 Report on Chinese Residents' Nutrition and Chronic Disease Status demonstrates that more than half of adult residents in China suffer from overweight and obesity, and the prevalence rate of children and adolescents under the age of 17 is close to 30% (State Council information office of China 2020). A variety of factors may trigger overweight and obesity, such as metabolic abnormalities, blood glucose abnormalities, intestinal flora disorders, and nutrient deficiencies. Similar to cardiovascular and cerebrovascular disorders, diabetes mellitus, hypertension, and other illnesses are frequently linked to overweight and obesity. In the list of the best diets in the United States published by the American authority in 2020, the Mediterranean diet (MD) ranks first for its healthy, light, simple, and nutrient-comprehensive food style. According to experts, MD is beneficial for fat and weight loss, management and prevention of diabetes, and heart health. At the same time, the diet pattern is easy to follow and suitable for long-term adoption.

In this paper, the MD model was selected to study its role in optimizing fat structure, controlling blood glucose, improving intestinal flora, supplementing deficient micronutrients, and other aspects of overweight-obesity intervention in adults over 18 years of age, as well as the therapeutic effects of MD in combination with exercise therapy on some common diseases in females. It provides a good research foundation for the optimization of future dietary habits, prevention and control of overweight-obesity, and treatment of overweight and obesity related female diseases.

 DOI: 10.1201/9781003587590-16

2 DEFINITION OF OVERWEIGHT AND OBESITY

The World Health Organization sets the standard for overweight and obesity based on body mass index (BMI) (BMI = weight/height squared [kg/m^2]). Adults (regardless of gender) are considered overweight when BMI ≥ 25 kg/m^2 and obese when BMI ≥ 30 kg/m^2. However, this standard serves as a general measure of the overweight and obesity situation within the population. Given the differences in gender, age, and physical fitness, individual cases of overweight and obesity must be specifically examined and analyzed. *The Chinese Recommendations for Adult Obesity and Overweight Prevention and Control* proposed a more suitable assessment standard for overweight and obesity in the Chinese population. According to this standard, a BMI of 18.5-23.9 kg/m^2 is considered normal weight, 24-27.9 kg/m^2 is classified as overweight, and greater than 28 kg/m^2 is categorized as obesity (China Obesity Working Group 2004).

Some studies have also used waist circumference (WC), waist-to-hip ratio (WHR, waist/hip circumference), and waist-to-height ratio (WHtR, waist/height) as assessment indicators of obesity. The specific criteria are as follows: (1) WC: male >90 cm, female >85 cm for abdominal obesity; (2) WHR: male ≥ 0.9, female ≥ 0.8 as abdominal obesity; and (3) WHtR: male or female ≥ 0.5 is considered abdominal obesity (Li 2021).

3 MEDITERRANEAN DIET

MD emphasizes a diverse selection of raw food ingredients, simplifying cooking methods, and minimizing the use of additives, with the aim of enabling people to consume a full spectrum of essential nutrients while preserving the natural flavors and nutritional value of the food. It also promotes moderation in the use of oil, salt, and sugar.

3.1 *Origin and dietary characteristics of Mediterranean diet*

MD, also known as the Cretan diet, originated in the 1940s and 1950s as a traditional diet in countries and regions around the Mediterranean, including Spain, southern Italy, and Greece. The diet guideline limits the consumption of red meat and sweets; recommends a moderate intake of poultry, dairy products, and eggs; encourages twice-weekly consumption of marine products; encourages consuming fresh fruits, vegetables, beans, and an appropriate amount of nuts every day, choosing whole grains and whole wheat for staple food as much as possible, and trying to choose vegetable oils (e.g., olive oil, rapeseed oil) instead of animal oils (e.g., lard, butter); advises drinking plenty of water and, if the doctor allows, a small amount of red wine with dinner.

3.2 *Role of Mediterranean diet in overweight and obesity*

3.2.1 *Optimize fat structure*

Overweight and obesity are often accompanied by fat accumulation and metabolic abnormalities, which can induce serious metabolic diseases, such as alcohol-unrelated fatty liver disease and atherosclerosis (Cui and Lv 2019). A review of the distribution of adipose tissue, inflammation, and its metabolic effects in the United States showed that the development of obesity arises due to the hypertrophy of dysfunctional adipose tissue, which produces an excess of preadipocytes that act as compensatory protectors against adverse metabolisms such as obesity and lead to the accumulation of fat in the ectopic sites of the liver, skeletal muscle, and pancreatic cells. The distribution of these fat accumulations is a significant factor in the emergence of overweight, obesity, and associated metabolic problems; it may also increase the risk of cardiovascular diseases (Chait and Hartigh 2020).

A cross-sectional clinical study in China investigated the relationship between eating habits, non-alcoholic fatty liver disease (NAFLD), and overweight and obesity in a rural provincial setting of Liaoning with 3308 participants. The results showed that the prevalence of NAFLD in the total sample was 39.9%. The prevalence of obesity in the study subjects was close to 50% when using BMI as the criterion, with a statistically significant correlation between obesity and NAFLD ($p<0.001$), regardless of whether BMI, WC, WHR, or WHtR was used as the evaluation index (Li 2021).

In the MD model, fat accounts for only 25%–35% of total energy intake, with 7%–8% coming from saturated fatty acid intake, primarily through the consumption of red meat and desserts. The remainder is provided by unsaturated fatty acids, with olive oil being a key source of monounsaturated and polyunsaturated fatty acids, mainly used to replace standard cooking oils, which is the central aspect of MD. In addition, foods rich in omega-3 and omega-6 polyunsaturated fatty acids, such as white meat, fish oil, seafood, and nuts, can significantly lower blood lipid and cholesterol levels and raise high-density lipoprotein levels (Pan and Li 2022). Therefore, MD, with its high-quality fat sources, has been shown to prevent and improve the occurrence of hypertension, NAFLD, and a variety of metabolic disorders.

3.2.2 *Control blood glucose*

The Chinese Guidelines for Medical Nutrition Therapy of Overweight/Obesity (2021) point out that both short-term low-carbohydrate and low glycemic index diets are beneficial for weight control and metabolic improvement. A randomized controlled trial divided 40 overweight young adults (average age: 26.4 years, BMI: 29.4 kg/m^2) equally into two groups to investigate the impact of dietary changes on food intake, body composition, and specific metabolic markers using real-time continuous glucose monitoring (rtCGM), low-glycemic index (GI), and glycemic load (GL) diets. The intervention group used the rtCGM system, enabling participants to monitor their blood sugar levels through instruments for 14 hours a day and adjust their dietary habits accordingly, whereas the control group did not use the rtCGM network. Both groups received nutritional guidance and information concerning low-GI and GL foods (Chekima *et al.* 2022).

The findings revealed a significant decrease in the total calorie consumption (average deviation: -3.6%, $p = 0.03$) and consumption of carbohydrates (average deviation: -15.2 g, $p = 0.04$) decreased obviously in the intervention group, which was significantly different from that of the control group; fasting blood glucose significantly decreased over time in the intervention group (mean change: 0.3 mmol/L), but was not significant in the control group; subjects in the two groups displayed significant decreases in their weight, BMI, and amounts of fat following the intervention; nevertheless, the intervention group's decreases were more apparent (Chekima *et al.* 2022). *The Chinese Expert Consensus for the Mitigation of Type 2 Diabetes published in 2021* states that obesity is strongly associated with type 2 diabetes mellitus (T2DM), with the prevalence of T2DM increasing with an increase in BMI. The prevalence of T2DM in obese individuals is three times higher than in those with normal body mass (Zou *et al.* 2021). A randomized trial in the UK found that for every 10% reduction in carbohydrate content as a proportion of total energy intake, 52 kcal/d more energy was expended. Compared to the high-carbohydrate diet group, stomach hunger hormone and levels of leptin were considerably lower in the low-carbohydrate diet group, suggesting that low-carbohydrate diets may increase energy expenditure, which may improve the success of obesity treatment (Ebbeling *et al.* 2018). Collectively these trials suggest that carbohydrate intake may be related to blood glucose levels and overweight and obesity.

MD promotes daily consumption of whole grains or whole wheat foods, most of which have a low glycemic index, making them less likely to cause significant fluctuations in blood sugar. By minimizing sugar intake while ensuring a well-rounded nutrient intake, the diet helps reduce hunger and appetite, promotes fat burning for energy, and ultimately supports achieving weight loss.

3.2.3 *Improve intestinal flora*

Intestinal flora, together with other tissues and organs in the human body, constitute a dynamic and balanced ecosystem, which jointly maintains the life activities and health of the organism. Intestinal flora is closely linked to digestion, absorption, and neuroimmune functions of the body, variations of which lead to the occurrence of several diseases. About two-thirds of the intestinal bacteria in adult intestinal flora belong to *Bacteroides* and *Firmicutes*, and about 15% to *Proteobacteria* and *Actinobacteria*. The intestinal flora is further categorized into probiotic, neutral bacteria, and pathogenic bacteria (Pan *et al.* 2021). Studies have shown that compared with the traditional Western diet, subjects taking MD have an increased abundance of enterobacteria, such as *Lachnoclostridium* and *Parabacteroides*, and produce more short-chain fatty acids (SCFA) and anti-inflammatory factors, which enhance insulin sensitivity, decrease inflammation, and support a healthy energy balance (Beam *et al.* 2021).

Chambers *et al.* (2015) used a randomized controlled trial in which 60 subjects were randomly assigned to the addition of 10 g of inulin-propionate ester test group and 10 g of inulin control group for a 24-week dietary supplementation study with compliance monitoring carried out every eight weeks. The results indicated that after 24 weeks, the test group lost more weight, but there was no statistically significant difference between the two groups in this regard (test group weight loss of 1.02 kg versus control group weight gain of 0.38 kg, $p = 0.099$). However, changes in intra-abdominal fatty tissue allocation were considerably less in the test group than in the control group ($p = 0.027$).

A systematic review included 72 animal studies and 15 clinical trials exploring the effects of probiotic supplementation on various aspects in overweight and obese hosts, with close to 85% of the animal studies demonstrating that probiotic supplementation reduces body weight gain and fat accumulation, and 8 of 9 clinical trials of probiotic supplementation given to obese adults showing that the effects of probiotics in reducing body weight, fat mass, and waist circumference were statistically significant (Ejtahed *et al.* 2019).

MD advocates a dietary pattern of high dietary fiber and recommends the consumption of whole grains and a rich variety of fruits and vegetables, which can promote the ecological balance and metabolism of human intestinal probiotic flora, regulate the health of the intestinal tract, reduce blood cholesterol and triglycerides, and ultimately achieve weight control.

3.2.4 *Supplement-deficient micronutrients*

Micronutrient deficiency is prevalent in the overweight and obese population before weight loss, and those with long-term illnesses, including T2DM and heart problems, are more likely to experience micronutrient deficiency. Multiple investigations have demonstrated that the significant dilution of fat, serum, liver, and muscle volume in obese individuals is likely a key reason for a higher incidence of vitamin D insufficiency in this population. However, there may still be other factors that cannot be excluded (Vranić *et al.* 2019). A diet high in fatty foods can lead to a deficiency of many vitamins, including folate, vitamin A, and vitamin C, as well as a decrease in the levels of fat-soluble vitamins. Continuous use of sugary drinks instead of milk and water can also result in inadequate absorption of calcium and vitamin D (Liu and Zheng 2022).

Some micronutrients, such as calcium and vitamin D, have also been shown to have a positive correlation between their supplementation and weight loss. A review included 17 randomized controlled trials, in which calcium supplementation resulted in fat loss ranging from 1 to 3.5 kg during caloric restriction in 5 trials, while the other 9 trials did not demonstrate any change (±0.7 kg) (Soares *et al.* 2011).

It has also been demonstrated that obese people who decreased their daily energy intake by 500–750 kcal and supplemented 1000 IU of vitamin D for one year lost 10% of their body weight, whereas there was no change in body weight in the control group who did not undergo the dietary intervention and exercise (Slusher *et al.* 2015). Furthermore, overweight and obese individuals who drank three servings of regular orange juice containing 100 IU of vitamin D_3 (110 kcal/serving) or low-calorie orange juice (50 kcal/serving), combined with a 500 kcal dietary restriction and walking exercise three days per week, had a 9% and 16% reduction in visceral adipose tissue (VAT), respectively, compared to control subjects who received unfortified orange juice, which showed only 4% and 5% reductions in VAT, respectively. It suggested that vitamin D_3 supplementation can help reduce VAT (Slusher *et al.* 2015).

MD recommends moderate consumption of nuts, fruits, vegetables, and dairy products, which are rich in vitamins and micronutrients that can affect overweight and obesity in different forms, for example, vitamin A is an important growth regulator of adipose tissue, vitamin A and B are involved in fat energy metabolism; calcium can limit the secretion of parathyroid glands; and zinc can regulate hormone secretion to affect the metabolism of adipose tissue. Moreover, a balanced intake of micronutrients is also necessary during and after weight loss to avoid micronutrient deficiencies or weight rebound brought by restrictive diets.

3.2.5 *Others*

MD recommends drinking more water, with 1.5–2L per person per day considered appropriate. Drinking water has the benefits of aiding digestion, promoting intestinal health, boosting metabolism, and circulating tissue fluids, which helps to prevent many diseases.

If your doctor allows it, drink a moderate amount of red wine with dinner. Red wine contains a large number of antioxidants, such as phenolics, tannic acid, flavonoids, and a variety of trace elements, which can eliminate or combat oxygen free radicals that help in anti-aging and disease prevention.

Proper physical activities can decrease the possibility of heart disease and prevent metabolic diseases such as obesity, diabetes, and hyperlipidemia. It can also help maintain healthy physiology, boost immunity, and energize.

4 MD COMBINED EXERCISE THERAPY INTERVENTION FOR FEMALE DISEASES

At present, the prevalence of overweight and obese patients has become common, the causes are complex, and the mechanism of disease has yet to be clarified. It is easy to rebound after weight loss. Women who are in the childbearing age, menopause, or other special stages, overweight and obesity have a certain degree of damage to their physical and mental health. Therefore, it is difficult to prevent its occurrence by a single activity only and requires a joint multidisciplinary intervention and lifelong management (Lu *et al.* 2020).

4.1 *PCOS of childbearing age*

The incidence of polycystic ovary syndrome (PCOS) is 6%~10% in women of childbearing age and pregnancy due to hormonal changes in the body, which may cause endocrine disorders, usually accompanied by hirsutism, irregular menstruation, infertility, or other symptoms. Additionally, persons with PCOS who are overweight and obese have an increased risk of developing T2DM, coronary artery disease, and uncommon uterine ovarian lesions (Xu *et al.* 2017). Currently, studies at home and abroad have shown that diet is associated with the occurrence of PCOS. MD, ketogenic diet, dietary approaches to stop hypertension, and low-GI diet can improve the prevalence of PCOS to varying degrees, whereas high-fat diet affects the ovarian function and the normal expression of ovulation genes, promoting the occurrence and development of PCOS (Li *et al.* 2022).

A Chinese clinical study included 64 obese PCOS patients to observe the changes in their body weight, BMI, and quality of life as measured by the PCOS patient quality of life questionnaire before and after a 4-, 8-, and 12-week intervention combining the MD with walking exercise (Xu *et al.* 2018). The study divided the samples into a test group and a control group (32 cases in each group) according to the randomized number method. Both groups received pharmaceutical treatment, with the test group receiving MD paired with walking exercise therapy as a foundation; it was also instructed and followed up to improve the adherence of the test group patients and to maintain their optimistic attitudes, while the control group was treated with a normal diet and exercise other than walking without any special instruction. After 12 weeks of intervention, the average weight of subjects in the test group decreased from 75.39 kg to 66.42 kg, while BMI decreased from 28.10 to 24.73, and the PCOS score increased from 19.35 to 29.35, all of which had a statistical significance of $P<0.05$ (Xu *et al.* 2018). Although the average weight of the control group decreased by about 2 kg, it was still statistically significant ($P<0.05$) compared with the test group (Xu *et al.* 2018). The conclusion shows that MD combined with walking exercise can improve the weight, endocrine, and metabolic disorders of PCOS patients.

4.2 *Obesity during menopause*

During menopause, estrogen levels in Chinese women decline, and ovarian function deteriorates, which not only causes physiological symptoms such as hot flashes, heart palpitations, and back pain, but also significant emotional fluctuations, including irritability, depression, and memory loss. Endocrine disorders and unhealthy lifestyles contribute to the rising prevalence of overweight, obesity, and T2DM in menopausal women. In the early stages, hyperinsulinemia may be an important cause and predictor of these diseases (Janssen 2021).

To further explore how diet combined with exercise affects obese menopausal women, particularly its influence on plasma insulin, a clinical study randomly and equally divided 48 obese menopausal women into a study group and a control group for a three-month observation period. Both groups received the same conventional medication and health education, but the study group additionally received dietary intervention (similar to MD) and exercise guidance (6-8h of aerobic exercise daily, such as swimming, running, and jogging, with exercise intensity adjusted according to individual conditions) to the study group (Xu 2021). The post-treatment results demonstrated that dietary and exercise interventions not only reduced menopausal symptoms like fatigue and depression but also led to significant improvements in BMI (26.45 in the study group versus 29.65 in the control group), lipid indices (unit mmol/L) (triglyceride: 1.08 in the study group versus 1.45 in the control group; high-density lipoprotein: 1.66 in the study group versus 1.32 in the control group; total cholesterol: 4.21 in the study group versus 4.88 in the control group), plasma insulin (unit Uu/ml) (17.05 in the study group versus 21.16 in the control group) showed a significant differences ($p < 0.05$). The study group's indexes greatly outperformed those of the control group (Xu 2021). This indicates that exercise and dietary interventions can effectively address obesity, improve lipid and insulin indexes, and have a significant therapeutic impact on the physical and mental health of menopausal women, thereby enhancing the quality of life of women.

5 CONCLUSION

With its dietary focus on low sugar, low fat, and high unsaturated fatty acid intake, along with increased consumption of fruits, vegetables, nuts, dairy products, and aquatic foods,

MD effectively lowers blood lipids, maintains stable blood glucose levels, and regulates intestinal health. By regulating lipid metabolism, lowering blood glucose concentration, and promoting the ecological balance of the intestinal flora, MD helps prevent fat accumulation, optimizes fat composition, and helps overweight and obese patients to control their body weight while forming healthy eating habits. Furthermore, since overweight and obesity are closely linked to many chronic diseases, particularly those affecting women, their treatment and prevention require long-term multidisciplinary intervention. The combination of MD and scientifically guided exercise has shown significant benefits in treating certain female health issues, helping to regulate hormones and improve overall quality of life.

In conclusion, while MD has proven effective in addressing overweight and obesity in adults, current research on its specific impact on various populations and its integration with other treatment approaches for chronic diseases remains limited. Studies often have small sample sizes and narrow scopes. Expanding sample sizes, increasing the number of clinical studies, and enhancing the value of the evidence base are necessary to further support MD's role in the diagnosis and prevention of obesity and chronic diseases in the future.

REFERENCES

Beam A., Clinger E. and Hao L. (2021). *Nutrients.* **13(8)**, 2795.

Cui L.M. and Lv N.Q. (2019). *Chin. J. Comp. Med.* **29(10)**, 22–25+111.

Chin. Prev. Med. **23(05)**, 321–339, (2022).

Chekima K., Noor M.I., Ooi Y.B.H., Yan S.W., Jaweed M. and Chekima B. (2022). *Foods*. 11(12), 1754.

Chambers E.S., Viardot A., Psichas A., Morrison D.J., Murphy K.G., Zac-Varghese S.E., MacDougall K., Preston T., Tedford C., Finlayson G.S., Blundell J.E., Bell J.D., Thomas E.L., Mt-Isa S., Ashby D., Gibson G.R., Kolida S., Dhillo W.S., Bloom S.R., Morley W., Clegg S. and Frost G. (2015). *Gut*. **64(11)**, 1744–54.

Chin. J. Front. Med. Sci. (Electron.Ed). **13(11)**, 1–55, (2021).

China obesity working group. *Acta Nutr. Sin.* **01**, 1–4, (2004).

Chait A. and den Hartigh L.J. (2020). *Front Cardiovasc Med.* **7**, 22.

Ebbeling C.B., Feldman H.A., Klein G.L., Wong J.M.W., Bielak L., Steltz S.K., Luoto P.K., Wolfe R.R., Wong W.W. and Ludwig D.S. (2018). *BMJ.* **363**, k4583.

Ejtahed H.S., Angoorani P., Soroush A.R., Atlasi R., Hasani-Ranjbar S., Mortazavian A.M. and Larijani B. (2019). *J. Funct. Foods.* **52**, 228–242.

Janssen J. (2021). *Int. J. Mol. Sci.* **22(15)**, 7797.

Li S., Cheng X.Z., Jiang X.T., Kuang H.Y. (2022). *J. Clin. Med. Pract.* **26(23)**, 113–118.

Li Y.B. (2021). *PhdThesis*, Shengyang.

Liu J. and Zheng X.L. (2022). *Chin. Gen. Pract. Nurs.* **20(03)**, 345–350.

Lu D.F., Yuan Z.F., Yang L.H., Jiang Y., Li M., Wang Y.Z., Jing L.L., Wang R.L., Zhang J.Q. and Guo X. H. (2020). *Chin. J. Diabetes.* **12(3)**, 163–168.

Pan J., Liu L.H. and Mou J.W. (2021). *J. Shandong Univ: Nat Sci.* **36(04)**, 337–365.

Pan Q. and Li Y.H. (2022). *Chin. J. Rural Med. Pharm.* **29(11)**, 72–76.

Soares M.J., Chan She Ping-Delfos W. and Ghanbari M.H. (2011). *Eur J Clin Nutr.* **65(9)**, 994–1004.

Slusher A.L., McAllister M.J. and Huang C.J. (2015). *Inflamm Res.* **64(8)**, 565–75.

State council information office of China. *Acta Nutr. Sin.* **42(06)**, 521, (2020).

Vranić L., Mikolašević I. and Milić S. (2019). *Medicina (Kaunas).* **55(9)**, 541.

Xu L., Liu H.H., Chen R.B., Li Z.Y., Song X.Y., Wang Y.Y. (2018). *J. Mod. Med. Health.* **34(21)**, 3305–3309.

Xu L., Wang H.X., Gong J.M. and Hou X.Y. (2017). *Matern. Child Health Care China.* **32(1)**, 122–124.

Xu Y.F. (2021). *J. Med. Theory Pract.* **34(07)**, 1247–1249.

Zou D.J., Zhang Z. and Ji L.N. (2021). *Chin. Gen. Pract.* **24(32)**, 4037–4048.

Biological Sciences and Environmental Health – Gao (Ed.)

Nutrition and dietary balance on growth and development of children and adolescents

Shengxue Li
Medical Department, Shenzhen University, Shenzhen City, Guangdong Province, China

ABSTRACT: From the perspective of children and adolescents, childhood is a golden period for physical and cognitive growth. Whether an adult has a healthy body, is competent in physical qualities, or maintains a stable mental state, these factors are closely related to their development during childhood and adolescence. Nutrition serves as the material basis for normal growth, development, and maturity. The concept of nutrition is broad, and it is inevitable that dietary balance must be discussed when studying nutrition. A normal diet can meet the body's calorie requirement, build up the body tissues, and maintain the proper functioning of the organs. Whereas a balanced diet goes further by combining the nutrients in appropriate proportions to better satisfy the body's needs and achieve a balance between supply and demand. Individuals can purposefully and selectively supplement specific nutrients through a rational diet.

1 INTRODUCTION

Nutrition, including vitamins, minerals, and proteins, is essential for human growth and development. A lack of nutrition will inevitably lead to imbalances in health and development, leading to various acute and chronic diseases. In 1986, British scholar Buck discovered that various cardiovascular and cerebrovascular diseases in adulthood may be linked to fetal underdevelopment in the womb. In addition, under malnutrition conditions, pregnant women may send warning signals to unborn fetuses, informing them that they are about to enter a harsh living environment. In response to these signals, the fetus adapts by lowering metabolic levels, becoming thinner and smaller in preparation for the anticipated post-birth food scarcity (Kathryn *et al.* 2022). From the perspective of children and adolescents, childhood is the golden period for physical and cognitive growth. Whether an adult has a healthy body, whether they will be able to cope with the physical demands of social life, and whether they will possess a stable state of mind are closely related to their development during childhood and adolescence. Nutrition forms the material basis for normal growth, development, and maturity.

The current generation of adolescents is growing up with unprecedented changes in the food environment, persistent nutritional problems, such as micronutrient deficiencies and food insecurity, and the rapid spread of overweight and obesity. The prevalence of childhood obesity continues to increase and may be accompanied by an increase in the incidence rate of obesity-related chronic diseases. Researchers compared the prevalence and severity of 14 chronic diseases between obese and non-obese adolescents aged 10–17, using data from the National Child Health Survey (NSCH) from 2018 to 2019. Through statistical methods such as chi-square tests and logistic regression, it was found that more than 85% of obese adolescents suffer from chronic diseases. Obese individuals are more likely to suffer from moderate-to-severe depression (Chen 2021). Despite these concerns, adolescence has been

DOI: 10.1201/9781003587590-17

largely neglected in nutritional research compared to other age groups, impeding the development of nutritional policies targeting adolescents (Sunaina and Pulkit 2021).

Between the ages of 12 or 13 and 17 or 18, individuals experience a leap in growth and development. During this period, brain development accelerates, endocrine activity becomes more pronounced, and metabolism is vigorous. Adolescents are typically energetic, lively, and active, with significant growth in large and small muscle groups, tissues, and organs leading to rapid physical changes. According to some data, between the ages of 12 and 18, the average weight increases by about 20 to 30 kg, and the average height increases by about 28 to 30 centimeters, with some individuals exceeding these averages. To support this rapid growth and ensure overall health, the supply of essential nutrients must be sufficient and well-balanced to promote healthy development and growth.

The impact of malnutrition on the human body is enormous. For instance, in the development of the nervous system of a child, a deficiency in certain key nutrients can lead to irreversible effects on the development of the brain, the proper formation of peripheral nerves, and the sensory sensitivity of the child. However, nutrition cannot be discussed in isolation. The concept of nutrition is broad, and when studying nutrition, the issue of dietary balance must inevitably be addressed. A normal diet can meet the body's caloric needs, support tissue growth, and maintain the normal functioning of organs. A well-balanced diet, however, goes a step further by ensuring that the nutrients are combined in the correct proportions to better meet the body's requirements, achieving a balance between supply and demand. This paper emphasizes the importance of achieving purposeful and selective supplementation of specific nutrients through a rational diet.

2 IMPACT OF NUTRITION AND DIETARY BALANCE ON THE NERVOUS SYSTEM

Nutrition and dietary balance play a crucial role in the development and function of the nervous system in children and adolescents. Adequate nutritional intake and a balanced diet provide essential nutrients that promote the growth and development of nerve cells while also supporting the normal function and overall health of the nervous system.

2.1 *Role of nutrients*

Key nutrients such as proteins, carbohydrates, and fats are essential for the normal growth and development of nerve cells. Protein is the main component of nerve cells, and an adequate supply of protein ensures the normal functioning and transmission of nerve cells. Carbohydrates serve as the primary source of energy for the brain, and an adequate intake helps meet the brain's energy demands to maintain its normal functions. Fats, on the other hand, are important components of the nervous system, especially brain fats that increase the speed and stability of transmission between neurons.

Vitamins and minerals are vital for the development of the nervous system in children and adolescents. Vitamins such as vitamin B-complex, vitamin C, and vitamin E support neuronal growth and differentiation while also helping maintain the normal function of the nervous system. Minerals such as iron, zinc, and calcium are key elements for the proper functioning of nerve cells; deficiencies in these minerals can lead to impaired nerve cell function. Additionally, omega-3 polyunsaturated fatty acids play a significant role in promoting the health and function of the nervous system.

In addition, dietary antioxidants play an important role in protecting the health of the nervous system in children and adolescents. Antioxidants help neutralize free radicals in the body and reduce the damage to nerve cells caused by oxidative stress, thus protecting the normal function of the nervous system.

2.1.1 *Supplementation and dietary preparation*

To ensure adequate vitamin intake, people should consume a variety of nutrient-rich foods. Carrots, sweet potatoes, green leafy vegetables, grains, meat, and a variety of fruits, as well as fish, egg yolks, and vegetable oils, are excellent sources of essential vitamins. For instance, citrus fruits, strawberries, and blueberries are a rich source of vitamin C; vegetable oils are a source of vitamin K; and fish is a source of vitamin D. Eating plenty of red meat, beans, nuts, and dairy products not only provides high-quality protein but also a variety of essential minerals such as calcium, magnesium, zinc, and iron. To supplement omega-3 polyunsaturated fatty acids, including alpha-linolenic acid, EPA, and DHA, it's important to include fish such as salmon, trout, and tuna in the diet, as well as plant-based sources such as flaxseed, flax oil, and walnuts. In China, the saying "eating more walnuts helps the brain" holds some truth, as walnuts indeed have brain-boosting properties.

Therefore, it is crucial to maintain a balanced nutritional profile at every meal. Meals should include staple foods rich in protein, such as red meat, eggs, or dairy products, alongside nutrient-dense green leafy vegetables, especially spinach. A well-rounded diet should also incorporate fruits, nuts, fish, and seafood between meals while ensuring moderation to avoid excess.

2.1.2 *Dangers of nutritional deficiency and dietary imbalance on neurodevelopment*

Poor dietary habits and malnutrition may negatively affect the nervous systems of children and adolescents. A lack of essential nutrients and unbalanced diets may hinder the growth and development of nerve cells, which in turn may affect the normal functioning of the nervous system. For instance, deficiencies in nutrients such as vitamin B complex and fatty acids can lead to poor development and abnormal functioning of the nervous system. Research has found that children aged 5 to 11 who have previously suffered from malnutrition have IQ scores 50% to 90% lower than children with sufficient nutrition supply. In addition, diets high in sugar and fat may cause obesity and metabolic syndrome, which in turn may adversely affect the health of the nervous system in children and adolescents. Additionally, iodine makes it necessary for the production of thyroid triiodothyronine (T3) and thyroxine (T4), both of which are essential for brain growth and development. Iodine deficiency during developmental stages can disrupt the functioning of the developing organism and impair nervous system excitability (Janet *et al.* 2004).

Therefore, to support the development and function of the nervous system and other aspects (such as the endocrine system) in children and adolescents, it is important to encourage the adoption of good dietary habits and a nutritionally balanced diet. This includes increasing the intake of proteins, carbohydrates, and fats, ensuring an adequate supply of vitamins and minerals, while reducing the intake of high-sugar diets and high-fat diets. By maintaining proper dietary nutrition and dietary balance, children and adolescents can be provided with essential nutrients to promote healthy neurological development and function.

3 IMPACT OF NUTRITION AND DIETARY BALANCE ON ENDOCRINE SYSTEM

3.1 *Impact of nutrition on endocrine system of adolescents and children*

In most developed countries, as well as economically advanced nations like China, obesity is the most common manifestation of how improper diet affects the endocrine system of adolescents. The incidence of overweight and obesity among adolescents in China has been steadily rising. According to experts at a press conference held by the National Health and Wellness Commission on July 13, 2021, nearly 20% of children and adolescents aged 6–17 years in China are overweight or obese. Obesity is a risk factor for many chronic diseases, including diabetes mellitus, hypertension, coronary heart disease, and malignant tumors. However, abnormal weight gain during the adolescent stage often goes unnoticed by parents due to the lack of obvious clinical symptoms.

Metabolic abnormalities in the adolescent stage mainly include dyslipidemia, hyperuricemia, and hypertension. In some obese adolescents, early glucose metabolism disorders, such as reduced glucose tolerance with insulin resistance, can be detected by OGTT (oral glucose tolerance test). As the body functions of adolescents are in the stage of growth and development, they have good compensatory mechanisms. As a result, even when relevant indexes are abnormal, they are often overlooked due to the lack of clear clinical symptoms (Sun 2022).

If overweight and obesity are caused by improper diet, their effects on the endocrine system of children and adolescents differ by gender. In boys, the predominant issue is genital dysplasia, manifesting as a shortened penis, partly accompanied by abnormal development of mammary glands. In girls, early menarche – commonly referred to as precocious puberty– is frequently observed, often accompanied by menstrual cycle disorders. As obesity progresses, polycystic ovary syndrome (PCOS) may develop. PCOS is a prevalent endocrine disorder characterized by symptoms such as menstrual irregularities, hirsutism, immature follicles, low estrogen levels, and high androgen levels, often accompanied by high blood sugar and abnormal insulin levels. In adolescent girls, PCOS frequently manifests as hirsutism, underdevelopment of secondary sexual characteristics, menstrual disorders, and even infertility. It is very common in adolescent girls. The disease is difficult to cure, mainly by drug treatment and dietary attention (Alesi *et al.* 2022). In addition, overweight girls tend to grow faster in height early on, but they are also prone to premature epiphyseal closure, which affects their final height. Treatment is challenging, relying primarily on medications and dietary management. Additionally, overweight girls may initially experience rapid height growth but are prone to premature epiphyseal closure, potentially limiting their final height. Therefore, it is important for children and adolescents to maintain a healthy body weight and intervene in the early stages of being overweight to prevent long-term complications.

3.2 *Nutrients and dietary combinations*

3.2.1 *Eating balanced meals of coarse and fine staple foods and adequate protein intake*

It is recommended to include coarse grains in each meal, as refined carbohydrates are absorbed quickly and tend to cause spikes in blood glucose and insulin levels. Consuming more coarse grains can slow down the rise of blood glucose and increase the intake of dietary fiber. Adequate protein intake is key to achieving dietary control; protein digestion and absorption take more time and energy than that of carbohydrates. Ensuring sufficient protein at every meal can slow down the overall absorption of food, preventing glucose and insulin peaks from a single intake of staple foods, and increasing satiety, which is more effective in achieving the goal of dietary control. For instance, breakfast can be accompanied by eggs and dairy, and lunch and dinner can be accompanied by meat, fish, and tofu dishes (Poutanen *et al.* 2022).

3.2.2 *Eating less, avoiding snacks, and staying away from sugary drinks*

With the rise in living standards, snacks have become more abundant, particularly refined high-carbohydrate and high-fat foods, which can easily lead to excessive energy and carbohydrate intake. The additives in snacks can also burden the health of adolescents and children, and many additive ingredients are difficult to metabolize. Beverages are especially popular among adolescents, but the sugar content in them is excessively high. Milk tea and coffee drinks, favorites among young people, are often consumed in uncontrolled amounts, which is concerning. It may cause diabetes and increase the risk of endocrine disruption (Sun 2022).

4 IMPACT OF NUTRITION AND DIETARY BALANCE ON LOCOMOTOR SYSTEM

Food nutrition and dietary balance significantly impact the physical health and motor system development of children and adolescents. Recent physical health monitoring among adolescents has shown that physical indicators such as endurance, strength, and speed continue to decline, and the rate of visual impairment remains high. The proportion of overweight and obese adolescents among urban residents has significantly increased, and the nutritional status of some rural adolescents urgently needs improvement. If these issues are not effectively addressed, they will seriously affect the healthy growth of adolescents and even affect the future of the country and nation. Children and adolescents are in a period of growth and development, and their bodies need sufficient nutrients to support the development and function of the motor system, including key nutrients such as calcium, vitamin D, and protein (Sun 2017).

4.1 *Bone development: Calcium and vitamin D*

Childhood and adolescence are critical periods for bone development, and calcium and vitamin D are key nutrients for bone health. Adequate calcium and vitamin D intake contribute to normal bone development and strength and reduces the risk of fractures. Calcium-rich foods include dairy products, tofu, and nuts, while vitamin D is primarily obtained from exposure to sunlight and certain foods such as fish and egg yolks. A study involving 100 children (from January 2019 to April 2020) used single- and double-number randomization method for grouping. The control group received regular clinical routine guidance intervention, while the experimental group also received vitamin D intervention. The results of the intervention of the children in the two groups were analyzed, which showed that the experimental group had significantly higher levels of 25-(OH)D3 after the intervention compared to the control group ($P<0.05$). Additionally, the experimental group exhibited improved bone metabolism indexes. This indicates that vitamin D intervention plays a crucial role in promoting children's growth and development, enhancing bone age and growth rate (Wang 2021).

4.2 *Protein for muscle development*

Protein is essential for muscle development and repair. Children and adolescents require sufficient protein to support their active lifestyles and athletic training. Rich sources of protein include meat, fish, poultry, pulses, dairy products, and nuts.

4.3 *Fat for joints and nerves*

A proper amount of healthy fats is also vital for the health of the locomotor system. Fats play a crucial role in maintaining joint lubrication and nerve conduction. Consuming foods rich in healthy fats, such as olive oil, fish, nuts, and seeds, can be beneficial to children and adolescents in terms of athletic performance and physical function.

According to current known theories, adipocyte transdifferentiation is an important regulatory mechanism for regulating adolescent sexual development and bone growth. By regulating white fat browning and Runx2 expression through PPARY, it can effectively stimulate hypothalamic GnRH to stimulate HPGA initiating development and influencing bone growth during adolescence. This aligns with modern research on "fat hypothalamic gonadal axis" and "pituitary bone axis" (Juan and Liu 2022).

4.4 *Other vitamins and minerals*

In addition to calcium and vitamin D, other vitamins and minerals are essential for the health of the locomotor system in children and adolescents. For instance, vitamin C contributes to the formation of collagen, which is beneficial for joint health, while vitamin E and zinc are important components for maintaining muscle and nerve function.

In summary, dietary balance and nutrient intake in children and adolescents are critical to the development and function of the locomotor system. A varied and balanced diet rich in proteins, carbohydrates, fats, vitamins, and minerals supports their athletic performance, promotes bone and muscle development, and maintains joint and nerve health.

5 ANALYSIS OF DIETARY GUIDELINES FOR CHILDREN AND ADOLESCENTS

Dietary guidelines are important policy tools for promoting optimal dietary patterns and healthy eating behaviors. Food education and nutritional literacy should be an integral part of quality education because all the nutrition people need comes from a variety of foods. Nutrition not only meets the requirement for growth and development of the body but it is also required for the development of the intellect. Insufficient or unreasonable nutrition in early life can directly affect adult health.

The Dietary Guidelines for Chinese School-Age Children (2022) highlight the following:

(i) Eating a good breakfast, choosing snacks reasonably, and cultivating healthy eating behaviors: While few primary and secondary school students skip breakfast, a closer examination reveals that nearly half do not consume a nutritionally adequate meal.
(ii) Drinking milk every day, keeping hydrated, avoiding sugary drinks, and prohibiting alcohol: Sugary beverages pose a significant problem in the diet of teenagers. The consumption of sugary drinks has risen among children and adolescents in recent years, with extensive evidence linking high added sugar intake to dental caries and increased risk of overweight and obesity. The World Health Organization also recommends limiting the intake of added sugars.
(iii) Regular monitoring of physical development to maintain appropriate weight growth: Whether it is malnutrition, micronutrient deficiencies, or overweight and obesity, the underlying issue often lies in unreasonable dietary practices. Overweight and obesity stem from too much energy intake, untimely consumption of food, and imbalanced nutrient intake. In some cases, obese children may not be overnourished; sometimes it is not overnutrition, but simply overenergized, leading to potential micronutrient deficiencies (Ma 2022).

The Greek 2014 National Dietary Guidelines for Infants, Children, and Adolescents (NDGGr) include food-based recommendations, food education, and health promotion information on (i) fruits; (ii) vegetables; (iii) milk and milk products; (iv) cereals; (v) red and white meats; (vi) fish and seafood; (vii) eggs; (viii) pulses; (ix) added lipids, olives, and nuts; and (x) added fats, olives, and nuts. (x) added sugars and salt; (xi) water and beverages; and (xii) physical activity. As a policy tool to promote healthy eating, the NDGGr has been disseminated in public schools throughout Greece (Kastorini *et al.* 2019). Various dietary guidelines for children and adolescents have been developed worldwide, all of which can be used as references.

6 CONCLUSION

Teenagers are the future of a nation, and it is of great significance to nurture the physical fitness and health of teenagers. The phenomenon of unbalanced nutrition and insufficient physical exercise among adolescents has become widespread, and the incidence of overweight and obesity is on a rapid rise. This has now become a public health issue, posing a significant challenge to the physical and mental well-being of adolescents in China. Diet and nutrition play a vital role in the process of growth and development of adolescents, closely linked to their overall physical condition. However, at present, the dietary behavior of Chinese adolescents requires improvement.

In China's metropolitan areas, favorable economic conditions often lead to excessive intake of common foods, resulting in nutritional imbalances among children. Parents frequently overlook reasonable dietary planning and fail to focus on the nutritional combination of meals, leading to diets high in sugar and fat. Over time, this surplus of nutrients can lead to nutritional imbalances. Some parents mistakenly believe that the more children eat, the better. More food intake is correlated with better health, leading to a cycle of indulgence. Additionally, children may develop picky eating habits, preferring foods they like while avoiding others.

Therefore, to address these issues, parents should ensure a balanced diet by thoughtfully mixing nutrients in the meal for their children. Parents should consistently include high-quality proteins, sufficient energy sources, and a variety of trace elements in the diet of teenagers and children. At the same time, various national policies should also emphasize the importance of nutrition and even implement regulations to require schools and social venues to strengthen the nutritional protection of young people and children. Such efforts will contribute to the continuous improvement of the overall quality of the population in the future.

REFERENCES

Alesi S., Ee C., Moran L.J., Rao V., Mousa A. (2022). *Adv Nutr. Aug* 1; **13(4),** 1243–1266.

Chen M.S. (2021). *Healthy Dietary Philosophy - Nutrition is Crucial Throughout Life*. **27 (2)**, Seal 2.

Janet B., Saskia O., Hughes D., Calvaresi E., Baghurst K. and Klinken J.V. (2004). *Nutrition Reviews*, **62(8)**, 295–306.

Juan D. and Liu LL. (2022). *Chinese Medical Journal*, **19 (27)**, 4.

Kastorini C.M., Critselis E., Zota D., Coritsidis A.L., Nagarajan M.K., Papadimitriou E., Belogianni K., Benetou V., Linos A. (2019). Greek National Dietary Guidelines Scientific Team. *Public Health Nutrition*, **22(14),** 2688–2699.

Kathryn K.E., Houtrow A. and Hall M., (2022). *Childhood Obesity*.

Ma G.S. (2022). *Chinese Food and Nutrition* **(06)**, 89.

Poutanen K. S., Kårlund A. O., Gómez-Gallego C., Johansson D. P., Scheers N. M., Marklinder I. M., Eriksen A. K., Silventoinen P. C., Nordlund E., Sozer N., Hanhineva K. J., Kolehmainen M. and Landberg R. (2022). *Nutr Rev.* May 9;**80(6)**,1648–1663.

Sun J. (2017). *Student Physical Health and Sports Physiology*.

Sun M.X. (2022). *Adolescent Health*, **20 (7),** 3.

Sunaina T. and Pulkit M. (2021). *International Journal of Adolescent Medicine and Health*, **34(6)**, 381–392.

Wang H. L. (2021). *Health Essentials* **19**, 27.

Biological Sciences and Environmental Health – Gao (Ed.)
© 2025 the Author(s), ISBN: 978-1-032-96016-6

Computational prediction of protein interactions using structural-based approaches

Zhuqin Li
Department of Biochemistry, University of Toronto, Toronto, Canada

ABSTRACT: Protein-protein interactions (PPIs) are pivotal for cellular functions, playing a fundamental role in processes ranging from signal transduction to structural support. Understanding these interactions on the molecular level is crucial for unraveling the molecular intricacies governing life's fundamental processes and for advancing fields like drug discovery. This review discusses computational methodologies designed to predict PPIs based on protein structures, offering a comprehensive survey of their principles, applications, and future directions. It introduces a repertoire of computational techniques, each addressing the challenge of deciphering protein interactions through distinct lenses. Template-based modeling, rooted in homology principles, emerges as a potent tool for predicting the tertiary structures of proteins. Docking simulations provide insights into the dynamic orientations of interacting proteins. Surface patch analysis captures intricate molecular attributes critical for interaction prediction. Conservation analysis, drawing on evolutionary cues, informs the identification of pivotal interaction sites. However, these computational methods are not without limitations. Because of the reliance they are on experimentally defined protein structures, many proteins, especially those engaged in transitory binding, are out of their grasp. Conformational shifts and the presence of intrinsically disordered proteins further challenge these methods. Nonetheless, the incorporation of machine learning and AI techniques offers promise in overcoming these limitations.

1 INTRODUCTION

Protein-protein interactions (PPIs) regulate a wide range of cellular activities, including structural support, signal transduction, mechanical mobility, and pathogen defense (Szilagyi and Zhang 2014). This intricate network of interactions, diverse and specific in nature, forms the bedrock of fundamental biological events (Szilagyi and Zhang 2014). Unraveling the dynamics of these interactions holds significance not only for decoding the mechanisms that drive cellular life but also for advancing fields such as drug discovery and therapeutic development.

Efforts to unravel the intricacies of the proteome have made remarkable progress. High-throughput screening techniques, including Yeast Two-Hybrid, Biomolecular Fluorescence Complementation, and Proximity-dependent Biotin Identification, play a pivotal role in identifying potential interaction partners (Szilagyi and Zhang 2014). However, these techniques afford insights into the "what" of interactions, leaving the "how" unresolved. The structural intricacies of protein interactions—how they interact at a molecular level—remain a fundamental question in understanding cellular processes (Szilagyi and Zhang 2014).

Individual protein structures have been revealed by structural methods like X-ray crystallography, nuclear magnetic resonance (NMR), and cryo-electron microscopy (cryo-EM). (Sunny and Jayaraj 2021; Xue *et al.* 2015). Yet, a gap persists in comprehending protein

 DOI: 10.1201/9781003587590-18

complex structures due to their transient and flexible nature, which defies traditional structural approaches (Sunny and Jayaraj 2021).

Herein arises the significance of computational approaches to predict the interactions. The two main types of computational methods are sequence-based and structure-based. The latter boasts higher accuracy owing to several advantages. Structure-based methods focus on identifying interfacial residues among surface residues, recognize spatial positions critical for macromolecular recognition, and provide geometric complementarity insight (Lee 2023). However, there is still limited studies focusing on the structure-based PPIs.

This review presents a comprehensive exploration of structure-based computational methodologies. Encompassing structural templates, docking simulations, surface patch analysis, and conservation analysis.

2 TEMPLATE-BASED METHOD

The basic concept of template-based modelling (TBM) is that homologous proteins with comparable sequences exhibit congruent structural conformations, and this principle is applied to predict the interaction interfaces. This paradigm was initially developed to predict the tertiary structure of single-chain proteins, and it has now expanded to include proteins with far-reaching homology (Szilagyi and Zhang 2014).

The TBM procedure encompasses five steps. First, identify one or multiple suitable templates. Second, align the target sequence with these templates. Third, create a preliminary target model. Four, carefully assemble the loops and termini that are missing. Lastly, the model is improved to produce an accurate prediction of the complete length of the atomic structure (Szilagyi and Zhang 2014).

This framework was expanded to include PPIs, and a template-based sophisticated modelling process was developed. This variation requires that existing structures (templates) relevant to the target sequences be identified. The process entails aligning the target sequences to the identified template, creating the structural scaffold of the target and template, and carefully injecting exact side-chain atoms into unaligned loop areas (Szilagyi and Zhang 2014).

The accuracy of a TBM prediction model is intrinsically tied to the precision of the identified template. To achieve this, TBM strategies employ three distinct methodologies for template identification: dimeric threading, monomer threading and oligomer mapping, and template-based docking (Szilagyi and Zhang 2014).

Dimeric Threading: This represents the earliest strategy, involving the alignment of both query proteins to the template protein complex with a known structure. The final model is scored based on threading alignment and interface evaluation scores (Szilagyi and Zhang 2014; Lu *et al.* 2002).

Monomer Threading and Oligomer Mapping: These strategies, involves individually threading protein chains (Chain A and Chain B) to identify the best-matched templates, ranking these templates based on alignment quality, identifying binding partners for Chain A from the templates, evaluating potential interactions by aligning the highest-scoring Chain B monomer models with Chain A's binding partner structures, then mapping the interactions between the Chain B and Chain A. (Szilagyi and Zhang 2014; Guerler *et al.* 2013).

Template-Based Docking: This approach incorporates structural alignment, recognizing commonalities between the query and template structures. It then identifies models for both monomers, aligning them with available complex structures in a library (Halperin *et al.* 2002; Szilagyi and Zhang 2014).

While TBM has revolutionized structural predictions, it is not without its limitations. The current library of complex structures is far from exhaustive, limiting the scope of proteins amenable to TBM approaches. TBM methods also face challenges in detecting distant homologous templates, particularly in the twilight-zone region where threading alignment accuracy decreases. Furthermore, TBM predictions frequently have gaps with missing residues or loops, including crucial functional regions, leaving incomplete, improved models of predicted complexes. Finally, the majority of TBM methods concentrate on predicting dimer structures, leaving the task of modeling multimolecular complexes, a prominent feature in cellular machinery, a challenge that awaits further exploration (Szilagyi and Zhang 2014).

3 DOCKING SIMULATIONS FOR INTERACTION PREDICTION

In addition to the template-based paradigm, there is also template-free method, enabling protein structure prediction without reliance on any reference. Within this realm, docking simulation stands as a noteworthy technique, specializing in predicting near-native orientations of interacting proteins (Halperin *et al.* 2002; Sunny and Jayaraj 2021).

Docking simulation's domain spans across oligomeric proteins, making it an encompassing method for various structural contexts. It can be divided into two primary categories: rigid-body docking and flexible docking, depending on the flexibility characteristics of the interacting proteins (Sunny and Jayaraj 2021). While rigid-body docking assumes that the molecules retain their structural rigidity during interaction, flexible docking acknowledges the dynamic nature of proteins, accommodating conformational changes during the interaction.

The docking process follows a general procedure comprising pose generation and scoring (Halperin *et al.* 2002; Sunny and Jayaraj 2021). In pose generation, the critical task is to enumerate potential binding poses of the interacting proteins. This phase is marked by the translation and rotation of these molecules, and it can be executed through either exhaustive or stochastic methods, depending on computational resources and objectives (Halperin *et al.* 2002; Sunny and Jayaraj 2021).

The second part, scoring, includes giving the created postures ratings based on a variety of factors. The distinctive properties of the proteins involved are critical for scoring effectiveness. There are many different docking scoring functions, and they can be categorised into groups including forcefield-based, knowledge-based, empirical, and consensus (Tsuchiya *et al.* 2022; Sunny and Jayaraj 2021).

Forcefield-based scoring encompasses intermolecular terms, such as van der Waals potential and electrostatic potential, coupled with intramolecular terms like bond angle, bond length, and dihedral angle (Sunny and Jayaraj 2021).

Empirical-based scoring functions rely on intermolecular interactions and changes in the accessible surface area of the proteins to compute scores (Sunny and Jayaraj 2021).

Knowledge-based scoring functions utilise current understanding of protein interactions to calculate statistically possible mean forces (Sunny and Jayaraj 2021).

Consensus-based scoring functions amalgamate various parameters, offering a holistic perspective on interactions (Sunny and Jayaraj 2021).

Diverse algorithms drive the computational machinery behind docking simulations:

Computational Geometric Algorithms trace a sphere over the proteins, generating surface paths fragmented into convex, concave, and flat regions. Alignment of these curved regions facilitates pose generation (Sunny and Jayaraj 2021).

Population Based Metaheuristic Algorithms harness inspiration from natural processes, working with candidate solutions. Notable examples include Genetic Algorithm, Flower Pollination Algorithm, Particle Swarm Optimization, and Glowworm Swarm Optimization (Sunny and Jayaraj 2021).

Monte Carlo (MC) algorithms introduce an element of randomness into the process, predicting probability values based on historical data. These algorithms excel in solving complex problems with deterministic methods falter (Sunny and Jayaraj 2021).

Graph-based algorithms represent data as graphs, allowing modeling of relationships between entities through vertices and edges (Sunny and Jayaraj 2021).

The future of docking simulations lies in overcoming bottlenecks, particularly in score calculation and refinement. Measures to reduce the conformational space and the inclusion of water molecules in scoring functions show promise in enhancing docking results. Combining information from diverse sources, including experimental techniques like X-ray crystallography, NMR spectroscopy, and proteomics, holds the key to addressing the flexibility challenge. As the computational landscape evolves, docking simulations continue to shape our understanding of molecular interactions, unveiling the intricate choreography of proteins in their dynamic partnerships (Sunny and Jayaraj 2021).

4 SURFACE PATCH ANALYSIS

The molecular surface analysis emerges as a potent tool to understand the protein interactions as a higher level representation (Zhu, Xiong and Kihara 2014). This representation conceptualizes proteins as continuous shapes, meticulously capturing both geometric and chemical attributes. These molecular surfaces serve as dynamic canvases imprinted with distinctive patterns of chemical and geometric features. These patterns serve as informative fingerprints, offering profound insights into a protein's interactions with other biomolecules (Gainza *et al.* 2019; Jones and Thornton 1997; Yin *et al.* 2009; Zhu, Xiong and Kihara 2014).

Distinctively, sites within proteins that orchestrate protein-protein interactions exhibit unique characteristics. Efforts have revealed that, to a discernible extent, these interaction sites can be differentiated from analogous patches on a protein's surface. It provides an insight into predicting protein-protein interaction (PPI) sites (Gainza *et al.* 2019; Jones and Thornton 1997). One notable attempt from 1997 leveraged six parameters—solvation potential, residue interface propensity, hydrophobicity, planarity, protrusion, and accessible surface area—to successfully predict PPI sites. This predictive algorithm operates in three stages: 1. Patch Evaluation for Individual Parameters. 2. Creating a Combined Score by Combining Several Parameters. 3. Picking the Best Patches (Jones and Thornton 1997).

Several algorithms were developed upon this pioneering attempt.

Three-Dimensional (3D) Zernike Descriptors: These descriptors provide a mathematical framework for capturing the shape and surface features of proteins in a manner that is invariant to their orientation, making them particularly useful for pattern recognition. These patches are characterized based on geometric shape, surface electrostatic potential, hydrophobicity, and concavity (Gainza *et al.* 2019; Jones and Thornton 1997).

Geometric Invariant Fingerprint (GIF) Descriptors: GIF descriptors encapsulate key geometric properties of protein surfaces, focusing on the distance-dependent distribution of curvatures from the center vertex. It enables the discrimination of various surface regions based on their shape characteristics. However, this technique can only effectively analyze surfaces with relatively simple topology (Gainza *et al.* 2019; Yin *et al.* 2009).

MaSIF (Molecular Surface Interaction Fingerprinting): A cutting-edge deep learning method, MaSIF revolutionizes molecular surface analysis by considering both geometric and chemical features. It divides a protein's surface into radial patches that overlap and have set geodesic radii. By putting these patches through application-specific neural network layers, MaSIF learns to incorporate the input features from these patches into numerical vector descriptors (Gainza *et al.* 2019).

The implications of molecular patch analysis extend far and wide. Molecular surface patterns identified through this analysis can empower protein design programs to optimize sequences, ensuring the display of patterns necessary for specific functional tasks. Also, this technique excels in pinpointing 'surface hot-spots'—regions of proteins that are more amenable to the design of new biologics for therapeutic applications (Gainza *et al.* 2019).

5 CONSERVATION ANALYSIS

The dynamic realm of protein-protein interactions is intricately influenced by the functional landscape of amino acid residues (Choi *et al.* 2009). This insight is corroborated by the reality that most residue mutations exert negative effects, particularly these in proximity to functional sites. Nature's evolutionary mechanisms underscore this significance, often favoring the elimination of mutations that undermine protein functionality (Choi *et al.* 2009; Vries *et al.* 2006).

Studies have illuminated a striking trend: proteins tend to exhibit greater structural conservation in their interfaces compared to the rest of their surface. This structural conservation extends to the very core of protein interactions. Intriguingly, it was observed that obligatory interfaces, critical for protein function, are significantly more conserved (at a rate of 77.18%) compared to transient interfaces (at a rate of 52.51%). Such insights into conservation patterns have transformative implications in understanding protein-protein interactions (Choi *et al.* 2009).

Incorporating conservation analysis, several prediction tools have emerged. One prominent computational tool that leverages conservation analysis is PINUP. This tool employs a scoring function that encompasses a multifaceted approach, considering side-chain energy, interface propensity, and residue conservation scores. Another influential player in the realm of conservation-guided analysis is WHISCY (Xue *et al.* 2015). This method computes a conservation score for each position within a Multiple Sequence Alignment (MSA) by aggregating evaluation from an altered Dayhoff matrix. WHISCY's calculation involves pairwise comparisons of each sequence in the MSA to a master sequence, considering the sequence distance between compared sequences (Vries *et al.* 2006; Xue *et al.* 2015). Notably, the combination of WHISCY with ProMate, an interface predictor, yields an increase in the correct prediction rates of both methods, showcasing the synergy of multiple approaches (Vries *et al.* 2006).

The utility of conservation analysis resonates across various facets of structural biology. In protein-protein docking, choosing near-native structures from the enormous pool of produced decoys is one of the main challenges. Conservation analysis can serve as a discerning filter, helping identify biologically relevant interactions amidst the noise of computational predictions. Beyond protein-protein interactions, the principles of conservation analysis extend to the domain of protein-ligand docking. By harnessing insights from structural conservation, researchers can refine and optimize protein-ligand docking results, enhancing the accuracy of drug discovery and development processes (Choi *et al.* 2009).

While conservation analysis offers profound insights, it's essential to acknowledge its limitations. Not all proteins exhibit uniformly conserved interfaces. Some proteins may have less conserved interfaces compared to the rest of their surface, reflecting the intricate nuances of molecular interactions. Also, a strong correlation exists between interface size and conservation. Proteins with smaller interfaces, particularly those under 1400 Å, may not consistently exhibit higher conservation levels than the rest of their surface (Choi *et al.* 2009).

6 CONCLUSION

In the evolving landscape of bioinformatics, computational methodologies have invigorated the study of protein-protein interactions. This review explored various approaches, revealing insights into the intricate realm of protein interactions.

Computational techniques such as docking simulations, surface patch analysis, conservation analysis, and template-based modeling have significantly enriched our comprehension of these interactions. The template-based methods, rooted in the principles of homology, have paved the way for accurate structural predictions. Docking simulations, on the other hand, have provided invaluable glimpses into the dynamic aspects of these interactions, enhancing our grasp of their spatial orientations. Surface patch analysis, by capturing the intricate attributes of molecular surfaces, has bestowed predictive capabilities of paramount importance. Conservation analysis, firmly grounded in evolutionary tenets, has elucidated critical interaction sites, transcending the confines of sequence-based methods.

Nonetheless, within the tapestry of these remarkable advancements, it must be acknowledged the constraints of structure-based predictions. While these methodologies offer invaluable revelations, their efficacy hinges on the availability of known protein structures. Countless proteins, particularly those engaged in transient binding, remain devoid of experimentally ascertained 3D configurations. The ever-present challenges of conformational shifts and the prevalence of disordered proteins compound the intricacies, curbing the scope of structure-based techniques.

Template-based methods, for instance, may struggle with incomplete libraries of known structures, particularly for multimolecular complexes. Docking simulations wrestle with the vast conformational space and are contingent upon the accuracy of scoring functions. Surface patch analysis, while offering insights into interaction sites, is limited by its effectiveness in differentiating true interaction patches from similar surface features. Conservation analysis, though insightful, may encounter proteins with less conserved interfaces.

Nonetheless, these limitations do not overshadow the immense potential of these techniques in advancing our understanding of protein interactions. Moreover, the landscape of structure-based prediction is evolving rapidly, with the infusion of machine learning and AI techniques to augment predictive accuracy. These advancements are poised to address some of the persistent challenges in the field, offering the promise of enhanced predictions and a broader application spectrum. The techniques introduced above not only hold the potential to predict protein-protein interactions but also offer avenues for exploring interactions with nucleic acids and ligands, thus extending their relevance in diverse research domains.

In conclusion, computational methods play a pivotal role in probing protein-protein interactions. Each technique uncovers unique facets of protein behavior. Moving forward, optimism must be balanced with caution to transcend current limitations. Through algorithms, structures, and evolving insights, the intricacies of protein choreography in life's symphony could be deciphered.

REFERENCES

Choi, Y. S., Yang, J.-S., Choi, Y., Ryu, S. H., and Kim, S. (2009). *Proteins: Structure, Function, and Bioinformatics*, **77**(1), 14–25.

de Vries, S. J., van Dijk, A. D. J., and Bonvin, A. M. J. J. (2006). *Proteins: Structure, Function, and Bioinformatics*, **63**(3), 479–489.

Gainza, P., Sverrisson, F., Monti, F., Rodolà, E., Boscaini, D., Bronstein, M. M., and Correia, B. E. (2019). *Nature Methods*, **17**(2), 184–192.

Guerler, A., Govindarajoo, B., and Zhang, Y. (2013). *Journal of Chemical Information and Modeling*, **53**(3), 717–725.

Halperin, I., Ma, B., Wolfson, H., and Nussinov, R. (2002). *Proteins: Structure, Function, and Genetics*, **47**(4), 409–443.

Jones, S., and Thornton, J. M. (1997). *Journal of Molecular Biology*, 272(1), 133–143.

Lee, M. (2023). *Molecules*, **28**(13), 5169.

Lu, L., Lu, H., and Skolnick, J. (2002). *Proteins: Structure, Function, and Genetics*, **49**(3), 350–364.

Sunny, S., and Jayaraj, P. B. (2021). *The Protein Journal*, **41**(1), 1–26.

Szilagyi, A., and Zhang, Y. (2014). *Current Opinion in Structural Biology*, **24**, 10–23.

Tsuchiya, Y., Yamamori, Y., and Tomii, K. (2022). *Biophysical Reviews*, **14**(6), 1341–1348.

Xue, L. C., Dobbs, D., Bonvin, A. M. J. J., and Honavar, V. (2015). *FEBS Letters*, **589**(23), 3516–3526.

Yin, S., Proctor, E. A., Lugovskoy, A. A., and Dokholyan, N. V. (2009). *Proceedings of the National Academy of Sciences*, **106**(39), 16622–16626.

Zhu, X., Xiong, Y., and Kihara, D. (2014). *Bioinformatics*, **31**(5), 707–713.

Biological Sciences and Environmental Health – Gao (Ed.)
© 2025 the Author(s), ISBN: 978-1-032-96016-6

The effects of circadian rhythm on the eye

Yangtao Du
Department of Biomedical Engineering, College of City University of Hong Kong, Hong Kong, China

ABSTRACT: Nowadays, the majority of species have circadian rhythms, which are produced by an internal biological clock with a 24-hour cycle rather than just by daily oscillations. The hypothalamus (SCN), which regulates circadian rhythms in peripheral organs in animals, serves as the primary pacemaker for circadian rhythms. The retina also has circadian clocks, which function independently of the SCN and control a variety of retinal physiologic processes. The ageing process of cone cells and the accelerated loss of cone cell structure, function, and viability are both accelerated by disruption of the retinal circadian rhythms. Melatonin has an impact on retinal cell health, hastening the ageing process and the onset of diseases like myopia in them. Dopamine is a crucial component of the retinal biological clock, which controls the circadian physiology of the retina, and it also plays a significant part in refractive development. In conclusion, melatonin and dietary restriction improve eye aging, fatigue, and myopia by affecting circadian rhythms and influencing the aging of photoreceptors in the eye.

1 INTRODUCTION

Almost all organisms on Earth have circadian rhythms. These rhythms are generated by a series of transcriptional and translational feedback loops (Takahashi 2017). Cellular metabolic functions are tightly controlled by circadian rhythms. The recent award of the 2017 Nobel Prize in Physiology or Medicine to Dr Jeffrey C. Hall, Dr Michael Rosbash and Dr Michael W. Young for the discovery of molecular mechanisms regulating circadian rhythms highlights the importance of circadian rhythms in controlling numerous body functions. The award emphasises the importance of circadian rhythms in regulating multiple body functions. Circadian rhythms play an important role in regulating multiple body functions. An important area of research is the investigation of circadian rhythms in the eye. Evidence to date suggests that dysregulation of circadian rhythms can lead to significant changes in function and health. This means that a "time-preserving system" may be effective in preventing age-related retinal-diseases.

The retinal circadian clock is the first circadian oscillator discovered in mammals. The retinal circadian clock's molecular mechanism is similar to that of circadian neurons, but apparently the retinal circadian clock is not as reliable. Some experiments show some other eyes' structures like cornea, also have circadian clocks that regulate important physiological functions. Interestingly, as in the case of the SCN, the neural retina appears to transmit optical information to other ocular structures via humoral signals. The purpose of this review is to describe the role of circadian rhythms in the control of ocular disease, aging, and longevity, as well as ways to improve circadian rhythms.

2 BACKGROUND

2.1 *Circadian rhythm*

Circadian rhythms are complex adaptations of animals to daily changes in a variety of environmental conditions (e.g., light, temperature, humidity, feeding conditions, intraspecific

 DOI: 10.1201/9781003587590-19

relationships, and natural enemies). Different organisms have distinctive circadian rhythms and can adapt to environmental conditions in complex ways. Circadian rhythms are approximately 24-hour oscillations in behaviour, cell physiology and biochemistry (Takahashi 2017). Circadian rhythms are generated by an internal clock that determines the time to pace gene transcription programmes and synchronise cellular physiology with daily environmental stresses. Circadian rhythms of activity are common in natural life; for example, most birds are particularly active during the day and are known as diurnal; other animals, such as bats and many other mammals, are active only at night and are known as nocturnal; and still others, such as flies, are active only at dawn or dusk.

Circadian rhythms in which animals alternate between activity and quiescence are often accompanied by changes in metabolic levels and changes in body temperature. In general, nocturnal animals have higher metabolic levels at night than during the day, and body temperature is slightly higher at night, while the opposite is true for diurnal animals. In addition, many physiological indicators have circadian activity rhythms, such as pulse, urine output, eosinophilic leukocytes, and adrenocorticosterone.

Based on circadian rhythms, insects can be classified as sunrise insects and nocturnal insects. Insects that are active during the day are called sunrise insects, such as butterflies, dragonflies, and step beetles; insects that are active at night are called nocturnal insects, such as most moths. Insects that are active only in low light are called low-light insects, such as mosquitoes, and they are usually active at dusk or dawn.

Since the length of day and night in nature varies with the seasons, the activity rhythms of many insects also show marked seasonality. The response of polymorphic insects to diurnal changes varies from generation to generation and is manifested in migration, mating, and reproduction.

Molecular clocks can control the production of downstream genes and help tissues to develop their own physiological rhythms (Rouyer 2015). In addition to the core pacemaker neurons that control the rhythm of muscle action, this feedback loop also affects peripheral tissues.

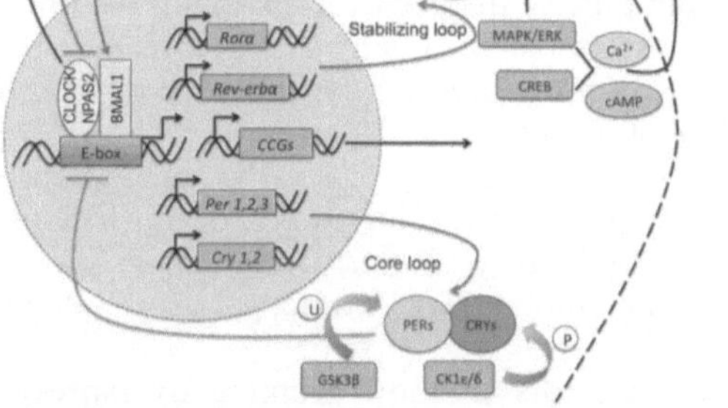

Figure 1. A series of transcriptional and translational feedback loops comprise the core molecular clock in mammals (Parekh *et al.* 2015).

Retinal ganglion cells (RGCs) process light as it travels through the eye and into the retina during the circadian rhythm of the eye, and these cells transmit all visual information. However, melanopsin, a photopigment, is present in 1-2 percent of these cells. Inner retinal photosensitive ganglion cells (ipRGCs) are the name given to this small subset of RGCs. Through the retinal hypothalamic tract, this light signal and the neurotransmitter glutamate reach the retina, where they play a role in the production of genes related to circadian functions.

The mammalian retina is approximately 200 micrometres thick. The perception of light by photoreceptor cells, cone cells and retinal ganglion cells is dependent on the retina. Unlike optic rod and cone cells, which are responsible for vision formation, ipRGCs do not form images but can interact with the SCN and other entities to influence various aspects of mammalian health. The circadian rhythm of the mammalian retina is independent of the main biological clock of the SCN. Therefore, disruption of the retinal biological clock may negatively impact ocular health.

2.2 *Melatonin*

One of the hormones secreted by the pineal gland of the brain is melatonin (MT). The chemical name for melatonin is N-acetyl-5-methoxytryptamine, commonly known as pinealotropin, melatonin, and melatonin. It is an indole heterocyclic molecule. Sympathetic stimulation will innervate the pineal cells, causing them to release melatonin after the hormone has been produced and stored in the pineal gland. Melatonin secretion has a clear circadian cycle, with night time secretion being active and daytime secretion being reduced (Martínez-Águila *et al.* 2021). Additionally, MT exhibits potent neuroendocrine immunomodulatory activity as well as free radical scavenging antioxidant capacity, suggesting that it may represent a novel strategy and method for antiviral therapy. The liver is where MT is finally metabolised, hepatocyte injury has an impact on the body's MT levels. Cellular receptors help in its action by mediating the action of melatonin. Mammalian membrane melatonin receptors for MT1 and MT2 have been described and cloned. the putative receptor for MT3 has been identified as quinone reductase 2, which has a lower melatonin affinity than MT1 and MT2 receptors.

There is a diurnal regularity to melatonin secretion. The activity of the enzyme in the pineal gland that produces melatonin rises after dusk as light stimulation falls, and the body's production of melatonin follows suit, peaking between two and three in the morning. The quality of sleep is directly influenced by melatonin levels at night. After the age of 35, the body's own melatonin secretion significantly decreased, on average by 10 to 15% every ten years, leading to sleep disorders and a variety of dysfunctions. Sleep reduction is one of the key indicators of the ageing of the human brain, as the pineal gland atrophy until calcification causes the biological clock rhythm to weaken or disappear. Therefore, adding melatonin supplements from outside the body can maintain the body's melatonin levels in a youthful state, adjust and restore the circadian rhythm, which not only improves the depth and quality of sleep but also, more importantly, the state of the body's overall functions, quality of life, and the rate of ageing.

The biggest difference with other sleeping pills is that melatonin is not addictive and has no obvious side effects. At night before going to bed orally 1∼2 tablets (containing about melatonin 1.5∼3 mg), usually twenty to thirty minutes to produce sleepiness, and the morning after dawn melatonin automatically expire, get up and do not have tired and sleepy wake up feeling.

In the human eye, MT2 receptors are more prominently expressed than MT1 receptors. The retina at the back of the eye contains melatonin receptors produced by photoreceptors. These receptors are found in the plexiform layer, ganglion cells, horizontal cells, amniocytes, rod photoreceptors, and horizontal cells.

2.3 *Dopamine and the circadian clock*

The most prevalent catecholamine neurotransmitter in the brain, which helps cells transfer impulses, is dopamine. This brain secretion delivers signals of excitement and joy and is connected to a person's eroticism and experiences. Parkinson's disease, schizophrenia, Tourette's syndrome, attention deficit hyperactivity syndrome, and the growth of pituitary tumours have all been linked to abnormalities in the control of the dopamine system.

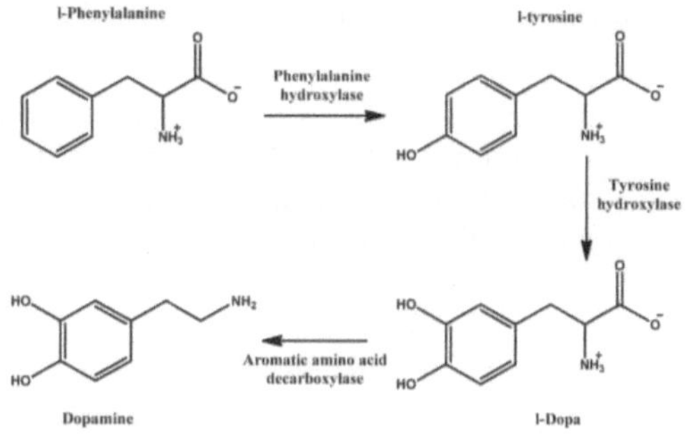

Figure 2. Dopamine synthesis pathway (Haddad *et al.* 2017).

Dopamine has -receptor agonism and some -receptor agonism. It can improve myocardial contractility, increase cardiac output, speed up heart rate with only a mild constriction of peripheral blood vessels, elevate arterial pressure, cause visceral vasodilatation, increase blood flow, and speed up glomerular filtration rate, resulting in an increase in urine volume and sodium excretion, and improve peripheral circulation. The heart rate is significantly influenced by the circadian system as well.

The circadian system also maintains adaptation to the external light-dark cycle and controls the sleep-wake cycle. Dopamine may be crucial to the circadian clock, as more and more research suggests.

Important parts of the circadian system include the retina and the SCN, both of which are involved in dopamine transmission. Dopamine is required by the retina to preserve vision and light sensitivity. Norepinephrine controls the amplitude of rhythmic clock expression and is a key regulator of circadian activity in the retina (Kim *et al.* 2017). This modulation may have an impact on the circadian clock nucleus. The rhythmic expression of the photosensitive pigment melanopsin and endogenous photoreceptor retinal ganglion cells, which are the primary photoreceptor cells responsible for light input to the circadian nucleus, are both regulated by DA via D2R. Retinal DA, a key regulator of non-visual light perception, may have an impact on how the oscillatory clock synchronises to light signals.

3 THE INFLUENCES OF CIRCADIAN RHYTHM ON THE EYE

3.1 *Myopia*

High myopia (6.00 diopters) interferes with television viewing and causes structural changes in the eye that raise the risk of diseases. Therefore, monitoring the progression of myopia during the growth phase of the eye is essential to prevent myopia from progressing to pathological myopia (Wildsoet *et al.* 2019). Weiss and Schaeffel were the first to describe the connection between chicken circadian rhythms and myopia development in 1993. They found that inducing myopia by depriving the eye of morphopia alters the axial growth cycle, in which growth remains constant during both day and night. A number of genes and clock-related neurotransmitters, such as melatonin and its receptor MT1, have since been found to be involved in the development of myopia.

In studies on animals, it was found that the presence of dopamine significantly slowed the development of myopia (Zhou *et al.* 2017). It should be remembered that the central nervous system, oscillates in opposite phases throughout the dopamine and melatonin circadian cycles. According to a recent study, myopic individuals have higher blood and saliva melatonin concentrations than mesopic individuals, although urine melatonin concentrations are lower. Like this, myopes also have reduced serum dopamine levels.

3.2 *Circadian rhythm regulation of eye lifespan under dietary restriction*

3.2.1 *Dietary restriction*

Dietary restriction (DR), which is defined as a reduction in all calories or some nutrients, is the best way to prevent disease and extend life. Given that OD increases the molecular clock's circadian transcriptional output and maintains circadian function with age, the mechanism by which OD benefits health and longevity may be intimately tied to circadian function. This is due to the fact that DR boosts circadian clock function in old age and enhances the molecular clock's circadian transcriptional output. A diet high in nutrients, on the other hand, inhibits circadian rhythms and speeds up ageing.

In this study, flies were performed to clarify the mechanisms of circadian rhythms induced in DR. A number of tests revealed that DR-fed flies had much higher expression of circadian processes in their eyes. The rhythmic expression of genes that produce proteins essential in light adaptation was especially enhanced by DR. The results suggest that CLK regulates transcription and CLK dysfunction accelerates age-related vision loss in photoreceptor cells as well as in whole neurons. A number of the ocular output genes of CLK, are likewise necessary for DR to postpone visual ageing and lengthen lifetime. Disruption of photoreceptor homeostasis also increases systemic immunological responses and shortens lifespan.

3.2.2 *CLK genes regulate eye vision, senility and longevity*

It is being investigated in several studies whether the eye's CLK-output genes affect aging-related vision deficits and lifespan. Researchers first looked at genes that displayed differential expression on DR in contrast to AL. Then, researchers looked at how the expression of a group of transcripts changed in nCLK-Δ1 fly heads (Stahl *et al.* 2017), choosing those whose DR is up-regulated with ageing. Retinene also contributes to the development of corneal nanocoatings, and its absence causes the deterioration of nanostructures and a reduction in anti-reflection properties (Kryuchkov *et al.* 2020). As a result of rhodopsin degradation in reaction to light, the sun encodes for a lysosomal tetraspanin that is mostly found in the retina and prevents photoreceptor degeneration. These results suggest a cooperative role for DR and CLK in the control of circadian genes specific to the eye that are involved in the inhibition of rhodopsin signalling and support earlier findings that lifetime extension with DR requires the presence of functional circadian clocks. (as shown in Figure 3)

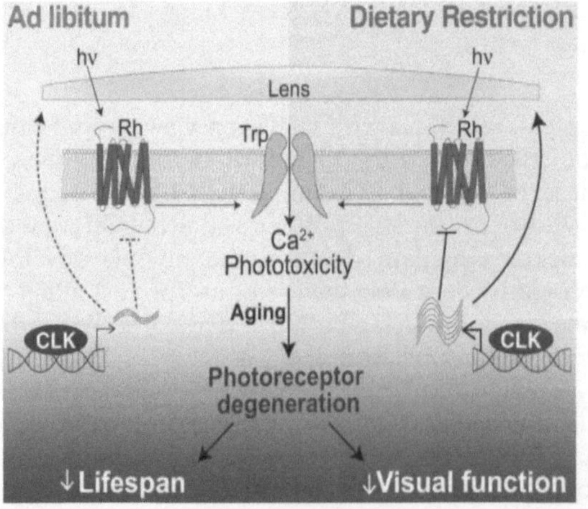

Figure 3. Dietary restriction extends lifespan by promoting rhythmic homeostatic processes in the eye (Zheng *et al.* 2020).

4 IMPROVEMENT

4.1 *Reduce the situation of myopia*

At the beginning of this century, the concept of using light to stop the development of myopia developed. The growth of the eyes in guinea pigs and chickens is reportedly greatly slowed by stimulating the retina with short-wavelength (blue) light as opposed to medium-wavelength (green) or long-wavelength (red) light, according to many authors. For the experiment, 20-day-old three-colored guinea pigs were split into four groups at random: control, defocused eyes, defocused eyes plus AA92593, and defocused eyes plus dimethyl sulphoxide (DMSO). -6.00D lenses were employed on the defocused eyes. Intravitreal administration of AA92593 increased axial length, decreased refractive index, decreased relative expression of the melanopsin protein in the retina, and increased melatonin levels in the unfocused group compared to the unfocused group, but had little to no effect on dopamine levels. These results suggest that retinal melanopsin suppresses lens myopia development in guinea pigs and that this inhibitory activity may be related to retinal melatonin (Zheng *et al.* 2020).

4.2 *Reduce eye strain and increase lifespan*

The experiment forced photoreceptor degeneration by knocking down *ATPα* in the eye and measured the expression of AMPs in the body to determine whether photoreceptor deterioration in Drosophila results in a systemic immune response. *ATPα* knockdown is used in the experiment as a model of photoreceptor ageing. Ocular *ATPα* knockdown rendered flies blind in comparison to control groups in both AL and DR conditions. As a result, DR does not reduce immune reactions when photoreceptor degeneration is triggered.

These findings provide credence to the idea that neuronal CLK function is required for the entire lifespan extension brought on by DR and show how crucial the transcription factor CLK's function in photoreceptors is for both organism survival and the preservation of visual function with ageing. According to our review, overexpressing CLK prevents age-related vision decreases whereas interrupting CLK activity in photoreceptors speeds up visual declines and shortens lifespan (Hodge *et al.* 2022).

4.3 *Limitation*

There is still much to discover about how the eye affects lifespan and whether these effects hold true for other organisms, with the most important question remaining whether these hypotheses hold true for humans. In the case of dietary restrictions, once researchers understand how photoreceptors can be used to maintain neuronal function throughout the aging process, experiments can look at targeting molecular clocks to slow aging. Once the experiments are concluded, humans could activate the biological clock within the eye to help maintain vision through diet, medication, or lifestyle (circadian rhythms) changes. How to apply these mammalian experimental data to improve human circadian rhythms, dietary restrictions related to eye aging and myopia is the next step in the experiment.

5 CONCLUSION

This review summarises the current information on the effects of circadian rhythms on the eye. Melanin and melatonin, among others, have significant effects on the eye, especially in myopia. Experiments have shown that myopia improves with reduced expression of the melatonin receptor MT1 and melatonin levels in the pineal gland. We have also identified circadian processes that are selectively enhanced in DR. The neuroprotective effect of DR on photoreceptors is mediated by the transcription factor CLK. Disruption of CLK function in photoreceptors contributes to vision loss and shortened life expectancy, whereas overexpression of CLK prevents age-related vision loss. Since CLK transcription regulates both diurnal and non-diurnal transcription, future studies should investigate whether diurnal regulation of these CLK genes is related to age-related eye health. could show whether it is associated with increased performance.

These researches could also look into whether CLK alone, as a transcription factor, mediates the advantages of DR on visual ageing and photoreceptor viability, or whether other factors, such as circadian clock function (rhythmic performance), are necessary.

REFERENCES

Haddad F., Sawalha M., Khawaja Y., Najjar A. and Karaman R. (2017). *Molecules.* **23(1)**:40.

Hodge B. A., Meyerhof G. T., Katewa S. D., Lian T., Lau C., Bar S., Leung N. Y., Li M., Li-Kroeger D., Melov S., Schilling B., Montell C. and Kapahi P. (2022). *Nat Commun.* **13(1)**:3156.

Kim J., Jang S., Choe HK., Chung S., Son GH. and Kim K. (2017). *Mol Cells.* **40(7)**:450–456.

Kryuchkov M., Bilousov O., Lehmann J., Fiebig M. and Katanaev V. L. (2020). *Nature.* **585(7825)**:383–389.

Martínez-Águila A., Martín-Gil A., Carpena-Torres C., Pastrana C. and Carracedo G. (2021). *Biomolecules.* **11(3)**:340.

Parekh P. K., Ozburn A.R. and McClung C. A. (2015). *Alcohol.* **49(4)**:341–9.

Rouyer F., (2015). Bull Acad. **199(7)**:1115–1131.

Stahl A. L., Charlton-Perkins M., Buschbeck E. K. and Cook TA. (2017). *Dev Genes Evol.* **227(4)**:271–278.

Takahashi J. S., (2017). *Nat Rev.* **18(3)**:164–179.

Wildsoet C. F., Chia A., Cho P., Guggenheim JA., Polling JR., Read S., Sankaridurg P., Saw SM., Trier K., Walline JJ., Wu PC. and Wolffsohn JS. (2019). *Invest Ophthalmol Vis Sci.* **60(3)**:M106-M131.

Zheng W., Chen Y., Zhou X.Z., Zhang X.Y., Chen Y.Y., Guan X.Y. and Mao J.F. (2020). *Optometry and Vision Science.* **97(7)**:489–495.

Zhou X., Pardue M. T., Iuvone P. M. and Qu J. (2017). *Prog Retin Eye Res.* **61**:60–71.

Chapter 3
Emerging therapeutic strategies and drug delivery

Biological Sciences and Environmental Health – Gao (Ed.)
 ISBN: 978-1-032-96016-6

Progress of application and off-target effects of CRISPR/Cas9

Tianren Shi
School of Science, Xi'an Jiaotong-Liverpool University, Suzhou, China

Zijian Zhong
Guangzhou Dublin International College of Life Sciences and Technology, South China Agricultural University, Guangzhou, China

ABSTRACT: Clustered regularly interspaced short palindromic repeats and CRISPR-associated protein 9 system (CRISPR/Cas9 system), as the third generation of gene-editing technology, develops from the immune system of archaea or some prokaryotes. Since it has advantages of high efficiency, easy design, and low cost to perform targeted gene editing, it has been widely regarded as a significant material resource, consistently leading to the development of a number of novel technologies, including safer and more precise base-editing technology based on CRISPR / Cas9 system, such as ABE and CBE. Improved CRISPR/Cas9-mediated gene editing technology has so far played a significant role in the diagnosis and treatment of illnesses, making it feasible to treat several uncommon or inherited diseases that were previously challenging to treat. For all that, the development of the CRISPR / cas9 system still faces some potential problems affecting its accuracy which is also urgent to be settled. This review systematically summarizes two base-editing techniques developed by CRISPR / cas9 and focuses on the practical utilization of CRISPR / Cas9 system in disease treatment and diagnosis. In addition, this review further discusses the problems faced by the current CRISPR / Cas9 technology and the corresponding improvement methods.

1 INTRODUCTION

Clustered regularly interspaced short pal-indromic repeats (CRISPR) is a versatile guard framework intervened by RNA in some archaea and microorganisms (Tiemin and Bo 2011). In order to protect themselves, bacteria and archaea will incorporate short fragments of unfamiliar nucleic acid into the host chromo-some toward one side of a monotonous component known as CRISPR (Zhou *et al.* 2023).

1.1 *Original process in bacteria*

A few indistinguishable rehashed DNA groupings which are isolated by exceptionally factor successions comprise the CRISPRs. These sorts of spacers begin from plasmids or either phage and keep up with the 'immunological memory' of prokaryotes. CRISPR-associated (Cas) genes encode conserved proteins, which together with CRISPRs constitute the CRISPR / Cas system and are responsible for protecting prokaryotic cells from invaders (Shuwen 2019). In prokaryotes, once a bacteriophage attacks a bacterium, its viral DNA will get into the bacteria and some of it will be injected into the bacteria genome between the repeated palindromic sequences, which will now be called spacer. Several different spacers potentially form different viruses caught in between repeated palindromic sequences

DOI: 10.1201/9781003587590-20

constitute the CRISPR array. This array will then undergo transcription to form pre-crRNA. Then the tracrRNA and protein cas9, a special kind of nucleases, will get involve into the process. tracrRNA can be complementary to the palindromic repetition, so it helps cas9 binding to crRNA. A complex of a crRNA, a tracrRNA and a cas9 protein will be formed by each spacer and the palindromic repeat attached to it. After that, the strand in between the complexes will be cut and the individual crRNA complexes are an effector complexes called surveillance complexes. When these complexes meet a section of viral DNA that has complementary base sequences, it will be paired with complementary, and a special period called PAM will be identified. Finally, the virus DNA will be cut at the PAM and loss of ability to continue transcriptional production of virus in the presence of Cas9. Thus, acting as a protection for bacteria (Wang and Doudna 2023).

1.2 *Process in genome editing*

crRNA and tracrRNA are two separate molecular entities, they can be synthesized into a single molecule called sgRNA in the laboratory to play a role in genome editing.

Scientists find the target DNA sequences which is about 20 base pairs and synthesize its complementary sequence into a sgRNA with cas9. The cas9 protein will search the PAM sites and bind by tracrRNA through base complementary pairing. When connection happens, cas9 will cleave two DNA strands by using its two domains. Ultimately, the DNA will be repaired by other nature enzymes.

2 BASE-EDITING BASED ON CRISPR/CAS9 SYSTEM

In addition to the advancements mentioned earlier, there have been further developments in CRISPR technology that have expanded its applications and improved its efficiency. With the aid of the ground-breaking technology known as base-editing, DNA sequences may be precisely edited without the need to introduce double-strand breaks (DSBs). Adenine base-editors (ABEs) and cytosine base-editors (CBEs) are the two primary categories of base-editors (Kantor *et al.* 2020).

2.1 *CBEs*

CBEs were initially created in 2016 and functioned by joining a protein called dCas9 with the cytosine deaminase enzyme APOBEC1. The fused enzyme, known as CBE1, deaminates cytosine to uracil in a targeted DNA region (Kantor *et al.* 2020). Uracil is identified as thymine during replication, causing a change from C-G to T-A. However, base excision repair (BER), a cellular repair mechanism that restores the edited base pair to its original state, limits the efficacy of CBE1 in human cells (Kantor *et al.* 2020). To overcome this limitation, subsequent generations of CBEs, such as CBE2 and CBE3, were developed. These improved versions incorporate an uracil DNA glycosylase inhibitor (UGI) or use Cas9 nickase (nCas9) to enhance editing efficiency by inhibiting the BER pathway. Further modifications and enhancements have been made to CBEs, such as the engineering of BE4-Gam and YEE-BE3, to additionally improve editing efficiency, reduce the formation of insertions and deletions, and narrow the scope of editing (Kantor *et al.* 2020). Moreover, alternative cytosine deaminase enzymes derived from various bacteria and engineered Cas9 variants have been investigated to broaden the targeting range of cytosine base editors.

2.2 *ABEs*

ABEs were developed to facilitate the transformation of adenine-thymine nucleotide pairs into guanine-cytosine nucleotide pairs within a DNA sequence. This allows for targeted editing of the genetic code. ABEs employ a Cas9 nickase (nCas9) linked to an engineered reverse transcriptase (RT) and a prime-editing guide RNA (pegRNA). The pegRNA is crucial to the prime-editing procedure as it directs nCas9 to the target sequence and functions as a template for RT to reverse-transcribe and edit the DNA (Kantor *et al.* 2020). The Escherichia coli tRNA adenosine deaminase enzyme (TadA), in an evolved form, was fused to nCas9 to produce the first-generation ABE, known as ABE1.2 (Kantor *et al.* 2020). This fusion protein enables an A-T to G-C transition by converting adenine to inosine, which is seen as guanine during DNA replication. Subsequent generations of ABEs, such as ABE7.10 and ABE8e, have been developed through protein engineering and directed evolution to enhance editing efficiency, broaden the targeting range, and improve compatibility with Cas9 homologs other than SpCas9.

Despite the capabilities of CBEs and ABEs, they are currently limited to certain types of base conversions and sequence contexts. Further optimization of the editing window size and expanding the targeting scope remains an area of active research.

To overcome this limitation, a new method called prime-editing was developed. Prime-editing utilizes an RT fused to nCas9 and a pegRNA to introduce precise edits beyond transition mutations (Kantor *et al.* 2020). The pegRNA contains the necessary sequence changes as well as complementary sequences to the target location. By instructing nCas9 to make a nick in the target DNA, the pegRNA enables reverse transcription (RT) to use the pegRNA as a template to reverse transcribe and alter the target DNA. The non-edited DNA strand is then repaired using the altered DNA strand as a template. In comparison to earlier base-editing techniques, the most recent generation of prime-editors, PE3, has shown the capacity to carry out all conceivable transition and transversion changes with high editing efficiencies and minimal off-target consequences (Kantor *et al.* 2020).

Nevertheless, since prime editing is still in its infancy, questions remain over its specificity and its unintended repercussions. More in vivo characterization is needed in order to fully use the possibilities of this technology.

3 APPLICATIONS OF CRISPR/CAS9

3.2 *CRISPR-driven cancer diagnostics*

Precision gene editing tools like CRISPR can be directed to selectively cut DNA at specific sites. This targeted cutting at repetitive DNA sequences called short tandem repeats that are found in microsatellites allows detection of cancer-linked changes. Looking for alterations in these repeated segments in tumors can help identify malignancies with high accuracy. When compared to sonication-based fragmentation, this method, known as STR-seq, exhibits greater precision and sensitiveness for microsatellite identification (Katti *et al.* 2022). Research using duplex sequencing with double-stranded DNA tags has shown that large DNA fragments spanning millions of bases can be cut out from the genome using Cas9 enzyme cleavage directed by CRISPR. In an ongoing clinical study detecting p53 mutations in ovarian cancer, CRISPR-duplex sequencing enables focused analysis of specific regions of the genome requiring only a small amount of DNA sample input (Katti *et al.* 2022). Other Cas enzyme-based CRISPR tools like Cas12 and Cas13 have been utilized for detecting cancer mutations in tumor biopsies, including methods such as selective high-efficiency reporter releasing (SHERLOCK) and DNA endonuclease-activated CRISPR signal amplifier (DETECTR). Simple and fast point-of-use diagnostic tests for SARS-CoV-2 infection have also been created using these CRISPR-Cas systems. Therefore, CRISPR technologies have some potential to be used as sensitive and individualized patients with cancer monitoring and detection systems.

3.2 *Ex vivo CRISPR-based therapies*

Ex vivo CRISPR-based therapies involve gene editing of T cells to knock out PD-1 and enhance their antitumor activity after adoptive transfer. Multiple clinical trials are underway for these therapies, with engineered CAR-T cells showing minimal adverse events (Weihua *et al.* 2023). For instance, a recent phase I trial from Penn Medicine used CRISPR/Cas9 to knockout PD-1 in T cells before infusing them into advanced cancer patients. Preliminary results demonstrated the therapy was well-tolerated without significant off-target effects (Figure 3). Engineered T cells persisted for months post-infusion with observed PD-1 knockout and tumor regression in some patients (Stadtmauer *et al.* 2020).

Various approaches have been taken, including targeting PD-1 alone or with endogenous TCR, and using Cas9 to enrich CAR expression at specific loci. A study showed that CRISPR-edited PD-1 knockout CAR-T cells had enhanced antitumor activity in mouse models (Weihua *et al.* 2023). While challenges exist in improving editing efficiency and quality control, ex vivo CRISPR gene editing demonstrates promise for advancing cell therapies. With progress in delivery techniques and precision, these therapies could transition from bench to bedside. But concerns over off-target effects, immunogenicity and manufacturing processes need to be addressed. Overall, ex vivo CRISPR editing of CAR-T cells is a remarkable innovation showing clinical potential for cancer immunotherapy.

3.3 *Preclinical potential of in vivo CRISPR therapies*

Clinical studies have employed precision genome editing with CRISPR-Cas9 to treat inherited single-gene disorders, especially sickle cell disease. Researchers successfully delivered Cas9 enzyme and guide RNA into patient cells using adeno-associated viruses to repair hemoglobin genes (Siwei *et al.* 2021). This demonstrates the potential of CRISPR-Cas9 in treating single gene inherited diseases. Additionally, some tumor-related genes have become targets for CRISPR cancer therapies. For instance, utilizing tissue-specific promoters to control Cas9 expression for tumor-selective delivery, or using CRISPR diagnostic tools to detect cancer mutations (Gootenberg *et al.* 2017; Wang *et al.* 2019). Although therapeutic efficacy requires further optimization, these studies exhibit the broad clinical prospects of CRISPR in medicine. In summary, CRISPR gene editing has revolutionary clinical application potential, but more research is needed to improve specificity and efficiency before it can be widely used for human gene and cell therapy.

4 PROBLEMS AND SOLUTIONS FOR CRISPR

4.1 *Off-target effects*

The primary challenge in CRISPR-Cas9 technology is the occurrence of off-target effects, where indels are frequently generated at unintended genomic locations. If sgRNA cannot form complementary base pairing with the right base sequence, it may cause some other sequences to be cleaved non-specifically, which is the cause of mutations (Zongfei *et al.* 2023). This effect is called the off-target effect. There are three main types of the wrong match: base mismatches at identical length, deletions of bases at off-target sites, and insertions of bases at off-target sites, and the mismatches are common in man-Malian cells (Zongfei *et al.* 2023). This poses a risk of unwanted mutations and toxicity, reducing the efficacy of editing.

Efforts have been made to address this challenge, the recognition ability of cas9 protein to target DNA is enhanced by modification, thereby reducing gene editing errors caused by off-target effects (Mengdan *et al.* 2021). Additionally, the characteristics of edited cells, such as cell number, type, generation, and expression patterns of genome editing systems, also affect target specificity. Additional study is required to improve the effectiveness and specificity of

CRISPR-Cas9 and lower the incidence of off-target effects. Currently, the cas9 protein has been modified primarily using two techniques.

Firstly, combining cas9 nickase mutants and coupled sgRNA into double-stranded DNA can break consistent with expectations (Ran *et al.* 2013). In this way, the off-target effect will be greatly weakened without attenuation the cutting efficiency because cas9 is a site-specific modification tool.

Second, by strictly cutting in the direction and base sequence indicated by sgRNA, dimeric RNA-guided Fokl nucleases (RFNs) can enhance the specificity of cas9 (Tsai *et al.* 2014).

4.2 *Low editing efficiency*

Ineffective editing presents the second difficulty. For the best therapeutic results, editing efficiency must be increased while off-target effects must be reduced. As a result, several strategies have been suggested to increase editing's effectiveness.

Non-homologous end-joining (NHEJ) and homology-directed repair (HDR), the two primary approaches for DNA double-strand break repair, have varying repair efficiencies in various cell types and stages. While HDR employs a DNA template to replace the target allele with an alternative sequence, NHEJ typically results in chimeras at cleavage sites. Delivering HDR templates into the nucleus is required. HDR templates are generally single-stranded oligonucleotides or plasmids. To do this, HDR templates have been sent using vectors created from viral or non-viral media. Promoting the co-delivery of Cas9 components/sgRNAs and HDR templates is one strategy to increase the effectiveness of HDR. This might be achieved by combining the nanocarriers used for HDR templates with Cas9 plasmids/proteins or sgRNAs.

Improvement of the specificity of sgRNA also makes the system function efficiently. Usually, 10 to 12 bases near PAM are called seed regions, which mainly determine the specificity of sgRNA and target recognition (Siyuan and Jianmin 2022). Some factors have been discovered that the frequency of off-target effect, or mutagenesis efficiency, is positively correlated with the content of C base and G base in the seed region and if three or more mismatches in the seed region of sgRNA and the target DNA sequence, the off-target effects die down and even disappear (Shuangjuan *et al.* 2021). So, increasing the content of C and G bases in the seed region of sgRNA may be an ideal way to overcome the influences of off-target effects (Shuangjuan *et al.* 2021).

4.3 *The fitness of edited cells*

The capacity of altered cells to adapt while being used poses a third difficulty. The likelihood of reaching the therapeutic threshold necessary for effective treatment results improves if the altered cells proliferate and adapt more readily than the unedited ones. On the other hand, if the editing process is inefficient or the modified cells are not adaptable, the therapeutic outcomes might not come out as anticipated. By growing the modified cells to the correct size before reinfusing them into patients, in vitro genome editing can partially overcome this difficulty.

Overall, if the problems described above are solved, CRISPR-based therapies will be more likely to succeed.

5 CONCLUSION

In conclusion, CRISPR/Cas9 has revolutionized genome editing and enabled major advances in biomedical research. The technology continues to evolve through engineering of Cas enzymes and guide RNAs to improve specificity while retaining on-target efficiency. Ex vivo cell therapies and CRISPR-based diagnostics are currently being tested in clinical studies, demonstrating the CRISPR tool's promise for precisely modifying the genome to produce therapeutic effects. Looking forward, further refinement of delivery methods and precision editing will be key to realizing the promise of CRISPR for in vivo gene therapies. Additional enhancements in specificity and efficiency of both Cas proteins and guide RNAs will help expand the versatility of CRISPR for research and therapeutic applications. With ongoing innovation in the CRISPR field, we are poised to unlock the full potential of programmable genome editing to combat human disease.

AUTHORS CONTRIBUTION

All the authors contributed equally and their names were listed in alphabetical order.

REFERENCES

Gootenberg, J.S., et al., (2017). *Science* 356, 438–442.

Kantor A., McClements ME., MacLaren RE., (2020). *Int J Mol Sci*, 21, 6240

Katti, A., Diaz, B. J., Caragine, C. M., Sanjana, N. E., and Dow, L. E. (2022). *Nat Rev Cancer*, 22, 259–279.

Mengdan M., Yubin Y., Yanping C., et al. (2021). *Life Science* 33, 1370–1381.

Ran, F.A., et al., (2013). *Cell*, 154, 1380–9.

Shuwen X. (2019). *Zhengzhou University*.

Shuangjuan L., Linjuan S., Qiyan L., et al. (2021). *Sichuan Zoology* 40, 622–631.

Stadtmauer, E.A., et al., (2020). *Science* 367.

Siwei Z., Frangoul H., Altshuler D. et al. (2021). *International Journal of Geriatrics* 42, 318.

Siyuan Z. and Jianmin Z. (2022). *China Science and Technology Information* 20, 29–31.

Tiemin L., Bo D. (2011). *Heredity* 33, 213–218.

Tsai, S.Q., et al., (2014). *Nature Biotechnology* 32, 569–576.

Wang JY. and Doudna JA., (2023). *Sci*, 379, eadd8643

Wang G., Chow R. D., Bai Z., et al. (2019). *Nat Immunol*, 20, 1494–1505.

Weihua J., GAO Yongshan, LIU Na, et al. (2023). *Chinese Journal of Gerontology* 43, 3483–3487.

Zhou XJ., Yang SQ., Zhang YW., et al. (2023). *Biotechnol Bull*, 39, 49–58

Zongfei Y., Lihan W., Chengcheng S., et al. (2023). *Journal of Shandong First Medical University, Shandong Academy of Medical Sciences* 44, 74–80.

Biological Sciences and Environmental Health – Gao (Ed.)

Exercise therapy for knee osteoarthritis: FITT-VP principle

Lilin Huang
Sport and Health Science Department, Nanjing Sport Institute, Nanjing, China

ABSTRACT: Knee osteoarthritis (KOA) is a chronic, progressing disorder. The primary causes of osteoarthritis include aging, trauma, strain, obesity, joint deformities, and other factors. The quality of life is significantly impacted by osteoarthritis. Exercise training seems to lessen pain, muscular weakness, joint dysfunction, and stiffness in those with knee osteoarthritis. However, there is no effective treatment for osteoarthritis. Surgery, physical therapy, exercise therapy, and medication are the three main treatments for knee osteoarthritis. In non-drug therapy, exercise therapy, as a physical therapy, has long been advocated abroad. Compared with other treatment methods, the advantage is that the side effects and adverse reactions are less, the patient acceptance is high, and the price is significantly lower than the surgical treatment. Exercise training techniques come in a variety of forms, including aerobic exercise, mind-body exercise, strength training, and aquatic exercise. In addition to serving as a resource for future research and clinical application of exercise training for the condition, we hope that this evaluation will assist patients in a range of situations obtain the best exercise treatment for knee osteoarthritis.

1 INTRODUCTION

KOA is a chronic complex disease involving the pathological changes of the whole knee joint caused by the damage and repair imbalance of the knee and surrounding tissues, which is the common osteoarthritis (Chen and Yu 2020). KOA is mainly found in elderly people, and the incidence of KOA in people over 75 years old is as high as 80 % respectively (Huang *et al.* 2022).

Osteoarthritis includes primary osteoarthritis and secondary osteoarthritis, according to the pathologic course. According to the pathophysiological mechanisms, primary osteoarthritis can be divided into three groups: type 1, which is genetically determined; type 2, which is oestrogen hormone dependent; and type 3, which is age-related osteoarthritis (Herrero-Beaumont *et al.* 2009).

Inflammation is a major factor in the emergence of KOA. The milieu inside the joint is gradually degraded when inflammatory molecules and cytokines are stimulated. Which causes synovial inflammation, remodeling of bone, bone breakdown, and osteophyte production, all of which affect the entire joint and cause discomfort, stiffness, edema, and a loss of regular joint function, and eventually the patient suffers from KOA (Zhang *et al.* 2023).

In clinic, drug therapy, physical factor therapy, and surgical treatment are usually used to treat KOA and have certain efficacy. However, there are a variety of adverse effects of drug treatment, and physical factor therapy also has certain limitations. Patients do not need surgery in the early stages of KOA, so finding a successful non-surgical treatment for KOA patients' symptoms is essential. A thorough analysis of exercise therapy for KOA revealed that it dramatically reduced joint pain and enhanced patients' quality of life and physical functionality (Mo *et al.* 2023). Through the patient's own strength, the assistance of a therapist, or the assistance of equipment, exercise training therapy seeks to improve the efficiency of any component of the body (Sheikh and Vissing 2019). In addition, exercise can

DOI: 10.1201/9781003587590-21

improve heart and lung function, increase muscle strength, increase physical stability, and promote mental health. As a result, exercise training therapy is quite important in the management of KOA. In order to offer a theoretical foundation for future study and implementation, this paper will particularly elaborate the exercise therapy of KOA and summarize the therapeutic effect of exercise therapy on KOA.

2 SYMPTOMS AND TREATMENT OF KOA

2.1 *Symptoms of KOA*

The symptoms that KOA patients typically suffer interfere with their regular activities. Pain, stiffness, decreased joint range of motion, and muscular weakness are the four major symptoms that predominate (Sharma 2021).

2.1.1 *Pain*

Pain is one of the common clinical manifestations in the vast majority of patients with KOA, initially mild to moderate and non-persistent; As the disease progresses, the pain may first affect using stairs and squatting down and standing up, and knee pain is usually worse with increased mobility (Wang and Yu 2019). Pain symptoms are further exacerbated by advanced disease progression, significantly affecting activities of daily living and even affecting sleep quality at night (Chen *et al.* 2023).

2.1.2 *Muscle weakness*

Patients with KOA frequently experience muscle weakness. Weakness brought on by muscle dysfunction may increase the possibility of developing KOA (Coudeyre *et al.* 2016). The reduction in extension and flexion strength is the most obvious sign of muscular weakening (Heiden *et al.* 2009). Aging and muscular dysfunction are both linked to muscle weakening, which can reduce knee stability and hasten the onset of KOA. When treating KOA, it's crucial to address muscle weakness, especially in the thigh muscles, such as quadriceps.

2.1.3 *Reduced joint motion*

Knee instability symptoms first and foremost emerge as restricted joint motion in the knee. Knee range of motion is narrowed in small areas in the end-range motion in the early stages of the disease. The joint range of motion decreases as KOA worsens (Taylor *et al.* 2014). Joint activity restrictions can become more severe over time if there are ongoing muscle weakening issues. Reduced range of motion can be caused by many factors, including pain, stiffness etc. One way to improve restricted joint mobility is to build up muscles.

2.1.4 *Stiffness*

Patients with KOA frequently complain of stiffness. People with KOA may have trouble moving their knee joints, especially in the morning, and their muscles may feel tight and tense, however this symptom can be relieved by stretching or activity. Knee osteoarthritis often lasts between a few minutes and 10 minutes, and seldom for longer than thirty. According to certain research, patients with KOA who have joint instability also experience knee stiffness as a compensatory and preventive mechanism (Gustafson *et al.* 2016).

2.2 *Treatment of KOA*

The treatment of KOA mostly adopts a comprehensive intervention program for symptoms. Stepwise treatment can be carried out according to the severity of the disease, generally following the order of basic treatment, drug treatment and surgical treatment.

Physical factor therapy is mainly used to use physical factors such as sound, light, cold, electricity, and force. The purpose of physical factor therapy is to improve local metabolism, accelerate the secretion of joint fluid, have a good effect on the improvement of joint interior, inhibit inflammation, and thus relieve the pain caused by the disease (Li *et al.* 2008).

Drug treatment for knee osteoarthritis can be divided into drugs that improve and suppress symptoms and drugs that improve symptoms and protect cartilage. At present, clinically, Western medicine is oral, and its effect is generally anti-inflammatory, inhibiting the development of inflammation. Such as: (1) antipyretic and analgesic drugs (2) nonsteroidal anti-inflammatory drugs (NsAIDs) (3) hyaluronic acid (HA) and so on (Wang and Yu 2019).

Exercise therapy, as a treatment modality for non-pharmacological treatment of KOA, is recommended by numerous medical guidelines at home and abroad. The primary types of exercise therapy used to treat KOA are aerobic activity, strength training, aquatic exercise, mind-body exercises, and others. Exercise training helps improve pain and range of motion in patients with KOA, improve physical function, and reduce the risk of cardiovascular disease.

Surgical treatment is mainly for patients with advanced knee osteoarthritis or patients who have serious clinical manifestations after ineffective physical therapy and drug treatment, and even seriously affect daily life. At present, there are three main surgical methods: (1) arthroscopic joint cavity cleansing (2) knee osteotomy (3) artificial joint replacement (Wang and Yu 2019).

In physical factor therapy, drug treatment, exercise therapy and surgical treatment, physical therapy is mainly used in the early and middle stages of patients, drug treatment runs through the middle and late stages, and surgical treatment is used as a last resort, but exercise therapy in physical therapy can run through the whole process of the treatment stage, including the recovery stage after treatment, and regular exercise can also prevent such diseases.

3 EXERCISE TRAINING FOR KOA

Exercise prescription follows the principle of FITT-VP, including frequency, F, intensity, I, time, T, type, T, volume, V, progression, P, this article will specifically elaborate on KOA exercise therapy from 6 aspects.

3.1 *Frequency, intensity and time*

FIT recommended for patients with KOA is summarized in Table 1 (Garber *et al.* 2011).

Table 1. FIT recommended for patients with KOA (Garber *et al.* 2011).

	Aerobic Exercise	Strength Training	Flexibility exercise
Frequency	3-5 days a week, varying in frequency with intensity. It is advised to engage in moderate exercise 5 days a week, vigorous exercise 3 days a week, or a combination of moderate and vigorous exercise 3 to 5 days a week.	Ideally, each major muscle group should be worked out twice a week.	Every day
Intensity	Moderate (eg, 40% to 59% HRR or VO,R) to high intensity (eg, 60% to B9% HRR or O,R) aerobic exercise is recommended for most	For beginners to intermediate exercisers looking to increase strength, use 60%-70% of the 1RM. For seasoned strength trai-	Movement within the range of motion (ROM) with tightness/stretching without pain. Slowly increase the range of motion of the joint

(*continued*)

Table 1. Continued

	Aerobic Exercise	Strength Training	Flexibility exercise
	adults; People with poor health are advised to engage in low-intensity (eg, 30%-39% HRR or O,R) to moderate-intensity aerobic exercise.	nees to increase strength, use 80% of the 1RM.	in the absence of pain.
Time	20 to 60 minutes of intense activity per day, or 30 to 60 minutes per day (150 minutes per week), is recommended.	8~12 repetitions 2~4 sets, including all large muscle groups	The dynamic movement reaches 10 times, and the static stretching is maintained for 10-30s

l-RM: 1 maximum number of repetitions; HRR: reserve heart rate; .ROM: range of motion of the joints.

3.2 *Type*

3.2.1 *Aerobic exercise and KOA*

The phrase "aerobic exercise" describes the prolonged, regular use of the body's major muscle groups when there is an adequate supply of oxygen. Aerobic exercise mainly includes walking, running, swimming, etc. According to studies, KOA has an impact on lower limb motor dysfunction as well as muscular strength and joint range of motion. It also lowers aerobic capacity (Abbasi 2017). Aerobic exercise benefits people with osteoarthritis by lowering pain, swollen joints, and other symptoms like restricted joint mobility in addition to enhancing cardiopulmonary function (Wellsandt and Golightly 2018).

Wallis *et al.* found that walking training for patients with KOA was not effective in relieving knee pain but reducing the risk of CVD (cardiovascular disease) (Wallis *et al.* 2017). Alghadir *et al.* found that walking upside down can better relieve pain and reduce dysfunction in patients with KOA, and can also improve the strength and function of the quadriceps (Alghadir *et al.* 2019).

At present, there are few clinical studies on running training for KOA patients, but the results of many animal experiments prove that low and moderate intensity running training can prevent chondrocytes loss and improve exercise performance. Moderate-intensity running training can reverse local inflammatory biomarkers in rats, regulate chondrocytes levels, prevent chondrocytes from loss, and improve gait and physical performance (Martins *et al.* 2019). Kim *et al.* discovered that whereas high-intensity running exercise is harmful, low-intensity running exercise has little repair impact (Chen *et al.* 2018).

Further study is required because there are no universal guidelines for the kind, degree, frequency, and length of aerobic activity in KOA patients. It's also important to remember that the majority of people can benefit from low- and moderate-intensity exercise, which can increase pain and create inflammation. Therefore, more study is required to determine the therapeutic effectiveness and safety of aerobic exercise in order to gather more persuasive data for the treatment of osteoarthritis.

3.2.2 *Strength training and KOA*

For individuals with KOA to regain their muscle strength, strength training is essential. Strengthening muscles, increasing muscle strength, enhancing joint stability, and delaying the progression of disease are the main goals of strength training. Currently, isometric, isotonic, and isokinetic training for the quadriceps muscles, the extensor muscles, represents the majority of the knee joint's surrounding muscles' strength training.

Isometric contracted muscles remain constant in length and muscle tone changes. In the treatment of KOA, quadriceps isometric exercise has been demonstrated to considerably reduce pain, enhance joint function and knee motor performance, improve quadriceps muscle strength and knee stability (Kang, Gong and Dai 2021). According to Huang *et al.*, quadriceps isometric contraction workouts significantly enhanced knee function and successfully reduced joint pain (Huang *et al.* 2018). Isometric exercise has been shown by Anwer *et al.* to considerably improve muscle strength in both male and female patients (Anwer *et al.* 2013). Isometric contraction can prevent joint wear since it does not result in joint activity, unlike isotonic or constant velocity contraction. Therefore, individuals with knee osteoarthritis who are unable to move their knee joint due to discomfort should particularly consider it. Isometric exercise can enhance both muscular function and strength in these patients.

Isotonic muscle training involves contracting the muscles while applying a fixed resistance load. Tanaka *et al.* found that KOA patients may effectively increase their muscle strength by low-load isotonic resistance exercise (Tanaka *et al.* 2018). One randomized controlled research found that centripetal and eccentric resistance training reduced knee osteoarthritis discomfort and enhanced muscle strength, but centripetal concentrated resistance training was more effective in lowering pain during walking and pain severity when stopping walking (Vincent and Vincent 2020). Patients with KOA can strengthen their muscles and experience pain relief via isotonic exercise. Both centripetal and eccentric anti-resistance exercises had comparable results. Depending on their specific circumstances, people can select from a variety of training modes. However, the optimal training movements, intensity, and frequency still need to be further studied.

Isokinetic strength training is a relatively recent method of building muscle, and it typically requires support from an apparatus. Coudeyre *et al.* found isokinetic training produced more noticeable gains in muscular strength assessments and femoral cartilage thickness than isometric and isotonic exercise (Coudeyre *et al.* 2016). According to one review, isokinetic strength training has a substantial impact on pain and impairment and can improve the development of dynamic strength in KOA therapy (Bahşi *et al.* 2022). Although isokinetic strength training equipment is expensive, difficult to use, and difficult to promote on a broad scale, it has a positive impact on pain reduction and muscle strength improvement in individuals with KOA.

In conclusion, strength training is a crucial component of exercise therapy training for KOA patients. A training method with significant clinical relevance is whole-body progressive strength training with a quadriceps focus. The results of various strength training alternatives vary, and the best training strategy is chosen based on the patient's disease stage and the available equipment.

3.2.3 *Aquatic exercise and KOA*

In order to train the human body, aquatic exercise therapy makes use of the buoyancy and resistance, pressure and temperature of the water, as well as other physical features. Boost cardiovascular health, mobility, and strength (Zhou *et al.* 2015).

In a randomized controlled trial in which 60 patients underwent 8 weeks of aquatic exercise training, it was shown that aquatic exercise reduced pain, improved limb function, and improved patients' quality of life (Taglietti *et al.* 2018). Another review showed that water sports had a better effect in the short term on disability, pain and quality of life reported by patients with KOA (Bartels *et al.* 2016).

Aquatic exercise may have a positive impact on pain, disability and quality of life in people with KOA. But whether aquatic training is a better long-term alternative to onshore training is unclear and further research is needed.

3.2.4 *Mind-body exercise and KOA*

The importance of mind-body mobility is emphasized in the 2019 Osteoarthritis Research Society International (OARSI) clinical guidelines, which also for the first time include mind-body exercises like tai chi and yoga in land-based exercise programs.

An additional meta-analysis of randomized controlled trials revealed that tai chi was clinically significant in improving pain, stiffness, and physical function in individuals with KOA (Kelley *et al.* 2022). One randomized controlled trial showed that tai chi exercises not only improved muscle strength and endurance in the upper and lower extremities, but also improved balance and functional performance in older adults (Li and Cheng 2019).

According to research by Lomgpre *et al.*, patients with KOA can benefit from yoga poses like lunging and squatting because they reduce knee joint adduction torque and increase quadriceps strength (Longpré *et al.* 2015). Yao *et al.* discovered that chair yoga has a beneficial impact on physical function and capacity for daily living in older women with KOA, which can slow the disease's progression (Yao *et al.* 2023).

It has been demonstrated that mind-body exercises, which are safe, simple, and generally slow with low joint impact and load, can treat KOA by reducing pain, enhancing physical function, improving quality of life, etc.

3.3 *Volume and progression*

The volume of exercise is determined by the frequency, intensity and time of exercise, that is, the FIT of training. The recommended amount of exercise for most adults is $\geq$ 500-1000MET-min/wk (Garber *et al.* 2011). This amount of exercise is approximately equivalent to moderate physical activity with an energy expenditure of 100okcal/wk, or moderate-intensity exercise of 150min per week (Garber *et al.* 2011). Specifically, the total amount of exercise is the sum of frequency, intensity, and duration, and the frequency, intensity, and duration have been described above, and the specific total amount of exercise should be formulated according to the severity of the patient's disease and tolerance to exercise.

The speed at which the exercise program progresses depends on the athlete's health, fitness, training response, and the purpose of the exercise program. To improve any of the FITT-VPs should follow the step-by-step principle of training. Gradually adjust the duration, frequency and intensity of the exercise to achieve the movement goal. A gradual exercise program can increase adherence and reduce the risk of skeletal muscle injury and adverse cardiovascular events.

4 CONCLUSION

The most effective exercise therapy for knee osteoarthritis is outlined in this review. Exercises that improve joint and physical function, reduce symptoms in KOA patients, such as aerobic activity, strength training, aquatic exercise, and mind-body activities. When formulating the FITT-VP exercise regimen, the functional status, health status, goals, etc. of KOA patients should be fully considered to ensure the effectiveness and safety of exercise therapy for KOA patients.

Exercise therapy for osteoarthritis does not yet have a single universal standard, and there are various ways to measure its effectiveness. In the future, more detailed clinical studies are necessary to explore the pathogenesis of KOA and the effects of various exercise prescription components on KOA. This will provide a scientific basis for the development of exercise therapies for KOA.

REFERENCES

Abbasi J. (2017). *JAMA* **318**, 2169.

Alghadir A.H., Anwer S., Sarkar B., Paul A.K. and Anwar D. (2019). *BMC Musculoskelet Disord* **20**, 159.

Anwer S., Equebal A., Nezamuddin M., Kumar R. and Lenka P. K. (2013). *Ann Phys Rehabil Med* **56**, 434.
Bahşi A., Altındağ Ö., Akaltun M.S., Aydeniz A., Avcı E.E., and Gür A. (2022). *Cureus* **14**, 28324.
Bartels E.M., Juhl C.B., Christensen R., Hagen K.B., Danneskiold-Samsøe B., Dagfinrud H. and Lund H. (2016). *Cochrane Database Syst Rev* **3**, CD005523.
Chen L. and Yu Y. (2020). *Adv Exp Med Biol* **1228**, 219.
Chen X., Fu H., Peng J., Wang W. and Zhai Q. (2023). *Orthopedics* **14**, 363.
Chen Z., Yan W., Mao Y., Ni Y., Zhou L., Song H., Xu W., Wang L., and Shen Y. (2018). *J Cardiovasc Transl Res* **11**, 230.
Coudeyre E., Jegu A.G., Giustanini M., Marrel J.P., Edouard P. and Pereira B. (2016). *Ann Phys Rehabil Med* **59**, 207.
Garber C.E., Blissmer B., Deschenes M.R., Franklin B.A., Lamonte M.J., Lee I.M., Nieman D.C. and Swain D. P. (2011). American College of Sports Medicine, *Med Sci Sports Exerc* **43**, 1334.
Gustafson J.A., Gorman S., Fitzgerald G.K. and Farrokhi S. *Gait Posture* **43**, 210.
Heiden T.L., Lloyd D.G. and Ackland T.R. (2009). *J Orthop Sports Phys Ther* **39**, 807.
Herrero-Beaumont G., Roman-Blas J.A., Castañeda S., and Jimenez S.A. (2009). *Semin Arthritis Rheum* **39**, 71.
Huang L., Guo B., Xu F. and Zhao J. (2018). *Int J Rheum Dis* **21**, 952.
Huang M., Chen J., Chen S., and Li Y. (2022). *Chin J Sports Med* **41**, 320.
Kang Z., Gong L. and Dai D. (2021). *Practical Gerontology* **35**, 1067.
Kelley G.A., Kelley K.S., and Callahan L.F. (2022). *Science Progress* **105**, 003685042210883.
Li J. and Cheng L. (2019). *Chin J Rehabil Med* **34**, 1304.
Li X., Liang W. and Liu X. (2008). *Chin J Bone Jt Injury* **23**, 598.
Longpré H.S., Brenneman E.C., Johnson A.L.M., and Maly M.R. (2015). *Clin Biomech (Bristol, Avon)* **30**, 820.
Martins J.B., Mendonça V.A., Aguiar G.C., da Fonseca S.F., Dos Santos J.M., Tossige-Gomes R., de S. Melo D., Oliveira M.X., Leite H.R., Camargos A.C.R., Ferreira A.J., Coimbra C.C., Poortmans J., Oliveira V.C., Silva S.B., Domingues T.E., Bernardo-Filho M. and Lacerda A.C.R. (2019). *Front Physiol* **10**, 1168.
Mo L., Jiang B., Mei T., and Zhou D. (2023). *Orthop J Sports Med* **11**, 23259671231172772.
Sharma L. (2021). *N Engl J Med* **384**, 51.
Sheikh A.M. and Vissing J. (2019). *Acta Myol* **38**, 215.
Taglietti M., Facci L. M., Trelha C. S., de Melo F. C., da Silva D. W., Sawczuk G., Ruivo T. M., de Souza T. B., Sforza C., and Cardoso J. R. (2018). *Clin Rehabil* **32**, 766.
Tanaka H., Ikezoe T., Nakamura M., Yanase K., Fujita K., Motomura Y., Kusano K., Araki K., Umehara J., Saeki J., Morishita K., and Ichihashi N. (2018). *Muscle Nerve* **57**, 83.
Taylor A.L., Wilken J.M., Deyle G.D., and Gill N.W. (2014). *J Orthop Sports Phys Ther* **44**, 273.
Vincent K.R. and Vincent H.K. (2020). *Am J Phys Med Rehabil* **99**, 932.
Wallis J.A., Webster K.E., Levinger P., Singh P.J., Fong C. and Taylor N.F. (2017). *Osteoarthritis Cartilage* **25**, 1969.
Wang B. and Yu N. (2019). *Chin J Jt Surg, Electron Ed* **13**, 124.
Wellsandt E. and Golightly Y. (2018). *Curr Opin Rheumatol* **30**, 151.
Yao C.T., Lee B.O., Hong H., and Su Y.C. (2023). *Healthcare (Basel)* **11**, 1024.
Zhang X., Zeng H., and Meng L. (2023). *Chin J Pain Med* **29**, 50.
Zhou Y., Lin H. and He C. (2015). *Chin J Rehabil Med* **30**, 1306.

Biological Sciences and Environmental Health – Gao (Ed.)

Engineered circular RNA: Emerging insights into cancer therapy

Huan Lin
Biological Sciences, Beijing Normal University, Beijing, China

ABSTRACT: Circular RNA (circRNA) is a single-stranded RNA molecule connected by covalent bonds in a circular shape. It is considered an emerging miRNA sponge with enhanced stability compared to its linear counterparts. CircRNAs play critical roles in cancer progression via the circRNA-miRNA-mRNA axis. CircRNAs can be engineered in vitro or in vivo to achieve temporary or long-term blockade of miRNAs, inhibiting their function. By taking advantage of the flexible design that can be directed against one or more targets, this technology could be used to suppress the overexpression of oncogenic miRNAs, providing a personalized approach to cancer. However, before engineered circRNAs enter clinical applications, several obstacles must be addressed: the development of design and production techniques, particularly for large-scale manufacturing, and the optimization of delivery systems. This review explores circRNAs' biological functions in cancer, synthesis and delivery systems, and preclinical studies on engineered circular RNA sponges to better understand their challenges and prospects as therapeutic tools for cancer.

1 INTRODUCTION

Cancer is defined as the irregular and uncontrollable division and growth of cells (Siegel *et al.* 2019). It is characterized by invasive and aggressive behavior, often associated with the metastatic nature and malignant phenotype of many cancer cells. Since 2000, the pace of development of therapeutic products in cancer has accelerated, with significant advancements in targeted therapies and biologics, especially gene therapy. This trend is largely driven by the challenges of metastasis, recurrence, and the heterogeneity of cancer cells, which render many conventional treatments ineffective for numerous malignancies (Sun 2015).

Circular RNA (circRNA) is a novel type of RNA that forms a closed loop, characterized by a covalent bond between its 3' and 5' ends. CircRNAs are highly abundant and evolutionarily conserved across species. Their functional significance has been unveiled by recent studies, even though they were initially regarded as byproducts of missplicing. As circRNAs are rich in microRNA (miRNA) binding sites, they usually function as miRNA sponges to regulate gene expression. The role of the regulatory mechanism has been demonstrated in a range of biological processes, including intercellular communication, differentiation and specification, and disease progression. Due to their stable circular structure and immunogenicity, circRNA-based targeted cancer therapies have emerged as a prominent area of research in recent years.

Studies have shown that therapeutic loss-of-function targeting specific miRNAs can be accomplished by utilizing engineered circRNA sponges, which further demonstrates the great promise of engineered circRNA as new tools in anticancer research (Liu *et al.* 2018). However, there are numerous limitations to overcome before circRNA therapy can be

DOI: 10.1201/9781003587590-22

effectively applied in clinical settings. For example, the synthesis technology of circRNA is still immature and needs optimization, as circularizing larger RNAs can be challenging. Additionally, circRNAs synthesized in vitro are often immunogenic (Chen *et al.* 2019; Liu *et al.* 2018). This review explores the biological functions of circRNAs in cancer, their synthesis and delivery systems, and preclinical studies on engineered circular RNA sponges, aiming to better understand their challenges and future prospects as therapeutic tools for cancer.

2 ENGINEERED circRNAs IN CANCER

2.1 *Biofunctions of circRNAs and circRNA-miRNA-mRNA Axis*

CircRNAs are highly versatile small molecules with great potential due to their unique structures that enable interactions with DNA, RNA, and even proteins. The number of identified human circRNAs has reached astonishingly over 100,000, making it challenging to summarize their functions with just one or two simple models. Generally, the biological functions and applications of circRNAs mainly encompass eight main aspects: RNA ligands, miRNA sponges, protein sponges, antisense circular molecules, innate immune activators, innate immune suppressors, protein translation, and biomarkers (Liu and Chen 2022). The following section will focus on their function as miRNA sponges.

Micro RNA (miRNA) is a type of small non-coding RNA that can suppress the translation or induce degradation of its target mRNAs (Tay *et al.* 2015). The interaction between circRNA and miRNA can be explained by the competitive endogenous RNA hypothesis. CircRNA interacts with miRNA via the miRNA response element, thereby inhibiting the binding of miRNA to mRNA. Consequently, the suppressive impact of miRNA on the expression of target genes is alleviated (Salmena *et al.* 2011). By associating the interactions between miRNA-circRNA and miRNA-mRNA, it is possible to construct a circRNA-miRNA-mRNA axis. Increasing research has shown that circRNAs are associated with substantial cancers, such as lung cancer, breast cancer, and hepatocellular carcinoma, highlighting their potential as therapeutic targets and diagnostic tools in the field of oncology. Leveraging the regulatory role of circRNAs in the axis can help explore their extensive application prospects.

2.2 *In vitro synthesis of circRNAs*

Efficient synthesis of circRNAs is the basis for understanding their functions and their biomedical applications. Historically, there have been three main methods for in vitro circRNA preparation, which include chemical-based chemical ligation, enzyme-based T4 ligase methods, and ribozyme-based Group I intron and Group II intron self-splicing systems, known as precursor introns for efficient circularization. Each method has its advantages and disadvantages since the ligation strategies vary significantly. Owing to low ligating efficiency and purity, the inability to synthesize circRNAs more than 80 nucleotides (nt) in length, and biosafety concerns, circRNA preparation using chemical ligation is not a widely adopted approach (Obi and Chen 2021). Although the Group I intron self-splicing system is widely used for in vitro circularization of RNA sequences up to 5 kb in length, it still exhibits immunogenicity (Lee *et al.* 2022; Wesselhoeft *et al.* 2018). Group II intron self-splicing systems do not introduce large fragments of exogenous residues, but they suffer from low circularization efficiency, making industrial production difficult (Chen *et al.* 2017). Traditional methods using T4 DNA or T4 RNA ligases with adapter sequences can achieve in vitro circRNA preparation but have low circularization efficiency, resulting in many byproducts and a complex purification process (Rausch *et al.* 2021). Therefore, new innovations are needed to improve existing circularization strategies, focusing on reducing immunogenicity, enhancing circularization efficiency, and increasing product purity. An efficient system for circRNA preparation developed by Cui *et al.* precisely reflects this research trend. It is based on a self-splicing ribozyme obtained from an enhanced *Tetrahymena thermophila* Group I intron and reportedly achieves significantly higher efficiency compared to the traditional method involving a flanking ICS-mediated approach (Cui *et al.* 2023).

2.3 *Potential therapeutic applications of circRNA sponges in cancer*

Compared to well-established cancer treatments or emerging cancer immunotherapy, circRNAs have unique advantages. While circRNAs exhibit high stability and resistance to degradation, leading to sustained miRNA sponge activity, they can also be engineered to specifically sequester and inhibit oncogenic miRNAs (Liu *et al.* 2018). Particularly, circRNAs have been shown to affect tumors and their microenvironment via the circRNA-miRNA-mRNA axis (Liang *et al.* 2020). Consequently, identifying circRNAs that act as miRNA sponges represents a promising breakthrough in the potential development of preventive and therapeutic approaches for cancer.

2.3.1 *Regulation of tumor progression*

Has_circ_0078710 functions as a sponge for miR-31 and has been found to up-regulate the expression of miR-31 target genes HDAC2 and CDK2. In both in vitro and in vivo experiments, it has been demonstrated that overexpression of has_circ_0078710 induces G1-M phase cell cycle progression to regulate tumor progression (Xie *et al.* 2019). In contrast to promoting tumor growth, circRNAs can also inhibit tumor occurrence, invasion, and metastasis by binding to multiple miRNAs. For instance, Wang *et al.* (2020) found that circ-CDYL regulates the expression levels of targeted TP53INP1 mRNA by binding to miR-190a-3p, thereby inhibiting the proliferation of breast cancer cells and inducing apoptosis.

2.3.2 *Regulation of tumor immunity*

Exosomal circRNAs play a significant role in intercellular communication, influencing both tumor immunosuppression and immunoenhancement. This includes their role in modulating immune and non-immune cells through direct or indirect pathways. For immunosuppression, circRNA-002178 could boost the PDL1 expression in lung adenocarcinoma cells by acting as a sponge for miR-34a. Additionally, it could be transported into T cells through exosomes secreted by tumors, leading to an increased PD1 expression by sequestering miR-28-5p, hence inducing CD_8^+ T cell depletion and suppressing their anti-tumor activity (Zhang *et al.* 2023). Whereas for immunoenhancement, exosomal hsa_circ_0004658 and circBTG2 have been shown to inhibit the progression of liver cancer and glioma through different molecular pathways. In the case of liver cancer, exosomal hsa_circ_0004658 acts via the miR-499b-5p/JAM3 pathway, while in glioma, circBTG2 hinders progression via the miR-25-3p/PTEN pathway (Shi *et al.* 2022; Zhang *et al.* 2022).

2.3.3 *Angiogenesis*

CircRNAs play a crucial role in antiangiogenesis. For example, circ-SHKBP1I has been shown to up-regulate the expression of AGGF1 through the miR-544a/FOXP1 or miR-379/FOXP2 pathway, further stimulating glioma angiogenesis (He *et al.* 2018). Moreover, research has revealed that circHIPK3 is downregulated in bladder cancer. Enforced overexpression of circHIPK3 effectively hinders the expression of heparanase and its downstream targets MMP-9 and VEGF via sponging miR-558, thereby significantly suppressing the migration, invasion, and angiogenesis of bladder cancer cells (Li *et al.* 2017).

3 RECENT PRECLINICAL RESEARCH ON ENGINEERED circRNAs

3.1 *Engineered circRNA sponges*

The dysregulation of miRNAs has been extensively observed in human cancers, leading to the development and optimization of miRNA sponge technology to achieve the loss of function of oncogenic miRNAs. As an alternative to linear sponges, circRNAs open a new way to sponge miRNAs with persistent effects. CircRNAs can be engineered with multiple bulged miRNA binding sites, which are complementary to miRNA targets, maximizing their capacity to regulate oncogenic mRNAs (Tay *et al.* 2015). Based on findings about specific mechanisms of miRNA dysregulation in human cancers, a growing body of research is focusing on the design, synthesis, and functional validation of circRNAs that sponge cancer-related miRNA targets.

For many human cancers, miR-21 has been validated as a promising therapeutic target, and that is where scientists have started exploring the great potential of engineered circRNAs (Pan *et al.* 2010). Lin *et al.* demonstrated that engineered circRNAs with multiple bulged miR-21 binding sites effectively suppressed the proliferation of gastric carcinoma cells and upregulated the expression of DAXX, a key tumor suppressor gene directly targeted by miR-21 (Lin *et al.* 2017). Similarly, a circular sponge containing seven miR-21 binding sites arranged in a tandem array was verified to have an anti-proliferative effect in lung cancer cells (Rama *et al.* 2022). Bayat *et al.* (2023) found that the introduced circular miR-21 decoy, CM21D, reduced the tumorigenesis of glioblastoma multiforme (GBM) by sponging miR-21. In the C6-rat GBM model, CM21D demonstrated superior suppression of tumor growth compared to the linear form, LM21D. Furthermore, an engineered circRNA that incorporates binding sites for both miR-21 and miR-93 effectively hinders the growth and movement of esophageal carcinoma cells, while facilitating programmed cell death (Wang *et al.* 2019).

However, for other miRNAs that are also important as part of the cancer progression, researchers have yet to develop and synthesize corresponding circular RNA sponges. This delay may be due to the unclear regulatory mechanisms of miRNAs in tumors and normal cells, as well as the difficulties in accurately designing miRNA binding sites and synthesizing them with high purity. It is worth noting that circRNAs also have a wide range of applications in other diseases. Lavenniah *et al.* (2020) reported that they engineered a circmiR sponge to specifically target known cardiac prohypertrophic miR-132 and -212. The introduction of this circmiR sponge led to a reduction in hypertrophic disease characteristics and preserved cardiac function in treated mice. Strong evidence suggests that engineered circular RNA sponges hold great promise as potential therapeutics in the future.

3.2 *Delivery systems of engineered circRNAs*

The development of circRNA delivery systems is crucial for harnessing the therapeutic potential of circRNAs and translating them into clinical applications.

3.2.1 *Lipid nanoparticles*

Lipid nanoparticles (LNPs) have become increasingly popular in gene therapy, particularly in the development of mRNA-based vaccines (Liu *et al.* 2022). The lipid-based nanoparticles have a hydrophobic core and a hydrophilic outer layer. The hydrophobic core encapsulates the therapeutic molecules, protecting them from degradation and facilitating their delivery, while the hydrophilic outer layer helps to stabilize the nanoparticles and enables them to interact with the cells of the body. In addition, the high biocompatibility, lack of immunogenicity, excellent cellular penetration and intracellular release capabilities, and ease of large-scale production make LNPs the most effective and preferred nanocarriers in current research on RNA delivery systems (Loan *et al.* 2023).

3.2.2 *Exosomes*

Exosomes are small, membrane-bound extracellular vesicles released by most cells, which contain various lipids, proteins, and nucleic acids derived from their cells of origin (Moon and Chang 2022). Owing to their inherent biocompatibility and low immunogenicity, exosomes can surpass diverse biological barriers and shuttle between different cellular environments rich in proteins, lipids, and genes, making them ideal nanocarriers for delivering synthetic RNA. Exosomes can be classified into natural and artificial types, with both types being limited in their large-scale production and clinical application due to high separation costs, low yield, low cargo loading efficiency, and harsh storage conditions (Loan *et al.* 2023).

3.2.3 *Viral vectors*

Plasmid vector and viral vector delivery are two commonly employed methods for achieving circRNA overexpression and are also commonly utilized for circRNA delivery systems (Katsushima *et al.* 2023). Unlike the low transfection efficiency of plasmid vectors, viral vector tools offer a more reliable method for efficient transduction in a wide range of cells and animals. However, when considering the delivery of a circRNA product, a significant limitation for clinical purposes arises from the requirement of a DNA intermediate for transcription and in vivo circularization of RNA (Loan *et al.* 2023). Moreover, despite notable advancements in procedures, adeno-associated virus stocks still retain considerable impurities, and failure to minimize them during production could lead to immunotoxicity when administering extremely high doses systemically (Penaud-Budloo *et al.* 2018).

In addition to these mainstream approaches, there are many transportation systems that deserve attention and development. For instance, polyethylenimine (PEI) is a cationic polymer that can bind with negatively charged DNA or RNA molecules, facilitating their transport into cells. Müller *et al.* (2020) demonstrated the effectiveness of PEIs in delivering circular RNAs and promoting their functionality in vivo. The advantageous biocompatibility of low molecular weight PEI F25-LMW, combined with its favorable characteristics, offers a platform for utilizing circRNAs in cancer therapy and optimizing nanoparticle properties. Moreover, it should be noted that advanced stimuli-responsive delivery systems safeguard the accurate transportation of dynamically active RNAs. For example, commonly used nanomaterials that respond to stimuli, such as pH-responsive, enzyme-responsive, and hypoxia-responsive nanomaterials, are well-suited for targeting tumor sites (Zhang *et al.* 2023).

3.3 *Adverse effects of engineered circRNAs in cancer treatment*

As an emerging therapy, engineered circRNAs face several challenges that need to be addressed. Although in vitro synthesis methods for circularization have been developed, there is still a need to upgrade their efficiency and the purity and immunogenicity of the resulting products. Circularization efficiency is greatly affected by genetic sequence and length, RNA structure, and the specific methods used, while purity of products faces the challenge of multiple purification processes. Moreover, for biomedical applications, scaling up production should be considered.

The debate is still ongoing as to whether circRNAs are immunogenic and whether this immunogenicity results from a lack of RNA modification (Chen *et al.* 2019; Chen *et al.* 2017; Liu *et al.* 2022). Although delivery vehicles such as LNPs have been widely applied, further research is still needed to optimize these nanocarriers for efficient and targeted delivery of circRNAs to specific cells or tissues. Notably, determining the most effective dosage and administration regimen remains a challenge, as the pharmacokinetics and in vivo distribution of circRNAs still require further study.

3.4 *Future directions for engineered circRNAs*

As sponges for miRNAs, circRNAs are trending toward a personalized RNA-based cancer therapy. Based on the circRNA-miRNA-mRNA axis, circRNAs with specific miRNA binding sites are specially designed for different types and stages of tumors. Achieving this, along with optimizing circRNA circularization efficiency, requires a deeper understanding of the miRNA dysregulation mechanisms in cancer, technological innovations, and even the incorporation of artificial intelligence. Apart from functioning as miRNA decoys, circRNAs can also encode, sponge proteins and even participate in RNA splicing and modifications. The protein-encoding function of circRNAs has been extensively explored, with applications in protein replacement therapy, circRNA vaccines, and cancer immunotherapy (Loan *et al.* 2023). In addition, it should be pointed out that engineered circRNAs in cancer treatment are still in their infancy. Many issues still require further research and validation: the huge differences in the immune response caused by the circRNA construction strategies, the effective targeting and regulation of circRNA expression, and their clinical application (Zhang *et al.* 2023). Furthermore, extensive preclinical and clinical trials are needed to evaluate the efficacy and safety of circRNAs in cancer therapy.

4 CONCLUSION

CircRNAs, which function as miRNA sponges possess abundant benefits, such as high stability, personalization potential, and lower immunogenicity, compared to protein-based therapies, making them a compelling and promising approach for addressing cancer. Studies described in this review indicate that there are primarily two categories of engineered circular RNA sponges. The first targets the identical miRNA and designs multiple binding sites on the circRNA to bind with the miRNA. The second involves engineering circRNAs to target different miRNAs, making them multifunctional. Validation of circular RNA sponges in current research has not yet reached the gene therapy trials for humans due to immature manufacturing processes, including design, in vitro synthesis, purification, and delivery. Thus, circular RNA sponges still have a significant journey ahead. Ultimately, circRNA unravels a new, exciting perspective in the field of RNA-based therapy with the potential to revolutionize personalized cancer treatment.

REFERENCES

Bayat H., Pourgholami M.H., Rahmani S., Pournajaf S., Mowla S.J. (2023). *Mol. Ther. Nucleic. Acids* **32**, 432–444

Chen Y.G., Chen R., Ahmad S., Verma R., Kasturi S.P., Amaya L., Broughton J.P., Kim J., Cadena C., Pulendran B., Hur S., Chang H.Y., (2019). *Mol. Cell* **76**(1), 96–109

Chen Y.G., Kim M.V., Chen X., Batista P.J., Aoyama S., Wilusz J.E., Iwasaki A., Chang H.Y. (2017). *Mol. Cell* **67**, 228–238

Cui J., Zhang L., Zhang Z., Luo X., Liu Y., Li C., Huang W., Zou L., Yu X., Xiao F. (2023). *Nucleic. Acids. Res* **51**(14), e78

He Q., Zhao L., Liu Y., Liu X., Zheng J., Yu H., Cai H., Ma J., Liu L., Wang P., Li Z., Xue Y. (2018). *Mol. Ther. Nucleic. Acids* **10**, 331–48

Katsushima K., Joshi K., Perera R.J. (2023). *Neurooncol Adv* **5**(1), vdad063

Lavenniah A., Luu T.D.A., Li Y.P., Lim T.B., Jiang J., Ackers-Johnson M., Foo R.S. (2020). *Mol. Ther* **28** (6), 1506–1517

Lee K.H. Kim S., Lee S.W. (2022). *Int. J. Mol. Sci* **23**(21), 13247

Li Y., Zheng F., Xiao X., Xie F., Tao D., Huang C., Liu D., Wang M., Wang L., Zeng F., Jiang G. (2017). *EMBO Rep* **18**(9), 1646–59

Liang Z.Z., Guo C., Zou M.M., Meng P., Zhang T.T. (2020). *Cancer Cell Int* **20**, 173

Lin C.W., Wang L.K., Wang S.P., Chang Y.L., Wu Y.Y., Chen H.Y., Hsiao T.H., Lai W.Y., Lu H.H., Chang Y.H., Yang S.C., Lin M.W., Chen C.Y., Hong T.M., Yang P.C. (2017). *Nat. Commun* **8**, 14502
Liu C.X., Chen L.L. (2022). *Cell* **185**(12), 2016–2034
Liu C.X., Guo S.K., Nan F., Xu Y.F., Yang L., Chen L.L. (2022). *Mol. Cell* **82**(2), 420–434
Liu X., Abraham J.M., Cheng Y., Wang Z., Zhang G., Ashktorab H., Smoot D.T., Cole R.N., Boronina T. N., DeVine L.R., Talbot C.C., Liu Z., Meltzer S.J. (2018). *Mol. Ther. Nucleic. Acids* **13**, 312–321
Liu X., Zhang Y., Zhou S., Dain L., Mei L., Zhu G. (2022). *J. Control Release* **348**, 84–94
Loan T., Chang K., James A., Li B. (2023). *Adv .Drug Deliv. Rev* **197**, 114826
Moon B., Chang S. (2022). *Cells* **11**, 316
Müller S., Wedler A., Breuer J., Glaß M., Bley N., Lederer M., Haase J., Misiak C., Fuchs T., Ottmann A., Schmachtel T., Shalamova L., Ewe A., Aigner A., Rossbach O., Hüttelmaier S. (2020). *NAR Cancer* **2**(3), zcaa014
Obi P., Chen T.G. (2021). *Methods* **196**, 85–103
Pan X., Wang Z.X., Wang R. (2010). *Cancer Biol. Ther* **10**(12), 1224–1232
Penaud-Budloo M., Francois A., Clement N., Ayuso E. (2018). *Mol. Ther. Methods Clin. Dev* **8**, 166–180
Rama A.R., Quiñonero F., Mesas C., Melguizo C., Prados J. (2022). *Int. J. Mol. Sci* **23**(6), 2963
Rausch J.W., Heinz W.F., Payea M.J., Sherpa C., Gorospe M., Le Grice S.F.J. (2021). *Nucleic, Acids. Res* **49** (6), e35
Salmena L., Poliseno L., Tay Y., Kats L., Pandolfi P.P. (2011). *Cell* **146**, 353–358
Shi L., Cao Y., Yuan W., Guo J., Sun G. (2022). *Cell Death Dis* **13**, 506
Siegel R.L., Miller K.D., Jemal A. (2019). *CA Cancer J. Clin* **69(1)**,7–34
Sun Y. (2015). *Med. Res. Rev* **35(2)**, 408–436
Tay F.C., Lim J.K., Zhu H., Hin L.C., Wang S. (2015). *Adv. Drug Deliv. Rev.* **81**, 117–127
Wang S., Liu F., Ma H., Cui X., Yang S., Qin R. (2020). *Clin. Breast Cancer* **20(5)**, 422–430
Wang Z., Ma K., Cheng Y., Abraham J.M., Liu X., Ke X., Wang Z., Meltzer S.J. (2019). *Lab Invest* **99**(10), 1442–1453
Wesselhoeft R.A., Kowalski P.S., Anderson D.G., *Nat. Commun* **9(1)**, 2629.
Xie B., Zhao Z., Liu Q., Wang X., Ma Z., Li H. (2019). *Gene* **683**, 253–261
Zhang F., Jiang J., Qian H., Yan Y., Xu W. (2023). *J. Hematol. Oncol* **16**(1), 67
Zhang L., Zhang J., Li P., Li T., Zhou Z., Wu H. (2022). *Cell Death. Dis* **13**, 32

Biological Sciences and Environmental Health – Gao (Ed.)

Application of nanomaterials in tumor microenvironment

Lingkai Zhang
China Pharmaceutical University, Nanjing, Jiangsu, China

ABSTRACT: Tumor microenvironment (TME) is primarily composed of immune cells, extracellular matrix, exosomes, and interstitial cells, making it a complicated system. The living environment of tumor cells is closely related to the occurrence, metastasis, and recurrence of tumors. Key characteristics of TME include hypoxia, low pH, high expression of H_2O_2 and glutathione, and immune suppression. These features can contribute to tumor metastasis, drug resistance development, and immune escape. Nanomaterials, as an emerging material, can not only regulate the TME in tumor therapy but also function as drug delivery systems to assist drug therapy. Modulating nanostructures can effectively improve the characteristics of the microenvironment, while nanodrug delivery systems can increase drug targeting, lower the occurrence of drug resistance, and reduce drug toxicity. This article reviews the applications of nanomaterials in these two areas and introduces the recent advancements and future prospects in the development of nanomaterials.

1 INTRODUCTION

Malignant tumors are one of the leading diseases threatening people's lives. Although current treatment methods have made significant progress, the limitations are still obvious. For some tumors that are difficult to treat, only conservative management can be used to prolong the lives of patients. As a closely related factor in tumor growth, tumor microenvironment (TME) often interacts with tumors, making it a viable target for the treatment of tumors. TME is mainly composed of immune cells, extracellular matrix, exosomes, and interstitial cells, forming a complex aggregate. The components of tumor environment tend to interact with each other, and they have a certain impact on the growth and development, deterioration, metastasis, and drug resistance of tumors. TME is characterized by low pH, high stiffness, high temperature, high expression of hydrogen peroxide (H_2O_2,) high levels of enzymes and glutathione (GSH), and severe hypoxia.

At present, numerous approaches have been proposed in the direction of TME, and nanomaterials have found applications in this area. Nanomaterials have the characteristics of strong modifiability, good biocompatibility, and flexible design. In practice, nanomaterials can be used to regulate TME, influencing the growth and progression of tumors, while responsive nanomaterials can serve as drug delivery systems, enhancing the specificity of drugs and precise control of drug dosage. This paper briefly summarizes the two primary applications of nanomaterials in TME, aiming to provide guidance to researchers in the field. The article will introduce these two application areas, focusing on their uses and limitations, and provide insights into future prospects.

DOI: 10.1201/9781003587590-23

2 MODULATING NANOSTRUCTURES

2.1 *O2*

Hypoxia, one of the main characteristics of TME, is often caused by abnormal development, uncontrolled division, and abnormal blood vessel formation near the tumor. Hypoxia can activate hypoxia-inducible factor (HIF) pathways for reverse use in tumor cells, such as PI3K/AKT/mTOR, MAPK, NF-kB, and other pathways related to hypoxia. These cytokines and signaling pathways activate genes, such as HIF and LOX genes, promoting tumor growth. Some studies have shown that the development of breast cancer is related to the inhibition of estrogen receptor 1 by HIF. Tamoxifen, a drug used for breast cancer, reduces HIF-1α levels by inhibiting mechanical induction of myosin-dependent contractile force and matrix stiffness (Cortes *et al.* 2019). In addition, this hypoxic microenvironment can also assist tumor cells in immune escape.

The current treatment plan for hypoxic microenvironment can be roughly divided into three stages: delivering oxygen to the interior of the tumor, generating oxygen inside the tumor, and regulating the hypoxic signaling pathway of the tumor. First, nanomaterials are used to introduce oxygen into tumor cells. In an experiment by Liu *et al.* polymeric nanoparticles coated with red blood cell membranes were synthesized (Gao *et al.* 2017). These nanoparticles achieved the goal of carrying oxygen by utilizing the efficient binding properties of fluorine atoms in PFC with oxygen. Due to the sensitivity of Bi_2Se_2 to near-infrared radiation, it can promote the release of oxygen in nanocarriers. This nanomaterial can be used in combination with radiotherapy to effectively improve the efficacy of radiotherapy. In addition, Yang *et al.* (2018) developed a multifunctional liposome, doxorubicin-loaded hemoglobin liposome (DHL), to reduce tumor hypoxia and chemotherapy resistance. In their experiment, hypoxic cells treated with DHL significantly reversed toward normoxic cells.

Second, hypoxia can be improved by transporting catalase or utilizing catalysis to produce O_2 from H_2O_2 within the tumor. In an experiment conducted by Mei *et al.* (2018), layered double hydroxides were used as the main structure, and monolayer hydrotalcite nanosheets were prepared by regulating the metal elements in the main layer and introducing metal ions such as cobalt and iron. This type of nanosheet can react with excessive H_2O_2 in TME, producing therapeutic reactive oxygen species (ROS) inside the tumor. In addition, manganese dioxide can also serve as an efficient H_2O_2 catalyst in nanomaterials. In their experiment, Liu *et al.* prepared manganese dioxide nanoparticles loaded with chloroprotein e6 (Ce6) with PEG modification, named Ce6@MnO_2 -PEG NPs, to enhance oxygen-dependent photodynamic therapy (Zhu *et al.* 2016). In addition to these, nanoenzymes with H_2O_2 catalytic properties are also a mainstream research direction now. Nanoenzymes can catalyze the activity of oxygen and H_2O_2 at acidic pH values, forming highly toxic ROS and killing tumor cells (Abdolahinia *et al.* 2022).

The third treatment strategy tends to use responsive nanodrug delivery systems to deliver drugs to the targeted locations of the signaling pathway. The hypoxic characteristics of TME are often linked to the drug resistance of tumors, and improving their hypoxic environment can to some extent alleviate the development of drug resistance.

2.2 *pH regulation*

According to the Warburg effect, even under aerobic conditions, tumor cells will convert a large amount of glucose into lactic acid through glycolysis. With the continuous accumulation of lactic acid, TME exhibits acidic characteristics. This mildly acidic environment is conducive to tumor invasion and metastasis. Also, the mild acidic nature of TME can cause reversible inactivation of tumor-infiltrating lymphocytes, while regulating the acidity of TME can restore the body's immune clearance function. Currently, there are two mainstream strategies to address this: (1) consuming excess H^+ in TME; and (2) inhibiting gene expression to reduce lactate production, thereby reducing H^+.

Som *et al.* (2016) prepared $CaCO_3$ nanoparticles, which when injected into mice, continuously consumed H^+ in TME. By modifying nanomaterials, tumor-target specificity can be achieved. $CaCO_3$ nanoparticles are also effective as responsive drug delivery systems, and their other uses will be discussed later. Zhang *et al.* (2019) utilized cationic lipid nanoparticle vesicles to encapsulate small interfering RNA, which reduced lactate production by decreasing the expression of lactate dehydrogenase, thereby improving the acidity of TME. Low pH levels in TME often have adverse effects on drugs, and regulating pH is beneficial for the effectiveness of drugs against tumors.

2.3 *Redox properties*

Compared to normal cells, there is more H_2O_2 in TME. In response to the damage caused by this strong oxidative stress, tumor cells produce GSH at levels 100 times higher than in the blood. Tumors can be treated by regulating their intrinsic redox balance. For this unique equilibrium, Gao *et al.* (2017) studied a Zr/Ce MOFs/DOX/MnO_2 composite material that not only regulates H_2O_2 and GSH in TME but also has a high drug loading capacity for doxorubicin. In addition, they synthesized a composite material of Prussian blue nanoparticles and zirconium-based metal-organic framework (UIO-66-NH_2), which was targeted and delivered to tumor cells to catalyze the production of O_2 and regulate the hypoxic environment (Haiqing 2022). This material can also achieve synergistic treatment of photothermal-promoted catalytic therapy under imaging guidance, improving the effectiveness of tumor treatment.

In the report by Li *et al.* they proposed a multifunctional therapeutic nanoassembly (PZTC/SS/HA) that encapsulates photosensitizer in Cu^{2+}-phenolic nanocapsules with disulfide bonds and hyaluronic acid (Sun *et al.* 2023). Around tumor cells, disulfide bonds can consume GSH, while phenolic nanocapsules can release photosensitizer and copper ions in acidic environments. Under the irradiation of near-infrared-II, copper sulfide photothermal nanoagent was generated. This innovative design forms a highly efficient combination therapy method.

2.4 *Immune system*

In TME, some differences from the normal cellular environment often lead to the resistance of tumor cells to the immune system. Tumor cells can not only evade immune detection but also promote their own growth and development through cytokines released by immune cells. Some literature categorizes them into direct and indirect immunosuppressive factors. The main representatives of direct immunosuppressive factors are M2 phenotype macrophages, myeloid-derived suppressor cells, Treg cells, adenosine, and tumor cells themselves. The immunosuppressive microenvironment created by these immunosuppressive factors has led to poor efficacy of some immunotherapies. Immune checkpoint blockade (ICB) therapy, an advanced means of resisting tumor progression, can activate those T cells and bypass immune evasion by tumor cells. However, for this complex immunosuppressive microenvironment, the objective response rate of ICB therapy is not ideal (Zhang *et al.* 2022). Additionally, immune checkpoint inhibitors may cause immune-related adverse events (irAEs). Nanomaterials can not only help improve the immunosuppressive microenvironment of tumors but also target the delivery of drugs to the interior of tumors, reducing the degree of side effects and playing an undeniable role in tumor treatment.

To address these issues, Wang *et al.* (2022) studied a type of PVA peptide conjugate. Under the influence of overexpressed TME matrix metalloproteinases in TME, this material can be decomposed and then self-assembled, forming nanofibers to help PD-L1 inhibitors accumulate at the tumor site. This shows the therapeutic feasibility of the strategy of in vivo recombination.

In the report by Yang *et al.* (2018), they discussed the current development status of iron-based nanomaterials. In the direction of immune regulation, iron-based nanomaterials can promote the polarization of TAMs (tumor-associated macrophages) phenotype and induce immunogenic death, and they can also collaborate with other immune cells for treatment. Fe_3O_4 can enter TAMs and be absorbed by lysosomes, with the released iron inducing TAMs to polarize toward the M1 phenotype. A large number of M1 phenotypes can also reshape the surrounding M2 phenotype through paracrine action (Fei *et al.* 2023).

3 NANODRUG DELIVERY SYSTEM

3.1 *pH response*

Acidic TME (pH 6.5–6.8) can serve as an effective target for tumor treatment. In response to this characteristic, a good nanodrug delivery system should not release its contents in a neutral environment of the blood system, but in the acidic TME. Currently, there are two main types of nanodrug delivery systems for pH response: protonation and chemical bond breakage.

Jafari *et al.* (2022) mention a graphene oxide nanomaterial based on pH response. They assembled graphene oxide and DOX into a hydroxyuronic acid chitosan-g-poly. In acidic environments, amine matrix substitution in the DOX structure results in the disappearance of hydrogen bonds between the DOX and graphene oxide. However, the pH in the TME considered is not low enough for this to be used as the main release method.

Doxorubicin is a traditional chemotherapy drug. The accumulation of it in the body can cause serious toxic side effects. There have been many studies on nanodrug deliveries targeting doxorubicin (Zhang *et al.* 2022). Many researchers have used pH-sensitive groups to bind doxorubicin to the nanoskeleton, which allows this system to release drugs in acidic TME.

3.2 *Redox response*

As mentioned earlier, there is an excess of H_2O_2 and GSH in TME. This subtle redox balance can also serve as a response site for the drug delivery system. For the strong oxidizing properties of ROS in TME, thioketal bonds are a good choice. For excessive GSH in the environment, disulfide bonds are currently a widely studied topic (Shen 2022). Additionally, Zhang *et al.* (2015) used phenylborate esters and β-cyclodextrin to synthesize ROS-responsive nanocarriers for in vivo delivery of the anti-tumor drug PTX.

3.3 *Others*

In addition to the two response types mentioned above, there are also ATP response types, enzyme response types, and hypoxia response types. Wang (2020), in his report, constructed an ovarian cancer microenvironment matrix metalloproteinases and ATP-responsive nanodrug delivery system. He embedded doxorubicin hydrochloride (DOX) into a DNA double helix structure rich in C⊠G base pairs to complete drug loading, improve its efficacy in the treatment of ovarian cancer, and reduce toxic side effects. At present, single-response nanosystems can no longer meet research needs, and more and more researchers are exploring multiresponse nanodrug delivery systems to achieve more accurate drug delivery and enhanced functionality.

4 RESTRICTION

4.1 *Modulating nanostructures*

In the modulation of nanostructures, the non-specific accumulation of metal-based nanoparticles in healthy tissues can cause systemic toxicity, and ensuring biosafety is challenging. Additionally, low tissue permeability prevents nanomaterials from infiltrating into tumor cells, making it difficult to fully utilize their potential.

4.2 *Nanodrug delivery system*

In the context of nanodrug delivery systems, rapid growth and mutation of malignant tumors make the tumor environment unpredictable and unstable, hindering precise drug release through responsive nanocarriers. For some protein drugs that need to function within cells, many reported nanodrug carriers still have defects in transmembrane transfer and lysosomal escape. Moreover, the production of multiresponse nanosystem carriers is relatively difficult, requiring significant time and financial resources for research.

4.3 *Common defects*

First, there are differences among different tumor patients, making it difficult to determine the applicability of treatments. Also, there are few clinical studies on related materials.

5 CONCLUSION

It is evident from the above discussion of the literature that research on regulatory nanomaterials focuses more on the properties of nanomaterials and nanomaterial matrices, while research on responsive nanomedicine delivery systems focuses on the chemical bonds between nanomaterials and drugs. Compared to regulatory nanomaterials, nanodrug delivery systems are more inclined toward the existence of auxiliary drugs, with some regulatory materials also playing the role of drug delivery systems. These two types of materials differ in their mechanisms, but some excellent nanomaterials can handle both tasks.

Current research is no longer limited to single functional nanomaterials. Nanomaterials that integrate diagnosis and treatment, as well as respond to and regulate the environment, are increasingly appearing in the literature. This is a sign of progress. As an emerging material, the potential of nanomaterials is undoubtedly immense. In tumor treatment, they are currently playing a more auxiliary role. However, their role cannot be underestimated, and their impact is significant in reducing drug toxicity. At the same time, they also allow some drugs that were originally limited to a type of cancer to expand their treatment scope. The most typical type is ICB inhibitors, which have poor therapeutic effects on solid tumors, but when paired with nanomaterials, they can also cause certain damage to tumor cells, which is one of the exciting characteristics of nanomaterials.

In addition, although nanomaterials have limitations in biocompatibility and their tissue permeability has not yet met the required standards, recent literature has shown progress in addressing these issues. It is believed that these challenges will be overcome in the future, and nanomaterial combination therapies may become a mainstream method of tumor treatment.

REFERENCES

Abdolahinia E., Fathi M., Pirdel Z., Jafari S., Samiei M., Adibkia K., Sefat F., Dizaj S.M., Sharifi S. (2022) *Open Nano* **8**, 100100

Cortes E., Lachowski D., Robinson B., Sarper M., Teppo J.S., Thorpe S.D., Lieberthal T.J., Iwamoto K., Lee D.A., Okada-Hatakeyama M., Varjosalo M.T., Hernández A.E. (2019). *EMBO Rep* **20**, e46557

Fei K., Chang G., Yan C. (2023). *Chinese Journal of Hospital Pharmacy* **43**, 458–463

Gao M., Liang C., Song X., Chen Q., Jin Q., Wang C., Liu Z. (2017). *Adv. Mater* **29**, 1701429

Haiqing G. (2022). Hubei University.

Jafari A., Chenab K., Malektaj H., Farshchi F., Ghorbani S., Ghasemiamineh A., Khoshakhlagh M., Ashtari B. (2022). *Flat. Chem* **34**, 100381

Mei X., Liang R., Wei M. (2018). *Handbook of the 14th National Bioinorganic Chemistry Conference of the Chinese Chemical Society*, **1**

Shen Q. (2022). Nanhua University.

Som A., Raliya R., Tian L.M. (2016). *Nanoscale* **8**, 12639–12647

Sun X., Liang X., Wang Y., Ma P., Xiong W., Qian S., Cui Y., Zhang H., Chen X., Tian F., Shi Y., Zheng F., Li L. (2023). *Biomaterials* **301**, 122263

Wang K. (2020). Tianjin Medical University

Wang T., He Z., Yuan C., Deng Z., Li F., Chen X., Liu Y. (2022). *J. Control. Release* **343**, 765–776

Yang J., Li W., Luo L., Jiang M., Zhu C., Qin B., Yin H., Yuan X., Yin X., Zhang J., Luo Z., Du Y., You J. (2018). *Biomaterials* **182**, 145–156

Zhang D., Wei Y., Chen K. (2015). *Advanced Healthcare Materials* **4**, 69–76

Zhang W., Guo H., Pan X. (2022). *Pharmaceutical Progress* **46**, 910–921

Zhang Y., Zhou R., Deng P. (2022). *Chemical Technology*, **30**-76P.

Zhang Y.X., Zhao Y.Y., Shen J.Z., *Nano Lett* **19**, 2774–2783 (2019)

Zhu W., Dong Z., Fu T., Liu J., Chen Q., Li Y., Zhu R., Xu L., Liu Z. (2016). *Adv. Funct. Mater* **26**, 5490–5498.

Biological Sciences and Environmental Health – Gao (Ed.)

BNCT: A promising treatment approach for head and neck cancer

Jinxiang Huang
Faculty of Science, The University of Hong Kong, Hong Kong, China

ABSTRACT: Head and neck squamous cell carcinoma (HNSCC) is a general term for cancers that develop on the epidermis of the oral cavity, pharynx, and larynx. The boron neutron capture therapy (BNCT) has been used to treat cancers, including head and neck cancer. The first step of the BNCT is the intake of boron atoms. Boron vectors, administered as boron drugs, are infused into patients. These vectors have a high affinity for cancer cell proteins, leading to the accumulation of boron in cancer cells, with the subsequent application of thermal neutron beams. The thermal neutrons are captured by boron atoms, initiating a fission process. The fission releases high linear energy transfer alpha particles and lithium atoms in opposite directions, which then destroy the cancer cells. Due to limited energy and precise targeting, BNCT minimizes damage to normal cells like most chemotherapies nowadays. However, there have been challenges in the application of the BNCT, including the experimental evaluation of compound biological effectiveness value and the creation of a new vector for boron. This review discusses the anticancer effects of the BNCT against HNSCC, focusing on the mechanisms and actions of the BNCT and the technical development of vectors and neutron sources. Ongoing clinical trials and challenges of recent research on BNCT are also discussed. Future studies are required to explore the application of BNCT beyond head and neck cancer to other types of cancers.

1 INTRODUCTION

Head and neck cancer is one of the most common malignant tumors (Bray *et al.* 2018). Of these, the pathological types of squamous cell carcinoma pose a significant public health threat. In China, the morbidity of head and neck squamous cell carcinoma (HNSCC) has been ranked sixth in incidence and seventh in cancer-related mortality (Bray *et al.* 2018). Statistically, the probability of encountering HNSCC in males is two to four times more than in females, particularly those addicted to alcohol or tobacco. Each year, approximately seven million patients suffer from HNSCC, with three million fatalities dying of HNSCC (Bray *et al.* 2018).

A new and effective treatment, boron neutron capture therapy (BNCT), has been developed to replace chemotherapy for head and neck cancer, which is highly toxic to human bodies. BNCT works by coupling boron atoms with cancer cells using boron vectors. When exposed to thermal neutron beams, the fission of the boron atom is activated to release an alpha particle and a lithium atom. The energetic alpha particle destroys the boron-coupled cancer cells without leaving excess energy to harm surrounding healthy cells (He, Yang and Kong 2022).

This review summarizes the action principles of BNCT, covering its basic theory, a brief introduction to the components of BNCT and their functions, as well as research related to vectors, neutron sources, accelerators, and treatment equipment for head and neck cancer. Additionally, it discusses clinical trials for treating head and neck cancer by BNCT,

DOI: 10.1201/9781003587590-24

compares BNCT with other therapeutic methods for HNSCC, and examines the limitations and challenges of BNCT.

2 ACTION PRINCIPLE OF BNCT

BNCT is a novel technique for the treatment of head and neck cancer. The mechanism involves accumulating a high concentration of boron-10B in cancer cells through a boron-based drug (He *et al.* 2022). The patient is then exposed to a thermal neutron beam from the neutron source. When the neutron is captured by the boron atom, fission occurs on the boron atom, releasing an alpha particle with high energy and a lithium-7 atom, which radiate in opposite directions to specifically target the cancer cells (He *et al.* 2022). The alpha radiation and lithium nuclei are high in linear energy transfer, ionizing adjacent tissue in the reaction site within a range of 5 to 9 micrometers (Jin *et al.* 2022). Since the range is relatively limited compared to human cells, the concentration gathering in the cancer cells should be high enough, which can be determined by the transport effectiveness of the boron vectors. However, this limited range ensures that the surrounding healthy cells would not be affected, provided the boron vectors accurately deliver boron to the cancer cells. Based on the mechanism, the key components of BNCT are the boron atoms, the vector of boron atoms, and the neutron source (He *et al.* 2022), which should be optimized based on different types and stages of cancer, conditions of patients, as well as other realistic factors.

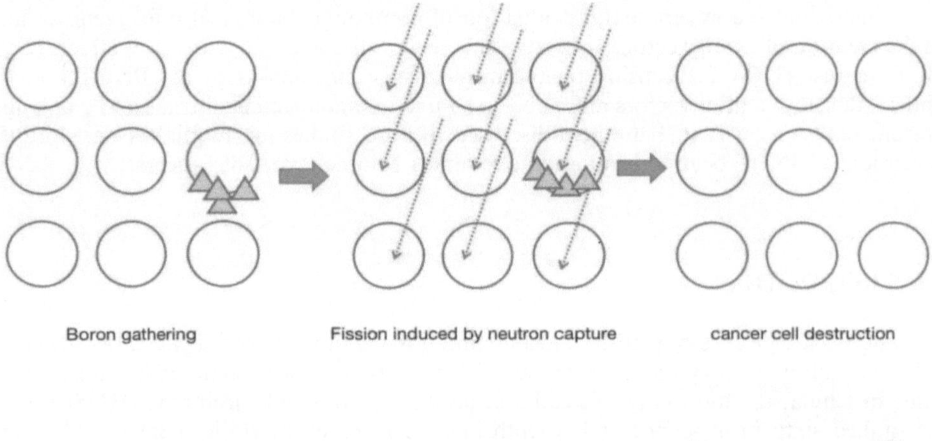

Figure 1. Mechanism of BNCT. Boron gathering can target cancer cells. Next, with the incident of thermal neutron beams, fission of boron atoms is induced. Alpha particles are released and destroy cancer cells. Figure credit: Original.

3 TREATMENT OF HNSCC WITH BNCT

3.1 *Vector of boron*

For treating HNSCC, the choice of boron vector is crucial. In recent times, mainly two types of vectors have been used, which include borocaptate sodium (BSH) and boronophenylalanine (BPA). The BSH vector comprising ten boron atoms is mainly used in the treatment of malignant cerebral glioma due to its polyhedral borocaptate structure (He *et al.*

2022). However, the ionic structure is not able to pass the blood-brain barrier. However, in some cases, cancer cells may destroy the blood-brain barrier, BSH remains unsuitable for transporting boron atoms to the HNSCC cells in the head when the blood-brain barrier is intact. BPA, synthesized by Snyder, utilizes the L-type amino transporters present in the human body for transporting boron atoms to the membranes of cancer cells (Miyabe *et al.* 2019), making it suitable for gathering boron atoms on HNSCC cells.

3.2 *Neutron source of BNCT*

After selecting the boron vector, the neutron source should be carefully considered. Traditionally, heated neutrons from nuclear reactors, produced as byproducts, have been used as a source for BNCT. However, due to the risks associated with nuclear reactors, including nuclear contamination, leakage, etc., most nuclear reactors are no longer permitted to be used (Kessler *et al.* 2014). To address this, the accelerator-based BNCT (ab-BNCT) was developed as an alternative to counter the problem of the lack of nuclear reactors. In this method, an accelerator is used to accelerate protons or deuterium ions to bombard lithium or beryllium, inducing fission in these metals and producing neutrons (He *et al.* 2022). One of the most reliable methods is bombarding lithium-7 with protons at an average energy of 2.5 MeV, generating neutrons with a maximum energy of 0.8 MeV, which is lower and safer than that produced by nuclear reactors. In addition to lower energy, accelerators offer advantages such as reduced radioactive waste, greater control, easier installation and maintenance, and lower cost compared to nuclear reactors (He *et al.* 2022).

3.3 *Procedures of BNCT*

With an appropriate choice of boron vector and source of neutrons, the first step of BNCT involves the intravenous administration of a boron drug. Patients receive a BPA solution via vein infusion over a specific period (Nakaxima 2022). The boron drug is transported through blood vessels approaching the blood-brain barrier, utilizing L-type amino transporters (LATs), which are sodium-independent and pH-neutral transport proteins. The LATs, which are responsible for transporting necessary amino acids, including phenylalanine, are abundant in brain microvascular endothelial cells. The phenylalanine ion component of BPA combines with LATs, allowing it to cross the blood-brain barrier, enter the central nervous system, and accumulate in the HNSCC cells (Nakaxima 2022).

After a period of slow infusion, a blood boron test is recommended to ensure that the boron atoms have properly targeted the cancer cells. To conduct the test, a fresh blood sample (half of a gram) of the patient is collected and mixed with beryllium solution and 0.1% Triton X-100 solution. The mixture is analyzed using specialized devices, such as the Agilent 5100 ICP-OES, aided by supporting software (Anttonen *et al.* 2023). Once the test confirms the proper orientation of the boron atoms, the proton accelerator device is triggered to generate a proton beam with an average energy of 2.5 MeV, which bombards metals, specifically lithium-7. This fission releases high-energy neutron beams that are directed toward the affected area by the neutron irradiation equipment. The boron atoms gathering on the cancer cells capture the beam of thermal neutrons and induce fission. An energetic alpha particle is emitted to destroy the cancer cells selectively since the strength of radiation is only sufficient to pass across one cell.

4 COMPARISON OF BNCT AND CETUXIMAB

Nowadays, cetuximab, a molecularly targeted drug for head and neck cancer, is widely used in a treatment called bioradiotherapy (BRT), which combines cetuximab with radiotherapy. Compared with chemotherapy, the cetuximab BRT reduces the effects of platinum accumulation but is less effective compared to BNCT. Additionally, BRT still carries the risk associated with radiotherapy, which can damage healthy cells indiscriminately. BNCT, on the other hand, neither has serious negative effects or toxins as CRT nor low effectiveness as BRT. Unlike BRT, which involves harmful emissions of gamma beams, BNCT uses safer thermal neutrons for boron fission (He *et al.* 2022). Thus, BNCT treatment poses less risk of radio side effects caused by gamma beams and offers a promising treatment with significant curative potential (Sakashita *et al.* 2015).

5 CHALLENGES FOR BNCT

5.1 *CBE value*

Despite the therapeutic effect of BNCT, there are challenges for its applications. One of the primary challenges for BNCT is the experimental evaluation of CBE value (He *et al.* 2022). During BNCT, cancer and normal cells are exposed to three different sorts of linear energy transfer (LET), which include high LET alpha particles, the low LET gamma beams during neutron capture, and the high LET protons from neutron capture by nitrogen atoms (He *et al.* 2022). Under the same physical condition, the high LET particles have higher biological effectiveness than the low LET particles. This phenomenon is called relative biological effectiveness (RBE). Evaluating the RBE of BNCT is essential for determining the safety and curative effect of BNCT. To evaluate the RBE accurately, the data of combined biological effectiveness and CBE must be determined (Fukuda 2021). Therefore, developing a reliable method to evaluate the CBE of cancer both clinically and experimentally is a significant step for the development of BNCT.

5.2 *Vectors of boron*

Another challenge in BNCT is developing new boron vectors. Two key aspects must be considered in the development of vectors. First, the vector must effectively target cancer cells and ensure a high concentration of boron on the cancer cells. The vector should be compatible with the human body and traced clearly in pharmacokinetics and pharmacodynamics, including factors such as metabolism, polarity, clearance, half-life, etc. In addition, to keep the boron concentration, each vector should take enough boron atoms and form stable bonds, such as a hydrolyzed chain (He *et al.* 2022). The second challenge is the potential toxicity of the vector itself. Although many large biological molecules can carry enough boron and form stable bonding, they can also be harmful by bonding to healthy cells, resulting in side effects similar to gamma radiotherapy.

Based on the two aspects, the number of boron vectors is extremely limited, indicating the relatively restricted use of BNCT in only a few types of cancers. Therefore, developing new vectors is essential to expanding BNCT's application to a wider range of cancers, although this requires advanced molecular techniques.

6 CLINICAL TRIALS FOR BNCT

6.1 *Application of BNCT on head and neck cancer*

Several clinical trials of BNCT on head and neck cancers have been approved. Hirose and his team applied BNCT to 21 patients with recurrent or locally advanced head and neck cancer (Hirose *et al.* 2020). The results showed a significant reduction in tumor size in all the patients, with no major side effects reported. After 90 days, some autoimmune encephalitis (AE) was observed, including alopecia, but no serious AE beyond grade 4 was detected (Anttonen *et al.* 2023). These data indicated that for patients with recurrent head and neck

R-SCC or R/LA-nSCC, BNCT is a promising treatment option with relatively low toxicity, as no severe AE typical of gamma chemotherapy was observed.

6.2 *Application of BNCT using CICS-1 accelerators*

Ongoing clinical trials are exploring the application of BNCT by CICS-1 accelerators. In one such trial, BNCT was used to treat angiosarcoma (ClinicalTrials.gov ID NCT05601232). Surgeries and chemotherapy have been proven ineffective for these patients. However, BNCT has shown the potential to prolong patients' lives, making it a promising treatment option (ClinicalTrials.gov ID NCT05601232). Therefore, BNCT could represent a breakthrough in the treatment of cancers more effectively and safely.

6.3 *Application of combined treatment of BNCT and Cetuximab*

Another noteworthy study is the coupled treatment of BNCT and Cetuximab. As previously mentioned, Cetuximab is less effective in cancer cell destruction. However, when combined with BNCT, a remarkable curative improvement in both the biological effects of Cetuximab and the physical effects of BNCT is expected to be observed (ClinicalTrials.gov ID NCT00927147). However, this research was interrupted due to the shutdown of the nuclear reactor used as a neutron source. With the development of ab-BNCT, it is expected that the study will be rerun with the support of an accelerator as a new source of neutrons.

Table 1. Clinical trials of BNCT.

Clinical trials	Objectives	Outcomes	Conclusion	Reference/ID
Application of BNCT in head and neck cancer	21 head and neck cancer patients treated with BNCT	Significant tumor size reduction. Only grade 4 or lower AE was observed.	BNCT is effective in cancer cell destruction with less side effects.	Hirose *et al.* 2020
Application of BNCT by CICS-1 accelerators	Patients who cannot be treated with other therapies received ab-BNCT	Patients' lives were prolonged	BNCT is a breakthrough for treating cancers untreatable with existing therapies.	ClinicalTrials.gov ID NCT05601232
Application of coupled treatment of BNCT and Cetuximab	Patients who cannot be treated by other therapies are treated by coupled treatment of BNCT and Cetuximab.	Research was interrupted due to shutdown of nuclear reactor as a source of thermal neutron	the research is expected to be rerun with the development of ab-BNCT recently.	ClinicalTrials.gov ID NCT00927147

BNCT = Boron neutron capture therapy.

7 CONCLUSION

Head and neck cancer is one of the most common types of malignant tumors worldwide. BNCT, a novel therapy that destroys cancer cells via alpha particles produced from neutron-capture-induced fission of boron atoms, is promising due to its few side effects, low radial toxicity, and higher safety compared with chemotherapy and surgeries. While technical challenges remain to be solved through further research, BNCT shows immense potential. Once these issues are resolved, BNCT could treat more sorts of cancers with a better curative effect compared to Cetuximab. In short, BNCT, with its effective BPA vector and accelerator-based technology, is already a mature treatment for HNSCC. Future advancements in boron vectors and proton accelerators may allow BNCT to treat most solid tumors.

REFERENCES

Anttonen A., Tenhunen M. and Joensuu H. (2023). *Cancer Biother. Radio*, **38**

Bray F., Ferlay J., Soerjomataram I., Siegel R. L., Torre L. A. and Jemal A. (2018). *CA Cancer J. Clin*, **68**, 394–424

Fukuda H. (2021). *Cells*, **10**

He H., Yang Y. and Kong L. (2022). *China Medical Equipment*, **19**, 164–168

Hirose K., Konno A., Hiratsuka J., Yoshimoto S., Kato T., Ono K., Otsuki N., Hatazawa J., Tanaka H., Takayama K., Wada H., Suzuki M., Sato M., Yamaguchi H., Seto I., Ueki Y., Iketani S., Imai S., Nakamura T., Ono T., Endo H., Azami Y., Kikuchi Y., Murakami M. and Takai Y. (2020). *Radiotherapy and Oncology*, **155**, 182–187

Kessler G., Veser A., Schlüter F., Raskob W., Landman C. and Päsler-Sauer J. (2014). *The Risks of Nuclear Energy Technology*

Miyabe J., Ohgakia R., Saito K., Wei L., Quan L., Jin C., Liu X., Okuda S., Nagamori S., Ohki H., Yoshino K., Inohara H. and Kanai Y. (2019). *Int. J. Pharm. Sci. Res*, **139**, 215–222

Nakaxima H. (2022). *Pharmaceutical Research Department*, YAKUGAKU ZASSHI, **142**, 155–164

Sakashita T., Homma A., Hatakeyama H., Furusawa J., Kano S., Mizumachi T., Iizuka S., Onimaru R., Tsuchiya K., Yasuda K., Shirato H. and Fukuda S. (2015). *Acta Oto-Laryngologica*, **135**, 853–858

Will H. Jin, C. Seldon, Butkus M., Sauerwein W. and Giap H. B. (2022). *Int. J. Part. Ther*, **9**, 71–82

Biological Sciences and Environmental Health – Gao (Ed.)

Lipid nanoparticle technology in liver-directed gene therapy

Wangwang Zhong
East China University of Science and Technology, Shanghai, China

ABSTRACT: Every year, approximately two million individuals pass away from liver diseases worldwide. Liver diseases such as hepatitis, hepatocellular carcinoma, hepatic veno-occlusive, and liver fibrosis, can be caused by genetic disorders. For nucleic acid drugs to be more clinically effective against liver diseases and to reduce side effects on the human body, it is crucial that they are delivered safely and efficiently to the target locations. Lipid nanoparticle (LNP) technology, the most mature non-viral delivery platform, has potential clinical applications in hepatic target locations. This review summarizes the difficulties in delivering nucleic acid drugs and recent studies about LNP technology in gene therapy, with a particular emphasis on the LNP-siRNA system used in liver-directed cells. Using ionizable lipids with suitable pKa as delivery systems to carry siRNA was found to be an effective solution for gene silencing in hepatocyte cells as the result of endocytosis and natural accumulated mechanism. Further research may focus on clinical applications of LNP technology in extrahepatic diseases.

1 INTRODUCTION

Worldwide, more than two million lose their lives because of hepatic diseases annually, including one million from cirrhosis and one million from hepatocellular carcinoma, viral hepatitis et al, which pose a huge threat to human health (Eaton *et al.* 2019). Diseases like hepatitis, cirrhosis, fatty liver disease and autoimmune liver disease are the most common liver disorders. They may significantly affect the liver's capacity in metabolism, detoxification, and synthesis of proteins, fats, and carbohydrates in addition to causing liver damage (Kang 2016). Furthermore, as more genetic causes or risk loci are discovered, a growing number of uncommon liver illnesses are getting recognized.

There have been significant attempts made to create drugs specifically for the liver as a result of unhealthy lifestyles, which largely pose a threat to the liver condition, considering the insufficient therapeutic effectiveness of presently existing medications. Due to the advancement of nucleic acid therapeutics, it is gradually becoming clinically feasible to treat some of rare liver disorders by focusing on their hereditary origins. Theoretically, nucleic acid treatments offer the possibility to adjust any piece of gene, both in RNA and DNA, compared to small molecule chemicals and biological products (Leone *et al.* 2022). To be more specific, the initial study mainly focused on the possibility to induce gene silencing by inhibiting the production of pathological or mutant proteins. However, for the situation of protein deficiencies, gene editing can play a role in repairing damaged genes. Moreover, gene expression can directly produce specific proteins to treat diseases. All the mechanisms above are able to run effectively in the liver as it is one of the organs with the most blood in addition to the regular pattern of human metabolism (first-pass elimination), which means that therapeutics can accumulate perfectly in the liver.

DOI: 10.1201/9781003587590-25

Delivery is the main issue hindering the clinical application of nucleic acid drugs. The key factors contributing to the problem of delivery include nucleic acids' physicochemical characteristics, rapid renal clearance *in vivo*, the elimination of serum nuclease activity, and the activation of innate immunity (Hope and Cullis 2017). For these reasons, nucleic acids may not accumulate in target tissues after systemic injection or enter target cells.

A range of delivery platforms were investigated in order to overcome these obstacles (Schaffer and Kotterman 2014; Vegas *et al.* 2013; Whitehead and Hajj 2017). Non-viral vector systems have the most potentials to deliver nucleic acid substances because of larger payloads, multi-dosing capabilities, ease of manufacture, flexibility of design and reduced immune responses. The LNP system, a liposomal system that contains lipids organized in a bilayer structure, is currently the most mature non-viral platform for enabling gene therapies (Dowdy and Springer 2018).

This review summarizes the difficulties of delivering nucleic acids and strategies to deliver nucleic acids by LNP technology, with a particular emphasis on the research about the LNP-siRNA system used in liver-targeted locations, and finally makes predictions for further applications of LNP technology.

2 LNP TECHNOLOGY FOR DELIVERING NUCLEIC ACID DRUGS

2.1 *Difficulties for delivery of nucleic acids*

It is apparent that unmodified nucleic acid substances have limited bioavailability as therapeutics becasue of poor activity and inability to accumulate at target sites. Precisely, for the naked DNA or RNA molecules, the serum nuclease activity and the activation of innate immunity represent first and second barriers respectively. Even after heavily modified, nucleic acids may be able to escape from immune system and serum nuclease, they are still subject to renal filtration as the third barrier (Dunbar *et al.* 2018; Witzigmann *et al.* 2019).

Predosing negatively charged polymers like dextran sulfate has been used to try to increase the bioavailability of nucleic acid medications (Takakura *et al.* 1995). However, this doesn't guarantee that the nucleic acids will preferentially concentrate at target areas. Internalization through endocytosis is problematic since the endocytic route ends in fusion with lysosomes, which break down nucleic acid substances. The DNA or RNA vectors need to avoid endosomes and enter the cell cytoplasm in order to maintain function constantly.

2.2 *Strategies for the delivery of nucleic acid drugs by LNP*

For a variety of uses, gene treatments enabled by LNPs are now being developed clinically (Table 1). However, in order to adapt LNP technology for genetic therapeutics, it was necessary to develop strategies for encapsulating RNA and DNA polymers into LNP systems effectively.

Table 1. Lipid nanoparticle (LNP) technology products approved by FDA and EMA in different development stages.

Product	Company/ Institution	Mechanism	Nucleic acid substances	Conditions	Administration Method	Development Stage
EDIT-301	Editas Medicine	Gene Editing	mRNA-Cas9	Transfusion Dependent Beta Thalassemia	i.v.	Phase II (Recruiting) NCT05444894
NTLA-2002	Intellia Therapeutics	Gene Editing	mRNA-Cas9	Hereditary Angioedema	i.v.	Phase II (Recruiting) NCT05120830

(*continued*)

Table 1. Continued

Product	Company/ Institution	Mechanism	Nucleic acid substances	Conditions	Administration Method	Development Stage
BNT111	BioNTech	Gene Expression	mRNA	Melanoma	i.v.	Phase I (Recruiting) NCT04526899
BNT142	BioNTech	Gene Expression	mRNA	Solid tumors	i.v.	Phase II (Recruiting)
mRNA-4157	Mordena TX	Gene Expression	mRNA	Melanoma vaccine	i.v.	Phase I (Recruiting) NCT03313778
Onpattro®	Alnylam Pharmaceuticals	Gene Silencing	siRNA-TTR	ATTRv amyloidosis	i.v.	Approved (2018)
Atu027	Silence Therapeutics	Gene Silencing	siRNA-PKN3	Pancreatic Cancer	i.v.	Phase I/II (Completed) NCT01808638
DCR-MYC	Dicerna Pharmaceuticals	Gene Silencing	dsRNA-MYC	Hepatocellular Carcinoma	i.v.	Phase Ib/II (Completed) NCT02314052

Previous studies have illustrated that LNP systems are a type of liposomal system that contain lipids organized in a bilayer structure. These systems have been used for the delivery of small molecular drugs, particularly in cancer treatment (Maeda 2012), which has led to improved tumor delivery and therapeutic benefits. In fact, the design criteria for LNP systems has been very reliably set up, so the optimization process for specific needs usually depends on the selection of the components and the techniques of production.

Emlpoying ionizable cationic lipids (i.e. DODAP and DODMA), in addition to the optimization of a method for ethanol-loading, has allowed for efficient encapsulation of genetic drugs into small LNPs with low surface charge. The ethanol-loading process was achieved under high-concentration ethanol conditions with mixing preformed LNPs containing ionizable cationic lipids and siRNA or oligonucleotides. This process has been further refined with techniques such as T-tube mixing and microfluidic mixing to achieve more rapid and controlled encapsulation. Several crucial performances for an *in vivo* delivery system contained nucleic acid drugs including rapid formulation, high encapsulation efficiency, adjustable size, stability, and low surface charge can be realized through modified processes.

Although it is very clear that the structure of LNP siRNA systems consists of a hydrophobic core of lipid-loaded oligonucleotides covered by PEG-lipid layers, the structure of LNP system to deliver mRNA is still being determined, but apparently the ethanol-loading technique has potential to be utilized to efficiently encapsulate mRNA and other negatively charged entities.

3 LNP TECHNOLOGY FOR LIVER-TARGETED GENE THERAPY

3.1 *Physiological structure and pathological changes of liver*

The liver, the most important organ for animals, has more than 500 functions such as immune responses, metabolism, and protein production. Liver cells can be generally divided into parenchymal and nonparenchymal cells. The parenchymal cells are the main cells that make up the liver and are highly differentiated cells. Non parenchymal cells of the liver include liver macrophages (i.e. Kupffer cells), hepatic stellate cells, liver related lymphocytes, and hepatic sinusoidal endothelial cells. Hepatocyte migration, proliferation, and differentiation are regulated by non-parenchymal cells through their interactions with hepatocytes. Non-parenchymal cells play a number of different tasks. They serve important roles in immunological responses, the pathophysiology of liver disorders, and the metabolic responses to potentially harmful substances. Particularly, they create a functional network with hepatocytes (Arias and Gissen 2015).

Pathological changes in the liver are morphological and structural changes in liver tissue that reflect the pathological process of liver disease. Due to a number of reasons, such as viral infection, excessive alcohol consumption, drug intoxication, malnutrition, and immune disorders, the liver can be damaged to varying degrees, leading to the onset and progression of liver diseases. Pathologic changes in liver pathology are the different types of lesions in these diseases. Pathological changes in liver pathology mainly include changes in the size, color, and hardness of the liver under visual observation, as well as histological and cytological changes. Histologic changes mainly include changes in terms of hepatocyte lesions, fibrosis, necrosis, and regeneration, whereas cytologic changes involve changes in a variety of cell types in the liver, such as hepatocytes, hepatic stellate cells, while cytologic changes involve disorders happened both in parenchymal calls and nonparenchymal cells (Li *et al.* 2017).

3.2 *LNP-siRNA system for liver-directed therapy*

Cullis PR et al firstly present the result of the remarkable *in vivo* activity that ionizable cationic lipids loading nucleic acid drugs are able to achieve through the mechanism of inducing gene silencing, which was achieved in hepatocytes after i.v. (Leone *et al.* 2022).

The study focused on the methods for adapting ionizable cationic lipids to the delivery of nucleic acid drugs, specifically siRNA, which bring out gene silencing effects in the liver. DLin-MC3-DMA is one of the most functional SNALPs for silencing targeted genes in the liver. It derived from the modification of a kind of Ionizable cationic lipid called DLinDMA (1,2-dilinoleyloxy-3-dimethylaminopropane). Due to the modification of the stucture and introduction of new groups (Figure 1), the ability of DLin-MC3-DMA to induce gene-silencing was improved by several thousand times from the potency demonstrated by LNP loading DLinDMA. The optimization process relyed on factors including the introduction of ether linkages, unsaturation of the acyl groups and the pKa of cationic lipids (Leone *et al.* 2022).

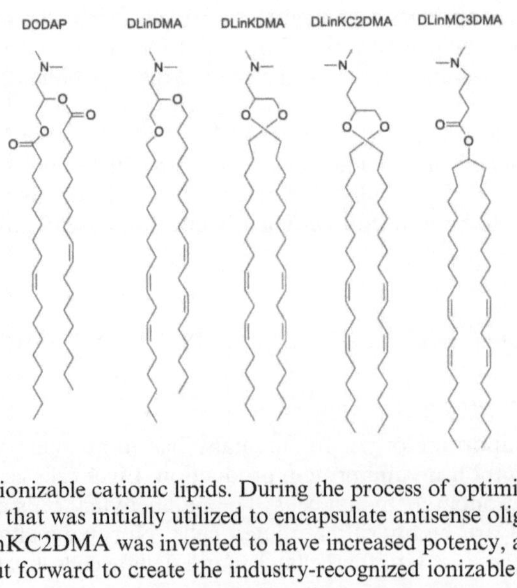

Figure 1. Evolution of ionizable cationic lipids. During the process of optimization, DLinDMA took the place of the DODAP that was initially utilized to encapsulate antisense oligonucleotides to increase potency. After this, DLinKC2DMA was invented to have increased potency, and a significant amount of synthesis work was put forward to create the industry-recognized ionizable cationic lipid DLinMC3DMA.

Among these factors, the pKa value is obviously crucial. The sufficiently high pKa values should be ensured, as once entering the endosomal it can meet the demand for providing a large number of proton pumps (cations) to combine with endogenous anions in the cytoplasm to destroy the bilayer membrane structure of the inclusion and release loaded siRNA. However, pKa should not be too high, as ionizable cationic lipids with relatively suitable pKa values may avoid elimination from the immune system in the body before reaching the target cells. Specificly, for the delivery of siRNA, ionizable cationic lipids with the pKa from 6.2 to 6.4 were found to be more suitable for hepatic gene silencing (Cullis *et al.* 1989).

According to the primary research, exogenous cationic lipids bind with endogenous anions in cells to construct a non-intact monolayer structure, ultimately releasing the nucleic acid substances carried by cationic lipids into the cells. It has already been proved some LNP systems encapsulating ionizable cationic lipids were found to be accumulated into targeted liver cells as the result of endocytosis (Akinc *et al.* 2010).

Besides the result of non-bilayer theory, which already well rationalize the optimization process of LNP delivery systems, the relative specificity towards liver cells is formed by the natural targeting mechanism due to the features of human metabolism. What is more, the adsorption ability of LNP siRNA systems on apolipoprotein E (ApoE) also has huge influence on the efficacy of gene silencing in hepatic cells. The results of many animal experiments indicated that the mechanism of LNP siRNA system targeting on liver cells is similar to some chylomicrons which adsorbs endogenous ApoE, inducing the uptake of ApoE receptors on the surface of liver cells and achieving the goal of entering liver cells.

In addition to cationic lipids, other LNP components, including PEG-lipid and cholesterol also affected the efficacy of the LNP-siRNA systems (Kruijff and Cullis 1978). The optimized LNP system containing the cationic lipid MC3, cholesterol, DSPC, and a rapidly dissociating $PEGC_{14}$-lipid showed high potency and excellent tolerability in preclinical models. This led to the invention of the first LNP-siRNA therapeutics Onpattro® whose main condition is hereditary amyloidogenic transthyretin (hATTR). The primary cause of this rare disease is some abnormal transthyretin (TTR) proteins, which are expressed by mutated genes. The disorder usually presents as progressive neuropathy and involves multiple organs. Onpattro® is able to prevent the production of abnormal TTR protein and the subsequent fibril formation. Therefore, patients with ATTRv amyloidosis, whose choices previously consisted only of TTR stabilizers or a liver transplant, now have access to an effective medication (Butler *et al.* 2016).

4 FUTURE DIRECTIONS

LNP systems that include nucleic acid drugs are designed to play a significant role in the emerging genre of drug delivery system which, by using highly targeted mechanisms, will be able to improve the bioavailability of *in vivo* metabolic processes meanwhile reducing side effects.

Nowadays, with the improvement of LNP siRNA systems, the research is not only limited in gene silencing and liver targeting. Current preclinical research has shown that these systems also have the potential clinical applications in extrahepatic target locations, such as brain, malignancies (Basha *et al.* 2016; Yamamoto *et al.* 2015) and the bone (Basha *et al.* 2016). siRNA employed for immunotherapy delivered by LNPs, which involves silencing genes in lymphatic system (Kedmi *et al.* 2018; Novobrantseva *et al.* 2012; Ramishetti *et al.* 2015; Veiga *et al.* 2019; Weinstein *et al.* 2016), is a prominent area of interest.

Another application of LNP technology, in addition to the delivery of siRNA, are also proven to be of substantial benefit for the approaches to deliver macromolecular substances. Especially for some big nucleic acid molecules like mRNA, they are not feasible to be modified or delivered by GalNAc systems. Effectively transfecting liver cells and inducing protein expression in the targeted organs with delivered LNP-mRNA opens the door to protein replacement treatment without compromising the genome. There is the study suggesting the possibility of using LNP systems to deliver specific mRNA, which can express human methylmalonyl CoA mutase (hMUT). It is able to constantly repaire the protein deficiency caused by methylmalonic acidemia, a kind of hereditary juvenile metabolic illness, in diseased mice (An *et al.* 2019).

Further application, for example stimulating the immune system to produce antibodies to combat chikungunya virus (Kose *et al.* 2019) and HIV (Pardi *et al.* 2017) provide additional ideas. It is important to note that employing LNP mRNA via i.e. to promote protein expression in immune system is becoming increasingly popular, particularly for developing (personalized) cancer immunotherapies (Kranz *et al.* 2016; Oberli *et al.*, 2017), which is similar to how LNP-siRNA works. Furthermore, LNP mRNA system also demonstrated its capacity for CAR-T therapies (Billingsley *et al.* 2020).

Overall, the development of LNP technology, specifically ionizable cationic lipids, made it possible for leading nucleic acid drugs to go into targeted locations and perform treating effects on different diseases beyond liver issues.

5 CONCLUSION

Every year, millions of patients suffer from liver diseases, and a certain number of these diseases are related to genetic causes. In recent years, some non-viral systems were invented for more options to deliver genetic drugs. Among them, LNP technology is obviously one of the most mature ones, which was initially investigated to deliver small molecule drugs. With subsequent developments, the siRNA LNP system has been shown as an effective solution for hereditary amyloidogenic transthyretin (hATTR) by the first marketing siRNA drug Onpattro® for preventing the production of abnormal Transthyroxine (TTR) in the hepatic cells. Additionally, recent research indicates that it can also provide guidance for various diseases that may be treated with gene therapy, such as cancer and brain diseases. Overall, LNP technology, which has the potential to become a leading non-viral delivery platform for curing indications related to genes beyond liver diseases, is worthy of promotion.

REFERENCES

Akinc A., De S., Qin J., Querbes W., Frank-Kamenetsky M., Jayaraman M., Rajeev K.G., Jayaprakash K. N., Qin L., Racie T., Sprague A., Dorkin J.R., Cantley W.L., Butler J.S., Zeigerer A., Fitzgerald K., Hope M.J., Fava E., Zerial M., Tracy M.A., Sah D.W.Y., Manoharan M., Koteliansky V. and de Fougerolles M.A.A. (2010). *Maier Mol. Ther. J. Am. Soc. Gene Ther.* **18**, 1357–1364

An D., Jacquinet E., Frassetto A., Eybye M., DeAntonis C., Milano J., Laureano R., Nguyen V., Milton J., Guey L.T., Sabnis S. and Lukacs C.M. (2019). *EBioMedicine*. **45**, 519–528

Arias I.M. and Gissen P. (2015). *J. Hepatol.* **63**, 1023–1037

Basha G., Cottle A., Scott W.R., Ordobadi M., Liu Y., Cullis P.R. and Wang H. (2016). *Mol. Ther. Nucleic Acids.* **5**, e363.

Basha G., Scott W.R., Ordobadi M., Cottle A., Wang H., Liu Y. and Cullis P.R. (2016). *Mol. Ther. Nucleic Acids.* **5**, e348

Billingsley M., Singh N., Ravikumar P., Zhang R., June C.H. and Mitchell M.J. (2020). *Nano. Lett.*

Butler J.S., Costelha S., Chan A., Willoughby J.L.S., Fishman S., Borland T.D., Foster D.J., Milstein S., Goncalves P., Qin J., Chen Q., Bettencourt B.R., Alvarez R., Sah D.W., Manoharan M., Fitzgerald K., Rajeev K.G., Meyers R.E., Saraiva M.J., Nochur S.V. and Zimmermann T.S. (2016). *Amyloid Int. J. Exp. Clin. Investig. Off. J. Int Soc. Amyloidosis.* **23**, 109–118

Cullis P.R., Bally M.B., Hope M.J., Madden T.D. and Mayer L.D. (1989). *Adv. Drug Deliv. Rev.* **3**, 267–282

de Kruijff B. and Cullis P.R. (1978). *Biochim. Biophys. Acta.* **513**, 31–42

Dowdy S.F. and Springer A.D. (2018). *Nucleic. Acid. Ther.* **28**, 109–118

Dunbar C.E., Joung J.K., Kohn D.B., High K.A., Sadelain M. and Ozawa K. (2018). *Science*. 359

Eaton J., Kamath P.S., Devarbhavi H. and Asrani S.K. (2019). *J. Hepatol.* **70**, 151–171
Hope M.J. and Cullis P.R. (2017). *Mol. Ther.* **25**, 1467–1475
Kang J.H., R.T. and M.M. (2016). *Criti. Rev. Biotechno.* **36**, 132–143
Kedmi R., Goldsmith M., Veiga N., Dammes N., Ramishetti S., Rosenblum D., Hazan-Halevy I., Leviatan-Ben-Arye S., Nahary L., Behlke M., Benhar I., Peer D., Harlev M. and Lieberman J. (2018). *Nat. Nanotechnol.* **13**, 214–219
Kose N., Sapparapu G., Fox J.M., Bombardi R., de Silva A.D., Tennekoon R.N., Elbashir S.M., Humphris-Narayanan E., Theisen M.A., Ciaramella G., Diamond M.S., Himansu S. and Crowe J.E. (2019). *Sci. Immunol.* **4**
Kranz L.M., Haas H., Diken M., Kreiter S., Reuter K.C., Loquai C., Meng M., Vascotto F., Fritz D., Hefesha H., Vormehr M., Grunwitz C., Hüsemann Y., Kuhn A.N., Selmi A., Buck J., Derhovanessian E., Attig S., Rae R., Diekmann J., Heesch S., Jabulowsky R.A., Hassel J., Grabbe S., Langguth P., Huber C., Sahin U. and Türeci Ö. (2016). *Nature.* **534**, 396–401
Leone R., Semple S.C., Lin P.J.C., Leone R. and Tam Y. K. (2022). *Pharmaceutics.* **14**, 398
Li Y., Xiao L., Zhang W., Gan J. and Xian J. (2017). *Chin. J. Hepatol.* **25**, 536–538
Maeda H. (2012). *J. Control. Release.* **164**, 138–144
Novobrantseva T.I., Wong J., Zafari M., Yucius K., Borodovsky A., Cullis P., Querbes W., Ruda V.M., Ge P., Milstein S., Speciner L., Manoharan M., Barros S., Basha G., Akinc A., Klebanov B., Donahoe J.S., Narayanannair Jayaprakash K., Jayaraman M., Duncan R., Bogorad R.L., Whitehead K., Love K., Nahrendorf M., Koteliansk V., Swirski F.K., Weissleder R., Levins C., de Fougerollesy A., Langer R. and Anderson D.G. (2012). *Mol. Ther. Nucleic Acids.* **1**
Oberli M.A., Dorkin J.R., Reichmuth A.M., Mitchell M.J., Jaklenec A., Fenton O.S., Anderson D.G., Blankschtein D. and Langer R. (2017). *Nano Lett.* **17**, 1326–1335
Pardi N., Shan X., Secreto A.J., Glover J., Debonera F., Yi Y., Ni H., Muramatsu H., Tam Y.K., Mui B.L., Shaheen F., Kariko K., Collman R.G., Danet-Desnoyers G.A., Hope M.J., Weissman D. and Madden T. D. (2017). *Nat. Commun.* **8**, 14630
Ramishetti S., Goldsmith M., Dykxhoorn D.M., Kedmi R., Sprague A.G., Leonard F., Godin B., Peer D., Gozin M. and Cullis P.R. (2015). *ACS Nano.* **9**, 6706–6716
Schaffer D.V. and Kotterman M.A. (2014). *Nat. Rev. Genet.* **15**, 445–451
Takakura Y., Kawabata K. and Hashida M. (1995). *Pharm. Res.* **12**, 825–830
Vegas A., Kanasty R., Anderson D. and Dorkin J.R. (2013). *Nat. Mater.* **12**, 967
Veiga N., Diesendruck Y., Ramishetti S., Behlke M.A., Goldsmith M., Rosenblum D., Benhar I., Peer D. and Elinav E. *Control. Release Off. J. Control. Release Soc.* **313**, 33–41
Weinstein S., Ramishetti S., Toker I.A., Hazan-Halevy I., Rosenblum D., Emmanuel R., Goldsmith M., Benjamini O., Abraham A., Raanani P., Nagler A., Bairey O., Peer D. and Lieberman J. (2016). *Natl. Acad. Sci. U. S. A.* **113**, E16–E22
Whitehead K.A. and Hajj K.A. (2017). *Nat. Rev. Mater.* **2**, 17056
Witzigmann D., Kulkarni J.A., Cullis P.R., Chen S. and Meel R. (2019). *Acc. Chem. Res.* **52**, 2435–2444
Yamamoto Y., Beraldi E., Leong J., Zhang F., Lin P.J.C., Kawai Y., Fazli L., Cullis P.R., Fraser R., Gleave M. and Katsumi H. *Clin. Cancer Res. Off. J. Am. Assoc. Cancer Res.* **21**, 4845–4855

Biological Sciences and Environmental Health – Gao (Ed.)
© 2025 the Author(s), ISBN: 978-1-032-96016-6

Role of AIM2 inflammasomes in insulin resistance

Anqi Sheng
Biological Science, University of California Davis, Davis, California, USA

Chunsheng Yang
Rosseau Lake College, Toronto, Canada

Xiaoyu Qiao
Ulink Beijing, Beijing, China

ABSTRACT: Inflammasomes are one of the most essential continents for innate immune defense. AIM2 inflammasomes recognize the secretion of double-stranded DNA (dsDNA) during pathogen invasion and cellular perturbations. The AIM2 recognition of dsDNA triggers the assembly of the inflammasome, which is a multiprotein oligomeric complex. This process leads to the production of bioactive interleukin-1β (IL-1β) and IL-18, as well as pyroptosis, a form of inflammatory cell death. In addition, the assembly of the inflammasome contributes to apoptosis, inflammation, and tumor regulation. Insulin resistance (IR) has been rising globally, and inflammasomes can directly or indirectly function in the insulin signaling pathway, affecting IR and type 2 diabetes mellitus (T2DM). Inflammasomes have high therapeutic potential as treatments for IR and T2DM. Compared to other inflammasomes, AIM2 is relatively less studied. This review focuses on the function of AIM2 inflammasomes and discusses their structure, function, mechanism, and relationship with IR, as well as their applications in treating various diseases or abnormal conditions. Relevant methods that could be used in this area are summarized. Further research is needed to explore the mechanisms and clinical applications of targeting AIM2 inflammasomes in the treatment of IR.

1 INTRODUCTION

The pancreas produces the hormone insulin, which reduces the concentration of blood sugar by facilitating glucose uptake into cells. Insulin resistance refers to an unsuccessful response of insulin by cells (Lebovitz 2001). When insulin binds with the insulin receptor, a series of proteins are activated, and translocation of vesicles with glucose transporter type 4 (GLUT4) is promoted. GLUT4 is an insulin-sensitive glucose transporter, which can be embedded in the cell's plasma membrane to transport glucose into the cell (Stöckli *et al.* 2011). However, when insulin resistance occurs, the number of GLUT4 transferred to the plasma membrane through insulin is significantly reduced. As a result, glucose transport into cells is impaired. To maintain a healthy blood sugar level, the pancreas must secrete more insulin to trigger the transportation of GLUT4.

The HIN-200 protein family includes Absent in Melanoma 2 (AIM2), which received its name from the lack of expression of the protein in melanoma. It typically consists of two components, an N-terminal PYD and a C-terminal HIN domain. AIM2 inflammasomes are composed of AIM2 protein along with pro-Caspase-1 and other associated components. The HIN domain can bind to PYD and get into a self-inhibitory state under a normal physiological condition. When double-stranded DNA (dsDNA) is detected, the pro-Caspase-1 is recruited via the adapter protein ASC (apoptosis-associated speck-like protein) by AIM2 protein, leading to the formation of functional AIM2 inflammasomes. This allows for the creation of fully functional AIM2 inflammasomes, which activate Caspase-1 and cleave

 DOI: 10.1201/9781003587590-26

pro-IL-1 and pro-IL-18. In addition, AIM2 inflammasomes accelerate the maturations of IL-1β and IL-18 to become fully functional to be released. Additionally, the cleavage of GSDMD by Caspase-1 triggers pyroptosis, a form of inflammatory cell death.

This review generalizes the introduction of AIM2 inflammasomes, their role in various diseases and conditions, and relevant research conducted both in vitro and in vivo.

2 STRUCTURE OF AIM2 INFLAMMASOME AND ITS COMPONENTS

2.1 *Structure of AIM2 inflammasome*

The AIM2 inflammasome is a cytosolic double-stranded DNA (dsDNA) sensor that signals downstream through the adaptor protein ASC, which contains a CARD (caspase-activation and recruitment domain) (Figure 1). The inflammasome detects DNA from both bacterial and viral sources simultaneously. The human coding gene AIM2 is located at 1q22 and is part of the PYHIN family (pyrin and HIN, commonly known as p200 proteins) (Cridland *et al.* 2012; Deyoung *et al.* 1997).

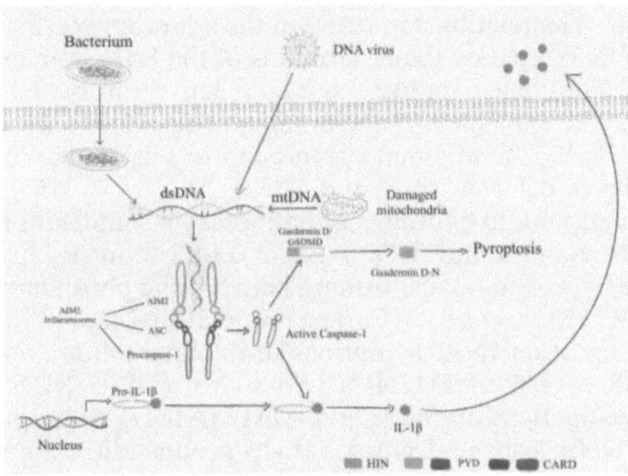

Figure 1. Structure and mechanisms of AIM2 inflammasomes. Figure credit: Original.

AIM2 consists of a long linker that binds the C-terminal HIN (hematopoietic, interferon-inducible, and nuclear) domain to an N-terminal PYD (pyrin domain). It is connected to ASC by a PYD-PYD isotypic contact, and the dsDNA can bind to the HIN domain without any sequence specificity. While the association with p202 (an additional PYHIN member) can inhibit AIM2-mediated inflammatory responses, the correlation between ASC activating procaspase-1 and AIM2 causes pyroptosis (Lu *et al.* 2023).

2.2 *Structure of AIM2 pyrin domain*

The AIM2PYD has the most variable PYD sequence known, with a small dynamic 3 helix and a longer 6 helix (Jin *et al.* 2013). Its electrostatic charge distribution is unusual, with charged residues covering most of its surface, which may lead to AIM2PYD self-association and AIM2-specific functions. AIM2PYD presents challenges in biophysical research because of its tendency to form large, insoluble oligomers in solution. To counter this, a maltose-binding protein tag is linked to prevent oligomerization (Lu *et al.* 2014). A specific mutation, F27G, has already been developed to balance the oligomerization, promoting a monomeric state. Human AIM2PYD, mouse AIM2PYD, and F27G mutant all share similar crystal structures, with an estimated 56% identical amino acid sequence. However, noticeable changes exist in the conformational arrangements of helices 2 and 3 (Jin *et al.* 2013).

2.3 *Structure of AIM2 HIN domain*

The HIN domain of AIM2 consists of over 200 amino acids and is composed of two tandem oligosaccharide-binding (OB) folds joined by a lengthy connection. The canonical OB folds are made up of five β-strands that form two sheets. The proximal OB1 fold includes β1, β4, and β5, which split into two shorter strands (Jin *et al.* 2012). Similarly, the distal OB2 fold (β1-β5) also exhibits the division of strand β5 into 2 inferior strands. The linker bridging OB1 and OB2 is approximately 30 residues long and folds into two α-helices. The two OB folds strongly engage with one another through conserved hydrophobic interactions. The HIN domains of IFI16, AIM2, and p202 are highly conserved and share the same topological configuration of OB folds (Jin *et al.* 2012).

3 MECHANISMS OF AIM2

3.1 *Interaction between dsDNA and HIN domain*

The N-terminal PYD of AIM2 links with dsDNA through electrostatic interactions along the DNA backbone, as shown by the structure of the AIM2HIN domain in the dsDNA complex (Lu *et al.* 2014). The relationship between the adaptor protein ASC and N-terminal PYD of AIM2 may be facilitated by the N-terminus of the HIN domain's distance from the DNA-binding surface. The innate immune system's activation by AIM2-induction in the presence of dsDNA may be explained by the binding of the HIN domain to either major or minor grooves of the DNA. The minimal size needed to initiate the induction of IL-1β by activated AIM2 is 80 bp of dsDNA (Fan *et al.* 2022).

Van der Waals interactions and hydrogen bonding play a significant role in DNA binding between the AIM2HIN domain and dsDNA. The α2-α3 loop residues participate in this binding, with bidentate hydrogen bonds forming between the phosphate groups of the DNA backbone and residue R311 (Lu *et al.* 2015). The minimal size needed for IL-1β induction by AIM2 activation is 80 bp of dsDNA. Mutations in the interaction areas, such as the OB1-linker and residue F165, decrease AIM2HIN's ability to bind to dsDNA (Lu *et al.* 2015).

Similar mutation investigations on full-length AIM2 (AIM2FL) have shown that defective binding of AIM2 with DNA leads to decreased IL-1β production, confirming the importance of the AIM2HIN domain in this process. An intact receptor binding surface is essential for the attachment to dsDNA and the subsequent immunological responses (Sharma 2021).

3.2 *AIM2 pyrin domain: HIN interaction*

AIM2 maintains the sensor in an autoinhibited state, which precludes PYD-mediated oligomerization and inhibits HIN:DNA binding without a ligand through intramolecular contacts between the PYD and HIN domains (Jin *et al.* 2013). According to docking analyses of crystal structures, the negatively charged helix α2 of the PYD is thought to be located near the interface of the PYD:HIN interaction. In addition, according to experiments using isothermal titration calorimetry, the PYD interacts with the HIN domain with a dissociation constant (Kd) of 23.5 μM, (Jin *et al.* 2013). It has also been demonstrated that the PYD and HIN domains cannot bind when acidic residues in helix α2 are altered. These findings demonstrate that electrostatic interactions between positively charged residues in the HIN domain and negatively charged residues in the PYD domain dominate the PYD-HIN interface. The negatively charged surface of AIM2PYD interacts with AIM2HIN and binds to ASCPYD, ensuring that dsDNA-activated AIM2 is the only time for downstream communication to the adaptor ASC (Sharma 2021).

3.3 *Mechanisms of regulation of AIM2*

Cellular homeostasis must be preserved through the control of inflammasome assembly. It has been observed that the mouse protein p202, which contains two HIN domains, binds to cytoplasmic dsDNA and prevents AIM2 activation. This binding is thought to balance the natural host defense and pathological DNA-induced inflammation (Roberts *et al.* 2009; Sharma 2021).

According to the crystal structure of the mouse p202-dsDNA complex, the p202HIN1 domain connects to DNA, while p202HIN2 interacts with AIM2 (Ru *et al.* 2013). Compared to AIM2, p202HIN1 total DNA binding affinity is increased due to the tetramer formation, which also creates an environment conducive to p202HIN1 binding to dsDNA (Yin *et al.* 2013). However, the linker bridging the two OB folds of p202 is not involved in DNA binding. A short sequence motif (MFHATVAT) that is buried in the center of the HIN domains of both proteins and used by p202HIN2 to interact with AIM2 is conserved in both proteins. Through homotypic PYD-PYD interactions, the downstream ASC is induced to polymerize by the upstream cytosolic dsDNA sensor AIM2, which further activates procaspase-1. Similar helical symmetry, overall dimensions, and subunit structure could be seen in the filaments produced by AIM2PYD and ASCPYD (Choubey *et al.* 2000).

According to EM findings and modeling studies, the AIM2PYD filament initiates the polymerization of the ASCPYD filament, causing the ASCPYD filament to localize near the end of the AIM2PYD filament (Ru *et al.* 2013). As a result, while ASCPYD has the ability to self-polymerize, the presence of AIM2PYD facilitates this process. Fluorescence polymerization assays imply that ASCPYD filament nucleation involves both AIM2PYD and the AIM2FL and dsDNA complex (Choubey *et al.* 2000). While it has been shown that the length of the self-association regulated by dsDNA and the spread of AIM2 and ASCPYD polymerization, all these molecules would speed up the assembly whether dsDNA is present or not. AIM2PYD, ASCPYD, and AIM2PYD-ASCPYD filaments are thought to exist in a three-stage continuous signal amplification that results from AIM2PYD-ASCPYD assembly (Yin *et al.* 2013).

3.4 *Relationship between insulin resistance and AIM2 inflammasome*

Research has shown a notable correlation between IR and AIM2 inflammasome. In T2DM patients, AIM2 expression is increased, and the level of mitochondrial DNA in the serum is elevated, which may be linked to the inflammatory process (Al-Kafaji *et al.* 2018). Damaged mitochondria can release a significant amount of mitochondrial DNA, thereby promoting the activation of AIM2 inflammasome and increasing IL-1 β levels (Figure 1). The expression of insulin resistance plays a critical role in the development and progression of T2DM (Bae *et al.* 2019).

In addition, the study also found that AIM2 has been implicated in various aspects of diabetes, including cardiomyopathy, macrophage aging, and systemic inflammatory status. For example, in ROS-mediated diabetes cardiomyopathy induced by high blood sugar, AIM2 is vital for the process of cardiomyocyte death and fibrosis through the GSDMD pathway. Inhibiting the expression of AIM2 can slow the progress of diabetes cardiomyopathy (Wang *et al.* 2019). Animal experiments have shown that AIM2 gene knockout mice (AIM2-/- mice) are more prone to obesity, impaired brown fat function, and elevated insulin levels (including IR) compared to wild-type mice. This may be related to the inhibitory effect of AIM2 on the encoding protein 202, which may prevent monocyte infiltration and adipogenesis, thereby improving obesity and metabolic abnormalities related to IR (Lu *et al.* 2023).

Another study suggested that AIM2 is highly expressed in neurons after trauma and is also associated with spinal cord ischemia-reperfusion. Through the study of a mouse ischemia-reperfusion model, it was found that AIM2 molecules played an important role in the abnormal dsDNA release induced by ischemia-reperfusion, triggering the activation of AIM2 inflammasome and regulating neuronal pyroptosis (Li *et al.* 2019).

4 AIM2 INFLAMMASOME FOR VARIOUS DISEASES AND UNUSUAL CONDITIONS

4.1 *Influence of AIM2 inflammasome on diseases*

AIM2 may affect many non-infectious diseases (Figure 2). For example, in inflammatory skin disorders, especially psoriasis and atopic dermatitis, a significant increase in AIM2 gene expression has been observed, suggesting a close relationship between AIM2 and the development of human skin diseases (Koning *et al.* 2012). The AIM2 inflammasome can recognize necrotic DNA in the kidneys and stimulate the release of IL-1 by macrophages β and IL-18, participating in the pathogenesis of chronic kidney disease. Additionally, AIM2 plays a vital role in atherosclerosis and cardiovascular diseases, especially in cytokine release, cell death, inflammatory reactions, and cell migration. Increased AIM2 expression and activation may be detrimental to cardiovascular disease progression. AIM2 also plays a complex role in neuroinflammation, which may be related to processes such as neuronal damage, morphological regulation, and behavioral changes. The function of AIM2 in chronic inflammatory diseases and cancer is controversial, as AIM2 may either promote tumor development or inhibit tumor growth, depending on the type of tumor, cellular environment, and specific mechanisms (Sharma *et al.* 2019).

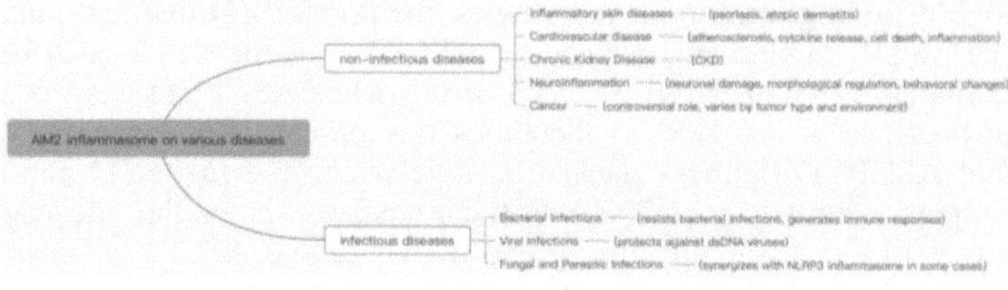

Figure 2. Effect of AIM2 inflammasome on infectious and non-infectious diseases. Figure credit: Original.

AIM2 may affect many diseases. For example, AIM2 inflammasome plays an important role in bacterial infections, and its activation helps the host resist bacterial infections and generate immune responses by recognizing and responding to intracellular events triggered by bacteria. The AIM2 inflammasome is crucial for immune protection by recognizing the presence of dsDNA viruses in the cytoplasm during viral infection (Sharma *et al.* 2019). This recognition leads to the binding of AIM2 with dsDNA, forming an inflammasome complex that drives febrile disease to provide host protection. Finally, although the exact functions and mechanisms of AIM2 in the immune response associated with fungal as well as parasitic infections are not yet clear, existing studies have shown that AIM2 may synergize with NLRP3 inflammasome in some cases and could be vital for immune protection (Cunha *et al.* 2017).

4.2 *Role of AIM2 inflammasome in insulin resistance*

Inflammasomes play a role in multiple physiological processes, such as fever, cell apoptosis, inflammation, and tumor regulation. Insulin resistance, a key component of metabolic syndrome, has been increasing in prevalence year after year. Inflammasomes are related to the initiation and development of metabolic diseases, as they affect the transmission of insulin signaling pathways and participate in the initiation of IR and T2DM.

AIM2 plays multiple roles in IR, and its relationship with different types of diabetes and related diseases is complex and requires further research. Studies have found that although AIM2 inflammasomes play a protective role against infections, they may play a harmful role in some aseptic diseases, such as chronic kidney disease, atherosclerosis, etc. Research has revealed that in subjects with T2DM, the expression levels and activity of AIM2 are elevated, together with upregulated circulating mitochondrial DNA (mtDNA) in monocytes. This elevation may be related to the inflammatory process in T2DM patients (Cataño Cañizales *et al.* 2018).

In addition, mitochondrial dysfunction is relevant to the pathogenesis of IR and T2DM. Damaged mitochondria release mtDNA, which triggers the activation of the AIM2 inflammasome and increases IL-1 β to contribute to the development of IR and diabetes. A high glucose environment induces impaired macrophage function through apoptosis that is related to cytoplasmic dsDNA/AIM2, causing accelerated aging and systemic inflammation. AIM2 also plays a role in diabetes cardiomyopathy through the GSDMD pathway, and its inhibition may help slow the progression of this condition.

AIM2 has a protective effect on metabolic syndrome. Research has found that AIM2 may improve obesity and IR by inhibiting the encoding protein 202 (p202) and improving brown fat function (Gong *et al.* 2019).

5 RELEVANT EXPERIMENTS ABOUT AIM2 INFLAMMASOME

5.1 *Improved heart failure by inhibiting AIM2 inflammasome activation through Probenecid*

IL-1β is an essential pathogenic component of cardiovascular diseases (Onódi *et al.* 2021). Inflammasomes, which are the principal producers of IL-1, offer intriguing new therapeutic targets for treating cardiovascular disorders (Testa *et al.* 1996). AIM2 inflammasomes, in particular, show increased activation in heart failure, with a similar activation pattern observed in end-stages of heart failure (Onódi *et al.* 2021). To reduce heart failure, it is important to inhibit the activation of AIM2 inflammasome, thereby decreasing the secretion and maturation of IL-1β (Testa *et al.* 1996). Probenecid, a drug used to treat chronic gout and gouty arthritis, can efficiently reduce the activation of AIM2 inflammasome in THP-1 monocytic cells and human AC16 cells, which in turn reduces cellular damage and improves cardiac function (Onódi *et al.* 2021).

Scientists have carried out a number of in vitro and in vivo investigations to support the aforementioned theory.

5.1.1 *In Vitro*

To confirm inflammasome activation in the interaction between immune cells and cardiac cells, human monocytic cell lines (THP-1) and human cardiac cells (AC16) were stimulated for 24 hours with poly (deoxyadenylic-deoxythymidylic) acid sodium salt [poly(dA:dT)], a particular AIM2 inducer, to study inflammasome activation in vitro. The results suggest that dsDNA and poly(dA:dT) can induce the activation of AIM2 inflammasome, with dsDNA being the primary trigger (Onódi *et al.* 2021).

5.1.2 *In Vivo*

To explore the mechanism of inflammasome activation, three pathologically different models of heart failure have been created, including volume-overload (AVS), pressure-overload (TAC), and post-infarction heart failure rat model (LAD), as shown in Figure 3 (Onódi *et al.* 2021).

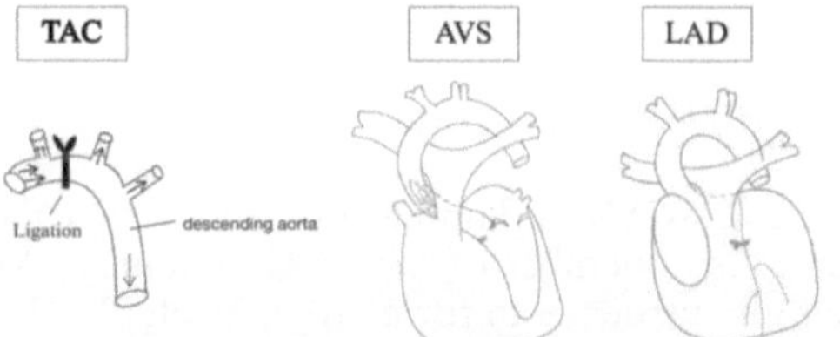

Figure 3. Diagram of pressure-overload (TAC), volume-overload (AVS), and post-infarction (left anterior descending, LAD) heart failure models. Figure credit: Original.

5.1.3 *Pressure-overload (TAC) model*

In the TAC model (Figure 3), a ligature is placed around the transverse aorta, reducing the flow velocity of the left ventricle. The limitation of the left artery will cause pressure overload, eventually causing cardiac dilation and heart failure. Compared with other heart failure models, the TAC model provides a more accurate simulation of ventricular hypertrophy and a more progressive progression of heart failure (Almeida *et al.* 2010).

5.1.4 *Volume-overload (AVS) model*

In the AVS model (Figure 3), aortic valve sclerosis involves a damaged valve from the heart to the body that acts improperly and even leaks blood. When the flow of blood out of the heart is blocked by a damaged valve, pressure can build up inside the organ and cause damage to the tissue. In the experimental AVS model, an artery and vein are surgically connected directly, avoiding the capillary bed. This causes the blood flow and pressure in the vein to increase, simulating the hemodynamic changes seen in some pathological situations (Farag *et al.* 2023).

5.1.5 *Post-infarction HF (LAD) model*

The left anterior descending (LAD) artery is the major coronary artery and travels through the anterior interventricular groove, next to the interventricular septum (Rehman *et al.* 2023). To simulate ventricular remodeling brought on by pressure and volume overload, permanent left anterior descending coronary artery closure in mice is typically performed (Muthuramu *et al.* 2014).

The results demonstrated a considerable increase in AIM2 expression in the TAC and LAD models. In line with the rise in inflammasome sensor expression levels, tissue IL-1 levels were elevated in both TAC and AVS animals, alongside an increase in the presence of monocyte/macrophage (Onódi *et al.* 2021).

5.2 *Basic protocol in inflammasome priming and activation in murine macrophages*

This experiment aims to find out how AIM2 inflammasomes are activated and mouse bone marrow-derived macrophages (BMDM) are primed. The study focuses on employing various Toll-like receptor agonists and TNF to stimulate the inflammasome in mouse macrophages, measure the maturation of interleukin (IL)-1 and IL-18 caused by inflammasome activation and pyroptosis, and induce AIM2 inflammasome activation with corresponding stimuli (Guo and Ting 2020).

5.2.1 *Experimental method*

The agonists for various Toll-like receptors first stimulate BMDMs, which then cause poly (dA:dT) transfection to stimulate the AIM2 inflammasome activation. The activation of inflammasomes is determined by using (1) ELISA to identify IL-1β as well as IL-18; (2) immunoblotting to detect cleaved IL-1β, IL-18, caspase-1, and gasdermin-D; (3) an LDH assay to measure pyroptosis; and (4) using an immunoblot of the active caspase-11 subunit p26 and a fluorescent substrate intensity measurement, the activation of caspase-11 in the presence of LPS is evaluated (Guo and Ting 2020).

6 CONCLUSION

The cytosolic dsDNA sensor, AIM2 inflammasome, signals to the adaptor protein ASC through a CARD domain. As a member of the PYHIN family, AIM2 faces challenges in biophysical research due to its tendency to form large, insoluble oligomers. The addition of an MBP tag to AIM2 helps prevent oligomerization, with a specific mutation F27G balancing oligomerization to monomer. The N-terminal PYD interacts with dsDNA, facilitating immune system activation. Mutations in AIM2 reduce its ability to bind, with downstream signaling occurring only after AIM2 is activated by dsDNA.

Studies have demonstrated that inhibiting the activation of AIM2 inflammasome can improve cardiac function and reduce cellar damage. In vitro and in vivo experiments have demonstrated a strong relationship between inflammasomes and cardiac function. One experiment was aimed to activate AIM2 inflammasomes and prime murine macrophages using Toll-like receptor agonists and TNF, which quantified inflammasome activation-mediated IL-1, IL-18, and pyroptosis.

The significance of AIM2 inflammasome in numerous diseases, its therapeutic potentials, and its interactions with other immunological pathways suggest important avenues for future research. Ongoing and future studies should focus more on comprehending the molecular mechanisms, regulatory pathways, and functional roles of AIM2 inflammasome in health and disease. This could lead to the successful development of targeted therapies that modulate AIM2 activity to treat a range of inflammatory disorders, autoimmune diseases, and even some types of cancer.

AUTHORS CONTRIBUTION

All authors contributed equally to this work, and their names are listed in alphabetical order.

REFERENCES

Al-Kafaji G. Aljadaan A., Kamal A. and Bakhiet M. (2018). *Exp. Ther. Med.* **16**, 1483–1492

Bae J. H., Jo S. I., Kim S. J., Lee J. M., Jeong J. H., Kang J. S. and Moon J. S. (2019). *Cells.* 8

Cataño Cañizales Y. G., Uresti Rivera E.E., García Jacobo R.E., Portales Perez D. P., Yadira B., Rodriguez Rivera J.G. and García Hernández M.H. (2018). *Iran. J. Immunol.* **15**, 142–155

Choubey D., Walter S., Geng Y. and Xin H. (2000). *FEBS Lett.* **474**, 38–42 (2000)

Cridland J.A., Curley E. Z., Wykes M. N., Schroder K., Sweet M. J., Roberts T. L., Ragan M. A., Kassahn K. S. and Stacey K. J. (2012). *BMC Evol. Biol.* 12, 140

Cunha L.D., Silva A.L.N., Ribeiro J.M., Mascarenhas D.P.A., Quirino G. F. S., Santos L. L. and Zamboni D.S. (2017). *Cell. Rep.* **20**, 794–805(2017)

de Koning H. D., Bergboer J. G., van den Bogaard E. H., van Vlijmen-Willems I. M., Rodijk-Olthuis D., Simon A., Schalkwijk J. and Koenen H.J.P. (2012). *Exp. Dermatol.* **21**, 961–964

deAlmeida A.C., van Oort R.J. and Wehrens X.H., *J. Vis. Exp.* 1729

DeYoung K.L., Ray M.E., Su Y A., Anzick S.L., Johnstone R. W., Trapani J.A., Meltzer P. S. and Trent J. M. (1997). *Oncogene.* 15, 453–457

Fan X., Jiao L. and Jin T. (2022). *Front. Microbiol.* **12**, 809412

Farag A., Mandour A.S., Hendawy H., Elhaieg A., Elfadadny A. and Tanaka R. *Front.* **10**

Gong Z., Zhang X., Su K., Jiang R., Sun Z., Chen W. and Muzumdar R. (2019). *Diabetologia.* **62**, 2325–2339

Guo H. and Ting J.P. (2020). *Curr. Protoc. Immunol.* **131**

Jin T., Perry A., Jiang J., Smith P., Curry J. A., Unterholzner L., Jiang Z., Horvath G., Rathinam V. A., Johnstone R. W., Hornung V., Latz E., Bowie A. G., Fitzgerald K. A. and Xiao T. S. (2012). *Immunity.* 36, 561–571

Jin T., Perry A., Smith P., Jiang J. and Xiao T.S. (2013). *J. Biol. Chem.* **288**, 13225–13235

Lebovitz H.E. (2001). *Exp. Clin. Endocrinol. Diabetes.* **109** S135–S148

Li X. Q., Yu Q., Fang B., Zhang Z. L. and Ma H. (2019). *Neuropharmacology.* **160**, 107661

Lu A., Kabaleeswaran V., Fu T., Magupalli VG. and Wu H. (2014). *J. Mol. Biol.* **426**, 1420–1427

Lu A., Li Y. and Yin Q. (2015). *J. Ruan. Cell Discov.* **1**,1–14

Lu S., Li Y., Qian Z., Zhao T., Feng Z. and Weng X., Yu L. (2023). *Front Immunol.* 14, 1052756

Muthuramu I., Lox M., Jacobs F. and De Geest B. (2014). *JoVE.*

Onódi Z., Ruppert M., Kucsera D., Sayour A. A., Tóth V.E., Koncsos G., Novák J., Brenner G.B., Makkos A., Baranyai T., Giricz Z., Görbe A., Leszek P., Gyöngyösi M., Horváth I.G., Schulz R., Merkely B., Ferdinandy P., Radovits T. and Varga Z.V. (2021). *Cardiovasc. Res.* **117**, 2639–2651

Rehman I., Connor C., Kerndt and Rehman A. (2023). *StatPearls.*

Roberts T.L., Idris A., Dunn J.A. and Kelly G.M. (2009). *Science.* **323**, 1057–1060

Ru H., Ni X., Zhao L. and Crowley C. (2013). *Cell Res.* **23**, 855–858

Sharma B.R., Karki R., and Kanneganti T. D. (2019). *Eur. J.Immunol.* **49**, 1998–2011

Sharma M. and de Alba E. (2021). *Int. J. Mol Sci.* **22**, 872

Stöckli J., Fazakerley D.J. and James D.E. (2011). *J. Cell Sci.* **124**, 4147–4159

Testa M., Yeh M., Lee P., Fanelli R., Loperfido F., Berman J.W. and LeJemtel T. H. (1996). *J. Am. Coll. Cardiol.* **28**, 964–971

Wang X., Pan J., Liu H., Zhang M., Liu D., Lu L. and An F. (2019). *Life. Sci.* **221**, 249–258

Yin Q., Sester D.P., Tian Y. and Hsiao Y.S. (2013). *Cell Rep.* **4**, 327–339

Biological Sciences and Environmental Health – Gao (Ed.)
© 2025 the Author(s), ISBN: 978-1-032-96016-6

Therapeutic effects and mechanisms of statins on depression patients

Yumin Hou
School of Chinese Medicine, Tianjin Univerity of Traditional Chinese Medicine, Tianjin, China

ABSTRACT: Depression, as the most common mental illness in life, often brings great suffering to patients. At the same time, the co-morbidity of depression and cardiovascular disease has created an unprecedented demand for new and more effective antidepressants with low side effects in the medical field. Recently, statins, as first-line drugs to cure cardiovascular disease, were found to be effective as antidepressants. Despite the fact that their exact mechanism of action is still unknown, the evidence shows that statins are strongly associated with anti-inflammation and the prevention of vascular lesions through immune regulation and anti-inflammatory effects, preventing depression by improving cerebrovascular lesions, increasing the hippocampus's brain-derived neurotrophic factor, etc. Simvastatin and atorvastatin are representatives of statins. There are many conjectures about its mechanism of action, and relevant clinical trials have also proved the effect of these two cardiovascular drugs on depression. Clinical trials of individuals with depression and cardiovascular disease also provide support for the antidepressant effects of statins by preventing new cardiovascular and depression events, alleviating symptoms, etc. Future research is necessary to clarify the molecular mechanisms of statins. Additional clinical studies are required to justify the use of statins for not only cardiovascular disease but also depression and related mental illness.

1 INTRODUCTION

Depression as a mental disease, is one of the most prevalent diseases (Ludka *et al.* 2013). Depression, as an emotional disorder, often brings great pain to patients and a great burden to society, which profoundly affects the quality of life of patients (Yu *et al.* 2019). At the same time, due to the increased risk of suicide and cerebrovascular disease brought about by depression, depression has gradually been regarded as a fatal disease. Statistics show that 14.3% of all deaths worldwide, or around 80,000 people per year, are caused by mental diseases (Walker *et al.* 2015). However, at this point, 30 to 40% of patients cannot be cured by first-line antidepressants, and need a change in therapy (Gaynes *et al.* 2009). However, the efficacy of current combination drugs has very limited clinical evidence and is accompanied by weight increase, cardiometabolic disruption, and nausea are significant adverse effects (Beach *et al.* 2014). This heralds the urgent need to develop new and more effective antidepressants with low side effects.

Cardiovascular disease is the disease with the highest morbidity and mortality in the world, which includes several important pathologies such as atherosclerosis (Gaziano *et al.* 2006). Recent studies show that patients with depression have higher death rates in the general population and are more prone to develop cardiovascular disease. Additionally, people with cardiovascular disease have a worse prognosis and are more likely to experience depression than people without it. According to a study, mortality triples in people with

 DOI: 10.1201/9781003587590-27

depression following acute myocardial infraction (Hare *et al.* 2014). The interaction between depression and cardiovascular disease not only aggravates the patient's condition but also increases the difficulty and challenge of treatment, causing a huge economic burden on patients and society. Ideally, a commonly used first-line cardiovascular drug would also reduce the risk of depression, which would greatly reduce the serious consequences of comorbidities.

Statins, sometimes referred to as 3-hydroxy-3-methylglutadiene-coenzyme A (HMG-CoA) reductase inhibitors, have been generally considered to be safe medications. Statins generally reduce the level of low-density lipoprotein and reduce the risk of atherosclerosis by inhibiting the enzymes that produce cholesterol in the body, and are widely used as first-line drugs to treat cardiovascular diseases (Lei *et al.* 2014). In addition, the pleiotropic effects of statins have also received extensive attention. Statins have been shown their anti-inflammatory, antioxidant, and neuroprotective properties and are considered to be potentially protective on neurobiological systems associated with depression, such as central nervous system neurotransmission (Otte *et al.* 2016).

Studies have shown that statins have the effect of reducing β-amyloid in Alzheimer's disease while improving the symptoms of multiple sclerosis (Gougol *et al.* 2015). In some animal studies, statins have also been proven to ameliorate depression-like behavior in mice. Even though the underlying mechanisms are still unclear, these clinical trials offer hope that statins may improve outcomes and recovery in patients with depression and comorbid cardiovascular disease. This review summarizes the molecular processes by which statins affect depression, how Simvastatin and Atorvastatin work, and relevant clinical studies.

2 MECHANISM OF ACTION OF STATINS ON DEPRESSION

2.1 *Immunomodulatory and anti-inflammatory effects of statins*

Research found increased levels of inflammatory markers such as C-reactive protein (CRP), tumor necrosis factor, and others in depression, indicating that inflammation may affect depression (Lei *et al.* 2014). The interplay of inflammation and the brain not only drives the development of depression but may lead to unresponsiveness to current antidepressant drugs (Miller and Raiosn 2016).

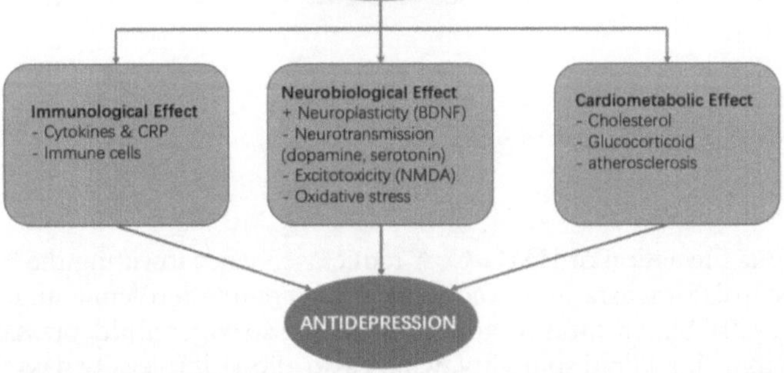

Figure 1. Mechanisms underpinning statins' depressive effects. Statins can achieve antidepressant effects by immunological effect, neurobiological effects, and cardioetabolic effects respectively. CRP, C-reactive protein; BDNF, Brain-derived neurotrophic factor; NMDA, n-methyl-d-aspartic acid. Figure credit: Original.

Statins have been shown to exert an anti-inflammatory and immunomodulatory effect (Figure 1) (Taniguti *et al.* 2019). Statins may have anti-inflammatory effects by lowering CRP (Ridker *et al.* 2001), decreasing oxidative stress, preventing pro-inflammatory cytokines from being expressed on monocytes, and blocking T-cell activation (Tousoulis *et al.* 2006). As a result, statins may lower the prevalence of depression, while clinical research is still being done to determine the precise mechanism.

2.2 *Reduce the incidence of depression by preventing atherosclerosis*

The antidepressant function of statins may be related to impact on atherosclerosis (Figure 1). First, The vascular depression hypothesis proposes that cerebrovascular diseases, such as microangiopathy, inflammation, and vascular inflammation, may induce depression, especially in the elderly population (Taylor, Aizenstein and Alexopoulos 2013). As an important symbol of the vascular depression hypothesis, cerebral arterial white matter lesions may lead to emotional and cognitive problems and increase the risk of depression by connecting neural networks in different brain regions. Second, it may induce depression by activating inflammation; at the same time, lesions may also play a role in the blood supply to the brain area, cause hypoxia in the brain tissue, and affect its function (Lassen and Christensen 1976). Statins are therefore extremely important for the prevention of depression and can enhance patients' quality of life by treating and preventing cerebrovascular disorders.

2.3 *Targeting brain-derived neurotrophic factor to treat depression*

Brain-derived neurotrophic factor (BDNF) is important in the survival, growth, and functional maintenance of neurons as a substance that preserves and elicits brain plasticity. Higher levels of BDNF are frequently linked to greater anxiety behaviors. Depression severity and BDNF levels are inversely associated with depressed people (Lee *et al.* 2007). Clinical studies have shown that with long-term treatment of depression, the level of serum BDNF in patients increases.

Statins' antidepressant effects were mediated through changes in glutamatergic transmission and increased expression of neurotrophic proteins associated with brain health (Figure 1) (Khoodoruth *et al.* 2022). Glutamatergic modulators have been utilized to elicit fast antidepressant effects in humans and preclinical models.

In conclusion, the controversial effects of statins have been demonstrated (Figure 1). At the same time, many antidepressant mechanisms of statins have neurobiological effects on inflammation, cerebrovascular diseases, BDNF, etc., and further *in vitro* and *in vivo* studies with different depression models are needed to prove the effectiveness and accuracy of their mechanisms.

3 EQUATIONS AND MATHEMATICS

3.1 *Simvastatin*

Simvastatin inhibits the action of HMG-CoA reductase, hence lowering the body's ability to synthesize cholesterol. Simvastatin is used to treat hypercholesterolemia and hyperlipidemia (Todd and Goa 1990). Simvastatin is thought to have a stronger antidepressant impact than other statins due to its high lipid solubility, which also allows it to easily pass the blood-brain barrier. The rationale behind the expected effect of simvastatin on depression can be explained in different ways.

Simvastatin reduces depressed behavior in mice brought on by chronic moderate stress (CMS) and lipopolysaccharide (LPS) (Yu *et al.* 2019). Microglia in the central nervous system are essential for preserving neuronal connections in the growing brain (Graeber 2010). Microglia are activated into different morphologies after being stimulated by LPS or CMS, and stimulate depressive episodes and activate related inflammatory mediators. LPS promotes pro-inflammatory polarization of macrophages and microglia, which in turn induces depression-like behavior after 24 hours (Dantzer *et al.* 2008). Simvastatin was added, and this reduced pro-inflammatory factors and blocked the NF-B signaling pathway (Yu *et al.* 2019). Simvastatin plays a comparable role to LPS in the CMS-induced depression paradigm. By blocking the NF-κB signaling pathway, it reduces neuroinflammation and ameliorates depressive-like symptoms like anhedonia, behavioral despair, and anxiety. Simvastatin, via engaging in the control of NF-κBp65, suppresses neuroinflammation, and as a result, improves depressed behavior primarily by reducing neuroinflammation.

Simvastatin was used in a study to prevent and treat mice with depressive behavior (Taylor *et al.* 2013). To measure the severity of the depressive behavior in the mice, methods including the forced swimming test (FST), the sucrose preference test (SPT), and immunohistochemical analysis were used. The findings demonstrated that oral simvastatin 20 mg/kg performed better in SPT, FST, and NSFT, indicating that it can prevent and treat neuroinflammation brought on by LPS and CMS (Taylor *et al.* 2013).

Statins can inhibit n-methyl-d-aspartic acid (NMDA) glutamate receptors *in vivo*. NMDA, a subtype of glutamate receptors is crucial to understanding the pathophysiology of depression and developing effective treatments. Statins may therefore function as NMDA antagonists to produce antidepressant effects.

3.2 *Reduce the incidence of depression by preventing atherosclerosis*

As another statin drug for treating high cholesterol and preventing cardiovascular disease, atorvastatin also shows potential antidepressant and anxiety effects in clinical research.

A trial employing atorvastatin to ameliorate anxiety and depression in mice by affecting -synuclein Ser129, NADPH oxidase 2 (NOX2)-mediated autophagy, as well as oxidative stress revealed that atorvastatin can decrease the expression of NOX2 (Yan *et al.* 2020), anxiety, depression, and exercise capacity are all improved by increasing the expression of LC3II/LC3I, promoting autophagic flux, and increasing the expression level of LC3 points. This suggests that atorvastatin may be identified as a NOX2 as a potential target and Drugs that improve clinical symptoms of Parkinson's disease (Yu *et al.* 2019).

Nitric oxide, one of the key neurotransmitters in the central system, exerts neuromodulatory effects, including depression and neurodegenerative diseases (Silva *et al.* 2000). Research has shown that the possible mechanism of atorvastatin's antidepressant effect is to increase the activity of PPAR_γ receptor and reduce the level of nitric oxide (Shahsavarian *et al.* 2014).

Additionally, a clinical investigation with 60 patients with major depressive disorder (MDD) that was double-blind and randomized revealed that when compared to the placebo group, cholesterol, triglycerides and low-density lipid (LDL) decreased, favorably affecting depressive symptoms in toxic MDD patients (Haghighi *et al.* 2014).

4 CLINICAL STUDIES SHOWING STATINS' ANTIDEPRESSANT EFFECTS

In this article, statins are systematically reviewed in randomized, double-blind, controlled studies that involve individuals with a variety of diseases, as well as different evaluation methods, trying to show the most representative and comprehensive effect of statins on anti-inflammatory effects (Table 1).

Table 1. Clinical trials of statins on depression severity in depressed and non-depressed patients.

Publication	Study Design	Population	Intervention	Follow-up	Outcomes
Molero *et al.* 2021	Historical cohort	1149384 non-depressed statin-users (age>/=15 years)	Statin	8 years	Diagnose of depression statin leads to lower chance of depression
Wium-Andersen *et al.*, 2017	Historical cohort	91842 ACS patients without depression	Statin	12 years	Diagnose of early (< 1 year) or late (1-12 years) depression; statin leads to reduced risk of depression
Kim *et al.* 2018	Cohort	711 ACS patients without depression	Statin	1 year	Diagnose of depression; statin leads to lower chance of depression
Ghanizadeh and hedayati 2013	RCT	68 MDD patients	Fluoxetine	6 weeks	HDRS decrease in depression scores was greater in treatment group
Abbasi *et al.* 2015	RCT	46 post CABG patients with depression	Sivastatin	6 weeks	HDRS decrease in depression scores was greater in treatment group
Kim *et al.* 2015	Cohort	300 depressed patients with ACS	Escitalopram	1 year	HDRS, BDI taking statins of patients showed higher response rates

RCT, or randomized controlled trial, stands for acute coronary syndrome. MDD, major depressive disorder; HDRS, short for Hamilton Depression Rating Scale, stands for coronary artery bypass graft. BDI, beck depression inventory.

An eight-year epidemiological study was conducted across Sweden, involving 1,149,384 non-depressed individuals over the age of 15 (Ljung *et al.* 2021). The experimental results show that statins were an extremely safe treatment option for treating certain mental illnesses, and would not cause mental illnesses such as suicide or anxiety disorders; and during the treatment period of statins, the risk of depression is significantly reduced (Ljung *et al.* 2021). Simvastatin have been thought to have greater anti-inflammatory and antidepressant effects due to its higher permeability of the blood-brain barrier (Lei *et al.* 2014).

The idea that post-ASC depression symptoms could be lessened by anti-inflammatory stems from the notion that accumulated low-grade inflammation may be a potential relationship between acute coronary syndrome and depression. Acetylsalicylic acid and statin use was linked to early post-ACS (within one year) depression only in people with ACS and a decreased risk of late (within 12 years) depression, according to a large cohort research involving ACS patients and non-ACS patients as control group with more than 90,000 patients for each group (Wium-Andersen *et al.* 2017). This study highlights the importance of statins in preventing new cardiovascular events and depression after ACS. Another study also demonstrated a similar conclusion (Kim *et al.* 2018), In a one-year follow-up, ACS patients using statins had a markedly lower risk of developing depression than ACS patients not taking statins. These trials show that statins are safe for people who are not depressed and have a great potential to lower the incidence of depression over the long and short term.

Additionally, statins are linked to decreased depression scores in people who are depressed, according to a number of cohort studies. In this randomized controlled trial of 68 depressed patients (Ghanizadeh and Hedayati 2013), after 6 weeks in the treatment group (fluoxetine plus lovastatin) and the control group (fluoxetine plus placebo), depression scores were presented in the treatment group A significantly more significant decrease was observed, although a downward trend was observed in both groups (12.8 ± 6.3 vs. 8.2 ± 4.0) (Ghanizadeh and Hedayati 2013). However, the limitation of this experiment is the small sample size. Thus, high dose, wide population, and long-term trial extension are required to be considered in the future. In a second randomized controlled trial, 46 patients with mild to moderate depression following coronary artery bypass surgery were compared to the antidepressant effects of simvastatin as well as atorvastatin (Abbasi *et al.* 2015). Clinically speaking, the simvastatin regimen is well tolerated and has better antidepressant effects than atorvastatin. Patients respond to the treatment more quickly as well, suggesting that it may someday replace atorvastatin as the medicine of choice for these conditions.

In addition, some studies have shown that the combination of statins and SSRIs has stronger antidepressant effects than SSRIs alone. Higher rates of depression remission were observed in patients treated with a combined regimen of escitalopram and a statin than in patients receiving escitalopram alone during the trial's one-year follow-up among 300 participants who had both depression and ACS (Kim *et al.* 2015).

5 CONCLUSION

In order to improve the harm caused by depression and cardiovascular diseases, statins, as the first-line drugs for the treatment of cardiovascular diseases, have been found to have certain antidepressant effects in recent studies. Even though the antidepressant mechanism of statins is not yet clear, it may include reducing depressive symptoms through immune regulation and anti-inflammatory effects, preventing depression by improving cerebrovascular lesions, furthermore enhancing brain-derived neurotrophic factor in the hippocampus to exercise its antidepressant effects, etc. Among them, simvastatin may have a stronger antidepressant effect due to its higher fat solubility; some clinical trials have also proved that simvastatin exerted an antidepressant effect in inhibiting inflammation and as an NMDA antagonist. Atorvastatin may inhibit NOX2 as a potential target to improve Parkinson's symptoms, increase the activity of PPARγ receptors and reduce nitric oxide levels to improve depression. Additionally, a number of clinical investigations have shown that statins may have a depression-preventive impact in patients who do not also have cardiovascular disease or depression as well as in those who have simply cardiovascular disease, depression, or both. effectiveness of antidepressants in comorbid individuals. At the same time, statins showed stronger antidepressant effects when combined with SSRIs than SSRIs alone. The discovery of the antidepressant effect of statins has brought great hope for improving the prognosis of patients with depression and cardiovascular disease comorbidities, and it is worthy of further and more in-depth research on its mechanism of action and clinical practice.

REFERENCES

Abbasi S.H., Mohammadinejad P., Shahmansouri N., Salehiomran A.. Beglar A.A., Zeinoddini A., Forghani S. and Akhondzadeh S. (2015). *J. Affect. Disord* **183**, 149

Beach S.R., kostis W.J., Celano C.M., Januzzi J.L., Ruskin J.N., Noseworthy P.A. and Huffman J.C. (2014). *J. Clin. Psychiatry* **75**, e441

da Silva G.D., Matteussi A.S., dos Santos A.R., Calixto J.B. and Rodrigues A.L., *Neuroreport* **11**, 3699

Dantzer R., O'Connor J.C., Freund G.G., Johnson R.W. and Kelley K.W. (2008). *Nat. Rev. Neurosci* **9**, 46

Gaynes B.N., Warden D., Trivedi M.H., Wisniewski S.R., Fava M. and Rush A.J. (2009). *Psychiatr Serv Wash DC* **60**, 1439

Gaziano T., Reddy K.S., Paccaud F., Horton S. and Chaturvedi V. (2006). *Disease Control Priorities in Developing Countries*, 2nd ed 33

Ghanizadeh A. and Hedayati A. (2013). *Depress. Anxiety* **30**, 1084

Gougol A., Zareh-Mohammadi N., Raheb S., Farokhnia M., Salimi S., Iranpour N., Yekehtaz H. and Akhondzadeh S. (2015). *J. Psychopharmacol* **29**, 575
Graeber M.B. (2010). *Science* **330**, 783
Haghighi M., Khodakarami S., Jahangard L., Ahmadpanah M., Bajoghli H., Holsboer-Trachsler E. and Brand S. (2014). *J. Psychiatr. Res.* **58**, 109
Hare D.L., Toukhsati S.R., Johansson P. and Jaarsma T. (2014). *Eur. Heart J* **35**, 1365
Khoodoruth M.A.S., Estudillo-Guerra M.A., Pacheco-Barrios K., Nyundo A., Chapa-Koloffon G. and Ouanes S. (2022). *Front. Psychiatry* **13**, 886918
Kim S.W., Bae K.Y., Kim J.M., Shin I.S., Hong Y.J., Ahn Y., Jeong M.H., Ahn Y., Jeong M.H., Berk M. and Yoon J.S. (2015). *Transl. Psychiatry* **5**, e620
Kim S.W., Kang H.J., Bae K.Y., Shin I.S., Hong Y.J., Ahn Y.K., Jeong M.H., Berk M., Yoon J.S. and Kim J.M. (2018). *Prog. Neuropsychopharmacol. Biol. Psychiatry* **80**, 250
Lassen N.A. and Christensen M.S. (1976). *Br. J. Anaesth* **48**,719
Lee B.H., Kim H., Park S.H. and Kim Y.K. (2007). *J. Affect. Disord* **101**, 239
Lei Q., Peng W.N., You H., Hu Z.P. and Lu W. (2014). *Pharmazie* **69**, 448
Ljung R., Köster M., Björkenstam E. and Salmi P. (2021). *Lancet Psychiatry* **8**, e2
Ludka F.K., Zomkowski A.D., Cunha M.P., Dal-Cim T., Zeni A.L., Rodrigues A.L. and Tasca C.I. (2013). *Eur. Neuropsychopharmacol.* **23**, 400
Miller A.H. and Raison C.L. (2016). *Nat. Rev. Immunol* **16**, 22
Otte C., Gold S.M., Penninx B.W., Pariante C.M., Etkin A., Fava M., Mohr D.C. and Schatzberg A.F., *Nat. Rev. Dis. Primers* **2**, 16065 (2016)
Ridker P.M., Rifai N., Clearfield M., Downs J.R., Weis S.E., Miles J.S. and Gotto Jr A.M. (2001). Air Force/Texas Coronary Atherosclerosis Prevention Study Investigators, *N. Engl. J. Med* **344**, 1959
Shahsavarian A., Javadi S., Jahanabadi S., Khoshnoodi M., Shamsaee J., Shafaroodi H., Mehr S.E. and Dehpour A. (2014). *Eur. J. Pharmacol* **745**, 52
Taniguti E.H., Ferreira Y. S., Stupp I.J.V., Fraga-junior E.B., Doneda D.L., Lopes L., Rios-Santos F., Lima E., Buss Z.S., Viola G.G. and Vandresen-Filho S. (2019). *Brain Res. Bull* **146**, 279
Taylor W.D., Aizenstein H.J. and Alexopoulos G.S. (2013). *Mol. Psychiatry* **18**, 963
Todd P.A. and Goa K.L. (1990). *Drugs* **40**, 583
Tousoulis D., Antoniades C., Koumallos N. and Stefanadis C. (2006). *Cytokine Growth Factor Rev* **17**, 225
Walker E.R., McGee R.E. and Druss B.G., *JAMA Psych* **72**, 334 (2015)
Wium-Andersen I.K., Wium-Andersen M.K., Jørgensen M.B. and Osler M. (2017). *Int. J. Cardiol* **246**, 1
Yan J., Huang J., Liu A., Wu J., Fam H., Shen M., Lai X., Ma H., Sun W., Yang J. and Xu Y. (2020). *Aging*, **13**, 831
Yu X.B., Zhang H.N., Dai Y., Zhou Z.Y., Xu R.A., Hu L.F., Zhang C.H., Hu H.Q., An T.Q., Tang C.R. and Lin G.Y. (2019). *J. Affect. Disord* **245**,939

Biological Sciences and Environmental Health – Gao (Ed.)

Anti-cancer effects and mechanisms of thymoquinone in gastric cancer

Mile Xue
Oakville Trafalgar, Ontario, Oakville, Canada

ABSTRACT: Thymoquinone, one of the major components of essential oils from a plant native to Southwest Asia, has been reported to have antioxidant and anti-tumor properties. In recent studies, scientists have shown that thymoquinone can be used as an anti-cancer drug in several cancers, such as breast, intestine, and gastric cancer. Thymoquinone may exert its anti-cancer effects not only through its anti-oxidant effects but also through several signaling pathways, including STAT3, PI3K/AKt/mTOR, PTEN, as well as TGF-β/Smad2/3. Researchers have also found that thymoquinone has tremendous potential in clinical trials. Advanced nanotechnology is now widely used in various fields, and nanotechnology was approved to be effective in the delivery of thymoquinone. This review summarizes the different pathways and related clinical trials. However, more in vitro and in vivo studies, as well as clinical trials of applications of nanotechnologies with thymoquinone, are required to prove the clinical values of thymoquinone.

1 INTRODUCTION

Stomach cancer occurs in many people. Whether hereditary or conventional, stomach cancer can affect a person's quality of life and lead to death in its later stages. In 2020, it was estimated that there would be more than 1 million new cases of stomach cancer worldwide, resulting in 700,000 deaths (Zhou *et al.* 2016). Thymoquinone is one of the most effective drugs to treat several types of cancer, such as breast, blood, and lung cancers.

Thymoquinone has antioxidant, anti-inflammatory, and anti-cancer properties. Thymoquinone inhibited the rise of miR-34a and decreased the concentration of Rac1. Thymoquinone can cause cell death and control the level of cell death. It can also reduce the phosphorylation of NF-κB and IKKα/β and reduce the activity of PI3K (National Center for Biotechnology Information 2004).

Furthermore, mechanisms of anti-cancer effects of thymoquinone also include pathways associated with 5-LO, COX, and PGD2. In an experiment with thymoquinone, researchers found that it inhibited the growth of gastric cancer cells and led to the death of gastric cancer tumors. It is concentration-dependent with autophagy (He *et al.* 2023). Transmission electron microscopy showed that the number of autophagosomes of gastric cancer cells increased after thymoquinone.

Clinical trials of treatment effects of thymoquinone have been approved on pathways, such as STAT3, and PI3K/AKt/mTOR, as well as its application in nanoparticle-based therapies.

This review summarizes the structure of thymoquinone, the mechanisms of its anti-gastric cancer effect, as well as related therapeutic strategies.

DOI: 10.1201/9781003587590-28

2 CHEMICAL STRUCTURE OF THYMOQUINONE

Thymoquinone is extracted from black grass with a molecular weight of 164.2 g/mol. The molecular formula is C10H12O2 (Sayed-Ahmed *et al.* 2010). To investigate the different chemical structures within a rock, the scientists employed three methods: high-resolution X-ray powder diffraction, Fourier transform infrared spectroscopy (FTIR), and thermogravimetric analysis. Research shows that triclinic unit cell has the following parameters: a = 6.73728 Å, b = 6.91560 Å, c = 10.4988 Å, α = 88.864 degrees, β = 82.449 degrees, γ = 77.0299 degrees, with a cell volume of 472.52 $Å^3$, and Z (the number of formula units per unit cell) equals to 2. Additionally, the researchers used FTIR to demonstrate absorption bands related to the carbonyl, carbon-hydrogen, and vinylic groups found in p-benzoquinone. In addition, according to the discontinuous reception (DRX) method, the gradual increase in the melting point and molecular bonding provides strong evidence for the emergence of the van der Waals model. The heat map indicates that thymoquinone can only exist as a triclinic crystal. Thymoquinone also contains PHD and RING finger domains-1, specifically UHRF1, which is a protein containing multiple domains.

3 MECHANISMS OF ANTI-CANCER EFFECTS OF THYMOQUINONE

Thymoquinone inhibits cancer through a number of different pathways, which include STAT3, PI3K, AKt, mTOR, PTEN, TGF-beta/Smad2, anti-oxidant, etc., as shown in Figure 1.

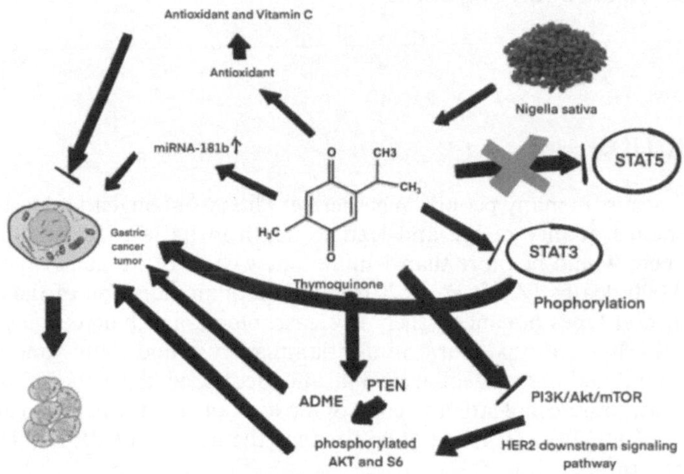

Figure 1. Mechanism of thymoquinone. Figure credit: Original.

3.1 *STAT3*

The cells of HGC27, BGC823, and SGC7901 were cultured using the external propagation method. They were treated with varying concentrations (0-125 μmol/L) of thymoquinone for 12 hours, 24 hours, and 36 hours (Ma *et al.* 2017). The control rate of cell increase or decrease was measured using the methyl thiazole tetrazolium method. A western blot assay was performed to analyze the protein expression of (STAT)3, p-STAT3, STAT5, and p-STAT5 signal transduction and transcriptional activation. Flow cytometry measures were used to assess the cell cycle and apoptosis (Bitarafan *et al.* 2018).

Comparison shows that thymoquinone can inhibit the phosphorylation of STAT3 and reduce the activity of STAT3, but not the phosphorylation of STAT5 (Bitarafan *et al.* 2018). In addition, according to the in vitro results, thymoquinone has a significant anti-tumor effect on mice with tumors.

This study provides sufficient evidence to demonstrate that the low STAT3 signaling pathway stimulates the death of gastric cancer cells with thymoquinone.

3.2 *PI3K/AKt/mTOR*

The way to test PI3K/mTOR involves using HER2-negative (MKN45) gastric cancer cell lines. Cell cycle progression, cell viability, and the HER2 downstream signaling pathway were detected and analyzed using the MTS assay, flow cytometry, and Western blotting (Zhu *et al.* 2015). Internally, the researchers used BEZ235 to study exosomes derived from patients with HER2-positive gastric cancer and to investigate the anti-gastric cancer activity of the AKt/mTOR pathway (Zhu *et al.* 2015).

The results showed that BEZ235 exhibited a stronger inhibitory effect than the strongly targeted drug trastuzumab in both external and internal body experiments. BEZ235 and trastuzumab showed some resistance. BEZ235 showed its anti-tumor properties in gastric cancer by inhibiting phosphorylated AKT and S6, inhibiting important HER2 downstream signaling pathways (Zhu *et al.* 2015).

This investigation showed that PI3K/AKt/mTOR can inhibit gastric cancer, and these important findings can be utilized to facilitate the design of future clinical trials.

3.3 *PTEN*

The study investigated the interaction between thymoquinone, its five derivatives, and phosphatase and tensin homolog (PTEN). The results of molecular docking showed that the binding energy of thymoquinone and PTEN was relatively suitable. In addition, molecular dynamics studies revealed that the molecular interaction between thymoquinone and the PTEN complex is extremely stable (Hokmabady and Fani 2022). The comparison of compounds in the study showed that the main effects of hydrogen bonding and chemical structure van der Waals interaction in the binding process of thymoquinone and PTEN conform to adsorption, distribution, metabolism, and excretion (ADME) (Hokmabady and Fani 2022).

As a result, PTEN may act as a target for drug development to inhibit gastric cancer. Further studies are required to elucidate the effects of thymoquinone on PTEN-related mechanisms.

3.4 *TGF-β /Smad2/3*

TGF-β/Smad2/3 plays a major role in gastric cancer. To demonstrate the relationship between miRNA-181b and the TGF-β-Smad2/3/4 pathway with epithelial-mesenchymal transition (EMT) in gastric cancer, researchers used wound healing and transwell assays to study cell migration (Al-Rawashde *et al.* 2022).

The scientists investigated the effects of TGF-β induction in human gastric cancer cells using miRNA-181b inhibitors to replace endogenous miRNAs. Expression levels of miRNA-181b, Timp3, and EMT-related markers were expressed by RT-PCR, and phosphorylated Smad2 and Smad4 were detected by Western blotting. The dual luciferase reporter gene assay confirmed the feasibility of miRNA-181b binding to Timp3 (Al-Rawashde *et al.* 2022).

It was reported that miRNA-181b could be inhibited by SD-208, which targets TGF-β-Smad2/3 and Smad4 signaling. This suggests that the TGF-β pathway can influence EMT in gastric cancer cells by enhancing miRNA-181b, which interacts with Timp3 through the Smad2/3/4 pathway (Al-Rawashde *et al.* 2022).

The experiment gives ideas for future research on targeting the TGF-β/Smad2/3 pathway.

3.5 *Anti-oxidant effect*

Anti-oxidant effects can be mediated through direct scavenging of free radicals, actions on mitochondria, or interactions with related enzymes. The study investigated the relationship between antioxidants and gastrointestinal cancers.

The effect of 4 ml per kg of thymoquinone on 200 ml per kg of diethyl nitrosamine (DENA), a potent liver cancer carcinogen, was studied in rats over seven consecutive days. Increased levels of total bilirubin and thiobarbituric acid reactive substances were observed (Kou *et al.* 2023). Thymoquinone supplementation attenuated DENA-induced liver cancer caused likely through its antioxidant signaling properties.

In addition, scientists have found that oral thymoquinone increases levels of detoxifying liver enzymes, glutathione transferase, and quinone reductase (Kou *et al.* 2023). This may also be a possible factor in the elimination of carcinogens by thymoquinone.

4 ANTI-CANCER EFFECTS OF THYMOQUINONE

Recent advancements in nanotechnology and the combination of thymoquinone with other anti-cancer drugs have expanded its clinical applications (Table 1). Nanotechnology enhances the bioavailability, delivery, and targeting capacity of thymoquinone while protecting it from nonspecific binding.

Table 1. Applications of anti-cancer drugs combined with thymoquinone.

Name of drug	Functions of drugs	Reference
Cisplatin	Pt-mediated DNA cross-linking damage (Alkyl-like mechanism)	Pazhouhi *et al.* 2016
Temozolomide (TMZ)	DNA damage is caused by alkylation and G2/M cell cycle arrest	Khalife *et al.* 2016
Tamoxifen (TAM)	Anti-estrogen	Dirican *et al.* 2015
Topotecan (TP)	Topoisomerase-I inhibitor	Şakalar *et al.* 2016
Paclitaxel (Pac)	To stabilize microtubule assembly and disrupt mitosis to affect spindle formation	Imani *et al.* 2017
Docetaxel	Microtubule disruptor	Farooqi, Attar and Xu 2022
MiR-34a	MicroRNA	Zhu *et al.* 2016

4.1 *Nanotechnology and its applications*

In biotechnology, nanotechnology is a technique that reduces the costs of medical delivery and production and improves outcomes through more efficient drug discovery, disease detection, and drug delivery. Currently, thymoquinone nanoparticles have more substantial clinical effects than thymoquinone alone, providing specific targets to help fight cancer in vitro and increasing replication and tumor distribution in vivo. In addition, thymoquinone is extremely unstable in aqueous solutions because of pH and light sensitivity, and oral administration can lead to enzymatic changes. In such cases, nanoparticle-targeted drugs are the best choice for thymoquinone delivery (Kohandel *et al.* 2021). Also, nanoparticles can develop multifunctional nanoparticle complexes that can deliver diagnostic and therapeutic agents to targeted sites. Nanoparticles can easily penetrate biological membranes and provide sustained release of thymoquinone.

So far, researchers have used thymoquinone nanoparticles in several cancers, such as stomach cancer, small bowel cancer, and lung cancer in rat models. In addition, scientists have also found that the nanoparticles have an inhibitory effect on *Escherichia coli*, *Staphylococcus aureus*, and *Salmonella typhi*, indicating that thymoquinone nanoparticles can effectively inhibit gastric cancer and play a protective role when taken orally.

Radiotherapy is a very old treatment for gastric cancer. High-energy ionizing radiation generated by radiation therapy can cause necrosis of tumor surface and internal tissues and inhibit microtumors and local lymph nodes (Kohandel *et al.* 2021). On the other hand, radiotherapy has some side effects. Improper treatment can cause radiation to spread throughout the body. Nowadays, radiotherapy is used only for advanced cases of gastric cancer. In this context, nanotechnology presents promising clinical applications, offering potential enhancements in targeting and minimizing side effects.

4.2 *Clinical applications*

Phototherapy is another approach for treating gastric cancer, with the advantage of being non-invasive and repeatable. Two main methods are photodynamic therapy (PDT) and photothermal therapy (PTT). In addition, nanoparticles can be used as a tool to deliver photosensitizers to tumor sites and change the location of tumors. Unlike radiation, light can be focused within a specific area, which also slows down damage to some healthy organs and improves safety (American Society of Clinical Oncology 2002).

In PDT, reactive oxygen species are generated by shining a laser at 808 nm onto the tumor surface, which helps in delivering agents like metformin and IR780 more effectively. Metformin directly inhibits complex I on the mitochondrial electron transport chain, reducing cellular respiration. Additionally, dimethyl double tiger induces tumor hypoxia, which further enhances the efficacy of PDT and PTT in gastric cancer treatment.

Trans endothelial transport via albumin-protein binding allows the nanoparticles to spread throughout the tumor tissue. These chemotherapies have been used in several different cancers, such as breast, kidney, and lung cancer. The nanoparticles were delivered to different tumor locations, which effectively inhibited the growth of gastric cancer tumors by releasing PTX with few side effects. Experimental reports have shown that tetrandrine can also enhance PTX to better inhibit tumors (American Society of Clinical Oncology 2002).

5 CONCLUSION

In summary, thymoquinone exhibits a structure with carbonyl, carbon hydrogen, and vinylic groups that contribute to its inhibitory effects against gastric cancer. Its anti-cancer mechanisms involve several pathways: (1) STAT3: thymoquinone inhibits phosphorylation of STAT3, thereby reducing gastric cancer tumor growth; (2) PI3K/AKt/mTOR: thymoquinone impacts cell viability and HER2 downstream pathways to inhibit gastric cancer progression; (3) PTEN: through ADME interactions, thymoquinone exerts inhibitory effects on gastric cancer; (4) TGF-β/Smad2/3: the role of thymoquinone in migration inhibition, which is an effective method for tumor suppression, was tested by wound healing and transpire invasion assays; and (5) Antioxidant effects: thymoquinone, alongside vitamin C, demonstrates potential in inhibiting tumor growth through its antioxidant properties.

Nanotechnology is a sophisticated technique to inhibit gastric cancer and can be used in clinical trials in several ways, such as transendothelial transport and photodynamic therapy. Thymoquinone has demonstrated several advantages in inhibiting gastric cancer. Despite the advances, further studies are needed to fully realize the potential of thymoquinone and nanotechnology in clinical applications. Thymoquinone has tremendous potential to become a highly effective treatment for gastric cancer.

REFERENCES

Al-Rawashde FA., Al-Wajeeh AS., Vishkaei MN., Saad HKM., Johan MF., Taib WRW. and Ismail I. (2022). *Pharmaceuticals (Basel)*. 8, 15(9), 1123

Bitarafan S., Yari M., Broumand MA., Ghaderian SMH., Rahimi M., Mirfakhraie R., Azizi F. and Omrani MD. (2018). *Cell J.* **20**, 564–568

Dirican A., Atmaca H., Bozkurt E., Erten C. and Karaca B. (2015). *Uslu R.Transl. Oncol.* **17**, 145–51

Farooqi AA., Attar R. and Xu B. (2022). *Int J Mol Sci.* 5, 23(11), 6311

He P., He Y., Liu J., Liu C., Baoping Y. and Dong W. (2023). *Phytother Res.* 37(8):3467–3480.

Hokmabady L. and Fani N. (2022). *J Mol Model.* 17 ;28(10) :321.

Imani S., Wei C., Cheng J.., Khan A., Fu S., Yang L., Tania M., Zhang X., Xiao X. and Fu J. (2017). *Oncotarget.* 28, 21362–21379

Khalife R., Hodroj M.H., Fakhoury R. and Rizk S. (2016). *Planta Med.* **82**, 312–21

Kohandel Z., Farkhondeh T., Aschner M. and Samarghandian S. (2021). *Biomed Pharmacother.* **137**, 111374

Kou B., Liu W. and Zhao W. (2023). *Oncol Rep.*

Living With Cancer, Physical, Emotional, and Social Effects of Cancer, (2002), available online at : https://www.cancer.net/about-us/cancernet-editorial-board

Ma J., Hu X. and Li J., *Oncotarget*. (2017)

National Centerfor Biotechnology Information ; 2004-. PubChem Compound Summary.

Pazhouhi M., Sariri R., Rabzia A. and Khazaei M. (2016). *Med. Sci.* 19, 890–898

Şakalar Ç., İzgi K., İskender B., Sezen S., Aksu H., Çakır M., Kurt B., Turan A. and Canatan H. (2016). *Tumour Biol.* 37, 4467–77

Sayed-Ahmed MM., Aleisa AM., Al-Rejaie SS., Al-Yahya AA., Al-Shabanah OA., Hafez MM. and Nagi MN. (2010). *Oxid Med Cell Longev*., 3(4) :254–61.

Wilson A.J., Saskowski J., Lalani AS. and Wass E. (2015). *Ovarian Res.* **28**, 8–46

Zhou Q., Zheng X., Chen L., Xu B., Yang X., Jiang J. and Wu C. (2016). *Cell Physiol Biochem.*, 39(2) :453–66.

Zhu WQ., Wang J., Guo XF., Liu Z. and Dong WG. (2016). *World J Gastroenterol.* 28, 4149–59

Zhu Y., Tian T., Zou J., Wang Q., Li Z., Li Y., Liu X., Dong B., Li N, Gao J and Shen L. (2015). *BMC Cancer* 15, 894.

Biological Sciences and Environmental Health – Gao (Ed.)

Therapeutic effects and mechanisms of compounds targeting ferroptosis in hepatic fibrosis

Yandi Ding
Biomolecular Science, School of Science and Environment, Griffith University, Brisbane, QLD, Australia

ABSTRACT: Liver fibrosis caused by various etiologies is a significant global health concern, intricately linked to the nosogenesis of liver diseases. The abnormal accumulation of hepatic stellate cells (HSCs) in the extracellular matrix (ECM) is a key contributor to liver disease development, exacerbating the process of fibrosis. Recent research has enhanced our understanding of the mechanisms underlying fibrosis, and a newly discovered mechanism known as ferroptosis, which induces self-apoptosis in HSCs. However, due to its intricate pathways, traditional monotherapy and drugs often struggle to modulate the corresponding signalling cascades effectively. Certain herbal extracts have demonstrated potent effects in animal experiments in mitigating fibrosis; however, the lack of clinical trial data has hindered the validation of their efficacy. This article aims to underscore the significance of Oroxylin A; Dihydroartemisinin; Curcumin; Tannic Acid and Celastrol by reviewing experimental findings and molecular biology mechanisms. By discussing these approaches, the paper emphasizes their potential importance as much-needed anti-fibrotic therapies. Further clinical trials are required to explore the practical applications of herb extractions.

1 INTRODUCTION

Ferroptosis is one of the forms that regulate apoptosis in cells. The primary manifestation of its action is the aggregation of cellular lipid peroxides and the dysregulation between oxidation and reduction (Pan *et al.* 2021). Ferroptosis is usually associated with amino acid and iron metabolism, ferritinophagy, and cell adhesion, as well as signalling pathways such as p53 and Keap1/Nrf2 (Pan *et al.* 2021). Multiple studies indicate a close correlation between iron autophagy and liver liver fibrogenesis. Liver fibrosis, as a worldwide health issue, has been affecting 80 billion people and kills 20,000 a year. Besides, chronic liver disease (CLD) stands as a major factor contributing to liver fibrosis (Parola and Pinzan 2019). Hepatic stellate cells (HSCs), catalyzed by the ongoing inflammatory response led by CLD, cause the excessive accumulation of extracellular matrix (ECM) within heterogeneous fibrogenic liver cell population, resulting in sustained activation of fibrosis and wound healing responses (Pan *et al.* 2021).

In recent years, many researchers have focused on pathways induced by drugs like Oroxylin A (Sun *et al.* 2023; Zhao *et al.* 2023), DHA (dihydroartemisinin) (; Dolivo *et al.* 2021; Zhang *et al.* 2021), curcumin (Zheng *et al.* 2022), tannic acid (Li *et al.* 2022), berberine, and celastrol (Luo *et al.* 2022) to induce iron-mediated cell death in HSCs, thereby reducing the excessive ECM accumulation and resultant liver fibrosis. The purpose of this paper is to overlook the role of ferroptosis in liver fibrosis, as well as relevant drugs to explore a novel avenue for treating liver fibrosis.

DOI: 10.1201/9781003587590-29

2 MECHANISMS

2.1 *Hepatic fibrosis*

Nowadays, liver disease is one of the deadliest causes in the world (Asrani *et al.* 2019). The potential causes of CLD are complicated. Some infections like hepatitis B and C are deadly to hepatic cells, alcohol ingestion may cause steatohepatitis, while those who do not drink can also catch fibrosis. Moreover, autoimmune and genetic disorders are other threatens to livers (Roehlen *et al.* 2020). Fibrosis of liver cells represents a representative progression of CLD.

Chronic liver diseases result in damage to liver tissues, leading to the formation of liver fibrotic scar tissue that replaces normal liver cell tissue. The excessive ECM generated from the activation of hepatic stellate cells (HSCs) is often considered a hallmark of liver fibrosis formation (Figure 1) (Li and Zhu 2023).

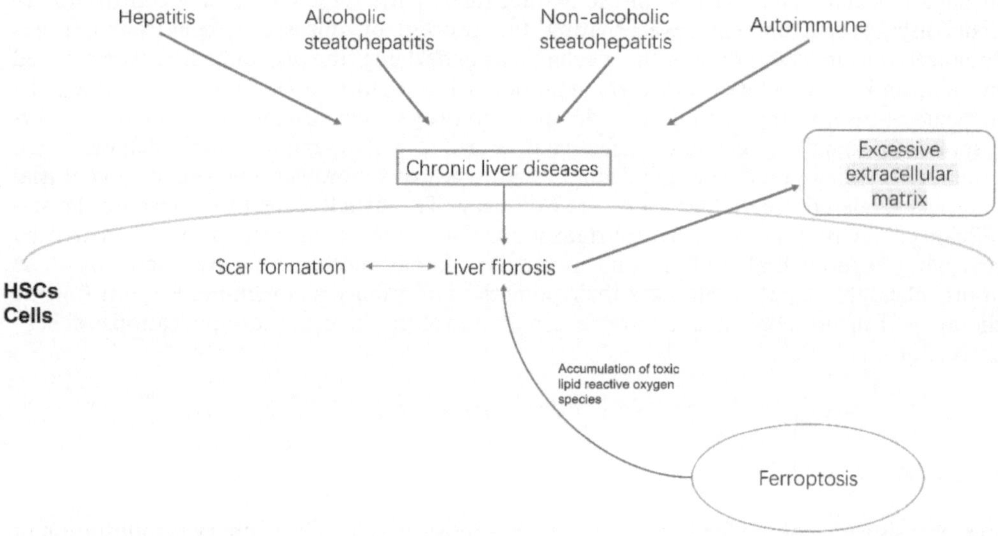

Figure 1. Mechanism of liver fibrosis and ferroptosis: Hepatitis and other external factors lead to chronic liver diseases. CLD may cause continuous damage on liver, which contributes to the formation of scars. Between the interaction of scars and fibrosis, excessive extracellular matrix is accumulated. Ferroptosis can be catalysed to enhance the apoptosis speed of HSCs, significantly reducing the fibrosis. Figure credit: Original.

2.2 *Ferroptosis in liver fibrosis*

Ferroptosis has a typical identity about the aggregation of toxic lipid reactive oxygen species (ROS), which is a way of iron apoptotic (Dixon *et al.* 2012). Inhibiting liver fibrosis can be achieved through the inactivation of HSCs and induction of HSC death. The majority of evidence points to the pharmacological effect of inducing HSC apoptosis through iron autophagy, particularly by specific drugs targeting specific pathways. The key critical of NCOA4 and FTH1 in ferroptosis has been mentioned in most of the literatures, and some research proved the effectiveness of targeted therapy for NCOA4 and FTH1 (Zhou *et al.* 2020). In summary, ferroptosis could potentially serve treat liver fibrosis as a fresh therapeutic strategy.

3 THERAPEUTIC EFFECTS OF DRUGS TARGETING INDUCING FERROPTOSIS OF HSCS

Recent research has mostly focused on identifying specific signalling pathways mediated by certain drugs that can cause ferroptosis in HSCs, thereby offering a potential avenue for treating liver fibrosis (Table 1). Some evidence has been proved with potential.

Table 1. Chemicals involved in the ferroptosis.

Name	PubChem CID	Molecular Formula	Pathways/Targeting	References
Oroxylin A	5320315	$C_{16}H_{12}O_5$	cGAS-STING	Sun *et al.* 2023; Zhao *et al.* 2023
Dihydroartemisinin	3000518	$C_{15}H_{24}O_5$	ROS-JNK1/2 dependent autophagy; NF-κB	Dolivo *et al.* 2021; Zhang *et al.* 2021
Curcumin	969516	$C_{21}H_{20}O_6$	Direct targeting NOCA4 and FTH1; LC3 - II and Beclin1 protein expression, reducing p62 protein expression	Tang *et al.* 2018; Zheng *et al.* 2022
Celastrol	122724	$C_{29}H_{38}O_4$	Peroxiredoxins (PRDXs); heme oxygenase 1 (HO-1)	Luo *et al.* 2022

Oroxylin A was approved to target the cGAS-STING pathway (Sun *et al.* 2023; Zhao *et al.* 2023). DHA has a decreasing in hepatic α-SMA and PDGF-B (Dolivo *et al.* 2021; Zhang *et al.* 2021). Curcumin increases the expression of NCOA1 and FTH4 mediates the degradation of FTH1 in autolysosomes (Zheng *et al.* 2022). Moreover, celastrol exerts an anti-inflammatory effect (Luo *et al.* 2022).

3.1 *Oroxylin A*

Oroxylin A is a flavone compound naturally found in various medicinal plants, including Scutellaria Baicalensis (Chinese skullcap) and Oroxylum indicum (Indian trumpet flower). Structure is known as $C_{16}H_{12}O_5$, and molecular weight is 284.26 g/mol.

Researchers found that Oroxylin A triggers senescence in HSCs by upregulating the expression of apolexis -related markers such as p16, p21, and HMGA1 (Sun *et al.* 2023). This is associated with a halt in the cell cycle and a decrease in telomerase activity, indicative of cellular aging. Oroxylin A affects the expression of NCOA4 (a protein involved in ferritinophagy) and FTH1 (a subunit of ferritin), with NCOA4 increasing and FTH1 decreasing dose-dependently (Zhao *et al.* 2023). NCOA4 siRNA interference was then conducted. When NCOA4 was knocked down, Oroxylin A's ability to induce senescence-related changes was attenuated, indicating that NCOA4 was involved in this process (Zhao *et al.* 2023). The team suggested that Oroxylin A can muted fibrosis indicators such as α-SMA and collagen 1 (Sun *et al.* 2023). This regulatory effect is hindered in the presence of siNCOA4, reinforcing the role of NCOA4 in Oroxylin A's actions.

Previous study proved that the cGAS-STING is known to trigger the expression of interferons, interleukins, and chemokines upon activation (Chen *et al.* 2018). The results in the production of cytokines, which can create conditions favourable for cellular senescence. Oroxylin A's pro-senescence effect is connected to the excitation of the cGAS-STING pathway. When cGAS is knocked down, Oroxylin A's ability to induce senescence-related changes is attenuated (Zhao *et al.* 2023). Some improvement in SA-β-gal expression (a senescence marker) is reduced in the existence of sicGAS. Similarly, the downregulation of p16 and p21 caused by Oroxylin A is reversed under the circumstances of sicGAS (Sun *et al.*

2023). These findings further contribute to understanding the mechanisms underlying Oroxylin A's anti-fibrotic and senescence-inducing properties.

3.2 *Dihydroartemisinin*

Artemisinin is a sesquiterpene lactone compound with an endoperoxide bridge. It was first identified in 1972 through the collaborative efforts of Project 523 in China, working alongside Dr. Tu Youyou. This compound was derived from the plant Artemisia annua (White *et al.* 2015).

Dihydroartemisinin (DHA) is also known as artenimol. Artenimol is an active metabolite of artesunate, with anti-malarial activity, and potential insulin sensitivity-improving, anti-inflammatory, immunomodulating and antineoplastic activities. The Molecular formula is known as $C_{15}H_{24}O_5$, and molecular weight is 284.35 g/mol.

DHA effectively mitigates hepatic fibrosis by instigating ferroptosis in HSCs. This therapeutic process revolves around DHA's capacity to induce the controlled death of activated HSCs through ferroptosis. However, the potential of DHA to induce ferroptosis is hindered by specific inhibitors of this process, namely ferrostatin-1 and liproxstatin-1 (Zhang *et al.* 2021). Notably, the engagement of autophagy appears to be intricately linked to DHA-induced ferroptosis. Manipulating the ATG5 protein, a vital component of autophagy, has significant implications: ATG5 siRNA obstructs DHA-triggered autophagy and consequent ferroptosis, while the introduction of an ATG5 plasmid amplifies DHA's impact on both autophagy and ferroptosis (Zhang *et al.* 2021).

In this complex mechanism, the upregulation of NCOA4 emerges as a pivotal player. NCOA4, a factor central to cellular processes, assumes a critical role in DHA-mediated ferroptosis. Silencing NCOA4 through siRNA compromises DHA-induced ferroptosis, whereas introducing an NCOA4 plasmid augments DHA's capacity to stimulate ferroptosis (Zhang *et al.* 2021).

In various animal pathological models, a decline in the synthesis of α-SMA and PDGF-B within the liver has been observed, accompanied by the restoration of peroxisome proliferator-activated receptor PPARγ expression. The alleviation of liver fibrosis is achieved through a concomitant decline in the expression levels of α-SMA, type I collagen, fibronectin, TGF-β RII, PDGF-RB, and EGFR. (Dolivo *et al.* 2021). Additionally, in a CCL4-induced hepatic fibrosis matrix, oral administration of DHA or artemisinin can mitigate liver damage, inflammation, and fibrosis through multiple mechanisms. These mechanisms include antagonizing the NF-κB signalling pathway, regulating the TLR4/MyD88/NF-κB signalling path, and inducing senescence in HSCs (Zhang *et al.* 2017).

3.3 *Curcumin*

Curcumin is a naturally occurring substance derived from the rhizome (root) of the turmeric plant, scientifically known as Curcuma longa. The Chemical formula is known as $C_{21}H_{20}O_6$, and molecular weight is 368.38 g/mol.

Western blot analysis revealed that curcumin exerted a significant inhibitory effect on P62 expression, while concurrently enhancing the expression of Beclinl and LC3II. Notably, curcumin upregulated the levels of ACSL4 and COX2 proteins, whereas it downregulated the expression of GPX4 and SLC7A11 proteins. Under transmission electron microscopy, distinct features of ferroptosis were observed, including the presence of vacuoles within cells, noticeable depression along the nuclear membrane, and a notable increase in autophagosome count following curcumin treatment (Stoyanovsky *et al.* 2019).

Moreover, curcumin induced a degradation process involving FTH1 within autolysosomes, facilitated by elevated NCOA1 and FTH4 expression. This degradation surpassing synthesis led to an overall reduction in FTH1 protein expression. Consequently, the substantial release of iron ions due to FTH1 degradation contributed to iron overload, initiating lipid peroxidation and ultimately triggering ferroptosis in HSCs (Zheng *et al.* 2022).

Curcumin treatment leads to a significant reduction in protein expression of TTC3 and Smads, accompanied by an upregulation of SMURF2 protein expression in liver cells, as demonstrated by gene binding heatmaps (Stoyanovsky *et al.* 2019). The mRNA levels of TTC3, SMURF2, and Smads are downregulated. The enhanced autophagy contributes to the suppression of TTC3, thereby augmenting the functionality of SMURF2. Importantly, SMURF2 effectively inhibits the formation of the Smad2/Smad3 complex, ultimately resulting in the inhibition of epithelial-mesenchymal transition (EMT) cascade in liver cells (Kong *et al.* 2020).

3.4 *Celastrol*

Celastrol was discovered from the root bark of Tripterygium wilfordi. Anti-inflammatory significance has been proved by studies (Deng *et al.* 2020; Tang *et al.* 2018). The structure is known as $C_{29}H_{38}O_4$, and molecular weight is 450.6 g/mol.

Celastrol treatment significantly suppresses the criterion of IL-1β, IL-6, IL-18, and TNF-α, when adding the amount of IL-10 and IL-13 in the fibrotic liver and sera, demonstrating potent anti-inflammatory properties. Significantly, celastrol effectively suppresses the mRNA and protein expression of α-SMA, fibronectin, and α(I) collagen in activated HSCs (Luo *et al.* 2022). Interestingly, compared to curcumin, celastrol treatment increases the expression of SIRT3, without affecting SIRT1 mRNA expression. Furthermore, celastrol enhances AMPK phosphorylation and effectively upregulates the expression of PGC-1α in activated HSCs. This results in a robust anti-inflammatory effect mediated by the AMPK-SIRT3 signalling pathway, ultimately showcasing the therapeutic potential of celastrol (Wang *et al.* 202).

One investigation unveiled that celastrol binds directly to the active cysteine sites of peroxiredoxins (PRDXs), including PRDX1, 2, 4, and 6, consequently inhibiting their anti-oxidative capabilities. Additionally, celastrol also targets heme oxygenase 1 (HO-1), leading to an elevation in its expression within activated hepatic stellate cells (HSCs). Lowering the levels of PRDX1, 2, 4, 6, or HO-1 in HSCs resulted in shifting degrees of increased level of ROS within cells, prompting iron-independent cell death (Luo *et al.* 2022).

3.5 *Other chemicals*

In the various herbal extractions explored, apart from celastrol, coincidentally all the other drugs, regardless of the specific signaling pathways they utilize, are associated with the induction of NCOA4 and FTH1. Although the discovery of ferroptosis began with the screening of small molecules targeting RAS mutations in 2007, over 16 years, a plethora of targets or proteins related to ferroptosis have been identified, including NCOA4, VDAC, System xc−, GPX4, HSPB1, TP53, Glutamine transporter, NFE2L2, lipoxygenases, ACSL4, FANCD2, PEBP1, NFS1, BAP1, OTUB1 etc. (Zhou *et al.* 2020). However, when it comes to ferroptosis-based treatments for liver fibrosis, NCOA4 appears to be an inescapable focus. The experimental content mentioned in the literature consistently demonstrates the therapeutic effects of the relevant drugs, and significant potential has been identified in relation to NCOA4. This highlights a concrete direction and approach for further in-depth research.

4 CONCLUSION

Considering the role of iron death that has been discovered in the pathogenesis of liver diseases, research on related drugs could represent a promising treatment target. Mechanism of ferroptosis has been proved through catalysing apoptosis of HSCs. Oroxylin A utilizes cGAS-STING to affect NCOA4 and FTH1 in hepatic cells. DHA triggered autophagy and consequent ferroptosis. Curcumin significantly decreases the protein expression of TTC3 and Smads. Celastrol has anti-inflammatory function mediated by AMPK-SIRT3 pathway.

Despite significant progress made in addressing liver fibrosis through iron death, the clinical application of related drugs is still in need of development. For instance, the targets of various drugs differ, and it's also uncertain in what specific pathological liver conditions or stages of diseases these drugs should be used.

REFERENCES

Asrani S.K., Devarbhavi H., Eaton J. and Kamath P.S. (2019). *J. Hepatol.* **70**,151–171

Chen W., Zhang Z., Yao Z., Wang L., Zhang F., Shao J., Chen A. and Zheng S. (2018). *Int. Immunopharmacol* **56**, 148–155

Deng Y., Luo H., Shu J., Shu H., Lu C., Zhao N., Geng Y., He X. and Lu A. (2020). *Chin. Med* **15**, 30

Dixon S. J., Lemberg K. M., Lamprecht M. R., Skouta R., Zaitsev E. M., Gleason C. E., Patel D. N., Bauer A. J., Cantley A. M. and Yang W. S. (2012). *B.* 3rd *Morrison, & B. R. Stockwell, Cell* **149**, 1060–1072

Dolivo D., Weathers P. and Dominko T. (2021). *Acta Pharm. Sin. B*, **11**, 322–339

Kong D., Zhang Z., Chen L., Huang W., Zhang F., Wang L., Wang Y., Cao P. and Zheng S. (2020). *Redox. Biol* **36**

Li L. and Zhu Z. (2023). *Front. Pharmacol* **13**

Li L., Wang K., Jia R., Xie J., Ma L., Hao Z., Zhang W., Mo J. and Ren F. (2022). *Redox. Biol* **56**

Luo P., Liu D., Zhang Q., Yang F., Wong Y. K., Xia F., Zhang J., Chen J., Tian Y., Yang C., Dai L., Shen H. M. and Wang J. (2022). *B* **12**, 2300–2314

Pan Q., Luo Y., Xia Q. and He K. (2021). *Int. J. Health Sci.* **18**, 3361–3366

Parola M. and Pinzani M., *Mol. Aspects Med*, **65**, 37–55

Roehlen N., Crouchet E. and Baumert T. F. (2020). *Cells* **9**, 875

Stoyanovsky D.A., Tyurina Y.Y., Shrivastava I., Bahar I., Tyurin V.A., Protchenko O., Jadhav S., Bolevich S.B., Kozlov A.V., Vladimirov Y.A., Shvedova A.A., Philpott C.C., Bayir H., and Kagan V.E. (2019). Free Radic Biol Med. **133**, 153–161

Sun Y., Weng J., Chen X., Ma S., Zhang Y., Zhang F., Zhang Z., Wang F., Shao J. and Zheng S. (2023). *Biomed. Pharmacother.* **162**, 0753–3322

Tang M., Cao X., Zhang K., Li Y., Zheng Q.Y., Li G.Q., He Q.H., Li S.J., Xu G.L. and Zhang K.Q. (2018). *Cell Death Dis.* **9**, 601

Wang S., Huang Z., Lei Y., Han X., Tian D., Gong J. and Liu M. (2022). *Front. Pharmacol* **13**

White N.J., Hien T.T. and Nosten F.H. (2015). *Trends Parasitol.* **31**, 607–610

Zhang Z., Wang X., Wang Z., Zhang Z., Cao Y., Wei Z., Shao J., Chen A., Zhang F. and Zheng S. (2021). *BioFactors* **47**, 1006–1016

Zhang Z.L., Yao Z., Zhao S.F., Shao J.J., Chen A.P. and Zhang F. (2017). *Cell Death Dis.* **8**

Zhao D., Gao Y., Su Y., Zhou Y., Yang T., Li Y., Wang Y., Sun Y., Chen L., Zhang F., Zhang Z., Wang F., Shao J. and Zheng S. (2023). **187**, 1043–6618

Zheng Y., Zhao T., Wang J., Jiang R., Huang J., Li W. and Wang J. (2022). *FASEB J*, **36**, 1

Zhou B., Liu J., Kang R., Klionsky D. J., Kroemer G. and Tang D. (2020). *Semin. Cancer Biol* **66**, 89–100

Biological Sciences and Environmental Health – Gao (Ed.)

Aβ in AD: Significance and potential as a therapeutic target

Junyao Zang
Department of Viticulture and Enology, University of California-Davis, CA, USA

ABSTRACT: Alzheimer's disease (AD) is an incurable neurodegenerative condition that deeply impacts cognitive function and behavior, presenting a substantial worldwide health concern. The amyloid hypothesis, a cornerstone of AD research, centers on the accumulation of Amyloid-beta (Aβ) peptides as a pivotal trigger in disease progression. We critically examined Aβ's intricate role in AD, exploring its generation, accumulation, and neurotoxic effects. Aβ peptides, derived from the Aβ precursor protein (APP), undergo enzymatic cleavage to form various variants, including the prominent Aβ42 and Aβ40. The accumulation of Aβ42/ Aβ40 in the brain is a hallmark of AD and is believed to drive disease development. We scrutinized the neurotoxicity of Aβ aggregation, emphasizing its potential to disrupt cellular function, induce oxidative stress, and prompt inflammation. Additionally, it explored the correlation between Aβ accumulation and cognitive decline, presenting evidence of their intertwined nature. This review highlights monoclonal antibodies as a targeted approach for AD therapy, investigating antibodies like lecanemab, aducanumab, and gantenerumab that aim to mitigate Aβ aggregation. It emphasized the challenges of designing effective drugs due to complexities in disease etiology, timing, blood-brain barrier permeability, and safety considerations.

1 INTRODUCTION

Alzheimer's disease (AD) is a progressive and irreversible neurological disorder that impacts the function of our brain, which leads to memory impairment, cognitive deterioration, perturbations in behavior. As per the World Health Organization (WHO), the global count of individuals affected by dementia stands at 55 million at present, with approximately 10 million new instances. Over 60% of dementia is AD and it is the most preeminent etiological factor of dementia among elders over 65 years old. Numerous research studies have been conducted on AD, and among the prevailing hypothesis, the amyloid hypothesis stands as a widely accepted explanation for the disease's cause. This paper aims to provide new researchers and students interested in AD with essential information about Aβ and its significance in the context of the disease. By delving into the fundamental aspects of Aβ's role, this resource seeks to offer a basic understanding of its implications in Alzheimer's pathology.

2 GENERATION AND ACCUMULATION OF Aβ

2.1 *What is Aβ?*

Amyloid-beta, often abbreviated as Aβ, is a short peptide consisting of 37 to 49 amino acid residues. It is derived from its precursor molecule, the beta-amyloid precursor protein (APP),

DOI: 10.1201/9781003587590-30

through a process known as protease cleavage. This enzymatic cleavage releases the Aβ peptide from the larger APP molecule.

The first discovery and identification of the Aβ peptide took place in 1984. This peptide was initially identified as a central component of meningovascular amyloid, a condition characterized by the abnormal deposition of amyloid proteins within the walls of blood vessels in the brain.

Of particular interest is a variant of Aβ known as Aβ42 and Aβ40, which contains 42 and 40 amino acid residues. Thes two specific variants have garnered considerable attention due to their association with AD, a devastating neurodegenerative disorder that affects memory, cognition, and behavior. The accumulation of Aβ42/ Aβ40 in the brain is a hallmark of AD and is believed to play a crucial role in the development and progression of the condition (Lewczuk *et al.* 2020).

2.2 *How is it generated?*

After years of extensive research, our understanding of Aβ has significantly deepened, leading to a better comprehension of its vital role in AD. Aβ is generated through a series of cuts on APP carried out by β-secretase and γ-secretase enzymes. APP is an essential trans-membrane protein found in numerous tissues, particularly concentrated in neuronal synapse. Multiple isoforms of APP are generated, varying in length from 695 to 770 amino acid residues. There are three common forms of APP: APP770, APP751, and APP695. In the human brain's neurons, the most abundant isoform is APP695, while APP770 and APP751 are mostly present on peripheral cells and platelets. The β-secretase enzyme triggers the initial cleavages of APP at the N-terminus of the Aβ sequence, resulting in the libration of secreted APP- β and left the C99 fragment within the membrane. Following this, the γ-secretase complex binds to the N-terminal C99 and performs an intramembranous cleave at the epsilon site, leading to the release of the C-terminal fragment and Aβ48. Aβ is mainly generated within endosomes, and release of Aβ from neurons is regulated by synaptic activity, both presynaptically. and postsynaptically.

3 NEUROLOGICAL TOXICITY OF Aβ ACCUMULATION

3.1 *Amyloid cascade hypothesis*

The amyloid cascade theory proposes that the root cause of AD is predominantly attributed to the buildup of Aβ protein within the brain. This protein tends to aggregate and give rise to structures known as amyloid plaques. Interestingly, individuals who maintain cognitive normalcy, yet exhibit the accumulation of Aβ in their brain, tend to display a heightened susceptibility to the development of cognitive impairments. This susceptibility is in stark contrast to individuals whose brains do not exhibit such an accumulation of amyloid. Out of the people who initially had good cognitive abilities and positive biomarkers, 34.4% showed a decline in cognitive function (measured by Clinical Dementia Rating $>$ 0). In comparison, only 8.4% of those with negative biomarkers had a similar decline in cognitive function (Long *et al.* 2022).

Aβ has the capacity to form different aggregative states, including oligomers, protofibrils, and amyloids fibrils (Figure 1) (Panza *et al.* 2019). Among these, amyloid fibrils hold particular significance due to their larger size, insolubility, and ability to accumulate into amyloid plaques.

Amyloid monomers are mostly nontoxic, but the aggregation of Aβ can cause damage to our brain. Several researches have shown that Amyloid beat oligomers are responsible for the damage to our brain. Aβ oligomers have the potential to form outside and inside cells. They exert harmful effects on neurons through various means. These include creating pores that lead to ion leakage, disturbing the balance of cellular calcium, and reducing membrane potential. Moreover, they can change membrane structure and function, leading to LTP suppression and neuronal death.

In ADs involving amyloid buildup, the harmful substances can come from two sources: deposits of amyloid fibrils that accumulate outside cells and affect brain function, or small groups of soluble proteins called oligomers (Evangelisti *et al.* 2016). In various neurodegenerative diseases linked to amyloid, these soluble oligomers can emerge during amyloid formation or be released by existing deposits, leading to problems in cells directly.

Even though the specific shape of these amyloid oligomers is important, it's not the only factor influencing their toxicity (Farrugia *et al.* 2020). The way these misfolded oligomers cause harm to cells appears to be connected to certain parts of their structure being exposed on the surface (Mannini *et al.* 2014), and their small size allowing them to move around rapidly.

Because of their misfolded nature and tendency to stick together, these amyloidogenic oligomers are harmful. Their unique structure leads them to interact abnormally with various components within cells, such as cell membranes, small molecules, proteins, receptors, genetic material, and cellular substances. These interactions can disrupt normal cell function and, over time, contribute to cell damage and cell death. Interestingly, many amyloid-related diseases also show signs of inflammation, possibly because the body's immune response reacts to the unfamiliar molecular structures produced during the amyloid buildup or to the products they generate.

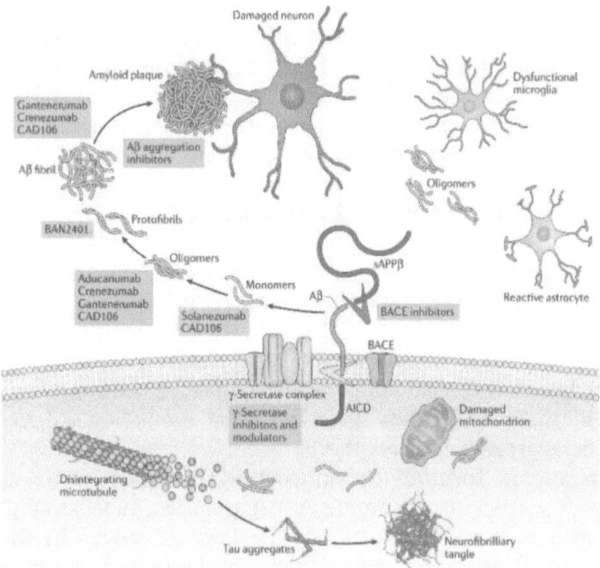

Figure 1. Formation of amyloid plaque.

3.2 *Correlation of Aβ and AD*

Amyloid plaques, renowned as significant markers of AD, prominently showcase the Aβ (Aβ) protein. Nevertheless, it's imperative not to disregard the point that these plaques also incorporate a plethora of other proteins in addition to Aβ. This diverse protein composition encompasses entities with diverse functions. Some of these proteins have direct interactions with Aβ, actively influencing the Aβ aggregation process and thus molding the formation of amyloid plaques (Wisniewski and Frangione 1992). Furthermore, the existence of proteins originating from microglia and astrocytes, the supportive cells encompassing and infiltrating the plaques, holds importance. These proteins possess the capability to impact glial function, potentially contributing to pathological glial reactions Another aspect of plaque makeup involves proteins embedded within dystrophic neurites, which are structurally compromised segments of nerve cells. These proteins offer insights into the fundamental factors behind the abnormal formation of neurotic plaques, which exhibit a more pronounced association with cognitive decline compared to diffuse plaques Conducting a comprehensive analysis of the proteins enriched within amyloid plaques could yield a more profound understanding of the mechanisms propelling the development of AD. This endeavor not only offers the potential to enhance comprehension but also to unveil new biomarkers and therapeutic targets for addressing AD.

There are two commonly observed neuropathological characteristics. One neurofibrillary tangle comprised of tau proteins that have undergone hyperphosphorylation, and the other one is amyloid plaques composed of amyloid β protein.

Yang found two types of Aβ42 filaments in brains of patients who have AD. Yang classified them as type I and type II Aβ42 filaments, which type I is found in brains of those with sporadic AD, while type II is found in those with familial cases of the condition (Yang *et al.* 2022). Instances of AD where Type I filaments were predominant saw individuals living to an older age at the time of death, in comparison to other cases of both Alzheimer's and non-Alzheimer's conditions where Type II filaments were more prevalent in the neocortex.

Oxygen stress is a significant factor in the pathogenesis of AD. Much evidence indicates that the accumulation of Aβ in AD disrupts normal mitochondrial dynamics, causing malfunction in mitochondria, which in turn triggers an excessive generation of reactive oxygen species (ROS). When ROS increases, it can trigger inflammation, elevated protease secretion, which all can contribute to cellular structure damage (Li *et al.* 2016). Consistently, across different transgenic mouse models of AD containing mutations of APP and PS-1, there was a consistent connection between the accumulation of age-related Abeta and heightened production of hydrogen peroxide and nitric oxide, along with increased oxidative changes in proteins and lipids. This correlation confirms the role of Abeta in driving oxidative stress. Mohmmad found 40% increased level of protein carbonyls (a sign of oxidation) in neuron cells with APP compared to wildtype neuron cells.

4 TARGET Aβ FOR DRUG DESIGN

Currently, there are four monoclonal antibodies in advanced clinical testing aimed at addressing Aβ-related concerns. These include lecanemab, aducanumab, gantenerumab, and donanemab. Each of these antibodies belongs to the monoclonal IgG1 category and is designed to target the aggregated forms of Aβ.

Lecanemab is an altered form of the murine mAb158 antibody, initially created at Uppsala University. It zeroes in on soluble Aβ aggregates, such as oligomers and protofibrils, showing a strong affinity. This antibody has been advanced by BioArctic and Eisai, and it demonstrated significant effectiveness in eliminating plaques and generating efficacy indications during a phase 2b clinical evaluation. The dosage of 10mg/kg biweekly is identified as effective with the least treatment emergent adverse event (TEAE), which is 39% among 161 patients (Swanson *et al.* 2021).

Aducanumab, formulated by Biogen, is a synthetic human antibody that binds specifically to amino acids 3–7 of the Aβ peptide. Its development faced a pause in 2019 due to initial data analysis from two phase 3 trials, which suggested the clearance and mitigation of neurotoxicity might not be achieved. However, further scrutiny of the data unveiled aducanumab bind to aggregated forms of Aβ, leading to its approval by the FDA in the USA in 2021. The relationship between dosage and exposure was consistently linear in both plasma and brain tissues following the prolonged administration of aducanumab in mice with plaques. Aducaneumab showed a dose-dependent reduction in Aβ levels within brain homogenates. This reduction reached up to 50% when compared to the control group (Sevigny *et al.* 2016). This impact was observable in the soluble Aβ40 and Aβ42 forms as individual molecules and in the combined structures, along with the non-dissolvable Aβ fibrils.

Gantenerumab, a product of Roche, emerged from a human combinatorial antibody library. It stands out as distinct from the other three antibodies due to its dual focus on both the 3-11 amino acids of N-terminal and 18-27 amino acids of mid-regions of the Aβ peptide (Bohrmann *et al.* 2012). Clinical trials involving gantenerumab experienced a setback in 2014 when two phase 3 trials were prematurely stopped following an interim analysis that revealed no significant efficacy regarding primary or secondary endpoints.

Aβ has been studied as a target for AD treatment. There are many forms of Aβ like monomers, oligomers, protofibrils, and insoluble fibrils. Since particular interest are oligomers and protofibrils, which are harmful, the removal of them could be effective in AD treatment. Lecanemab, Aducanumab, and Gantenerumab are antibodies that can be bound to Aβ. All three of the antibodies have a low affinity to monomers, but LEcanemab and aducanumab exhibited less potent binding to monomers in comparison to gantenerumab. Lecanemab demonstrated a tenfold higher binding affinity to protofibrils when contrasted with fibrils, whereas aducanumab and gantenerumab displayed a greater binding affinity to fibrils rather than protofibrils (Söderberg *et al.* 2023).

5 CHALLENGES AND CONSIDERATIONS IN Aβ DRUG DEVELOPMENT

Drug development for Alzheimer's disease is an intricate and multifaceted challenge, marked by a web of interconnected factors that collectively impede progress in the quest for effective treatments. At the core of this formidable challenge lies the enigmatic nature of the disease itself. Alzheimer's, a complex neurodegenerative disorder, continues to shroud its intricate mechanisms in mystery, leaving researchers grappling with a formidable obstacle. This knowledge gap not only hampers our ability to understand the root causes of Alzheimer's but also presents a formidable hurdle in developing precise, targeted therapies to combat the disease effectively.

5.1 *Diagnosis*

One of the most pressing concerns in Alzheimer's drug development is the persistent difficulty in diagnosing the disease at an early stage. Typically, Alzheimer's remains elusive until its later stages when significant brain damage has already taken its toll. This late diagnosis poses a twofold challenge: it not only limits the window of opportunity for intervention but also complicates the development of drugs designed to halt the disease's progression before it gains a foothold or, ideally, prevent symptoms from manifesting altogether.

Compounding these challenges is the critical absence of reliable biomarkers for Alzheimer's disease. These diagnostic indicators, capable of accurately detecting the disease and tracking its progression, remain frustratingly scarce. Without robust biomarkers, identifying suitable candidates for clinical trials becomes a formidable task, and assessing the effectiveness of potential treatments becomes an imprecise endeavor, further clouding the drug development landscape.

5.2 *Blood-brain barrier*

Furthermore, the presence of the blood-brain barrier adds another layer of complexity. This naturally occurring defense mechanism zealously guards the brain, restricting the passage of many substances, including potential drug candidates. Overcoming this formidable obstacle and crafting drugs that can successfully traverse the blood-brain barrier to reach their intended targets within the brain stands as a pivotal challenge in the field of Alzheimer's drug development.

5.3 *Other concerns*

The complexity of Alzheimer's is further underscored by its lack of uniformity. The disease manifests in various subtypes and exhibits variations in its presentation and progression from person to person. This inherent heterogeneity necessitates the development of treatments capable of addressing the diverse facets of Alzheimer's, making it even more challenging to find a one-size-fits-all solution.

The global aging population exacerbates the situation, as the prevalence of Alzheimer's disease is projected to surge in the coming years. This escalating caseload not only intensifies the urgency to find effective treatments but also complicates the process of conducting clinical trials and providing care for the growing number of affected individuals.

Moreover, the intricate interplay between genetics and Alzheimer's disease remains a subject of ongoing exploration. While certain genetic factors are known to elevate the risk of developing Alzheimer's, the precise role and mechanisms of these genetic influences continue to evolve. This knowledge gap complicates efforts to develop personalized treatments tailored to an individual's genetic profile.

Ethical considerations loom large in the realm of Alzheimer's drug development, particularly when it comes to testing potential treatments on vulnerable populations, such as individuals with advanced cognitive impairment. The ethical implications of informed consent, ensuring the well-being of participants, and the potential risks and benefits of experimental treatments are complex and require careful navigation.

6 CONCLUSION

In conclusion, the pursuit of effective Alzheimer's disease treatments centered around targeting Aβ proteins presents a formidable scientific and medical challenge. Aβ, derived from the beta-amyloid precursor protein (APP), plays a pivotal role in the pathology of Alzheimer's, particularly Aβ42 and Aβ40 variants, which accumulate in the brain and are strongly associated with the disease.

Understanding the generation and accumulation of Aβ is critical for drug development. Aβ is generated through enzymatic cleavage of APP, with β-secretase and γ-secretase enzymes playing key roles. This process occurs mainly within endosomes, and its regulation is influenced by synaptic activity.

The neurological toxicity of Aβ accumulation is a central focus of Alzheimer's research, and the amyloid cascade hypothesis posits that Aβ buildup is a primary driver of the disease. Aβ can aggregate into various forms, including amyloid plaques, which have been linked to cognitive decline. Additionally, Aβ oligomers, small soluble proteins, are recognized as particularly harmful to brain cells, as they can disrupt normal cellular function and lead to cell damage and death.

The correlation between Aβ and Alzheimer's is intricate, involving the complex composition of amyloid plaques and their interactions with various proteins, glial cells, and dystrophic neurites. This multifaceted relationship offers opportunities to better understand the disease and identify potential biomarkers and therapeutic targets.

Efforts to target Aβ for drug development have led to the investigation of monoclonal antibodies like lecanemab, aducanumab, gantenerumab, and donanemab. These antibodies are designed to bind to aggregated forms of Aβ, particularly oligomers and protofibrils. Clinical trials have shown promise in reducing Aβ levels, but challenges remain in optimizing dosages and addressing potential side effects.

However, Alzheimer's drug development is rife with challenges and considerations. The late diagnosis of the disease, the lack of reliable biomarkers, and the presence of the blood-brain barrier make drug development complex. Additionally, Alzheimer's heterogeneity, the aging population, genetic factors, and ethical concerns further complicate the path toward effective treatments.

REFERENCES

Bohrmann, B., Baumann, K., Benz, J., Gerber, F., Huber, W., Knoflach, F., Messer, J., Oroszlan, K., Rauchenberger, R., Richter, W. F., Rothe, C., Urban, M., Bardroff, M., Winter, M., Nordstedt, C. and Loetscher, H. (2012). *Journal of Alzheimer's Disease : JAD*, 28(1), 49–69.

Evangelisti, E., Cascella, R., Becatti, M., Marrazza, G., Dobson, C. M., Chiti, F., Stefani, M. and Cecchi, C. (2016). *Scientific Reports*, 6, 32721.

Farrugia, M. Y., Caruana, M., Ghio, S., Camilleri, A., Farrugia, C., Cauchi, R. J., Cappelli, S., Chiti, F., and Vassallo, N. (2020). *Scientific Reports*, 10(1), 17733.

Lewczuk, P., Łukaszewicz-Zając, M., Mroczko, P., and Kornhuber, J. (2020). *Pharmacological Reports: PR*, 72(3),528–542.

Li, R., Jia, Z. and Trush, M. A. (2016). *Reactive Oxygen Species* (Apex, N.C.), 1(1), 9–21.

Long, J. M., Coble, D. W., Xiong, C., Schindler, S. E., Perrin, R. J., Gordon, B. A., Benzinger, T. L. S., Grant, E., Fagan, A. M., Harari, O., Cruchaga, C., Holtzman, D. M., and Morris, J. C. (2022). *Brain: a Journal of Neurology*, 145(12), 4506–4518.

Mannini, B., Mulvihill, E., Sgromo, C., Cascella, R., Khodarahmi, R., Ramazzotti, M., Dobson, C. M., Cecchi, C. and Chiti, F. (2014). *ACS Chemical Biology*, 9(10), 2309–2317.

Panza, F., Lozupone, M., Logroscino, G., and Imbimbo, B. P. (2019). *Nature Reviews. Neurology*, 15(2), 73–88.

Sevigny, J., Chiao, P., Bussière, T., Weinreb, P. H., Williams, L., Maier, M., Dunstan, R., Salloway, S., Chen, T., Ling, Y., O'Gorman, J., Qian, F., Arastu, M., Li, M., Chollate, S., Brennan, M. S., Quintero-Monzon, O., Scannevin, R. H., Arnold, H. M., Engber, T., and Sandrock, A. (2016). *Nature*, 537(7618), 50–56.

Söderberg, L., Johannesson, M., Nygren, P., Laudon, H., Eriksson, F., Osswald, G., Möller, C. and Lannfelt, L. (2023). *Neurotherapeutics : The Journal of the American Society for Experimental NeuroTherapeutics*, 20 (1), 195–206.

Swanson, C. J., Zhang, Y., Dhadda, S., Wang, J., Kaplow, J., Lai, R. Y. K., Lannfelt, L., Bradley, H., Rabe, M., Koyama, A., Reyderman, L., Berry, D. A., Berry, S., Gordon, R., Kramer, L. D. and Cummings, J. L. (2021). *Alzheimer's Research & Therapy*, 13(1), 80.

Wisniewski, T., and Frangione, B. (1992). *Neuroscience Letters*, 135(2), 235–238.

Yang, Y., Arseni, D., Zhang, W., Huang, M., Lövestam, S., Schweighauser, M., Kotecha, A., Murzin, A. G., Peak-Chew, S. Y., Macdonald, J., Lavenir, I., Garringer, H. J., Gelpi, E., Newell, K. L., Kovacs, G. G., Vidal, R., Ghetti, B., Ryskeldi-Falcon, B., Scheres, S. H. W. and Goedert, M. (2022). *Science (New York, N.Y.)*, 375(6577), 167–172.

Biological Sciences and Environmental Health – Gao (Ed.)
© 2025 the Author(s), ISBN: 978-1-032-96016-6

Current status and challenges of CAR-NK in the treatment of gynecological cancer

Zhuoting Zhang
Biomedical Science (Department), City University of Hong Kong, Hong Kong, China

ABSTRACT: Gynecological cancers, including the ovarian, cervical, endometrial, and breast cancers, account for a large proportion of female cancer patients and significantly contribute to the worldwide cancer burden. Currently, the main treatments for these cancers are surgery, chemotherapy, and radiotherapy, while immunotherapy is being developed as a treatment with better efficacy and fewer side effects. As an innovative cancer immunotherapy method. In recent years, CAR-NK therapy has received many attention, because it can address some of the limitations of CAR-T therapy with some unique advantages in terms of the preparation, efficacy, and safety. Research on CAR-NK therapy for blood cancers or various types of solid tumors has been widely reported, however, there is still a lack of a unified overview of the current research status of CAR-NK treatment of gynecological cancers. Therefore, this article classifies and summarizes relevant research on the gynecological cancers, and discusses current status, challenges, and potential improvements.

1 INTRODUCTION

The gynecologic cancers, mainly including ovarian, cervical, and endometrial cancers have a serious impact on women's health and longevity. According to the reports of WHO in 2020, these three categories of cancer combined account for nearly 15% of all newly diagnosed cancers in global women, and it is noteworthy that cervical and ovarian cancers account for the 4th and 8th largest number of cancer deaths in women patients, with a combined total of 12.4% of cancer deaths. Meanwhile, far more than any other type of cancer, breast cancer is the largest category of cancer deaths in women globally in 2020 with 2.26 million new diagnoses. Breast cancer will also be covered as a gynecologic cancer in this article because less than one percent of breast cancers occur in male patients, and it is the cancer with the highest number of new cases and deaths among women cancer patients worldwide. These gynecological cancers drastically reduce women's fertility and survivability and impose a significant financial burden on them. Current treatments regarding gynecologic cancers include surgery, chemotherapy, and radiation therapy, but all of these treatments have some limitations, such as poor effectiveness in treating metastatic cancer or advanced tumors and various side effects.

As research related to cancer treatment continues progressing, immunotherapy of cancer is playing an increasingly important role in cancer treatment, with particular advances in the therapy of metastatic cancers. Therefore, the treatment of gynecologic cancers through immunotherapeutic approaches that include adoptive cell therapy (ACT), immune checkpoint inhibitors(ICI), CAR-T, and CAR-NK to improve cure rates is an important and promising direction for cancer therapy. CAR-T therapies are effective in treating blood cancers: Since 2017, the FDA has approved six CAR-T treatments that are mainly for B-cell-related blood cancers, but CAR-T therapies are also associated with adverse effects (National Cancer Institute 2022). The advantage of CAR-NK over CAR-T is that non-autologous NK cells can also be used, such as NK-92 cell lines, which effectively avoids GVHD and CRS, and allows for a much shorter manufacturing cycle for CAR-NK (Pan

 DOI: 10.1201/9781003587590-31

et al. 2022). Therefore, CAR-NK therapy has had some clinical trials in recent years as a way to overcome some of the shortcomings of CAR-T used to treat cancer.

Currently, research and clinical trials on CAR-NK are mainly focused on leukemia, especially on B-cell malignancies, while fewer studies have been conducted on the treatment of gynecological cancers that are mainly about CAR-NK for ovarian and cervical cancer. Due to the lack of an overall summary of the status and challenges of CAR-NK to treat gynecologic cancers, this article will describe the mechanism of CAR-NK for treating gynecologic cancers, the current status of the research situation, current challenges and potential improvements, and look forward to the development of this therapeutic approach.

2 CAR-NK MECHANISMS

The mechanisms of action of CAR-NK primarily involve cytotoxicity: CAR-NK cells can activate the cytotoxic responses by recognizing tumor-specific antigens (TSAs) through CARs. These responses include the release of cytotoxic granules, production of cytokines, and induction of apoptosis, ultimately leading to the death of tumor cells. Another mechanism is immunomodulation: NK cells possess immunomodulatory functions and can produce various cytokines to regulate immune cell activities. By modulating the activity and balance of immune cells, CAR-NK cells enhance overall immune responses and improve the ability to combat tumors.

CAR-T therapy utilizing autologous T cells of patients to express CARs for targeting and eliminating cancer cells has shown favorable efficacy in certain hematologic malignancies. However, it faces limitations when applied to solid tumors as follows (Pan *et al.* 2022). First, the complex tumor microenvironment makes manufacturing and amplification of CAR-T cells difficult, limiting the availability of a sufficient number and quality of them. Second, solid tumors often lack clearly defined TSAs, preventing CAR-T cells from targeting tumor cells, and resulting in suboptimal therapeutic outcomes. Third, the limited tumor infiltration of CAR-T cells restricts their interaction and killing efficacy against tumor cells. Fourth, solid tumors can create an immunosuppressive tumor microenvironment (TME), consisting of immune inhibitory cells and molecules, which dampens CAR-T cell activity, thus limiting the therapeutic response. Fifth, antigen escape: tumor cells may evade CAR-T cell targeting by altering antigen expression or selectively inhibiting antigen presentation. Last, CAR-T therapy may cause excessive releases of inflammatory cytokines that lead to CRS and neurotoxicity (Pan *et al.* 2022).

CAR-NK therapy offers several advantages that can compensate for some disadvantages of the CAR-T therapy. First, allogeneic NK cells or preexisting cell lines can be used to construct CAR-NK, eliminating the need for patient-derived cells and simplifying the manufacturing process without GVHD (Wang *et al.* 2020). Second, multi-faceted killing mechanisms of CAR-NK including with CAR and without CAR recognition of targets. The CAR can recognize TSAs, while the activation receptors on NK cells can trigger cytotoxic responses, enhancing the killing capacity against cancer cells. Third, CAR-NK therapy carries a lower risk of CRS and neurotoxicity compared to the CAR-T cell therapy since the effector functions of NK cells can be regulated without requiring additional stimulation. Fourth, it can reduce the immune escape (Li *et al.* 2022).

In summary, CAR-NK therapy offers advantages such as simplified manufacturing, multi-faceted killing mechanisms, lower toxicity, and reduced immune escape, providing a potential new strategy for gynecologic cancer treatment.

3 CURRENT STATUS OF CAR-NK RESEARCH ON GYNECOLOGIC CANCERS

3.1 *Ovarian cancer (OC)*

OC has greatest mortality rate of any gynecologic malignancy and even after surgery and multiple drugs of chemotherapy, there is still a high rate of recurrence. Considering cancer stem cells (CSC) are crucial for development of metastases and chemoresistance that may lead to high recurrence in ovarian tumors, the CSC markers CD133, CD24, and CD44 have received attention as the potential particular targets of CAR-NK used to treat ovarian cancer. Research demonstrated that anti-CD133-CAR NK cells displayed the ability to effectively kill ovarian tumors in both primary OC cells and CD133-positive OC cell lines, and the results of the experiment indicated that NK cells maintained to be active and cytotoxic when exposed to cisplatin and that consecutive application of cisplatin and CAR-NK had the most potent killing effect (Klapdor *et al.* 2017). Research of NK-92 cells modified with anti-CD24-CAR revealed that the cells had significant cytotoxic effect on the primary OC cells and CD24-expressing OC cell lines. Furthermore, to minimize potential off-target effects, the dual-CAR was developed against cells that expressed both CD24 and mesothelin in vivo (Klapdor *et al.* 2019). In 2021, a study of CD44-specific CAR-NK demonstrated that the cells displayed a killing effect against ovarian tumors in vitro and the combination of cisplatin and CD44-CAR-NK cells achieved the most effective anti-tumor result (Klapdor *et al.* 2021). These several CAR-NK therapies targeting markers of CSC are potentially promising and effective treatments for preventing ovarian cancer recurrence and provide research directions for further clinical studies.

Considering folate receptor alpha (αFR) overexpression accounts for 90% of OC, anti-αFR CAR-NK was constructed and the third-generation (αFR-28BBζ) CAR showed better cytotoxicity against αFR-positive OC, providing foundational information for further clinical investigation (Ao *et al.* 2019).

Mesothelin (MSLN) is overexpressed in ovarian cancer, therefore MSLN-CAR-NK was constructed and both in vitro and in vivo experimental results displayed potent and specific anti-tumor activity, indicating mesothelin is a promising target for CAR-NK to treat OC (Cao *et al.* 2020).

Since the human leukocyte antigen G (HLA-G) is over-expressed in the OC and has been associated with immune tolerance and tumor escape, it was used as a way to perform specific recognition to disrupt immunosuppressive mechanisms in OC. The HLA-G signal that inhibits NK function can be changed into an activation signal by the anti-HLA-G CAR, causing a cytotoxic killing response in vitro, reduction of tumor development in vivo, and extension of lifespan in mice. When this treatment is used in combination with low-dose chemotherapy, it can promote further tumor ablation (Jan *et al.* 2021).

3.2 *Cervical cancer*

Cervical cancer ranks fourth in the number of deaths among women cancer patients, with around 90% of patients coming from low- and middle-income countries, imposing a heavy financial strain on patients' families and society. In cervical cancer immunosurveillance, NK cells are crucial, but immune escape mechanisms in the cervical cancer microenvironment can limit NK cell activity by the cytokines expression and changes in ligands of tumor (Gutiérrez-Hoya and Soto-Cruz 2021). Therefore, a research investigated the prostate stem cell antigen (PSCA) as a target recognized by CAR-NK cells to strengthen activity to treat cervical cancer. The result demonstrated that CAR-NK cells targeting PSCA exhibit potent anti-cancer activities against PSCA-positive cervical tumors. Additionally, they successfully infiltrated tumor tissues, promoting the release of TNF-α and IFN-γ which are anti-tumor cytokines (Gutiérrez-Hoya and Soto-Cruz 2021). The study suggests that this CAR-NK as a therapeutic strategy holds promise for treating cervical cancer.

3.3 *Breast cancer (BC)*

BC occurs most commonly in women cancer patients with a low survival rate, representing a global health challenge. Overexpression HER2 has been associated with this cancer, and studies have shown that HER2 is overexpressed in 25-30% of breast cancer patients (Valabrega *et al.* 2007). The NK-92/5.28.z cell line, a stable clone of HER2-specific

CAR-NK-92 cells, was developed and efficiently lysed HER2-expressing cancer cells in vitro and showed specific antitumor activity in vivo (Schönfeld *et al.* 2015). NK-92/5.28.z cells created by Nowakowska's team are clinically useful, showing specific potency against HER2-positive targets that are commonly resistant to NK-cell cytotoxicity (Nowakowska *et al.* 2018). The NK-92 cells were able to specifically enhance the breakdown of HER2-expressing human tumors and reduce cancer metastasis in mice (Liu *et al.* 2015). Thus, HER2 is expected to be used as a target for the effective treatment of BC.

For triple-negative breast cancer (TNBC), studies related to the CAR-NK targeting the EGFR and tissue factor (TF) have been reported. A poor prognosis was associated with the overexpression of EGFR, which was present in 45% to 70% of TNBC patients, according to the EGFR-associated gene expression profile. EGFR-CAR-NK cells was proved effective in identifying and eliminating EGFR-overexpressed breast cancer cells, significantly extending mouse survival time and preventing tumor growth, showing a promising treatment option for TNBC patients (Liu *et al.* 2020). A study found that TF is an effective marker in 50-85% of the TNBC patients, and then TF-targeted CAR-NK cells with co-expressed CD16 and FcγIII were developed and tested for mediating ADCC (Hu 2020). The results showed that they have the ability to destroy TNBC cells in vitro and that L-ICON increased their potency. They also showed therapeutic effects in both cell lines and patient-derived mouse models of transplanted TNBC (Hu 2020).

The main treatment for ER-positive breast cancer is anti-estrogens administered as hormone therapy, and fulvestrant is the only anti-estrogen medicine currently clinically licensed that causes ER degradation, but fulvestrant resistance exists in some breast cancer patients. To overcome drug resistance, Lin *et al.* developed CAR-NKs that specifically target B7-H6 and assessed them in tumors that have developed fulvestrant resistance (Lin *et al.* 2021). The outcomes demonstrated that these CAR NK cells successfully promoted the death of drug-resistant BC cells, which was amplified by the increase of B7-H6 expression in the cell surface. This strategy offers a novel therapeutic approach to overcome drug resistance in breast cancer.

In addition, it is mentioned that NK cells expressing both CAR and IL-15 showed highly activity of selectiving cell-killing against BC cells that expressed epithelial cell adhesion molecule (EpCAM) (Sahm *et al.* 2012).

The following Table 1 summarizes the various targets for CAR-NK treatment of ovarian, cervical, and breast cancers with the in vitro or in vivo experiments, which show favorable application prospects.

Table 1. Current status of CAR-NK research on gynecologic cancers.

Cancer type	Target	NK source	Reference
Ovarian cancer	CD 133	NK-92	Klapdor *et al.* 2017
	CD 24	NK-92	Klapdor *et al.* 2019
	CD 44	NK-92	Klapdor *et al.* 2021
	α FR	NK-92	Ao *et al.* 2019
	Mesothelin	iPSC-NK or NK-92	Cao *et al.* 2020
	HLA-G	PB-NK	Jan *et al.* 2021
Cervical cancer	PSCA	NK-92	Gutiérrez-Hoya *et al.* 2021
Breast cancer	HER2	NK-92/5.28.z or NK-92	Schönfeld *et al.* 2015 Nowakowska *et al.* 2018 Liu *et al.* 2015
	EGFR	PB-NK	Liu *et al.* 2020
	TF	NK-92	Hu 2020
	B7-H6	NK-92	Lin *et al.* 2021
	EpCAM	NK-92	Sahm *et al.* 2012

4 CURRENT CHALLENGES AND POTENTIAL SOLUTIONS TO CAR-NK FOR GYNECOLOGIC CANCERS

CAR-NK for gynecologic cancers has been studied such as ovarian, cervical, and breast cancer, but there are currently no CAR-NK studies for endometrial cancer. Although the mortality rate of endometrial cancer is not as high as these three cancers, its negative impact on women's fertility and health still should not be underestimated. Moreover, as there is a poor survival rate of late-stage endometrial cancer, and the main treatment is chemotherapy at present, there is still a need for a more effective treatment with fewer side effects, and CAR-NK may provide a new option for future research on treatments.

CAR-NK cell immunotherapy is still at an early stage of research and therefore faces some challenges that need to be further investigated and improved, such as optimal sources and preparation strategies for NK cells used to construct CAR-NK, and the most appropriate signaling domains for CAR triggering that remain to be elucidated. Some CAR-NK therapeutics have progressed and verified safety in human clinical trials, proving that the clinical use of CAR-NK has a promising future. For example, CD33-CAR-NK-92 for patients with refractory and relapsed AML has been proven to be safe, but for gynecological cancers has only been subjected to some in vitro experiments or in vivo experiments in mice, and further studies are needed to increase the security and efficacy of CAR-NK to treat gynecologic cancers (Tang *et al.* 2018).

Although CAR-NK has many advantages to compensate for the disadvantages of the CAR-T, there are still some limitations of CAR-NK that are comparable to CAR-T that need to be further resolved, like the NK cells are not the predominant immune cell type present in the TME, so NK cell functions may be suppressed by the immunoinhibitory TME when infiltrating the tumor sites (Pan *et al.* 2022). One potential treatment to address this problem is CAR-macrophages, as macrophages are one of the major infiltrating cells in TME. According to preclinical research, a clinical study using CAR macrophages against HER2-expressing solid tumors with potential anticancer efficacy is now in progress. CAR macrophages are being developed as antigen presenters, TME modifiers, and immunostimulators for enhancing anticancer immunity (Pan *et al.* 2022).

5 CONCLUSION

The article focuses on the current status of research on CAR-NK for gynecological cancers, with the corresponding CAR target types for each of these cancers and the findings of related experiments. Little research has been done on using CAR-NK to treat endometrial cancer, indicating a potential direction for CAR-NK research. Research on CAR-NK in gynecological cancers is relatively scarce, focusing on in vitro experiments and in vivo experiments in mice with certain progress, and further clinical trials in humans are needed to develop the application of it in the treatment of gynecological cancers. At the same time, there are limitations of CAR-NK that need to be further investigated and addressed, and CAR-macrophages may be a potential improvement.

REFERENCES

Ao X., Yang Y., Li W., Tan Y., Guo W., Ao L., He X., Wu X., Xia J., Xu X. and Guo J. (2019). *J Immunother.* **42**(8), 284–296.

Cao B., Liu M., Wang L., Liang B., Feng Y., Chen X., Shi Y., Zhang J., Ye X., Tian Y., Zhi C., Li J., Lian H., Wu Q. and Zhang Z. (2020). *Biochem Biophys Res Commun.* **524**(1), 96–102.

CAR T Cells: Engineering Immune Cells to Treat Cancer. (2022, March 10). National Cancer Institute.

Gutiérrez-Hoya A. and Soto-Cruz I. (2021). *Cells.* **10**(11), 3104.

Hu Z. (2020). *Sci Rep.* **10**(1), 2815.
Jan C. I., Huang S. W., Canoll P., Bruce J. N., Lin Y. C., Pan C. M., Lu H. M., Chiu S. C. and Cho D. Y. (2021). *J Immunother Cancer.* **9**(10), e003050.
Klapdor R., Wang S., Hacker U., Büning H., Morgan M., Dörk T., Hillemanns P. and Schambach A. (2017). *Hum Gene Ther.* **28**(10), 886–896.
Klapdor R., Wang S., Morgan M. A., Zimmermann K., Hachenberg J., Büning H., Dörk T., Hillemanns P. and Schambach A. (2021). *Biomedicines.* **9**(10), 1339.
Klapdor R., Wang S., Morgan M., Dörk T., Hacker U., Hillemanns P., Büning H. and Schambach A. (2019). *Int J Mol Sci.* **20**(3), 660.
Li H., Song W., Li Z. and Zhang M. (2022). *Front. Immunol.* **13**, 992232.
Lin Y. Z., Lee C. C., Cho D. Y., Wang Y. L., Chen C. Y., Weng C. Y., Chiu S. C., Hung M. C. and Wang S. C. (2021). *Am J Cancer Res.* **11**(9), 4455–4469.
Liu H., Yang B., Sun T., Lin L., Hu Y., Deng M., Yang J., Liu T., Li J., Sun S. and Jiao S. (2015). *Oncol Rep.* **33**(1), 95–102.
Liu Y., Zhou Y., Huang K. H., Fang X., Li Y., Wang F., An L., Chen Q., Zhang Y., Shi A., Yu S. and Zhang J. (2020). *Cell Prolif.* **53**(8), e12858.
Nowakowska P., Romanski A., Miller N., Odendahl M., Bonig H., Zhang C., Seifried E., Wels W. S. and Tonn T. (2018). *Cancer Immunol Immunother.* **67**(1), 25–38.
Pan K., Farrukh H., Chittepu V. C. S. R., Xu H., Pan C. X. and Zhu Z. (2022). *J Exp Clin Cancer Res.* **41**, 119.
Sahm C., Schönfeld K. and Wels W. S. (2012). *Cancer Immunol Immunother.* **61**(9), 1451–1461.
Schönfeld K., Sahm C., Zhang C., Naundorf S., Brendel C., Odendahl M., Nowakowska P., Bönig H., Köhl U., Kloess S., Köhler S., Holtgreve-Grez H., Jauch A., Schmidt M., Schubert R., Kühlcke K., Seifried E., Klingemann H. G., Rieger M. A., Tonn T., Grez M. and Wels W. S. (2015). *Mol Ther.* **23**(2), 330–338.
Tang X., Yang L., Li Z., Nalin A. P., Dai H., Xu T., Yin J., You F., Zhu M., Shen W., Chen G., Zhu X., Wu D. and Yu J. (2018). *Am J Cancer Res.* **8**(6), 1083–1089.
Valabrega G., Montemurro F. and Aglietta M. (2007). *Ann Oncol.* **18**(6), 977–984.
Wang W., Jiang J. and Wu C. (2020). *Cancer Lett.* **472**, 175–180.

Biological Sciences and Environmental Health – Gao (Ed.)
© 2025 the Author(s), ISBN: 978-1-032-96016-6

PROTAC: A promising treatment for hepatocellular carcinoma

Minxi Li
Applied Biology and Biotechnology, Department of Applied Biology and Chemical Technology, The Hong Kong Polytechnic University, Hong Kong, China

ABSTRACT: The high prevalence and unfavourable prognosis of hepatocellular carcinoma (HCC) provide a substantial worldwide health burden. Despite advances in therapy, the development of efficient therapeutics for HCC is still a critical major unmet need. The targeted protein degradation approach, known as proteolysis targeting chimeras (PROTACs), has become apparent as a potential option in the field of cancer therapy, including HCC. This review aims to summarize the current understanding of PROTAC-based therapies for HCC. PROTACs refer to a category of small molecule compounds that possess the ability to enlist E3 ubiquitin ligases in order to target specific proteins for degradation through the ubiquitin-proteasome system selectively. By eliminating disease-driving proteins, PROTACs offer a novel therapeutic approach with potential advantages over traditional inhibitors. Several PROTACs have been developed and evaluated for HCC, targeting various oncogenic proteins involved in HCC pathogenesis, including BRD4, Bcl-xL, EGFR, and FKBP12. Preclinical studies have shown promising anti-cancer activity of PROTACs in HCC models, resulting in reduced tumor growth and improved survival rates. Additionally, combination therapies involving PROTACs have exhibited synergistic effects with existing standard-of-care treatments, providing a potential avenue for enhanced therapeutic outcomes. While PROTAC-based therapy shows great potential for HCC treatment, several challenges still need to be overcome, including identifying optimal target proteins and further optimizing PROTAC compounds. Additionally, issues such as drug delivery and resistance mechanisms need to be addressed for successful translation into clinical practice.

1 INTRODUCTION

Hepatocellular carcinoma (HCC) constitutes approximately 90% of all instances of liver cancer (Singal *et al.* 2020). It ranks as the fourth most prevalent cause of cancer-related mortality on a global scale (Singal *et al.* 2020). The occurrence of HCC has witnessed a significant threefold growth over last forty years. Projections indicate that the United States will observe the emergence of around 41,210 new instances of HCC by the year 2023. Although early-stage HCC can be treated with local resection or liver transplantation, the majority of cases are typically detected in the advanced stage and require chemotherapy (Singal *et al.* 2020). Approved drugs such as sorafenib, levatinib, cabozantinib and regorafenib have been shown to improve the survival of patients with HCC (Singal *et al.* 2020). However, sorafenib often produces a poor tumour response, whereas levatinib and regorafenib have been associated with the development of drug resistance and complications related to hypoxia (Singal *et al.* 2020). Due to chemotherapy suffers from limitations such as poor selectivity and drug resistance, there is an increasing interest in targeted cancer therapy, especially new targets and small molecule inhibitors (SMIs), which have gained attention as a potential solution. Nevertheless, drug resistance remains a major challenge in targeted therapy. Therefore, new targeted HCC treatments are needed.

In recent years, a new strategy called protein hydrolysis-targeted chimeras (PROTAC) has emerged. PROTAC are molecules that degrade specific proteins via the E3 ubiquitin ligase

 DOI: 10.1201/9781003587590-32

(E3) pathway (Qi *et al.* 2021). They use appropriate junctions to link the target protein (POI)-binding ligand to E3. This technology has the potential to address the limitations of conventional drug therapy. However, there is a lack of a complete account of the research and treatment associated with PROTAC for HCC. Therefore, this article focuses on the advantages and research progress of PROTAC technology for the treatment of HCC.

2 ADVANTAGE OF PROTAC

The basic mechanism of PROTAC involves a bifunctional molecule known as a chimera (Qi *et al.* 2021). The mechanism of action of PROTAC is shown in Figure 1. The PROTAC chimera consists of three main components including a target protein ligand (TP ligand), an E3 ubiquitin ligase ligand (E3 ligase ligand), and a chemical connector. Initially, the chimaera forms a complex by binding to both the target protein and the E3 ubiquitin ligase. The TP ligand establishes an interaction with the target protein, while the E3 ligase ligand establishes an interaction with the E3 ligase, hence facilitating the spatial closeness between the target protein and the E3 ligase. Due to this proximity, the E3 ligase transfers the ubiquitin molecule to the target protein for labelling. Subsequently, the cell's proteasome machinery recognises and breaks down the polyubiquitinated target protein. The application of PROTAC demonstrated efficacy in bringing down the level of target proteins, resulting in good therapeutic effects.

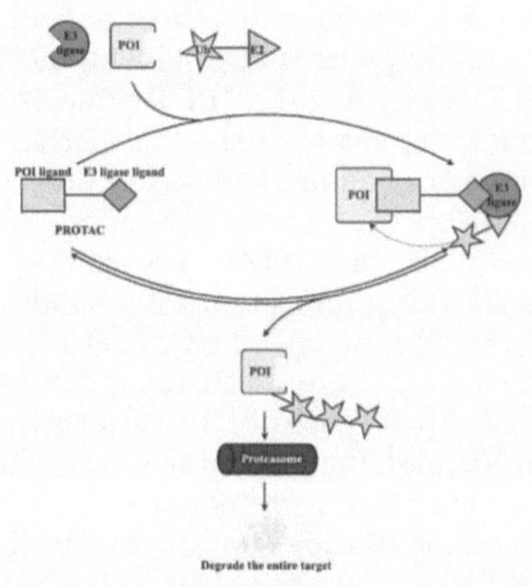

Figure 1. Mode of action of PROTACs. (Original).

PROTAC technology has several advantages over traditional drug development methods (Qi *et al.* 2021). Initially, PROTACs can achieve more complete and sustained inhibition of target proteins and reduce off-target effects. Because PROTACs are designed to selectively degrade specific target proteins within the cell. This targeted protein degradation approach has advantages over traditional approaches that typically involve inhibiting or blocking protein activity. In addition, PROTACs minimise off-target effects on other non-disease related proteins. This selectivity reduces the risk of adverse side effects associated with conventional drug therapies and may reduce drug resistance. Second, PROTACs can be designed as small molecules, making them orally bioavailable. This route of administration provides convenience and improves patient compliance compared to intravesical or other parenteral routes. Notably, PROTAC can be combined with other drugs or therapies to target multiple pathways or overcome resistance. This flexibility allows for personalised and tailored treatment approaches.

3 TARGETING HCC WITH PROTACS

The specificity of PROTAC for HCC cells depends on the design and selection of TP ligands and E3 ligase ligands in PROTAC chimeras. To achieve specificity for HCC cells, the TP ligand should be selected to selectively bind target proteins that are overexpressed or aberrantly regulated in HCC cells compared to normal cells. This could be a protein involved in promoting proliferation, survival or other disease-specific pathways in liver cancer cells. Similarly, the E3 ligase ligand should be selected to interact with an E3 ubiquitin ligase that is present or highly expressed in HCC cells but minimally or not expressed in normal cells. This ensures that PROTAC chimeras can selectively recruit the E3 ligase to target proteins in liver cancer cells. By combining these two factors, PROTAC chimeras can be designed to specifically target recognised target proteins in HCC cells without harming normal cells. This specificity in targeting HCC cells improves the therapeutic index and reduces potential off-target effects on healthy tissues. It is important to note that the selection of target proteins and E3 ubiquitin ligases as well as the optimisation of the PROTAC design need to be thoroughly investigated and validated to ensure efficacy and specificity. The specificity of PROTAC for HCC cells may also be affected by other factors such as cellular uptake and metabolism as well as the microenvironment of the tumour.

3.1 *BET family proteins*

The Bromodomain and Extra-Terminal Structural Domain (BET) proteins constitute a cohort of epigenetic regulators that significantly influence gene expression regulation (Qin *et al.* 2018). The protein family in comprises BRD2, BRD3, BRD4, and components specific to the testis, known as BRDT (Qin *et al.* 2018). BET proteins have garnered considerable attention as potential therapeutic targets for various cancers. This is mostly due to their significant participation in the underlying mechanisms of these diseases.

Current BET degradants developed using the new approach of the PROTAC concept include dBET1, ARV-771, ARV-825, and MZ1. The compounds dBET1 and ARV-825 were developed by integrating JQ-1, in conjunction with thalidomide, which acts as a ligand for cereblon (Winter *et al.* 2015). The identification of JQ-1 as a strong and selective inhibitor of BET proteins has significantly advanced research on BET proteins as potential therapeutic targets (Winter *et al.* 2015). These BET degraders have demonstrated their efficacy in inducing BET protein degradation, inhibiting cancer cell growth, and promoting apoptosis to a greater extent than their corresponding BET inhibitors (Lu *et al.* 2015). Specifically, dBET1 showed superior efficacy compared to JQ-1 in inhibiting tumor growth in an acute leukemia mouse model (Winter *et al.* 2015). Furthermore, ARV-771 effectively inhibited tumor growth in a mouse model of desmoplasia-resistant prostate cancer xenograft (Lu *et al.* 2015). Overall, the aforementioned research present persuasive findings that support the potential efficacy of small molecule BET degraders in the therapeutic management of diverse human cancer and associated disorders.

However, there are limited studies demonstrating that BET-PROTAC can degrade BET family proteins and therapy HCC. In a recent study, the researchers Zhang *et al.* have made a significant finding on the involvement of BETd-260 in the promotion of apoptosis, which is critical for the anti-HCC efficacy (Raina *et al.* 2061). Apoptosis, the regulation of the intrinsic pathway of cell death involves the participation of many proteins from the Bcl-2 family and the inhibitor of apoptosis (IAP) family. Through RNA-seq RT-PCR and protein blotting, the researchers found that BETd-260 is highly effective in inhibiting the expression of Bcl-2 and Mcl-1, two key proteins involved in apoptosis resistance in HCC cells (Raina *et al.* 2061). Interestingly, the study additionally demonstrated that HCC cells with higher levels of Mcl-1, particularly in the HepG2 and BEL-7402 cell lines, exhibited increased resistance to apoptosis (Raina *et al.* 2061). This observation indicates that Mcl-1 has a substantial influence as a resistance determinant in the aforementioned cell lines. Additionally, BETd-260 was found to a considerable decrease in the levels of XIAP and c-Myc expression within the HCC cells, unlike the effects of JQ1 alone (Raina *et al.* 2061). Furthermore, Deng *et al.* discovered that ARV-771 also induces the degradation of BRD2, BRD3, and BRD4 proteins (Deng *et al.* 2022). In a similar manner, the compound ARV-771 was observed to trigger apoptosis in HCC cells by the downregulation of Bcl-2 and Bcl-xL proteins, both of which are recognised as mitochondria-associated anti-apoptotic proteins (Raina *et al.* 2061). Meanwhile, researchers demonstrated that ARV827 can also selectively degrade the target BRD4 protein to sustainably inhibit c-Myc expression in HCC (Raina *et al.* 2061).

These findings indicate that the complete depletion of BET proteins, achieved by using BET-PROTAC, is more effective in HCC than simple BET inhibition. This may be due to the potent apoptotic cell-killing effect of BET-PROTAC. The induction of apoptosis in HCC cells has been demonstrated by BETd-260 by its targeting of numerous genes associated with apoptosis. Therefore, BET-PROTAC has great potential as a unique agent for addressing the issue of apoptosis resistance in HCC.

3.2 *FKBP12*

RC32 was synthesised through the conjugation of rapamycin and pomalidomide, demonstrating notable efficacy and in vivo applicability. The efficacy of RC32-induced FKBP12 degradation in HCC cells was characterised by Zhong et al (Zhong *et al.* 2022). The degradation of FKBP12 protein produced by RC32 was found to be quite rapid, with FKBP12 being almost completely degraded within 4 to 6 hours (Zhong *et al.* 2022). Furthermore, it is worth noting that the degradation of FKBP12 induced by RC32 exhibited a high degree of specificity, as only FKBP12 was affected at low concentrations (Zhong *et al.* 2022). In addition to in vitro, the modulatory effect of RC32 on ferredoxin was verified in vivo. The FKBP12 protein underwent total degradation in liver samples after a 12-hour timeframe subsequent to the administration of RC32 (Zhong *et al.* 2022). Collectively, the findings of this study provide confirmation that the compound RC32, which functions as a degrader of FKBP12, effectively regulates the expression of feromodulin in vitro and in vivo. Moreover, this approach demonstrates promise as a therapeutic method due to lack of immunosuppressive effects.

3.3 *Bcl-xL*

Yang *et al.* report the identification of a novel compound called 753b (Yang *et al.* 2023). It functions as a strong hepatophilic senescent agent by targeting BCL-xL through the use of PROTAC technology. They discovered that 753b exhibited selective clearance of senescent hepatocytes in both old and STAM mice (Yang *et al.* 2023). However, its efficacy in eliminating a broad spectrum of senescent cells (SnCs) was observed solely in vitro experiments (Yang *et al.* 2023). This is partially attributed to the lack of effective enrichment of 753b in the liver following intraperitoneal injection. In addition, the administration of 753b therapy shown significant efficacy in mitigating the progression of HCC in STAM mice (Yang *et al.* 2023). The results of this study indicate that 753b exhibits promise as an innovative treatment option for HCC.

3.4 *EGFR*

The involvement of epidermal growth factor receptor (EGFR) in the proliferation and spread of HCC carries considerable importance. Shi *et al.* conducted a study where they created PROTAC17 and examined its effects on HCC-827 cells (Shi *et al.* 2022). The findings revealed that PROTAC17 demonstrated strong antiproliferative activity and effectively degraded EGFR (Shi *et al.* 2022). However, PROTAC could lead to unintended degradation of non-target proteins, which may cause toxicity and limit its application in clinical settings. Hypoxia, a characteristic feature of most solid tumors accompanied by increased nitroreductase (NTR) levels, inspired the researchers to develop an NTR-responsive PROTAC that specifically degrades POIs in tumor tissues (Harris 2002). Building upon these findings, Shi *et al.* synthesized PROTAC17-1 by incorporating a nitroimidazole component onto PROTAC17 (Shi *et al.* 2022). The synthesis of PROTAC17-1 was a significant milestone since it was the first instance of utilising the Von Hippel-Lindau (VHL) E3 ligase ligand doped with a caging moiety to create an NTR-responsive PROTAC. The activation of PROTAC17-1 was verified by the researchers, demonstrating its ability to be activated in the presence of NTR. This activation resulted in the release of the active component PROTAC17, with the highest level of release observed at a concentration of 8 μg/mL NTR. Furthermore, the administration of PROTAC17-1 resulted in the targeted degradation of the EGFR protein within tumour tissues (Shi *et al.* 2022).

4 COMBINED USE OF PROTAC AND HCC DRUGS

4.1 *Sorafenib*

Due to the limited effectiveness of sorafenib as a targeted agent for advanced HCC, there is a need to find a compound that can enhance its efficacy. Sorafenib primarily targets the Raf-1 and B-Raf kinases, as well as their downstream effectors such as the MEK/ERK and p38 MAPKs (Zhu *et al.* 2017). Building on previous research which indicated that the activation of these signaling pathways limits the effectiveness of ARV-771, investigate the combination of sorafenib and ARV-771 in HCC cells. The combined administration of ARV-771 and sorafenib demonstrated a synergistic effect in efficiently inhibiting the proliferation of HCC (Deng *et al.* 2022). This finding provides evidence for the adoption of a novel technique that involves the integration of the respective benefits of two drugs as a viable strategy for the treatment of cancer.

4.2 *GALARV*

Additionally, ARV is a molecule that needs to be stronger and better soluble in water, posing challenges in developing an effective parenteral formulation for its administration. However, due to its potential in treating HCC, there exists a requirement for the creation of formulations to enhance the transport of substances within the human body. Nanoparticles have demonstrated the ability to enhance the bioavailability of medicinal medications while concurrently mitigating their systemic toxicity. In particular, liposomes are versatile drug delivery systems composed of natural phospholipids that are biocompatible, non-immunogenic, and biodegradable. They have advantages such as enhancing drug solubility, prolonging drug circulation in the body, providing sustained release, and protecting against drug degradation. In order to enhance the specificity of liver cancer cell targeting and reduce unintended impacts on non-targeted cells, liver-targeted carriers have been engineered through surface modifications utilising chemicals such as galactose. Galactose exhibits a distinct ability to selectively identify and bind to the asialoglycoprotein receptors (ASGPR) that are prominently present on the external membranes of hepatocytes, hence facilitating a very effective mode of transportation to the liver. In Aishwarya *et al.*' study, galactosylceramide was used as a ligand to target ASGPR and employ galactosylated nanoliposomes incorporating ARV (GALARV) (Saraswat *et al.* 2022). GALARV would extend their circulation time and enhance their accumulation within the matrix of liver tumours (Saraswat *et al.* 2022). This strategy would enable the targeted delivery of antiretroviral drugs specifically to the liver while minimising any potential adverse effects on non-target tissues. GALARV was shown to exhibit significant in vitro cytotoxicity and apoptotic effects in HCC cells, and also exhibited significantly higher intracellular concentrations of antiretroviral, showed good physical stability and negligible hemolysis. Also, there is significant down-regulation of the target BRD4 protein, apoptotic Bcl-2, survivin proteins and oncogenic c-Myc (Saraswat *et al.* 2022). The findings of this study indicate that

GALARV represents a newly developed targeted nanotherapeutic approach utilising PROTAC technology for the treatment of HCC.

5 CONCLUSION

Based on the novel technology of PROTAC, several groups have reported the synthesis of PROTAC molecules targeting BET family proteins. Notably, preclinical studies have shown that BET-PROTAC is capable of completely eliminating BET proteins from HCC. In addition, several groups have reported a novel PROTAC named ARV, which achieves its effective and long-lasting BRD4 protein degradation. It can be seen that the potential advantages of PROTAC technology may compensate for the shortcomings of conventional drugs in treating HCC, thus facilitating its rapid development. The field of PROTAC-based HCC therapeutics could develop the development of novel PROTAC molecules, working towards the discovery and design of new PROTAC molecules targeting different key proteins involved in HCC. This could involve the identification of specific protein targets that play a key role in tumour growth, metastasis and treatment resistance and developing PROTACs that efficiently degrade these targets. In addition, PROTAC delivery systems could be optimised. The development of an efficient PROTAC delivery system is essential to ensure its targeted delivery to liver cancer cells while minimising off-target effects. Strategies to enhance the stability, biodistribution and cellular uptake of PROTAC can also be investigated. Interestingly, combining PROTAC-based therapies with other therapeutic modalities (e.g., chemotherapy, targeted therapies, or immunotherapies) could be explored to enhance therapeutic efficacy. Synergistic effects can be achieved by simultaneously targeting different pathways or overcoming mechanisms of therapeutic resistance. Combination therapies may improve treatment outcomes and patient response. Overall, PROTAC is a promising treatment modality that has been extensively studied and is expected to improve outcomes and prognosis for patients with HCC.

REFERENCES

Deng Y., Yu C., Chen L., Zhang X., Lei Q,, Liu Q. Q., Cai G., and Liu F., (2022). Front. *Pharmacol.*, **13**, 858901–858901

Harris A. L., (2002). Nat. Rev. *Cancer*, **2**, 1, 38–47

Lu J., Qian Y., Altieri M., Dong H., Wang J., Raina K., Hines J., Winkler J. D., Crew A. P., Coleman K., and Crews C. M., (2015). *Chem. Bio.*, **22**, 6, 755–763

Qi S. M., Dong J., Xu Z. Y., Cheng X. D., Zhang W. D., and Qin J.J., (2021). Front. *Pharmacol.*, **12**, 692574–692574

Qin C., Hu Y., Zhou B., Yang C. Y., Liu L., McEachern D., Fernandez E., Przybranowski S., Wang M., Stuckey J., Meagher J., Bai L., Chen Z., Lin M., Yang J., Ziazadeh D. N., Xu F., Hu J., Xiang W., Huang L., Li S., Wen B., Sun D., and Wang S., (2018). *J. Med. Chem.*, **61**, 15, 6685–6704

Raina K., Lu J., Qian Y., Altieri M., Gordon D., Rossi A. M. K., Wang J., Chen X., Dong H., Siu K., Winkler J. D., Crew A. P., Crews C. M., and Coleman K. G., (2016). *PNAS*, **113**, 26, 7124–7129

Saraswat A., Vemana H. P., Dukhande V. V., and Patel K. (2022), *Heliyon*, **8**, 1, e08702–e08702

Shi S., Du Y., Zou Y., Niu J., Cai Z., Wang X., Qiu F., Ding Y., Yang G., Wu Y., Xu Y., and Zhu Q. (2022), *J. Med. Chem.*, **65**, 6, 5057–5071

Singal A. G., Lampertico P., and Nahon P. (2020), *J. Hepatol.*, **72**, 2, 250–261

Winter G. E., Buckley D. L., Paulk J., Roberts J. M., Souza A., Dhe-Paganon S., and Bradner J. E., (2015). *Science*, **348**, 6241, 1376–1381

Yang Y., Jn-Simon N., Hu W., Zhang P., Zheng G., Pi L., He Y., and Zhou D., (2023). *Cancer Res.*, **83**, 2, B009

Zhong T., Sun X., Yu L., Liu Y., Lin X., Rao Y., and Wu W. (2022), *STTT*, **7**, 1, 163

Zhu Y. J., Zheng B., Wang H. Y., and Chen L., (2017). *Acta Pharm. Sin. B*, **38**, 5, 614–622

Biological Sciences and Environmental Health – Gao (Ed.)
© 2025 the Author(s), ISBN: 978-1-032-96016-6

Testing therapies in nebulin nemaline myopathy model

Hans Fu
Life Sciences, University of Toronto, Toronto, Canada

ABSTRACT: Nemaline myopathy (NM) is a hereditary disorder chiefly marked by muscle debility and the manifestation of nemaline bodies or rods within muscle tissues. Among several identified genetic culprits, mutations in the NEB gene, responsible for the nebulin protein, are particularly significant. While the genetic roots of NM are increasingly understood, concrete therapeutic solutions for nebulin-driven NM remain elusive. This review embarks on an exhaustive exploration of potential treatments tailored for nebulin-associated NM. It outlines the multifaceted methodologies employed to investigate these therapies, spanning from in-depth animal model studies to human clinical trials. Furthermore, this review will highlight contemporary therapeutic advances, encompassing gene therapy, pharmacological strategies, rehabilitative therapy, and stem cell applications, underscoring both their merits and constraints. Recognizing the intricate interplay of opportunities and challenges in NM treatment research, this narrative aims to consolidate knowledge, portraying a consolidated roadmap of the strides taken, obstacles encountered, and the potential path forward. Ultimately, the objective is to furnish researchers and medical professionals with an integrated perspective on the evolving therapeutic horizons for nebulin nemaline myopathy.

1 INTRODUCTION

Nemaline myopathy (NM) encompasses a group of inherited muscle disorders, characterized by the distinct presence of nemaline bodies or rods within muscle cells (Bodkin *et al.* 2022). Clinically, NM demonstrates a wide variability - from pronounced neonatal forms resulting in respiratory complications to more subtle variants with gradual progression over years.

While multiple genes have been implicated in NM's etiology, mutations in the NEB gene, responsible for producing the nebulin protein, stand out prominently. Nebulin is integral to muscle fiber function and structure. It orchestrates the alignment of the actin-myosin complex, pivotal for muscle contraction. Disruptions in the NEB gene compromise this intricate mechanism, leading to the hallmark muscle weakness and rod structures seen in NM patients (Braga *et al.* 2022).

Despite strides in elucidating NM's genetic intricacies, therapeutic avenues remain limited. Currently, patients grapple with symptomatic treatments, devoid of interventions targeting NM's core pathology. The task at hand for the scientific and medical community is to pivot from understanding NM at a molecular level to devising actionable therapeutic strategies (Chung *et al.* 2002).

In this review, they embark on a detailed exploration of therapies for nebulin-related NM. By delving into emerging treatments, their methodologies, and inherent challenges, the goal is to present a comprehensive snapshot of the ongoing endeavors and potential breakthroughs in the NM therapeutic domain (Chung *et al.* 2002).

 DOI: 10.1201/9781003587590-33

2 METHODOLOGICAL APPROACHES TO TREATMENT

The path towards deciphering and potentially addressing nebulin-associated NM is mapped by a variety of methodological approaches. From live animal model studies to detailed ex vivo cell culture, and zebra fish investigations and the rigorous scrutiny of clinical trials, these methodologies have been pivotal in enhancing the grasp on the disease's pathophysiology and prospective treatments (Coors *et al.* 2017).

2.1 *Animal models*

Nemaline myopathies are a varied collection of hereditary muscle diseases primarily characterized by skeletal muscle weakness; in some severe cases, these conditions can lead to early mortality shortly after birth. Roughly half of the instances of this disease can be attributed to mutations in the gene responsible for producing nebulin, a protein essential for the proper function of muscle thin filaments. Despite the gravity of this illness, effective treatments are notably lacking, and research focused on potential therapies remains limited. Some individuals with nemaline myopathy have resorted to using supplements such as L-tyrosine, even though the scientific basis for their efficacy is scant.

To investigate possible therapies, biologists created a zebrafish model that mimics nemaline myopathy due to a mutation in the nebulin gene. These engineered zebrafish display characteristics like the formation of electron-dense nemaline bodies and diminished muscle functionality, mirroring symptoms observed in human patients. Leveraging this model, they evaluated the effectiveness of four supplements—L-tyrosine, L-carnitine, taurine, and creatine—that some patients are currently taking on their own initiative. Unfortunately, the examination of changes in muscle pathology and mobility following these treatments showed no significant enhancement in muscle function (Labeit and Ottenheijm 2011).

Zebrafish were cared for in accordance with established guidelines (Labeit and Ottenheijm 2011). By using two zebrafish strains: Tg(neb+/–; Lifeact-eGFP) and an ENU-induced neb mutant line (sa906), acquired from the Zebrafish International Resource Centre. Nebulin genotyping was conducted using allele-specific PCR through KASP technology (Geneworks) (Coors *et al.* 2017).

In toxicology studies involving wild-type fish, all measurements were normalized to control fish that were treated with water supplementation within the same experimental replicate. The D'Agostino and Pearson test was applied to verify data normality. For normally distributed data in the toxicology studies on wild-type fish, one-way ANOVA was performed with Dunnett's correction for multiple comparisons. In cases where data did not pass the normality test, the data log-transformation, which did not result in normally-distributed data. Consequently, data from all replicates were combined, and a Kruskal-Wallis test was conducted with Dunn's test correction for multiple comparisons (Coors *et al.* 2017).

For swimming performance and muscle fiber area analysis in the NEB nemaline myopathy model, measurements were normalized to average values from water-supplemented neb+/+ siblings. Data normality was again verified using the D'Agostino and Pearson test. A normally-distributed data was analyzed using either an unpaired t-test or one-way ANOVA with Dunnett's correction. For non-normally-distributed data, researchers attempted normalization by removing outliers through the ROUT method (Q=1%) or by log-transforming the data. In both instances, the data remained non-normally distributed, leading us to pool the data from all replicates and apply a Kruskal-Wallis test, followed by Dunn's correction for multiple comparisons.

2.2 *Clinical trials*

Clinical trials represent the apex of NM research and are conducted under stringent regulatory frameworks. These include ethical considerations, FDA approvals, and oversight by Institutional Review Boards (IRBs).

Clinical trials stand as the capstone of therapeutic research, offering a rigorous framework to evaluate prospective treatments within the human population. In the context of nebulin-associated NM, designing and executing such trials requires an intricate blend of scientific rigor, ethics, and adaptability, given the disease's unique challenges and complexities.

At the forefront are the structured phases that characterize clinical trials. These phases, beginning with Phase I, which focuses on safety and dosage, transition to Phase II where preliminary efficacy is gauged in a smaller patient group. Phase III involves large-scale evaluations, confirming the drug's efficacy across a broader spectrum of patients (Telfer *et al.* 2011). Occasionally, post-market studies or Phase IV come into play, offering long-term insights after the treatment has been approved and is in public use (Labeit and Ottenheijm 2011).

Especially pertinent to NM, with its genetic intricacies, are gene therapy trials. These represent a beacon of hope but are also strewn with challenges. Ensuring precise and effective gene delivery to targeted muscle cells, managing potential unintended genetic consequences, and instituting robust long-term safety monitoring are all part of the meticulous planning required (Braga *et al.* 2022).

Further complexity arises from NM's heterogeneous nature. This variability necessitates adaptive trial designs, where patient groups might be segmented based on genetic mutation types, disease severity, or age of onset. As a result, outcomes become multifaceted, relying on both tangible biomarkers and subjective patient-reported outcomes.

To encapsulate, clinical trials for nebulin-associated NM demand a holistic, flexible approach, balancing scientific precision with patient-centric considerations, all aiming to bring forth efficacious and safe treatments (Laplante and Sabatini 2012).

3 INTERVENTIONS

3.1 *Gene therapy*

Nebulin Mutation in Zebrafish Alters RNA and Protein Expression acquired adult zebrafish carrying a specific mutation in the neb gene from the Sanger Institute Zebrafish Mutation Project. Identified as IVS43+1G>A, this mutation is located in a critical splice donor site, anticipated to disrupt the splicing of exon 43. This particular exon has a human NEB equivalent, exon 78, known for its mutations in nemaline myopathy cases. When bred these carrier fish, and generated embryos—referred to as neb embryos—with both evident motor deficiencies and atypical physical appearances. These neb embryos appeared at a proportion of 28.7% (38 out of 132), aligning with Mendelian expectations (Moreno *et al.* 2023).

Impact of the Mutation on RNA Processing of Nebulin was investigated the RNA samples from neb and control embryos to examine the effects of this mutation on the RNA processing of nebulin. Using reverse-transcriptase PCR (RT-PCR), and found that RNA from control embryos produced a strong band of the expected molecular size along with a larger and a smaller one. In contrast, neb embryo RNA revealed a faint band of the expected size and a more prominent smaller band missing exon 43. These results imply that the G>A mutation causes the skipping of exon 43, although a trace amount of normal RNA is still present, suggesting that exon 43 splicing isn't fully eliminated (Moreno *et al.* 2023).

To gain further insights into how this mutation influences Nebulin protein levels, using executed western blot tests. In control siblings, these tests yielded a high molecular weight band (>500 kDa), while in neb embryos, no such band appeared. These findings, consistent across two different Nebulin antibodies, indicate the absence or truncation of Nebulin protein in neb embryos. Further, motor activity in the developing neb embryos. During the first 48 hours after fertilization, no distinguishing features or behaviors were observed between neb and unaffected sibling zebrafish. This was further confirmed by evaluating spontaneous coiling, a typical motor action that occurs between 20 and 28 hours post-fertilization. No variations were noted in the offspring from neb +/- crosses, even though approximately 25% should theoretically exhibit the neb phenotype.

3.2 *Molecular interventions*

The intricacies of nebulin-associated NM, especially its cellular disruptions, have directed attention to interventions at the molecular level. These interventions aim to alleviate symptoms by either targeting the direct implications of NEB gene mutations or addressing secondary cellular disruptions associated with NM. One primary manifestation of NM is weakened muscle contractility. To address this, researchers have explored agents that can enhance the strength and duration of muscle contractions. Calcium plays a central role in muscle contraction, and thus, molecules like ryanodine receptor stabilizers have been studied. By influencing calcium release in muscle cells, these agents have shown potential in boosting muscle strength and endurance (Bodkin *et al.* 2022). Preliminary studies in cellular and rodent models have indicated improved muscle performance, but translating this to human trials is an ongoing effort.

Muscular disorders, including NM, often lead to increased oxidative stress, which exacerbates muscle damage and fatigue. Consequently, a therapeutic angle has been to employ antioxidants and agents targeting mitochondria, the cell's energy-producing centers. By reducing oxidative stress, these molecules can potentially slow muscle degradation and improve overall muscle health. Early trials with specific antioxidants have shown a decrease in markers of oxidative damage and improved muscle function in NM models (Bodkin *et al.* 2022).

At the cellular level, mutations in the NEB gene can disrupt various signaling pathways and metabolic processes essential for muscle maintenance. Intervening in these pathways can be a potential therapeutic strategy. For instance, mTOR signaling, which plays a crucial role in muscle growth and repair, has been a target of interest. Drugs modulating this pathway could restore some aspects of muscle function in NM (Powers *et al.* 2016).

Chronic inflammation, a frequent accompaniment of muscular disorders, can aggravate NM symptoms. Anti-inflammatory agents, both steroidal and non-steroidal, have been explored as potential therapeutic agents. By reducing inflammation, these drugs aim to preserve muscle integrity and function (Bodkin *et al.* 2022).

One intriguing area of molecular intervention is the promotion of muscle regeneration. Molecules that can stimulate satellite cells, the primary cells responsible for muscle repair and regeneration, are being researched. Enhancing the muscle's intrinsic ability to repair could offer a long-term strategy for managing NM.

In essence, molecular interventions for nebulin-associated NM represent a diverse array of strategies. These approaches, grounded in the detailed understanding of cellular disruptions caused by NEB gene mutations, offer hope for a multi-pronged therapeutic regimen. As research advances, a combination of these molecular interventions, tailored to individual patient needs, might emerge as the standard of care for NM (Romero *et al.* 2013).

3.3 *Protein modulation*

Proteins, as the primary workhorses of cells, play pivotal roles in ensuring optimal cellular function. In nebulin-associated NM, the compromised function of the nebulin protein, due to mutations in the NEB gene, instigates a cascade of cellular disruptions. Given this central role of proteins, strategies have emerged aiming to modulate protein behavior or function, seeking to alleviate the deleterious effects of these genetic aberrations (Sanoudou *et al.* 2006).

Every protein needs to assume a specific shape or conformation to be functionally active. Mutations can sometimes lead to misfolded proteins, which are often non-functional or even detrimental to cellular health. Chaperone therapies introduce molecules that assist proteins in achieving their correct conformations. By aiding the correct folding of the nebulin protein or other related proteins, chaperones can potentially restore some degree of muscle function.

Preliminary research has shown that specific chaperones can increase the stability and function of mutated nebulin in cell culture models.

Nature often has redundancies. In the context of muscle function, other proteins might compensate, albeit not perfectly, for the loss of nebulin's function. Therapeutic strategies have been developed to upregulate or promote the activity of these compensatory proteins. The idea is that even if nebulin is not functioning correctly, boosting the function of related proteins might offset some of the muscle weaknesses seen in NM. Experimental studies have identified a few proteins, such as nebulette, that might serve this compensatory role when upregulated.

The functionality of a cell is based on an intricate network of protein interactions. By targeting and modulating specific protein-protein interactions that are disrupted in NM, therapeutic benefits might be realized. For instance, molecules that enhance the interaction between actin and myosin, the primary proteins involved in muscle contraction, might be beneficial in the context of nebulin-associated NM.

Another avenue of interest is the stabilization of the nebulin protein itself or other closely associated proteins. By introducing molecules that bind and stabilize these proteins, their functional lifespan in cells might be extended, leading to improved muscle function.

In cases where mutated nebulin or other aberrant proteins are harmful to cells, strategies to selectively degrade these proteins have been explored. By removing harmful protein species, cellular health might be improved, leading to better muscle function.

In summation, protein modulation represents a nuanced and targeted approach to managing nebulin-associated NM. By delving deep into the molecular intricacies of muscle cells, researchers aim to harness the potential of protein-based interventions, offering hope for more effective therapies that address the root causes of NM.

3.4 *Physical and supportive therapies*

While groundbreaking molecular, genetic, and protein-based therapies promise to target the underlying causes of nebulin-associated NM, the immediate well-being and quality of life of patients are often significantly augmented by physical and supportive therapies. These therapies, which address the physical manifestations and complications of NM, are indispensable in offering holistic care.

Physical therapy remains a cornerstone in managing muscular disorders. Tailored to the specific needs and progression of each patient's condition, it aims to maintain and possibly enhance muscle strength and flexibility. Specialized exercises and routines can mitigate muscle atrophy and help in maintaining joint mobility. Further, physical therapy provides strategies to prevent or address complications such as contractures, which are common in NM.

Nebulin-associated NM, particularly in its severe forms, can lead to compromised pulmonary function. As muscles involved in respiration weaken, patients might face difficulties in breathing, especially during sleep. Non-invasive ventilation, including the use of BiPAP or CPAP machines, can be crucial in ensuring adequate oxygenation. Moreover, respiratory physiotherapy exercises can help maintain lung function and teach patients techniques to clear airway secretions.

Given the metabolic demands of muscles and potential feeding difficulties in some NM patients, nutritional support becomes paramount. Dieticians can design high-protein, nutrient-rich diets that cater to the specific needs of NM patients. In cases of severe dysphagia, alternative feeding methods, such as gastrostomy tubes, might be considered.

The muscle weaknesses accompanying NM can lead to skeletal abnormalities, such as scoliosis. Orthopedic interventions, ranging from bracing to surgical corrections, might be required. Moreover, assistive devices like wheelchairs or walkers can aid in mobility, enhancing the independence and quality of life for patients (Sewry *et al.* 2019).

In cases where facial and throat muscles are affected, speech therapy can be instrumental in improving communication and swallowing. Occupational therapy, on the other hand, assists patients in mastering daily living skills, ensuring they can navigate their environments and perform essential tasks with minimal challenges.

Living with a chronic muscular disorder like NM can pose significant emotional and psychological challenges. Counseling, support groups, and cognitive-behavioral therapies can play vital roles in addressing the emotional well-being of patients, helping them cope with the psychological implications of the disease.

To conclude, while advancements in targeted therapies provide hope for addressing the root causes of nebulin-associated NM, physical and supportive therapies remain indispensable. These interventions, tailored to the unique needs of each patient, ensure that while strive for a cure, the daily lives of patients are as fulfilling and uncomplicated as possible.

3.5 *Future prospects and emerging therapies*

The therapeutic landscape for nebulin-associated NM is continually evolving, driven by advancements in genetic, molecular, and biomedical research. As I understand of the disease deepens, several promising avenues emerge that offer potential solutions for this challenging condition.

The breakthroughs in genome editing technologies, especially the CRISPR/Cas systems, have opened new horizons for genetic disorders like NM. While still in nascent stages for muscular disorders, there is hope that precise genome editing can correct the specific mutations causing NM, offering a definitive solution.

As the field of nanotechnology grows, so does its applicability in medicine. Nanomedicines, or therapies at the nanoscale, could allow for targeted drug delivery, potentially enhancing the effectiveness of molecular interventions while minimizing side effects.

The potential of stem cells in regenerating damaged tissue is being fervently researched. For NM, introducing healthy muscle precursor cells derived from stem cells might offer a method to replace damaged muscle fibers, rejuvenating muscle tissue.

Advances in genomics and proteomics suggest a future where treatments are tailored to individual genetic profiles. For NM patients, this could mean therapies specifically designed based on their unique NEB mutations (Coors *et al.* 2017).

In essence, the horizon of NM treatment is expansive, and with each scientific breakthrough, the hope for effective therapies and, ultimately, a cure becomes more tangible.

4 CHALLENGES IN THERAPEUTIC INTERVENTIONS

In the pursuit of efficacious treatments for nebulin-associated NM, scientists, clinicians, and patients face numerous challenges. These hurdles span a wide spectrum, from fundamental scientific intricacies to broader societal and ethical considerations (Laplante and Sabatini 2012). Understanding these challenges is crucial, as it paves the way for developing better-informed strategies and highlights areas that require greater focus and resource allocation.

4.1 *Scientific and technical challenges*

The intricate nature of nebulin-associated NM brings forth a multitude of scientific and technical challenges. These difficulties underscore the complexity of developing treatments for genetic disorders and highlight the importance of continued research and innovation.

The human NEB gene is one of the largest genes, comprising an intricate arrangement of exons and introns. Its sheer size makes it particularly challenging for gene therapy approaches. Efficiently encapsulating, delivering, and ensuring the expression of such a large gene without compromising its function requires precise and advanced methodologies. Current viral vectors have payload limitations, making it a daunting task to introduce the entire NEB gene.

Different patients may carry various mutations within the NEB gene, leading to a spectrum of clinical manifestations. This genetic heterogeneity demands a tailored approach to treatment. Designing therapies that can cater to each specific mutation or develop broad-spectrum solutions that account for this diversity is a challenging endeavor.

Laboratory success doesn't always equate to clinical efficacy (Telfer *et al.* 2011). While a therapeutic approach might demonstrate promise in petri dishes or animal models, human biology presents its own unique challenges. Factors such as immune responses, metabolic differences, or simply the intricacies of human musculature can impede the translation of benchtop findings to bedside applications.

Any intervention at the genetic or molecular level carries the risk of unintended consequences. Ensuring specificity, where the treatment targets only the defective components without affecting healthy cellular processes, is of paramount importance. The culmination of these challenges underscores the necessity for rigorous research, collaboration, and innovation in their pursuit of treatments for nebulin-associated NM.

4.2 *Clinical and logistical challenges*

Navigating the realm of clinical practice and treatment logistics for nebulin-associated NM presents its own set of complications. These challenges emphasize the need for a multifaceted approach that considers not just the biological aspect of the disease, but also the broader infrastructure supporting patient care.

Recognizing NM in its initial stages can be problematic. Its early symptoms, often subtle and potentially resembling other neuromuscular disorders, can lead to either misdiagnoses or delays in intervention. A timely diagnosis is essential as it opens the door for early therapeutic interventions, potentially leading to better outcomes and patient prognosis (Sztal *et al.* 2018).

With the introduction of newer therapeutic approaches, especially those that intervene at the genetic or cellular level, understanding their prolonged effects becomes crucial. Monitoring patients over extended periods post-treatment is necessary to ensure no latent adverse outcomes or complications arise, demanding extended resources and commitment.

Efficiently delivering treatments, especially at the cellular level, to affected muscle tissues poses significant challenges. Overcoming biological barriers, optimizing drug delivery systems, or ensuring gene therapies reach their intended targets requires sophisticated techniques and careful planning.

After receiving treatment, patients require ongoing observation to assess the therapy's efficacy, potential side effects, and overall well-being. Establishing and maintaining robust monitoring mechanisms can be resource-intensive (Telfer *et al.* 2011).

NM's effects aren't just limited to muscle tissues. Managing the disease holistically requires the coordinated effort of pulmonologists, cardiologists, nutritionists, and more, demanding an integrated healthcare approach.

Addressing these clinical and logistical challenges requires a blend of medical expertise, strategic planning, and patient-centered care. The goal remains to ensure that each patient receives timely, effective, and comprehensive treatment for nebulin-associated NM.

4.3 *Ethical and societal challenges*

Nebulin-associated NM, like many rare genetic conditions, introduces a series of ethical and societal dilemmas. As the scientific community progresses in its understanding and potential treatment modalities, these challenges often become more pronounced, requiring careful consideration and community engagement (Sewry *et al.* 2019).

As treatments, especially experimental ones, present unknown risks, obtaining informed consent becomes a paramount concern. This process isn't just about legal documentation but ensuring that patients, or their guardians, fully grasp the implications, risks, and potential outcomes of a therapy. For a disease as intricate as NM, conveying these nuances transparently and understandably can be challenging.

Cutting-edge therapies, while groundbreaking, can come with a high price tag. The ethical challenge lies in ensuring that treatments are available to all who need them, irrespective of socio-economic backgrounds. Health inequalities can become glaringly apparent, especially when access to potentially life-changing treatments is restricted by financial constraints.

For many affected by NM, any hint of a new therapy can bring immense hope. However, there's an ethical responsibility to present the reality of the situation. Overhyping experimental treatments or not adequately addressing their limitations can lead to false hope and potential disillusionment.

As genetic testing becomes more prevalent, concerns about data privacy emerge. Ensuring that an individual's genetic data remains confidential and isn't used discriminatively, especially by entities like insurance companies, is a pressing societal concern. Tackling these ethical and societal challenges requires a blend of medical ethics, societal engagement, regulatory oversight, and a commitment to fairness and justice in healthcare (Laplante and Sabatini 2012).

4.4 *Regulatory and policy challenges*

The path to realizing effective treatments for nebulin-associated NM is not only paved with scientific and clinical hurdles but also encounters significant regulatory and policy obstacles. These challenges often dictate the speed and manner in which new therapies reach the patients (Labeit and Ottenheijm 2011).

Regulatory bodies, such as the FDA, serve as gatekeepers to ensure that newly developed therapies are both safe and effective. However, the rigorous approval processes can be time-consuming. For conditions like NM, where timely interventions can be crucial, waiting for prolonged approval processes can be particularly frustrating for patients, caregivers, and researchers.

Use Occasionally, drugs or therapies approved for one condition show promise for another, like NM. Using treatments "off-label," or outside their approved indications, introduces both regulatory and ethical complexities. It also raises issues regarding insurance coverage and cost reimbursements (Laplante and Sabatini 2012).

NM's rarity amplifies the importance of global research collaboration. However, collaborating across borders means navigating a maze of varied regulations, clinical trial standards, and data-sharing policies. These differences can slow down research momentum and complicate international cooperative efforts.

As the healthcare landscape becomes more patient-centric, integrating patient voices into regulatory decisions is essential. Yet, striking a balance between patient advocacy and rigorous scientific scrutiny can be challenging. Addressing these regulatory and policy challenges necessitates a harmonized global effort, transparent communication, and a commitment to patient welfare and safety (Laplante and Sabatini 2012).

5 CHALLENGES IN THERAPEUTIC INTERVENTIONS

Nebulin-associated nemaline myopathy (NM) epitomizes the profound intricacies often associated with rare genetic disorders. Its multifaceted nature demands an integrated and relentless pursuit of understanding and intervention. This review has endeavored to shed light on the comprehensive efforts, breakthroughs, and impediments encountered in the therapeutic journey, painting a picture of both promise and challenge.

There's heartening progress in the arena of methodologies. The growth and adoption of various models, from animals to sophisticated cell cultures, offer invaluable perspectives on NM's molecular intricacies. Concurrently, the emergence of diverse therapeutic avenues, spanning from gene-centric approaches to protein adjustments, are at different developmental stages, with each holding a unique potential to address the disease's core challenges. Yet, these scientific leaps are only meaningful if they can be seamlessly translated into tangible patient benefits, accentuating the paramount importance of clinical studies and practical applications.

Nevertheless, the path to a definitive solution is interspersed with obstacles. The landscape is riddled with ethical concerns, regulatory nuances, logistical complexities, and overarching research considerations, necessitating a harmonious collaboration among researchers, healthcare professionals, and regulatory bodies.

To conclude, while the quest for a consistent, impactful treatment for nebulin-associated NM continues, the united endeavors of the international scientific and medical realms provide a glimmer of hope. This journey underscores the significance of resilience, inventive thinking, and cooperative spirit when addressing medical complexities.

REFERENCES

Bodkin C., Comer A., Felker M., Gutmann L., Jones KA., Kincaid J., Payne K. K. and Skinner B. (2022). *Seminars in Neurology*, **42**, 716–22

Braga L., Conte Filho C. and Mota F. (2022). *Therapeutic Advances in Rare Disease*, **3**, p.263300402211008

Chung C., Chu A. and Chung B. (2002). *Frontiers in Public Health*, **10**, p.1028545

Coors M., Bauer L., Edwards K., Erickson K., Goldenberg A., Goodale J., Goodman K., Grady C., Mannino D., Wanner A., Wilson T., Yarborough M. and Zirkle M. (2017). *Translational Science of Rare Diseases*, **2**, 175–94

Labeit S., Ottenheijm C. A. C., Granzier H. (2011). *The FASEB Journal*, **25**, 822–29

Laplante M. and Sabatini D. M. (2012). **149**, 274–93

Moreno M., Artilheiro C., Fonseca S., Camelo G., de Medeiros C., Sassi C., de Andrade F., Donkervoort S., Silva S., Dalfior-Junior L., Abath-Neto L., Reed C., Bönnemann C. and Zanoteli E. (2023). *Neurology. Genetics*, **9**, p. e200056

Powers K., Lynch S., Murphy T., Reid B. and Zijdewind I. (2016). *Medicine & Science in Sports & Exercise*, **48**, 2307–19

Romero B., Sandaradura A. and Clarke F. (2013). *Current Opinion in Neurology*, **26**, 519–26

Sanoudou D., Corbett A., Han M., Ghoddusi M., Nguyen T., Vlahovich N., Hardeman C., Beggs H. (2006). *Human Molecular Genetics*, **15**, 2603–12

Sewry A., Laitila M. and Wallgren-Pettersson C. (2019). *Journal of Muscle Research and Cell Motility*, **40**, 111–26

Sztal E., McKaige A., Williams C., Oorschot V., Ramm G. and Bryson-Richardson J. (2018). *Acta Neuropathological Communications*, **6**

Telfer R., Nelson D., Waugh T., Brooks V. and Dowling J. (2011). *Disease Models & Mechanisms*

Tudur Smith C., Williamson R. and Beresford W. (2014). *Best Practice & Research Clinical Rheumatology*, **28**, 247–62

Westerfield M. (2007). *The Zebrafish Book*.

Biological Sciences and Environmental Health – Gao (Ed.)
© 2025 the Author(s), ISBN: 978-1-032-96016-6

Systematic study of treating strategies targeting Alzheimer's disease

Wenhui Ding
AP Center Wuxi Tianyi High School, Wuxi, China

ABSTRACT: The formidable threat posed by Alzheimer's disease (AD) looms large over humanity, demanding the utmost attention. Regrettably, as of now, a definitive cure for this debilitating ailment remains elusive. Within the pages of this academic publication, this paper embarks on an exhaustive exploration of Alzheimer's disease, spanning its pathological underpinnings to its clinical manifestations. In this article it traverses the landscape of theoretical conjectures, therapeutic interventions, and the promising trajectory of future research, amalgamating the wealth of previous scientific insights with contemporary societal observations, then meticulously structured into three pivotal sections, each shedding light on a distinct facet of Alzheimer's disease. First the prevailing hypotheses that have engrossed researchers, providing a comprehensive overview of the multifaceted etiology of AD are discussed. Subsequently, the mainstream pharmacological approaches and meticulously dissecting the mechanisms of drugs which designed to alleviate the burden of this ailment are presented. Chart of select drugs' historical evolution and feedback which garnered from their clinical application are elucidated to lend context to the narrative. Furthermore, the societal repercussions of Alzheimer's disease are illuminated, exploring its profound impact on individuals, families, and communities. The efficacy and utility of existing drugs are assessed while casting a discerning eye on the contemporary landscape of drug development in the AD domain, drawing insights from the 2023 AD drug development pipeline. The aspiration is not only to provide a compendium of knowledge but also to inspire a broader perspective on AD drug development—one that transcends the mere quest for pharmacological efficacy to encompass the holistic well-being of those affected by this relentless malady.

1 INTRODUCTION

Alzheimer's Disease (AD) is a serious psychiatric disorder which will cause gradual loss of memory, impairment in daily functioning, and predisposition to dependence and disability.AD was first discovered in 1906 by the pioneering German psychoneurologist Alois Alzheimer, and it has been eponymously associated Epidemiologically, the incidence of AD is high, but it is difficult to diagnose, with its prevalence escalating as individuals age. Regrettably, it has become the first and most lethal disease in some countries. Moreover, the incidence of AD in men and women varies according to hormonal and other factors. Research has indicated that although estrogen prevents the development of AD, the incidence of AD in women is still significantly higher than that in men. One possible explanation for this phenomenon is that women possess a broader knowledge base than men, but undergo a more rapid decline in memory.

There are several theories on the origin of AD, but they are all still up for debate in the academic world.

1.1 *Aβ hypothesis*

The most popular hypothesis in current AD research now is the Aβ hypothesis, which is supported by the observation that Y-secretase produces Aβ during intracellular shearing and this Aβ is released outside the cell, accumulating in the brain to form protein plaques.The blood-brain barrier is comprised of astrocytes, pericytes, and brain microvascular endothelial cells (BMECs), and Aβ disrupts BMECs and the tight junctions (TJ) and associated

DOI: 10.1201/9781003587590-34

proteins, leading to loss of integrity of the Blood-brain barrier (Wang *et al.* 2021). However, this hypothesis has undergone revisions in recent years, with emerging evidence challenging its validity. For example, some experiments have demonstrated that Aβ is actually a product rather than a causative agent of AD (Thomas *et al.* 2020). Furthermore, many drugs employing Aβ as a therapeutic target have failed in pre-market screening, and the effects of the existing approved drugs remains uncertain. Consequently, the accuracy and credibility of the Aβ hypothesis are still in need of further sustantiation.

1.2 *The cholinergic hypothesis*

The second hypothesis is the cholinergic hypothesis, representing the earliest hypothesis, postulated by Deutsch back in the 1970s and subsequently explored by later scholars. Cholinergic is an indispensable substance for the brain's ability to transmit information and regulate various neurological functions through the modulation of acetylcholine receptors (Li *et al.* 2018). This cholinergic system plays a fundamental role in governing attention, sleep patterns, and sensory processes. Acetylcholinesterase (AchE) in the brain, however, breaks down Ach, leading to a decrease in Ach in the brain. This decline in Ach levels could potentially lead to cognitive deficits in the brain, as Ach levels have a positive impact on learning and memory processes (Xu *et al.* 2015). As a result, the majority of drugs that use the cholinergic hypothesis as a mechanism are directed to reduce the degradation of AchE for Ach in the brain. While some drugs have been produced and shown to be effective in improving memory, their actual effect is limited, tends to be most pronounced in the early and middle stages. In the advanced stages, when synaptic transmission function is severely compromised, these drugs may not yield significant reversals in cognitive decline (Martorana *et al.* 2010).

1.3 *Tau protein hypothesis*

The third hypothesis in AD research is the tau protein hypothesis, which is the main component of cellular filamentous deposits in the brains of AD patients, Tau protein accumulation undergoes a three-dimensional stacking process during the onset of AD, similar to Aβ. However, this hypothesis suggests that there exist minimal differences in outcomes between Aβ amyloid and Tau proteins, and some studies have indicated a synergistic relationship between Aβ amyloid and Tau proteins (Huang *et al.* 2022). Efforts in drug development aimed at targeting Tau proteins mainly include strategies such as inhibiting the over phosphorylation of Tau proteins, preventing the aggregation of Tau proteins, and promoting the catabolism of Tau proteins, etc. However, it's important to note that the development of Tau protein-related drugs is still at an early stage, and there are no drugs that have been approved for use yet.

1.4 *Metal ion disorder hypothesis*

Human cells need metal ions to function properly, and disordered ions can lead to toxins and dysfunction, resulting in neuronal death. Disorders involving iron and copper have the potential to lead to such outcomes, with iron overload related to late AD damage, while iron deficiency may be associated with the early AD formation. Iron is essential for normal brain function, but too much of it can build up in the brain, producing toxins that have the potential to cause brain cell death (Wang *et al.* 2020). Zinc, on the other hand, exerts an influence on neuronal activity, as it is predominantly found in synaptic vesicles within glutamatergic nerve endings, where it is released to regulate a variety of biological functions (Wang *et al.* 2020). Complexes formed by copper and Aβ aggregates penetrate neurons, setting off oxidative stress within different neuronal subregions. Despite the fact that copper is observed to be enriched in areas where amyloid plaque accumulates in the brain, patients with AD often exhibit reduced copper levels in various brain regions, including cerebral cortex, frontal cortex, amygdala, and hippocampal regions, with decreases of up to 50% compared to normal brains (Wang *et al.* 2020). Calcium is another important element for neural growth, differentiation, and learning and memory processes. However, excessive calcium levels are often shown to be toxic to cells and contribute to psychiatric disorders such as AD (Wang *et al.* 2020). Disruptions in metal ion homeostasis in the brains of AD patients may also amplify the toxicity of Aβ, against which metal chelators and natural antioxidants play a significant protective role (Chen *et al.* 2023).

1.5 *Threats of AD to human health*

The treatment landscape for AD faces significant challenges, with the majority of available medications offering relief from symptoms but not a cure. Moreover, the symptoms are not obvious in the early stage, which can be easily mistaken for the natural aging process. Therefore, many elderly people suffering from AD are neglected. By the time AD is detected, the disease is already in an advanced stage, requiring prolonged and demanding care from family members, and very few medications are available to alleviate the condition. AD patients gradually lose their ability to perform daily activities, making caregiving a formidable task. The families not only have to face the financial strain of expensive medical expenses, but also to bear the emotional burden of witnessing their loved ones' decline. These circumstances can lead to anxiety and emotional breakdowns among family members. The family of Li Meng, Zhao Qiu Rong, and Chen Zhanqing is an example of the difficulty of care, huge spending and little hope. Consequently, the development of a drug that can effectively treat this without drastic side effects could take the pressure off society as a whole.

1.6 *A global overview of AD drugs today and major R&D advances*

Based on the variety of hypotheses about the etiology of AD nowadays, the direction of drug development is common knowledge in every field, but such a wide spread makes the success rate very small. Currently, the only FDA-approved drugs marketed for AD treatment include Donepezil, Revastigmine, Galantamine, Menantine, and Aducanuma. With the exception of Menantine and Aducanumab. Among these, the first four drugs are AchE inhibitors, which are valuable for improving memory and cognitive impairments in AD patients. (Figure 1) However, they cannot slow down the progression of the disease, and at the same time, all the various drugs have different side effects, which can have some other effects on the body of the patients, especially the elderly. Tacrine was once approved for use, which showed promising treatment efficacy but had to be taken off the market for the strong hepatotoxicity that can cause acute liver injury and associated adverse effects. However, the above are only reflections derived from social observation, and there is no experimental proof.

While new drugs are constantly being developed, the challenges of clinical testing, safety, and efficacy have led to a low success rating. According to statistics, only 2.7% of AD drugs have successfully passed clinical trials and been translated into practical treatment, while the rest have been declared failures at different stages. Some of the drugs can be effective, but then they are abandoned because their side effects lead to other serious illnesses or discomforts.

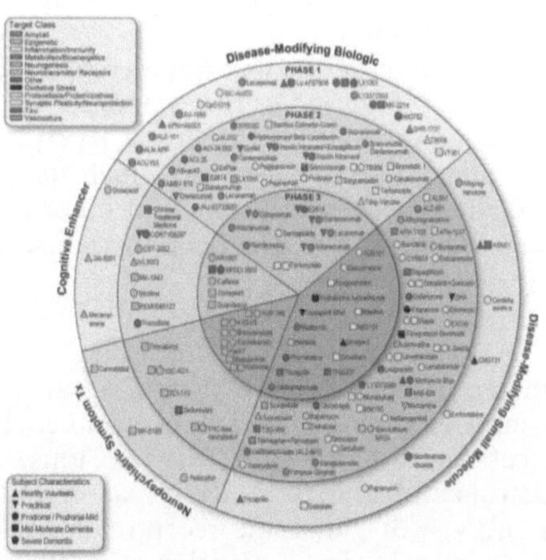

Figure 1. Overview of drug development for AD in 2023 (Raskind and Peskind 2000).

2 MAIN BODY

Main Mechanisms of Action of AD Drugs Donepezil, Revastigmine, Galantamine, Menantine, and Aducanumab, which are widely available on the market, have been developed based on different hypotheses.

2.1 *AchE inhibitors*

AchE is a key enzyme in biological nerve conduction, as it plays a central role in in degrading Ach, thereby preventing single transmission between the neurons. Therefore, cholinergic transmission has been demonstrated to improve the patient's cognitive and memory functions (Xu *et al.* 2015), thereby allowing improvements in behavior and memory.

Donepezil, Rivastigmine, and Galantamine all belong to the class of AchEIs, each of them has different mechanisms of action.

2.1.1 *Donepezil*

The primary drug for treating AD is thought to be donepezil, a second-generation AChEI. Due to donepezil's reversible binding to acetylcholinesterase and its suppression of acetylcholine's hydrolysis, acetylcholine levels at synapses are elevated (Xu *et al.* 2015). The medicine is generally well tolerated and the neurological system and gastrointestinal tract are only temporarily affected by modest cholinergic side effects.

2.1.2 *Rivastigmine*

Rivastigmine operates as a pseudo-irreversible inhibitor of AChE and butyrylcholinesterase (BuChE), blocking ACh metabolism by adhering to the two active sites, anion and ester sites of AChE.

Rivastigmine dissociates more slowly than AChE, so it is called pseudo-irreversible (Xu *et al.* 2015). Nausea, vomiting, indigestion, exhaustion, anorexia, and weight loss can occur after taking the medication orally.

2.1.3 *Galantamine*

For mild to severe instances of AD, galantamine is typically used as the first line therapy. Cholinergic dysfunction is a hallmark of Alzheimer's disease.

According to one theory, the disease's cognitive abnormalities are a result of this dysfunction. This theory served as thc foundation for the use of galantamine as a cholinergic enhancer in Alzheimer's disease therapy.

By blocking the enzyme acetylcholinesterase, which is in charge of acetylcholine hydrolysis, galantamine increases the quantity of acetylcholine that is available for synaptic transmission (Raskind and Peskind 2000).

When it binds to the allosteric region of the nicotinic receptor, galantamine also produces a structural change in the receptor (Raskind and Peskind 2000). This allosteric regulation increases the acetylcholine responsiveness of the receptor. Acetylcholine release is increased by the stimulation of presynaptic nicotinic receptors, which further increases acetylcholine availability (Farlow 2003). Galantamine stood out from other medications due to its dual mode of action, which included competitive acetylcholinesterase suppression and allosteric nicotinic modulation.

2.1.4 *NMDAR antagonist*

The NMDA receptor is an ion channel protein that plays an important role in synaptic plasticity, learning by allowing ions through the cell membrane. However, overactivation of the receptor leads to an excessive influx of Ca2+(calcium ions), leading to excitotoxicity, which may have other detrimental effects. Luckily, as a low-affinity noncompetitive antagonist of NMDAR, a subtype of glutamate receptor, memantine provides a remedy. This medication reduces the neurotoxic hyperactivation of glutamatergic systems that occurs in AD patients. Because it inhibits excitatory receptors without affecting typical synaptic transmission, the medication is reliable and widely tolerated. Memantine's low affinity allows it to be swiftly ejected from the NMDAR receptor by high glutamate concentrations, preventing long-term blockage over time (Camps and Muñoz-Torrero 2002). In essence, Memantine offers a relatively gentle therapeutic approach with a very low probability of inducing neurotoxic effects, making it a promising option for managing AD-related excitotoxicity.

2.2 *Aβ- antagonist*

The third method of treating Alzheimer's disease is based on the widely accepted Abeita theory. FDA-approved Aducanumab is the first medication to use this strategy. It is a monoclonal IgG antibody that is believed to decrease the course of Alzheimer's disease by binding to the amyloid beta protein at the third and seventh amino acids (Miguel *et al.* 2022). Aducanumab's conjugation to amyloid beta is thought to speed up the removal of A aggregates by triggering microglial phagocytosis, according to research. Due to its affinity for A aggregates and binding stoichiometry, aducanumab is the only antibody that prevents secondary nucleation, which refers to the development of oligomers on the fibril surface, and hence inhibits the A aggregation process in addition to scavenging.

3 DESCRIPTION OF SEVERAL APPROVED DRUGS FOR AD

3.1 *Donepezil*

Eisai embarked on pioneering development of donepezil in 1983. A significant milestone in this developmental journey was reached in 1989, when Phase I clinical trials of Donepezil hydrochloride was initiated in Japan, followed by the Phase I clinical trial in the United States in 1991. Clinical phase II trials began in 1992 and phase III trials began in 1994, while phase III trials were conducted in patients with mild and moderate AD, comparing a placebo group with a donepezil hydrochloride group (5mg and 10mg once a day). These double-blind controlled trials involved approximately 150 patients and spanned durations of 12 and 24 weeks, respectively. The results of the final trial were made public in September 1995 with minimal side effects, leading to an application to the FDA in Japan in March 1996. And in November 1996, the FDA granted approval for Donepezil as a treatment for AD (Sugimoto *et al.* 1999). The cholinesterase is bound by donepezil and is reversibly deactivated, which prevents acetylcholine from being hydrolyzed. Acetylcholine concentrations at cholinergic synapses rise as a result. While donepezil has the benefit of improving cognitive function, it also has the drawback of possibly causing ADHD. Pervasive Developmental Disorder and Anorexia Nervosa.

3.2 *Aducanumab*

Aducanumab stands as a groundbreaking achievement, representing the first FDA-approved drug for Ad in approximately two decades. Its mechanism of action is centered on mitigating brain toxins by reducing the concentration of Aβ in the brain. Aducanumab had a bumpy road to development. Biogen first developed the drug and Eisai joined the development in 2017, after two clinical trials, an independent committee concluded that Aducanumab would not achieve the expected results, so these trials were stopped in 2019, however, the trials were later resumed and the FAD announced an accelerated approval issued in 2020, which is generally used to approve some drugs for the treatment of risky diseases (AMERICA BRAIN FUNDATION 2022). In May 2015, Aducanumab was studied in a Phase I study in 25 patients with mild-to-moderate AD in Japan by increasing the dose to 6 mg/kg. Two phase III efficacy trials were started in August of the same year. After the approval, there was no shortage of criticism in the market, mainly because the drug did not have enough evidence in the clinical phase to show that it could reduce the level of beta-amyloid plaques in the brain. Other things are that the FDA expert advisory committee charged that one-third of the patients had serious complications because of the drug, etc.. All of these protests made the drug Aducanumab full of uncertainty. So the end result is that while the FDA approved Aducanumab, the European Medicines Agency (EMA) and Japan's Health Ministry rejected Biogen's application.

Here are the detailed timelines:

- In 2012, Biogen started the PRIME Aducanumab study.
- Biogen reports that PRIME has entered Phase III as of 2014.12.
- Presentation of data in 2015 at the AD/PD conference.
- Phase I, 2015.5. Japan study included 25 individuals and 6 mg/kg.
- 2015.7 Following a trial, it is suggested to REDUCE the A level using data from 6mg/kg monitored over a year.
- 2015.8 There are two Phase III efficacy trials and two Phase 221 efficacy trials.
- 2016: Biogen announces its use of the metered titration protocol in Phase III and publishes PRIME data indicating that it reduces ARIA-E.
- 2017, 2018 Aducanumab's usefulness in reducing the rate of cognitive performance is announced by Biogen.
- Biogen announced the trial's termination on March 3, 2019.
- Biogen declared that the interim futility analysis was inaccurate on 2019-10-22.
- 2020, 3,27 In order to reopen the Aducanumab trial in 2020, Biogen submits a biologics license application to the FDA.
- FDA review is still not approved in 2020, 11, or 6 due to public protest and FDA objection.
- 2021, 6, 7 The FDA approved aducanumab via the agency's accelerated approval procedure, which needs strong proof of efficacy on an intermediate marker (amyloid elimination), reasonable possibility of a significant therapeutic benefit, and other criteria.
- 2021, 6 In order to assess Aduhelm's bioavailability following subcutaneous injection with intravenous infusion in 30 healthy volunteers, Biogen started Phase 1 research. healthy participants. In October 2021, the trial was supposed to come to a close.
- The Health Ministry of Japan issued negative efficacy data for A on December 22, 2021. In October 2021, the trial was supposed to come to a close.
- The U.S. Centers for Medicare and Medicaid Services (CMS) only allowed clinical studies to be covered for A starting in 2022.
- The FDA-required Phase 4 confirmatory trial, known as ENVISION, starts in 2022, with findings anticipated in 2026.

4 DISCUSSION

4.1 *Shortcomings of AD pharmaceuticals*

AD presents a formidable challenge due to its elusive etiology, absence of reliable experimental models,and resultant uncertainty in guiding pharmaceutical research, resulting in a high failure rate, poor results, and a difficult pharmaceutical process. Existing drugs are not sufficiently effective in treating AD, further complicating efforts to achieve breakthroughs with existing drugs. But perhaps an alternative perspective warrants consideration: since it is a mental illness, could psychological interventions be a viable avenue for prevention and intervention?

Some investigations emphasize the significance of understanding homeostasis as the key to treating AD. Some antioxidant molecules in some certain species, such as curcumin and the pineal hormone, can cross the BBB and inhibit the aggregation of Aβ, suggesting potential therapeutic value. Extracting medicinal ingredients from plants like ginkgo may offer an approach to avoid the drastic side effects associated with chemical drugs (Kastenholz *et al.* 2009).

In contrast to Western medicine, traditional Chinese medicine has unique features. Alzheimer's disease was recognized by ancient Chinese doctors as early as 100 years ago, developing their distinct treatment protocols. Because ancient Chinese doctors believed that it was caused by blood stasis that blocked the brain, forgetfulness, and a lack of kidney essence, the medications used by Chinese medicine to treat dementia were a different approach than the modern medications that are specifically designed to treat the nervous system (Howes *et al.* 2017).

However, music therapy has actually been experimentally proven to alleviate most mental illnesses and has shown improvement in orientation and memory for AD patients, to whatever degree. There have also been experiments that show the emotions of AD patients are important and giving them encouragement and freedom would be more important than taking medication. This would be a more relaxing therapy for both the patient and their families. Depression and anxiety would also be reduced. However, this therapy can only be properly carried out in a form of comfort, as the patient's condition will continue to deteriorate until a truly effective medicine is developed (Beata *et al.* 2023).

5 CONCLUSION

This study combines the various speculations and solutions for Alzheimer's disease from the 20th century to the 21st century, introduce the old and new hypotheses of Alzheimer's disease such as the Aβ hypothesis and the cholinergic hypothesis in detail, and summarize the characteristics of different drugs such as donepezil and aducanumab, and clearly demonstrate their pharmacological logic. Although there is no cure for AD so far, scientists are still working tirelessly to probe deeper and deeper, developing one new drug after another. But as long as the cause of Alzheimer's disease has not been fully recognized, all the drugs cannot stand firm. Continue to guess, grope, and learn from failures is important to success. This is a difficult process, there's a lot to do in the future, and the scope of research and concern about Alzheimer's disease should be extended to a wider range. Medical causes and drug innovations are only one part of the equation, but the social aspects of mental and human health are also important to consider. Only in this way human will be able to come closer to the full picture, achieve a balance and accelerate the search for the perfect cure.

REFERENCES

AMERICA BRAIN FUNDATION, Accelerated Approval Program, 12 1 (2022)

Beata B-K., Wojciech J., Johannes K., Piotr L. and Barbara M. (2023). *International Journal of Molecular Sciences.* 24 2

Camps P., Muñoz-Torrero D. (2002). *Mini Rev Med Chem.* 2 1

Chen LL., Fan YG., Zhao LX., et al. (2023). *Bioorg Chem.* 131:106301.

Farlow MR. (2003). *Clin Pharmacokinet.*42, 15

Howes MR., Fang R. and Houghton PJ. (2017). *Int Rev Neurobiol.*135

Huang Q., Liao C., Ge F., et al., (2022). *Journal of Neurorestoratology*

Kastenholz B., Garfin DE., Horst J. and Nagel KA., (2009). *Amyloid,* 16 2

Li X., Yu B., Sun Q., Y. et al. (2018). *Proc. Natl. Acad. Sci. USA* 9,115

Martorana A., Esposito Z. and Koch G. (2010), *CNS Neuroscience & Therapeutics,* 16

Miguel V., Vítor S., Cristina M. and Silvestre S., (2022). *Clinical Interventions in Aging,* 17

Raskind MA., Peskind ER. and Wessel T. (2000), *Neurology.* 27,54,12

Sugimoto H., Yamanishi Y. and Ogura H., (1999). *Yakugaku Zasshi* 119 2

Thomas KR., Bangen KJ., Weigand AJ., Edmonds EC., Wong CG., Cooper S., Delano-Wood L. and Bondi MW., (2020). *Neurology.* 28,94(4)

Wang D., Chen F., Han Z., Yin Z., Ge X. and Lei P. (2021). *Front. Cell. Neurosci,* 19,15

Wang L., Yin YL., Liu ZX., et al. (2020). *Transl Neurodegener.* 3,9,10.

Xu M., et al., (2015). *Nat Neurosci* 18

Biological Sciences and Environmental Health – Gao (Ed.)

Microbes and Alzheimer's disease

Hairuo Sun
School of Chemistry and Chemical Engineering, China University of Petroleum, Shanghai, China

ABSTRACT: Alzheimer's disease (AD), a widespread neurodegenerative condition, continues to affect numerous individuals worldwide, and its underlying causes remain incompletely understood. In recent years, an increasing body of scientific research has shed light on the presence of diverse pathogenic oral microbial populations within the oral cavity of AD patients. These bacteria appear to have a noteworthy impact on the development of AD. Furthermore, extensive studies have demonstrated the influential role of the gut-brain axis, wherein the gut microbiota can modulate brain health and development. Probiotics, living microorganisms beneficial to human health, play a pivotal role in maintaining the equilibrium of intestinal microecology. This review offers a comprehensive review of global research conducted over the past five years, focusing on the relationship between oral and intestinal flora and AD. Additionally, it examines recent advancements in combining probiotics with other drugs to ameliorate AD. These findings present novel avenues for both the prevention and treatment of AD.

1 INTRODUCTION

In recent years, with the increase in human life expectancy, the challenge posed by an aging population has grown more pronounced. Numerous diseases significantly impact the well-being and quality of life of middle-aged and elderly individuals, with neurological conditions being particularly prevalent in this age group. These conditions include AD and Parkinson's syndrome. AD, also known as senile dementia, is a widespread neurodegenerative disorder affecting individuals worldwide. According to the International Dementia Association, the current global count of individuals living with dementia exceeds 55 million, and this number is projected to reach 152 million by 2050, equivalent to one person developing dementia every three seconds (Scheltens *et al.* 2021).

Consequently, the situation regarding AD disease is particularly dire. The pathogenesis of AD disease is highly intricate and not yet fully elucidated. Several pathogenic hypotheses exist, including the amyloid cascade hypothesis, neuroinflammation hypothesis, mitochondrial damage hypothesis, among others (Breijyeh and Karaman 2020; Younkin 1998). Currently, the concept of the "microbial-gut-brain axis" has gained prominence, and numerous studies have demonstrated that the gut microbiota plays a pivotal role in regulating gut-brain function (Narengaowa *et al.* 2021). The sympathetic and parasympathetic branches of the autonomic nervous system have the capacity to impact the enteric nervous system circuit, resulting in alterations in intestinal motility. These changes affect the delivery of prebiotics such as resistant starch and dietary fiber, as well as other essential nutrients for intestinal microbes, into the small intestine and colon, thereby influencing the balance of the gut microbiota (Zhuang *et al.* 2018). Consequently, regulating and intervening in the composition and function of gut microbes represents a novel

 DOI: 10.1201/9781003587590-35

approach to improving neurological diseases and developing corresponding preventive and treatment strategies. Furthermore, an increasing number of scientists have confirmed the presence of various oral pathogenic microbial populations in the brains of AD patients, and reducing these microbial populations has been shown to effectively mitigate the progression of the disease.

Probiotics encompass a broad category of living microorganisms beneficial to the human body, including lactic acid bacteria, bifidobacteria, and more, which function as probiotics by modulating the balance of the gut microbiota. Several studies have indicated that AD can be effectively prevented and ameliorated through the consumption of specific probiotics (Den *et al.* 2020; Naomi *et al.* 2021). A growing body of research underscores the intricate connections between oral and gut microbiota and AD. This paper provides a review of studies conducted over the past five years that have explored the impact of oral and intestinal flora on AD.

2 THE PATHOLOGIES OF AD

2.1 *The cause of AD*

The etiology of AD is multifaceted, and its onset arises from the intricate interplay of numerous factors. In recent years, considerable scholarly scrutiny has been dedicated to the realms of genetics, neurotransmitter theory, viral infections, and immunology in the pursuit of a deeper understanding of this affliction.

2.1.1 *Genetic factors*

AD exhibits a propensity for familial clustering, with approximately 20% of patients manifesting a positive family history, thereby conferring a heightened risk of the ailment upon their first-degree relatives. Molecular biology investigations have divulged the presence of aberrant gene loci on chromosomes 21, 19, 14, and 1 (Younkin 1998). These implicated genes encode the following proteins: β-amyloid protein (β-AP), apolipoprotein E (ApoE), procasein-1 (PS-1), and presenilin protein 2 (PS-2), respectively (Younkin 1998). Mutations in these genes, along with alterations in peptide composition, are intricately associated with the onset of AD.

β-AP is generated through the anomalous cleavage of β-amyloid precursor protein (β-APP) and constitutes the primary constituent in the formation of amyloid plaques. The ApoE gene ranks among the most pivotal genetic factors influencing the aging process, with the risk of developing familial AD and sporadic AD contingent upon the quantity of ApoE4 allele present (Younkin 1998).

2.1.2 *Cholinergic hypothesis*

Alterations in neurotransmitter systems are pivotal in the context of AD, encompassing the acetylcholine system, monoamine system, amino acids, and neuropeptide transmitters. Among these, the reduction in choline acetyltransferase and acetylcholine transmitters stands out as a significant contributor to AD pathogenesis. Neuropharmacological investigations have unequivocally validated the diminished activity of acetylcholine transferase in the cerebral cortex and hippocampus of AD patients. This reduction directly impacts the synthesis of acetylcholine and impairs the functioning of the cholinergic system.

Furthermore, AD patients exhibit notable decreases in somatostatin, corticotropin-releasing factor, and norepinephrine levels, while the activity of dopamine hydroxylase is markedly diminished.

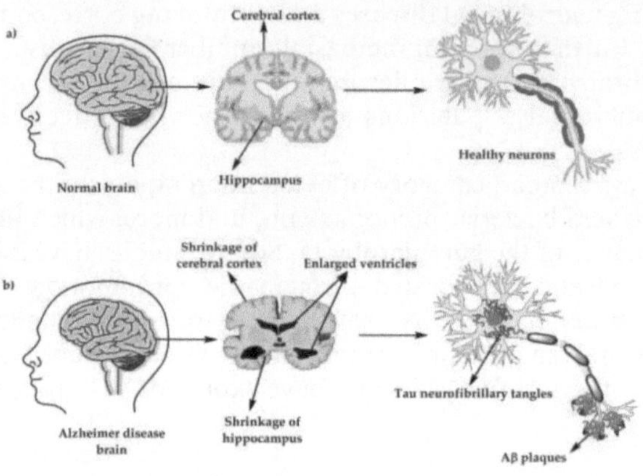

Figure 1. Comparing the physiological structures of neurons in (a) healthy and (b) AD Brains (Breijyeh and Karaman 2020).

2.1.3 *Amyloid hypothesis*

In 1991, scholars introduced the amyloid protein hypothesis, proposing that the accumulation of beta-amyloid protein (βA) in the brain may be the fundamental trigger for AD as shown in Figure 1. This theory was substantiated by the discovery that the pre-amyloid protein gene (APP) resides on chromosome 21, and individuals with trisomy 21 syndrome (Down syndrome) carry an extra set of chromosome 21 genes (Breijyeh and Karaman 2020). Additionally, apolipoprotein E, a prominent genetic risk factor for AD, has been implicated in the buildup of amyloid proteins in the brain. Consequently, it was postulated that beta-amyloid is the root cause of AD. Subsequent support for this hypothesis emerged from experiments involving transgenic mice, where researchers introduced a mutated version of the human APP gene. These mice exhibited the formation of fibrillar amyloid plaques, brain pathological changes akin to AD, and spatial learning deficits.

However, a vaccine designed to clear amyloid plaques, initially promising in early human trials, failed to yield significant improvements in dementia patients. As a result, researchers shifted their focus towards non-fibrillar beta-amyloid oligomers, particularly amyloid-derived diffusible ligands (ADDLs). These toxic oligomers bind to receptors on nerve cells' surfaces, disrupting synaptic structures and, consequently, neuronal communication.

It is worth noting that one of the receptors for beta-amyloid protein oligomers may be prion proteins, the same proteins implicated in diseases such as BSE (bovine spongiform encephalopathy) and Creutzfeldt-Jakob disease, suggesting potential connections between the pathogenesis of these neurodegenerative disorders and AD.

In 2009, an updated version of the hypothesis emerged, based on new research indicating that another beta-amyloid-related protein might be the primary culprit in AD. This research suggested that a pruning mechanism associated with amyloid proteins during rapid brain growth in early life might be reactivated during the aging process in old age. Activation of this mechanism was found to result in neural damage in Alzheimer's patients. N-APP, the amino-terminal fragment of APP, closely related to beta-amyloid protein, is cleaved from APP by the same enzyme. When N-APP binds to the neuroreceptor death receptor 6 (DR6), which is abundant in areas of the human brain susceptible to AD, it triggers a self-destructive pathway. This mechanism may become compromised in older brains, leading to brain damage. In this model, beta-amyloid proteins appear to play a secondary role by inhibiting synaptic function.

2.1.4 *Tau hypothesis*

The Microtubule-Associated Protein Theory proposes that AD development is significantly influenced by abnormal microtubule-associated proteins. In this model, hyperphosphorylated Tau proteins begin to aggregate with other Tau proteins, leading to the formation of neurofibrillary tangles within nerve cells. This aggregation causes the microtubules within the nerve cells to deteriorate, disrupting the intracellular transport system. Consequently, this breakdown in biochemical communication between nerve cells ultimately results in nerve cell death, as illustrated in Figure 1.

2.1.5 *Virus infection*

Previous studies have demonstrated that a virus capable of causing brain tissue abnormalities in sheep can induce the formation of characteristic amyloid plaques in the brains of small white mice. In vitro experiments have further revealed that herpesvirus infection can lead to a reduction in the levels of acetylcholine transferase in chromaffin cells, specifically PC12 cells. These findings suggest that viral infections may be a potential contributing factor to the development of AD (Naseri *et al.* 2019).

2.1.6 *Metal action*

In certain AD patients, the concentration of aluminium in the brain has been found to be significantly elevated, reaching levels 10-30 times higher than those observed in a normal brain. Moreover, the accumulation of aluminium within the core of senile plaques (SP) has been noted when dementia occurs. These observations have led to speculation about the potential relationship between aluminium and dementia. However, it remains unclear whether aluminium is a cause or an effect of dementia (Wang *et al.* 2020).

The exact role of aluminium in the pathogenesis of AD is still a subject of ongoing research and debate. While some studies have suggested a possible association between aluminium exposure and the development of AD, the evidence is not yet conclusive. It is important to note that the accumulation of aluminium in the brain may be a consequence of the disease process rather than a direct cause.

Further research is needed to better understand the relationship between aluminium and dementia, including whether aluminium plays a causative role in the development of the disease or if its presence is a secondary effect. Researchers continue to investigate the potential contributions of various factors, including genetics, environmental exposures, and lifestyle, to the onset and progression of AD.

2.1.7 *Immune dysfunction, free radical damage*

Immune dysfunction and the detrimental effects of free radicals have been associated with the onset and development of AD. Notably, studies have revealed that individuals with AD exhibit elevated levels of brain reactive antibodies, which were approximately 20% higher than those observed in the control group. This finding suggests that the increased presence of autoantibodies in AD patients may contribute to neuronal loss and the aging process.

The role of the immune system and its components in AD is a complex and evolving area of research. It is believed that chronic inflammation and immune system dysregulation may exacerbate neurodegenerative processes in the brain, potentially contributing to cognitive decline and neuronal damage seen in AD (Morales *et al.* 2010).

Furthermore, the involvement of free radicals, or reactive oxygen species, is thought to lead to oxidative stress, which can cause cellular damage and has been implicated in the pathology of AD.

Research into the interactions between the immune system, free radicals, and neurodegenerative diseases like AD is ongoing and aims to better understand the mechanisms involved and identify potential therapeutic targets.

2.1.8 *Other hypotheses*

Another hypothesis posits that AD may stem from age-related disruptions in myelin within the brain. This theory suggests that the release of iron ions during myelin breakdown may exacerbate damage, and the imbalance in myelin repair homeostasis may foster the buildup of beta-amyloid proteins and Tau proteins in the brain. Oxidative stress and disturbances in the regulation of biological metals may also hold significance in the pathological changes observed in AD patients (Morales *et al.* 2010).

Notably, AD patients exhibit a substantial loss—approximately 70%—of cells responsible for norepinephrine production in the locus coeruleus. In regions like the neocortex and hippocampus, norepinephrine serves not only as a neurotransmitter but also diffuses through varicose veins, acting as an endogenous anti-inflammatory agent for nerve cells, glial cells, and the microenvironment surrounding blood vessels (Morales *et al.* 2010). Research has indicated that norepinephrine stimulates microglia in mice. These findings imply that the degeneration of the locus coeruleus may contribute to the accumulation of beta-amyloid protein in the brains of AD patients.

2.2 *The sign and symptom of AD*

2.2.1 *Memory impairment*

The earliest sign of AD often manifests as memory-related issues, specifically encompassing forgetting and forgetfulness.

"Forgetting" pertains to the difficulty in retaining and recalling new information or knowledge, and it is closely associated with cortical dysfunction. This means that the brain regions responsible for processing and storing new memories are affected, leading to deficits in the ability to learn and remember recently acquired information.

On the other hand, "forgetfulness" involves deficits in recalling information from the past, which is referred to as distant memory. This aspect of memory loss is associated with subcortical dysfunction. Initially, AD may present with impairments in short-term memory, where individuals struggle to remember recent events or information. As the disease progresses, it can lead to deficits in long-term memory, making it challenging for individuals to recall experiences, facts, or knowledge from their distant past. Ultimately, as the disease advances, both short and long-term memory impairments can coexist, significantly affecting an individual's ability to retain and retrieve information from various time periods in their life (McCormick *et al.* 1994).

2.2.2 *Cognitive impairment*

Cognitive impairment involves the ability to acquire and utilize knowledge. This encompasses both verbal and non-verbal skills, the capacity to retain new information, and the ability to retrieve knowledge from an extensive knowledge base. Cognitive dysfunction plays a pivotal role in diagnosing dementia, including AD. Notably, non-verbal cognitive impairments tend to manifest more rapidly and at an earlier stage than verbal impairments. In the early stages of AD, individuals may experience difficulties with calculations, exhibit poor judgment, struggle with generalization, become easily distracted, and develop left and right agnosia. These cognitive challenges become increasingly pronounced as the disease progresses.

2.2.3 *Aphasia*

Language changes serve as sensitive indicators of cortical dysfunction. Aphasia is a common and distinctive symptom of AD, distinguishing it from other causes of dementia. In AD, oral comprehension progressively deteriorates, although the ability to repeat information remains relatively preserved until the late stages (Nicholas *et al.* 1985). Syntax and pronunciation of language also tend to remain intact until the advanced stages, while semantic aspects gradually decline. Aphasia in AD can manifest as difficulty in finding words, spontaneous language redundancy, inability to name objects, glass aphasia, and a gradual development of paraphasia. In the middle and late stages of the disease, patients may exhibit various pronounced speech disorders, including imitating language, repeating words and phrases spoken by others, hyperglossia (repeating one's own words and expressions), poly-terminal syndrome (repeating the final part of a word), and, in the late stage, dysarthria (unintelligible speech) or even mutism (silence).

2.2.4 *Impairment of visuospatial skills, agnosia and apraxia*

In the early stages of AD, impairments in visuospatial skills are more prominent compared to other forms of dementia. These impairments can manifest as difficulties in tasks such as copying graphics or engaging in structural work, connecting tests and pendulum blocks, or solving puzzles. Approximately one-third of AD patients experience visual agnosia, facial agnosia, issues with body orientation, visual spatial agnosia, geographic disorientation, and these difficulties tend to worsen with the progression of the disease (Nicholas *et al.* 1985). AD patients may also display various forms of apraxia, including structural apraxia, clothing apraxia, ideomotor apraxia, ideational apraxia, walking apraxia, and apraxia of speech.

3 ORAL MICROBIOTA AND AD

3.1 *Oral microbial population*

The oral microbiome consists of a diverse array of microorganisms that inhabit the human mouth, including bacteria (e.g., Porphyromonas gingivalis), spirochetes (e.g., Treponema), viruses (e.g., herpesvirus), fungi (e.g., yeast), and more (Kolenbrander 2000). Research has highlighted the role of the oral microbial population in inducing various oral infectious diseases, including caries, pulpitis, periodontal disease, wisdom tooth pericoronitis, and jaw osteomyelitis, all of which pose significant threats to oral health. For instance, gram-negative bacteria like Porphyromonas gingivalis can thrive in gum and periodontal tissues, triggering host immune responses that result in chronic inflammation, characterized by gum swelling, the formation of periodontal pockets, and eventual loss of periodontal support tissues.

Moreover, the composition of oral microbial communities has a close relationship with systemic diseases, such as cancer, diabetes, rheumatoid arthritis, cardiovascular diseases, and premature births. This connection arises from the unique anatomical location of the oral microbiome, its metabolites, movement patterns, and the inflammation it can induce. The structural characteristics of oral microbial communities can serve as essential markers for assessing oral and systemic health. In recent years, increasing attention has been given to exploring the link between the oral microbial population and the pathogenesis of AD. Oral diseases like periodontal disease have been associated with the occurrence and progression of AD.

Oral microbial populations can enter the bloodstream due to various factors, including infection, trauma, or medical interventions. They may breach the blood-brain barrier and directly access the brain, producing toxic substances that trigger inflammation. This inflammation can lead to the deposition of Aβ, hyperphosphorylation of tau proteins, and ultimately result in irreversible damage to neurons, potentially leading to neuronal apoptosis. Understanding how oral microbial populations enter the brain and cause neuronal damage has become a focal point in understanding the pathogenesis of AD. Subsequent sections will delve into different pathways of microbial entry into the brain and the mechanisms underlying neuronal injury.

3.2 *Theoretical basis of the effect of oral microbial population on AD*

Oral microbial populations can infiltrate the brain through two primary avenues. Firstly, during instances of temporary bacteremia, such as dental treatments, tooth extraction, and gum abscesses, oral bacteria can gain access to the bloodstream and subsequently migrate into the brain. Secondly, these microbes may find their way into the brain through the trigeminal nerve, olfactory nerve, and facial nerve, which are connected to the central nervous system. Once the oral microbial population breaches the blood-brain barrier, it can trigger immune responses and the body's defense mechanisms against infection. This, in turn, can stimulate the activation of peripheral immune cells and exert regulatory influence on the occurrence of brain injuries, autoimmunity, and neurological conditions. As a result, oral microbial populations and the immune system can wield significant influence over neurodevelopmental, psychiatric, and neurodegenerative diseases. This process primarily encompasses two distinct mechanisms: the direct injury pathway and the indirect injury pathway (Sureda *et al.* 2020).

3.2.1 *Direct damage pathways*

As individuals age, there is an observed increase in the permeability of the blood-brain barrier among elderly patients. Consequently, pathogenic microorganisms can more readily breach this barrier, gaining access to brain tissue where they can directly interact with neurons. This interaction leads to the activation of the inflammatory cascade, resulting in direct harm to the central nervous system.

On one hand, when bacteria enter brain tissue, their secreted virulence factors can trigger the activation of Toll-like receptors 2 (TLR-2) and TLR-4, initiating the classical endogenous immune signaling pathway. This activation prompts microglia to release inflammatory cytokines such as tumor necrosis factor-α (TNF-α), interferon-γ (IFN-γ), and other molecules, thereby inciting an inflammatory response. On the other hand, inflammatory reactions within brain tissue can be induced by the activation of the complement system (Narengaowa *et al.* 2021).

Furthermore, researchers have identified an outer membrane protein called porin on the surface of gram-negative bacteria. The biological function of these porins is associated with the transport of small solutes, facilitating the movement of such solutes from the bacterial cytoplasm to the exterior of the cell membrane. This mechanism regulates the passage of small solutes across the cell membrane and influences cell metabolism. This may be one of the contributing factors to the induction of neuron apoptosis by bacteria. Pathogenic bacteria in the brain disrupt the integrity of nerve cell outer membranes, allowing the movement of materials between neurons. This, in turn, triggers the deposition of amyloid-beta (Aβ) and leads to neuronal damage (Abbayya *et al.* 2015).

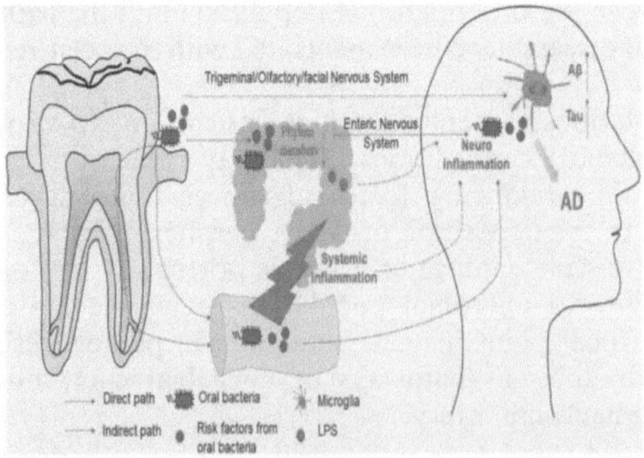

Figure 2. Illustrating the routes of oral and intestinal microbiota entry into the central nervous system (Narengaowa *et al.* 2021).

3.2.2 *Indirect injury pathway*

Oral microbial populations indirectly influence AD by releasing bacterial toxins, outer membrane vesicles (OMV), and pro-inflammatory factors that enter the brain through the bloodstream. For instance, Gram-negative bacteria have the capability to secrete OMVs with a diameter ranging from 20 to 250 nm, which are rich in lipopolysaccharide (LPS) and carry specific active membrane proteins. It has been substantiated that OMVs produced by Gram-negative bacteria can modulate the immune response, potentially serving as a means by which oral pathogens indirectly participate in the immune reactions within the nervous system.

Additionally, pathogenic microorganisms and their metabolites can induce alterations in the body's inflammatory response and immune defenses, elevating the levels of inflammatory factors in the circulatory system and instigating or amplifying the inflammatory cascade within brain tissue. Inflammatory factors released by pathogenic microorganisms, such as interleukin-1β (IL-1β), IL-6, and TNF-α, possess direct neurotoxic effects. The sustained, chronic inflammatory response within brain tissue further exacerbates the accumulation of Aβ, the hyperphosphorylation of tau protein, and disruptions in the blood-brain barrier's permeability. This hinders the efflux of Aβ from the central nervous system to the periphery, thereby increasing Aβ deposition within the central nervous system and ultimately leading to neuronal damage, as shown in Figure 2 (Narengaowa *et al.* 2021).

In summary, oral microbial populations can have a dual impact: firstly, they can breach the blood-brain barrier, inciting immune cascade reactions, and directly harm the nervous system; secondly, they can release pro-inflammatory factors and OMVs that affect neurons, causing indirect harm. Nevertheless, the relative significance of these two modes of action remains to be fully elucidated.

4 INTESTINAL MICROBIOTA AND THE PATHOGENESIS OF AD

4.1 *Intestinal flora and the gut-brain axis*

The gut microbiota is vital in numerous critical physiological functions, including food digestion, metabolism, immune responses, and the regulation of inflammation. Simultaneously, it has become increasingly evident that the gut microbiota can significantly impact the onset and progression of various mental disorders, such as anxiety, depression, autism, schizophrenia, and neurodegenerative diseases. Research has generated compelling evidence highlighting the intricate connection between microbiota, the gastrointestinal system, and the brain, commonly termed the "brain-gut axis." This axis signifies a two-way communication network between the brain and the gut, wherein alterations in the structure and makeup of intestinal flora can directly or indirectly influence the central nervous system (Narengaowa *et al.* 2021).

4.2 *Changes of intestinal microflora in AD patients*

The research findings have indicated significant differences in the intestinal microbial composition between AD patients and normal elderly individuals. At the phylum level, there was an increase in the abundance of Bacteroidetes and a decrease in the abundance of Actinomyces. At the genus level, there was an increase in the numbers of Bacteroides and Ruminococcus, along with a decrease in the numbers of Clostridium trichoides. A cross-sectional study has revealed that AD patients exhibit an elevated proinflammatory microbiome, suggesting that changes in cognitive function may be closely linked to systemic inflammation originating from the proinflammatory microbiome in the gut.

Pathogenic bacteria such as Escherichia coli possess the ability to secrete amyloid proteins, which share structural and immunogenic similarities with the abnormal misfolded

β-amyloid proteins commonly associated with AD. These amyloid proteins can activate cells to release inflammatory factors, exacerbating the inflammatory response within the AD-afflicted brain. Moreover, alterations in the structure of the intestinal flora often lead to the production of enteritis cytokines, which can induce neuroinflammation via factors like blood endotoxins. Cyanobacteria within the intestinal flora can severely impair neurological function, serving as a key factor in the development of AD (Zhuang *et al.* 2018). The disruption of the gut microbiota balance reduces the expression of gamma-aminobutyric acid and brain-derived neurotrophic factor in the brain, while also affecting tryptophan metabolism. This cascade of effects ultimately results in central nervous system dysfunction, personality changes, cognitive impairment, and may even contribute to the development of AD.

4.3 *Study on probiotics ameliorating AD*

Presently, a substantial body of animal and clinical research has demonstrated that probiotics and their metabolites have the potential to ameliorate AD and other neurodegenerative conditions through various mechanisms, including the regulation of the immune response, maintenance of intestinal microecological balance, and antioxidative actions. Furthermore, probiotics can serve as adjunct therapies to enhance the effectiveness of other AD treatments. As a promising avenue for AD mitigation, it is imperative that probiotics are thoughtfully designed and subjected to extensive clinical investigations to ensure their safe, efficacious, and disease-specific preventive roles (Naomi *et al.* 2021).

To advance this approach, modern food and bioengineering technologies are being leveraged to explore and expand the potential of a new generation of probiotics. These efforts are complemented by research methodologies aimed at elucidating the internal molecular mechanisms by which probiotics influence intestinal microecology and contribute to AD improvement. Based on this evolving understanding, the development of novel drugs and treatment modalities represents a critical direction for the future of AD prevention and management (Den *et al.* 2020; Naomi *et al.* 2021).

5 CONCLUSION

The aforementioned review underscores a robust and intricate relationship between oral and intestinal flora and AD, a relationship deserving of further exploration. There exist both direct and indirect pathways through which disturbances in oral flora can potentially contribute to the onset and progression of AD.

In the direct pathway, oral bacteria have the capability to infiltrate brain tissue via two primary routes: the circulatory system and nerves. This invasive journey culminates in the precipitation of Aβ proteins or the initiation of brain neuroinflammation, resulting in direct damage to neurons. The consequences of this direct neuronal damage are believed to be significant in the development and exacerbation of AD.

The indirect pathway involves the ability of oral bacteria to induce systemic inflammation. This systemic inflammation, in turn, can lead to damage in brain vessels, ultimately contributing to the pathogenesis of AD. This intricate cascade of events highlights the multifaceted nature of the relationship between oral flora and AD.

On the other hand, the gut microbiota plays a pivotal clinical role in maintaining overall health, and its dysregulation has been linked to various central nervous system disorders, including AD. In the realm of preventive measures, individuals can consider incorporating probiotic supplements into their daily routines. These probiotics serve to preserve the diversity of gut flora and enhance the population of beneficial microorganisms. In doing so, they promote optimal intestinal function and, importantly, mitigate the risk of AD.

A plethora of scientific studies has demonstrated the potential of probiotics and their metabolites to ameliorate AD and other neurodegenerative diseases. Their mechanisms of action include the regulation of immune responses, the maintenance of intestinal microecological balance, and providing antioxidant benefits, among others. Additionally, probiotics have emerged as valuable adjuncts to conventional anti-AD medications, enhancing their overall efficacy.

As a potential strategy for AD mitigation, it is imperative that probiotics are meticulously designed, and a substantial number of clinical trials are undertaken to ensure their safe, effective, and specific preventive role. Leveraging modern food and bioengineering technologies, researchers can develop a new generation of probiotics and associated research methods. This will aid in clarifying the intricate molecular mechanisms underpinning their regulation of intestinal microecology and their capacity to improve AD outcomes. Such endeavors represent a crucial and promising avenue for the future prevention and treatment of AD.

REFERENCES

Abbayya K., Puthanakar N.Y., Naduwinmani S. and Chidambar Y.S. (2015). *NAJMS*, **7**, 241

Breijyeh Z. and Karaman R. (2020). *Molecules*, 25 , 5789

Den H., Dong X., Chen M. and Zou Z. *Aging*, (2020). **12**, 4010

Kolenbrander P.E. (2000). *Anne Rev Microbiol* , **54**, 413

McCormick W.C., Kukull W.A., van Belle G., Bowen J.D., Teri L. and Larson E.B. (1994). *J Am Geriatr Soc*, **42** ,517

Morales I., Farías G. and Maccioni R.B. (2010). *Neuroimmunomodulat*, **17**, 202

Naomi R., Embong H., Othman F., Ghazi H.F., Maruthey N., Bahari H. (2021). *Nutrients*, 14, 20

Narengaowa, Kong W., Lan F., Awan U.F., Qing H. and Ni J. (2021). *Front.Cell.Neurosci*, **15**, 633735

Naseri N.N., Wang H., Guo J., Sharma M. and Luo W. *Neurosci Lett*, (2019), **705** , 183

Nicholas M., Obler L.K., Albert M.L. and Helm-Estabrooks N. (1985). *J Speech Lang Hear R*, **28** ,405

Philip Scheltens, Bart De Strooper, Miia Kivipelto, Henne Holstege, Gael Chételat, Charlotte E Teunissen, Jeffrey Cummings and Wiesje M van der Flier, (2021). *Lancet.*, **397**, 1577

Sureda A., Daglia M., Castilla S.A., Sanadgol N., Nabavi S.F., Khan H., Khan H., Belwal T., Jeandet P., Marchese A., Pistollato F., Forbes-Hernandez T., Battino M., Berindan-Neagoe I., D'Onofrio G. and Nabavi S.M. (2020). *Pharmacol Res*, **151**, 104582

Wang L., Yin Y.L., Liu X.Z., Shen P., Zheng Y.G., Lan X.R., Lu C.B. and Wang J.Z. (2020). *Transl Neurodegener*, **9,** 1

Younkin S. G., (1998). *J. Physiol. Paris*, **92**, 289

Zhuang Z.Q., Shen L.L., Li W.W., Fu X., Zeng F., Gui L., Lü Y., Cai M., Zhu C., Tan Y.L., Zheng P., Li H. Y., Zhu J., Zhou H.D., Bu X.L. and Wang Y.J. (2018). *J Alzheimers Dis*, **63**, 1337

Chapter 4
Microfluidics, wearables, and medical devices

Biological Sciences and Environmental Health – Gao (Ed.)

Application of wearable somatosensory devices in VR/AR

Zhenzheng Dong
Telecommunications Engineering with Management Major, Beijing University of Posts and Telecommunications, Beijing, PR China

ABSTRACT: Virtual reality (VR) and augmented reality (AR) technologies are currently used extensively across a wide range of industries. In order to improve user experience and realize more natural human-computer interaction, new forms of interaction are becoming more and more in demand. The use of wearable somatosensory devices in the contexts of virtual reality and augmented reality is examined in this research study, along with its prospective uses and effects. The article first introduces the working principle and key technologies of wearable somatosensory devices, including sensors, data processing and gesture recognition. Then, the application fields of wearable somatosensory devices in VR and AR are elaborated, such as games, training, medical treatment and interaction design, etc. Finally, the future development prospects of wearable somatosensory devices in VR and AR are summarized. The study presented in this paper is very important for the use of wearable somatosensory technology in VR and AR. This article will help to improve user experience, realize more natural human-computer interaction, and promote the development of VR and AR technology, providing a better way for various fields.

1 INTRODUCTION

The application of wearable somatosensory devices in the fields of virtual reality and augmented reality has become a hotspot. Amidst the swift progression of VR and AR technologies, people's demands for more immersive and intuitive interaction methods and more natural human-computer interaction experience continue to increase. As an innovative way of interaction, wearable somatosensory devices can provide a more intuitive and natural interaction experience, so it has received extensive attention and research.

VR technology allows people to fully immerse themselves in a virtual environment, creating realistic sensations and experiences. However, traditional interaction methods, such as external controllers such as keyboards, mice, and joystick controllers, limit the direct interaction between users and the virtual environment to a certain extent, and cannot meet users' expectations for free and intuitive interaction. In order to solve this problem, wearable somatosensory devices came into being. Wearable somatosensory devices perceive the user's body movements, gestures and postures through sensor technology, and convert them into digital signals to realize interaction with VR/AR systems. This enhanced and instinctive method of interaction empowers users to engage with the virtual environment in a more seamless manner, ultimately enhancing user experience and active involvement (Kim *et al.* 2017; Wang *et al.* 2021).

VR and AR technologies have demonstrated significant potential and promising application prospects in the domains of gaming, education, healthcare, and design (Perez and Zeadally 2021; Wegen *et al.* 2023). These technologies can provide an immersive experience, bringing users from the real world into a virtual environment or blending virtual elements

DOI: 10.1201/9781003587590-36

into real scenes. In the field of games, wearable somatosensory devices can provide a more realistic and immersive gaming experience; in terms of training, it can simulate real scenes to help users with skill training and practice; in the medical field, wearable somatosensory devices can be used for rehabilitation training and treatment, Provide more efficient, personalized medical care. In terms of interaction design, wearable somatosensory devices can break the limitations of traditional interfaces and achieve more intuitive and free interaction methods.

Although wearable somatosensory devices have great potential and broad application prospects in VR/AR, they still face some challenges. First of all, the accuracy and response speed of sensors need to be continuously improved to ensure that user actions can be accurately captured and presented. Second, the comfort and use experience of the device needs to be continuously improved to increase user acceptance and comfort for long-term wearing. In addition, the cost of wearable somatosensory devices is also a consideration, and the manufacturing cost needs to be reduced so that more users can benefit from this technology.

This thesis aims to deeply discuss the application of wearable somatosensory devices in VR/AR. Through the analysis of relevant research and practical application cases, this article will discuss the impact of wearable somatosensory devices on VR/AR interactive experience, as well as its specific applications in the fields of games, education, medical care and industry. At the same time, the article also discusses the challenges faced by current wearable somatosensory devices, and proposes the direction of improvement and development. Through in-depth research in this field, we hope to provide useful enlightenment and guidance for the further development and application of wearable somatosensory devices in the field of VR/AR.

2 WORKING PRINCIPLE OF WEARABLE SOMATOSENSORY DEVICES

The working principle of wearable somatosensory devices is based on various sensor technologies, such as accelerometers, gyroscopes, and magnetometers. These sensors can capture user motion and posture information (Wang *et al.* 2023). Through the integration of sensor data, wearable devices have the capability to interpret the user's real-time movements and gestures. This article next introduces some common sensors for wearable somatosensory devices.

An accelerometer (as shown in Figure 1) is a sensor that measures the acceleration of an object and is often used to detect an object's linear acceleration and gravitational acceleration. It senses changes in the user's acceleration, such as gait, running or jumping. A gyroscope is a sensor that measures the angular velocity of an object and is used to detect the speed of rotation and rotation of an object. It can sense the user's rotation and posture changes, such as turning around, sit-ups, and other actions. A magnetometer is a sensor that measures the strength of the magnetic field around an object, which can be used for positioning and orientation awareness. It can help determine the position and orientation in space (Wang *et al.* 2023).

These sensors work by collecting user motion data and transmitting it to the processing unit of the wearable device. The processing unit analyses and interprets sensor data using algorithms and models to recognize user actions and gestures. For example, by combining accelerometer and gyroscope data, the user's gait can be detected, and the number of steps can be estimated; by combining gyroscope and magnetometer data, the user's rotation angle and direction can be determined.

In addition, positioning and tracking technologies also play an important role in wearable somatosensory devices. By combining sensor data and localization technologies, wearable devices can track the user's position and movement path in space in real-time, enabling more precise motion analysis and localization functions (Ali *et al.* 2023).

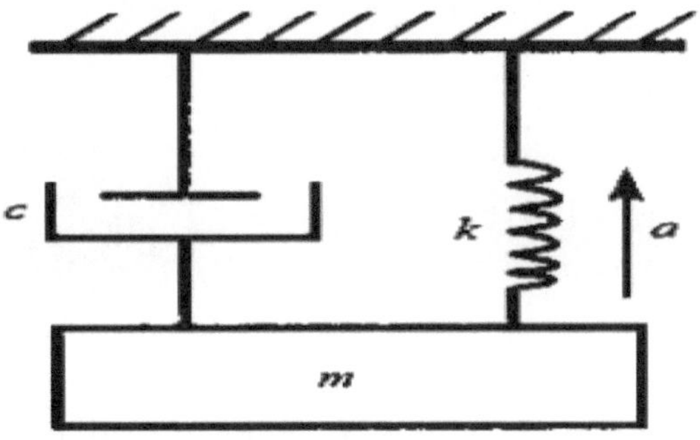

Figure 1. Accelerometer schematic diagram (Picture credit: Original).

3 APPLICATION OF WEARABLE SOMATOSENSORY DEVICES

The article mainly discusses three application aspects of wearable somatosensory devices: motion tracking, tactile feedback, and physiological parameter monitoring.

3.1 *Motion tracking*

Motion tracking is the basic function of wearable somatosensory devices, which can convert the user's physical motion into digital input to control virtual objects in the VR/AR environment. For example, the tracker of the HTC Vive can track the user's head and hand movements and translate these movements into perspective and gesture changes in the virtual reality (VR) environment.

HTC Vive system ensures precise representation of the users' actions and postures within the virtual environment through the following methods:

Head pose tracking: HTC Vive headset (as shown in Figure 2) has multiple built-in sensors, including gyroscopes, accelerometers, and magnetometers, to track the pose and movement of the user's head. These sensors detect head rotation, tilt and roll to accurately track the orientation and position of the user's head within the virtual space (Niehorster *et al.* 2017).

Controller tracking: HTC Vive system uses hand-held controllers as a tool for users to contact with the virtual world. Each controller has built-in sensors, including accelerometers and gyroscopes, that track the controller's position and attitude. The system utilizes infrared beams emitted by the base station to establish precise calculations of the controller's position and orientation within the virtual environment. By interacting with these infrared beams, the system accurately determines the controller's spatial data in the virtual space.

Base Station tracking: HTC Vive system uses a "Lighthouse" base station for precise location tracking. These base stations are placed in the room's corners or at appropriate locations and emit infrared beams to scan. The controller and headset sensors receive the beam and communicate with the base station. The device can precisely locate and orient the controller and headset by calculating the temporal and angle differences of the beams.

HTC Vive system can accurately capture and present the user's actions and postures in the virtual environment through above head posture tracking, controller tracking, and base station tracking technologies. This enables users to interact with the virtual world naturally and intuitively, enhancing the realism and interactivity of immersive VR experiences . For example, when using the HTC Vive system to play the Beat Saber game, by wearing a Vive helmet and using the handle, the player uses a virtual lightsaber to cut through the blocks, and at the same time, moves according to the rhythm of the music, so that the player feels that he has entered a world full of music and light and shadow.

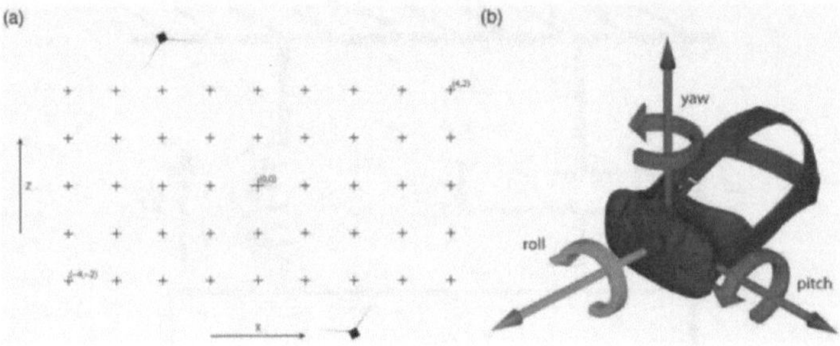

Figure 2. HTC Vive headset schematic diagram (Niehorster *et al.* 2017).

3.2 *Tactile feedback*

The tactile feedback function of the wearable somatosensory device enhances the user's level of immersion within the VR/AR environment by simulating the tactile stimulation in the real world (Wegen *et al.* 2023). For example, HaptX Glove (as shown in Figure 3) is a glove with a tactile feedback function, which uses micro-bubbles and force feedback actuators to simulate tactile stimulation, enabling users to "feel" the shape, texture, and weight of virtual objects (Pooryousef *et al.* 2019).

HaptX Glove is an advanced haptic feedback glove that provides a realistic tactile and force feedback experience. It uses several techniques and principles to achieve this:

Pressure sensor array: HaptX Glove has a large number of pressure sensors distributed in key parts of the glove, such as fingers and palms. These sensors measure the distribution and changes in pressure when the hand comes into contact with an object.

Tactile feedback: HaptX Glove uses pressure sensors and control algorithms to simulate objects' tactile sensations and surface details. When the hand is in contact with a virtual object, the glove will sense the pressure and shape of the object's surface through the sensor and generate corresponding tactile feedback, allowing the user to feel the object's hardness, texture, and shape.

Force feedback: Apart from haptic feedback, the HaptX Glove is capable of delivering force feedback as well allowing users to feel the weight, resistance, and movement of objects. Active force controllers inside the glove apply force and resistance, simulating what it's like to interact with virtual objects.

Motion Capture: The HaptX Glove also features motion capture, which tracks the movement and posture of the user's hands. By capturing and tracking hand movements, the HaptX Glove can precisely translate the player's gestures and actions into the virtual scene. This enables a deeply immersive interactive experience by accurately mapping real-world hand movements to the virtual environment.

Using these above technologies and principles comprehensively, HaptX Glove can provide a highly realistic haptic and force feedback experience. Thanks to it, users can interact with things in a virtual environment, feel real touch and force changes, and amplify the immersion and interactivity of applications in the realm of virtual and augmented reality.

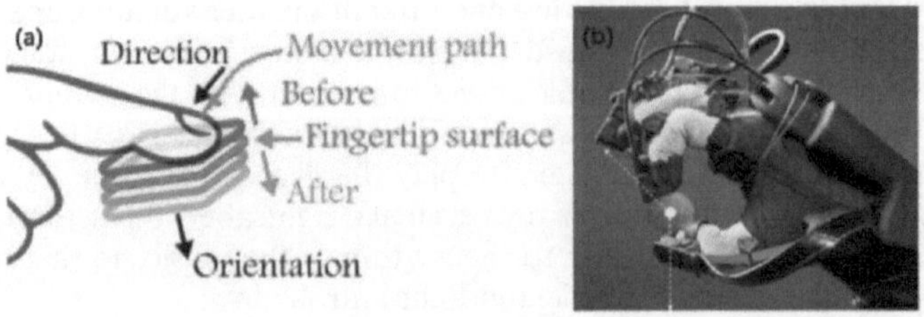

Figure 3. HaptX Glove schematic diagram (Alcaide 2021).

3.3 *Physiological parameter monitor*

Physiological parameter monitoring is a new application field of wearable somatosensory devices, which can monitor the user's heart rate, skin conductance, eye movement and other physiological parameters to provide a deeper immersive experience (Ali *et al.* 2023). For example, the Neurable headset (as shown in Figure 4) monitors the user's brain waves and uses them to control virtual objects in a VR environment (Alcaide 2021).

Each earpad of the headphones has 10 electrodes in addition to reference and ground electrodes. The ear cushions are surrounded by these dry, active electrodes, which are made of a conductive mesh substance. The headphone is designed to capture and interpret the user's brain activity through electroencephalography (EEG) signals, enabling interaction with virtual reality (VR) and augmented reality (AR) environments. The Neurable headphones (as shown in Figure 4) works as follows:

Electroencephalogram sensors: The Neurable headband touches the user's scalp with multiple EEG sensors to measure brain electrical activity. These sensors record electrical activity in the cerebral cortex, including neurons' electrical signals and brain waves.

Signal Acquisition and Processing: Sensors in the headband transmit EEG signals to an internal signal processing unit. Here, the signal is filtered, amplified and digitized to extract useful EEG features.

Brain-computer interface algorithms: Headphones uses advanced brain-computer interface algorithms to analyse EEG signals and convert them into understandable instructions. These algorithms can identify specific patterns and pattern changes in brain activity to infer a user's intent and focus of attention.

Interacting with virtual and augmented reality environments: By analysing EEG signals, Enten headphones are able to interact with virtual and augmented reality environments in real time (Alcaide 2021). Users can control objects in the virtual scene, perform gesture recognition or perform specific operations through ideas or concentration.

The underlying principle of the Enten headphones revolves around the gathering and analysis of EEG signals, which are subsequently utilized to interpret the user's brain activity. This interpretation makes it easier to interact naturally with virtual and augmented reality situations. This brain-computer interface technology provides people with a novel and intuitive way of interacting, translating human thoughts and intentions into actions and behaviours in a virtual environment.

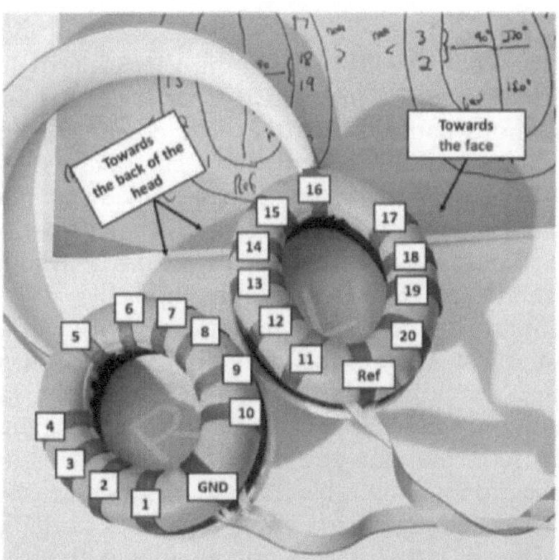

Figure 4. Enten headphones prototype (Alcaide 2021).

4 FUTURE DEVELOPMENT

Wearable somatosensory devices will continue to usher in technological development and innovation in the future. The following are possible technological trends:

Miniaturization and integration: In the future, wearable somatosensory devices will tend to be smaller and lighter in design to improve wearing comfort and portability. Furthermore, integrating sensors and processing units will further enhance the performance and functionality of devices (Perez and Zeadally 2021; Roggio *et al.* 2021).

High precision and low latency: Future wearable somatosensory devices will pursue higher motion capture accuracy and real-time performance to provide a more accurate and natural interactive experience. This may involve higher-resolution sensors, more powerful data processing capabilities, and optimized algorithms.

Multi-modal perception: Future development trends may include integrating multiple sensors to achieve more comprehensive user motion and environmental perception. By combining multiple modal information such as vision, sound, and touch, wearable somatosensory devices can provide richer and more realistic virtual and augmented reality experiences.

With the popularization and wide application of wearable somatosensory devices, user privacy and security issues have become particularly important. Here are the related challenges and solutions:

Data privacy protection: User data collected by wearable somatosensory devices may contain sensitive information, such as body movements and physiological indicators. Protecting the privacy and security of these data will be a key issue, requiring strict data protection policies and encryption measures (Chen *et al.* 2020).

User authentication and access control: To prevent unauthorized access and use, wearable somatosensory devices require effective authentication mechanisms and access control strategies to ensure that only legitimate users can use the device and related functions.

Security vulnerabilities and attack prevention: Wearable somatosensory devices, as IoT devices, may face security vulnerabilities and potential network attacks. Researchers and manufacturers need to strengthen the security design and vulnerability repair mechanism of devices to ensure the safety of users' data and devices (Wang *et al.* 2014).

5 CONCLUSION

The application of wearable somatosensory devices in VR/AR is of great significance. It can provide a more intuitive and immersive interactive experience, enabling users to interact with the virtual environment more naturally. In the field of games, wearable somatosensory devices can make games more exciting and real, and increase users' sense of participation. In the field of training and medical treatment, it can provide a more realistic simulation environment to help users perform skill training and medical treatment. In terms of interaction design, wearable somatosensory devices can break the traditional interface restrictions and achieve more direct and free interaction methods.

However, the application of wearable somatosensory devices in VR/AR still faces some challenges. First, the cost and stability of the technology remain issues, limiting its adoption in large-scale applications. Secondly, security and privacy issues also need further research and improvement. In addition, the accuracy and real-time performance of data is also a key issue to achieve precise pose recognition and motion tracking.

To sum up, the application of wearable somatosensory devices in VR/AR has great potential. With the further development and improvement of technology, it can be expected to be widely used in the field of virtual reality and augmented reality.

REFERENCES

Alcaide R., (2021). *Attention-based Artificial Intelligence for the Detection of COVID-19 From Chest X-ray Images*, Available online at: https://doi.org/10.1101/2021.06.21.448991.

Ali A., Ashfaq M., Qureshi A., Muzammil U., Shaukat H., Ali S., Altabey W. A., Noori M., Kouritem S. A. (2023). *Sens.* **23**, 6586.

Chen S., Zhu X., Zhang H., Zhao C., Yang G. and Wang K. (2020). *IEEE Trans.Sustain.Comput*, **5**, 526.

Kim M., Jeon C. and Kim J. (2017). *Sens.* **17**,1141.

Niehorster D. C., Li L. and Lappe M. (2017). *I-Perception*, **8**.

Perez A. J. and Zeadally S. (2021). *Sens.* **21**, 6828.

Pooryousef V., Brown R. and Turkay S., (2019). *ACM CHISIG*, 433.

Roggio F., Ravalli S., Maugeri G., Bianco A., Palma A., Di Rosa M. and Musumeci G. (2021). *WJO.* **12**, 467.

van Wegen M., Herder J. L., Adelsberger R., Pastore-Wapp M., van Wegen E. E. H., Bohlhalter S., Nef T., Krack P. and Vanbellingen T., (2023). *Sens.* **23,** 1563.

Wang B., Yu S., Lou W. and Hou Y. T., (2014). *IEEE INFOCOM*, 2112.

Wang X., Yu H., Kold S. and Rahbek O. (2023). *BIR.* **3**.

Wang Y., Wang Y., Chen J., Yang J., Jiang T. and He J. (2021). *Sens.* **21**, 1582.

Biological Sciences and Environmental Health – Gao (Ed.)

Wearable devices for electrocardiogram signal acquisition

Weiqi Wang
Electronic, Electrical and Systems Engineering, University of Birmingham, Birmingham, UK

ABSTRACT: With the development of society, an increasing number of people are suffering from cardiovascular diseases, which have become one of the leading health concerns worldwide. Cardiovascular diseases pose a serious threat to people's health and lives. To address this, the electrocardiogram (ECG) was developed to detect and monitor the electrical activity of the human heart and help doctors diagnose and prevent heart disease. A wearable device for ECG signal acquisition has also been invented to monitor heart conditions in real time.

This article introduces the background of ECG, explains its principles, and finally analyzes its practical applications. It explains the principles, applications, and precautions of wearable ECG devices. While wearable devices have already become part of a large number of patients' lives, there are still many aspects that need to be improved. The article concludes with an objective analysis of the current state of wearable devices for ECG collection.

1 INTRODUCTION

The heart functions as the power source of the human body, facilitating blood circulation and ensuring the supply of oxygen necessary for maintaining normal functions of the body. According to Khan *et al.*, cardiovascular diseases are life-threatening and have a significant negative impact on human health. Cardiovascular diseases account for approximately one-third of deaths globally, with over 70% of those at risk having such risk factors. The United Nations estimates that by 2050, one in six people will be over 65, up from one in eleven in 2019 (Khan *et al.* 2020), further contributing to the increasing frequency of such diseases globally.

An electrocardiogram (ECG) is a non-invasive test that detects the electrical activity of the heart, enabling doctors to diagnose arrhythmias or other heart conditions. However, traditional ECG signal acquisition devices are large, difficult to carry, and expensive, presenting significant limitations. Therefore, portable ECG monitoring devices, which can be easily monitored in real time, have been developed. Among these wearable ECG monitoring devices, smartwatches are the most popular.

Wearable devices for ECG collection have several advantages. Wearable ECG monitoring devices enable timely heart monitoring, preventive care for high-risk groups, and real-time tracking of patients' conditions. Besides, real-time ECG monitoring can be used for clinical diagnosis and early detection and diagnosis of heart diseases such as arrhythmia. In addition, these devices can also be used to monitor the treatment effects of cardiac patients, providing more accurate medical decision-making and personalized treatment plans.

In short, cardiovascular disease has become a critical health issue that cannot be overlooked. Despite the considerable human and financial resources dedicated to addressing heart disease, many patients still die of heart disease every year. Therefore, integrating ECG signal acquisition devices into patients' lives has become increasingly important. However,

 DOI: 10.1201/9781003587590-37

traditional ECG monitoring devices are bulky and expensive, leading to the growing trend of developing and popularizing wearable ECG signal collection devices. This article discusses the meaning and principles of ECG and wearable ECG signal acquisition devices, as well as their inadequacies.

2 ANALYSIS OF ELECTROCARDIOGRAM

ECG, which demonstrates the activity of the human heart, was invented more than a hundred years ago by Dutch physiologist Willem Einthoven. The ECG signal provides information about the condition of the heart and various parameters that allow doctors to quickly identify cardiac conditions and accurately diagnose cardiac issues, leading to better treatment outcomes. The invention of ECG has greatly improved patient survival rates.

ECG generates a kind of electric signal that tracks the heartbeat. The signals are generated as tiny electric potentials produced by cardiac tissue, which create an electric signal detected by ECG electrodes. The small signals are amplified and recorded as an ECG. Specialized cells in the sinoatrial node (SA node) often generate electrical activity spontaneously and exhibit automation. The electrodes in the heart's cell produce the electric current, where the outer surface of the cell walls is positively charged in a normal resting state. As a result of the reversal of this charge, the outside of the cell wall becomes negatively charged, which spreads as electrical pulses to neighboring cardiac tissues. ECG serves multiple functions, such as detecting ischemia and myocardial infarction, arrhythmia, and conduction disturbances (Wasimuddin 2020).

Wang *et al.* (2012) noted that the ECG is a weak, bipolar signal of low frequency, normally ranging between 0.05 and 100 Hz, with the most common range being 0.05-35 Hz. Besides, its amplitude ranges from 10 μV to 4 mV, with an average value of 1 mV.

Cardiovascular disease can lead to a series of heart-related conditions, including arrhythmia, which in severe cases can even lead to sudden death. According to Fong and Chung (2015), the number of annual deaths from cardiovascular diseases is projected to increase from 17 million in 2008 to 25 million in 2030. Therefore, the prevention and diagnosis of cardiovascular diseases has become extremely important. ECGs are especially common now as they allow doctors to make early predictions and diagnoses based on ECG signals.

Non-contact ECG monitoring technology has been developed and is now widely used for long-term monitoring, drastically reducing death rates among heart disease patients. Traditional ECG devices often use Ag/AgCl electrodes coated with an electrically conductive adhesive to ensure close contact with the patient's skin. However, this may cause discomfort. Non-contact ECG signal collection devices measure biological signals through an insulating material, such as clothing, without directly touching the skin. This method allows for more comfortable monitoring, minimizes discomfort, and reduces the potential negative impact on the patient's quality of life.

Plesnik *et al.* (2010) demonstrated that an ECG signal collection system has a comparatively simple structure and components. However, due to its highly sensitive nature to external interference, the measuring circuit is prone to noise and other disturbances, making it essential for the system to have excellent quality and effective connections. This sensitivity results when the ECG signals are obtained from the surface of the skin, particularly when ECG signals are remotely monitored. To address the noise issue, a suitable analog circuit may be used to eliminate most of the noise before digital signal processing. The conceptual architecture of the ECG signal acquisition and remote monitoring system typically involves several steps (Figure 1): electrode analog signal acquisition, signal amplification, bandpass filter signal processing, and analog-to-digital signal conversion. Three types of electrodes are also used to capture other biological signals such as electromyography, electroencephalography, etc.: wet electrodes, dry electrodes, and insulated or capacitive electrodes.

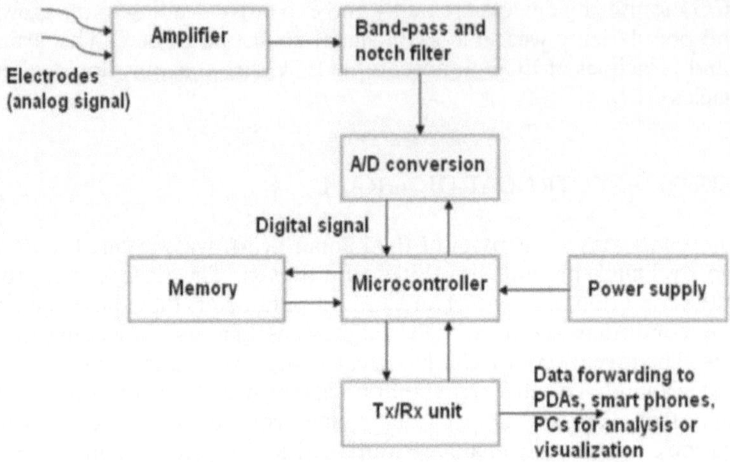

Figure 1. ECG signal acquisition and remote monitoring system architecture (Plesnik *et al.* 2010).

3 ANALYSIS OF WEARABLE DEVICES ON ELECTROCARDIOGRAM

Wearable devices that can collect ECG signals are becoming more and more important due to their convenience and constant monitoring ability. Over the past few years, cardiac health monitors have grown in popularity as heart disease remains the leading cause of death worldwide. These wearable devices are small, low-power, lightweight, and interoperable with different mobile devices and communication networks. In addition, it allows for real-time signal processing. Zhang *et al.* (2015) highlighted that ECG is considered the gold standard physiological signal for wearable heart health monitoring because of its numerous meaningful temporal, spatial, spectral, and statistical characteristics.

Noureddine *et al.* demonstrated that the hardware system of the wearable device for ECG signal acquisition consists of three layers, as shown in Figure 2. The sensor layer comprises a biological amplifier and a bandpass filter. The communication layer is composed of a Bluetooth module. The processing layer includes a microcontroller, whose role is to capture and digitize ECG signals, connect with Bluetooth devices, and transmit proper data as instructed. For ECG signal processing algorithms, refer to Belgacem *et al.* (2011).

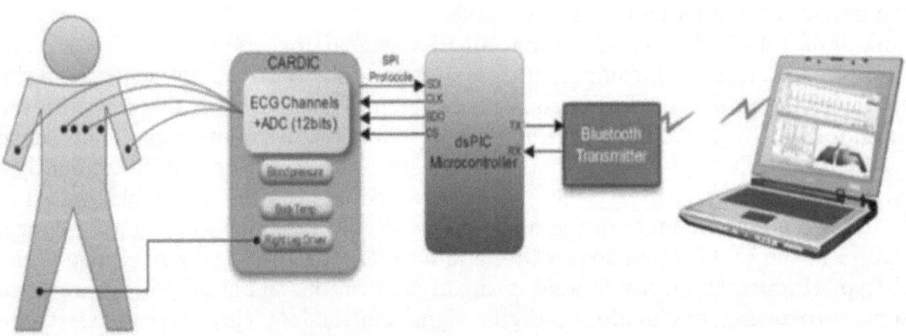

Figure 2. The overall hardware system (Belgacem *et al.* 2011).

Noureddine *et al.* show that wearable devices for ECG acquisition are analyzed in three main sections. First, ECG collection is designed to capture analog ECG in digital form so that it can be stored and analyzed. This is accomplished through a separate hardware collection unit, built on an embedded system that synchronizes with MATLAB for automatic data storage. The hardware collection section is composed of a microcontroller, a Bluetooth transmitter, and a low-power multisensor front-end acquisition system. The ECG processing and PC-based data collection systems have become increasingly popular over the past ten years as a result of the growing usage of microcontrollers as front-end programmable devices. A microcontroller is chosen as a preferred device due to its advantages, including low cost, programmability, affordability, and fast processing capabilities. Prior to digitizing, the sensor output is amplified, and the microcontroller generates a communication protocol for transferring data to a standalone PC. The wireless revolution has introduced a host of new radio devices with a host of stringent requirements, such as having to be smaller, lighter, wider in bandwidth, and more cost-effective. The integration of radio frequency systems onto a single chip is now a reality for such systems (Belgacem *et al.* 2011). There are several precautions for wearable devices that collect ECG signals.

3.1 *Aesthetics*

Aesthetics has become a key factor in the mainstream acceptance of wearable devices, particularly in the context of human-computer interaction studies. As interest in the design and aesthetics of wearable technology grows, it is evident that these devices must go beyond being simply functional and visually appealing. The design of wearable technology should also consider the relationship between technology and its physical, cultural, and social meaning (Jarusriboonchai and Häkkilä 2019).

3.2 *Easy to use and comfortable*

Wearable devices must offer simple interaction options and present the desired feedback clearly to enable users to interact more efficiently. The usability of the device is enhanced with a straightforward, simple, and intuitive interface that helps increase user engagement. The wearer is sufficiently comfortable that they do not feel the device for some time. Comfort considerations include acceptable temperature, texture, shape, weight, and tightness (Motti and Caine 2014).

3.3 *Security and privacy*

According to Baig *et al.* (2013), the key element for wearable devices is the safety and confidentiality of patient data. As wearable devices become more widely used, it is possible to obtain and record the information of the patient by electronic means. This includes a patient's biometrics, health records, and other sensitive personal information. The data is crucial for patient safety, individual privacy, and the overall welfare of society. Ensuring the protection of patient privacy and personal information in today's large data-intensive information environment has become a pressing issue. With the rise of big data, artificial intelligence, and 5G technologies, it has made it easier for people to collect their personal information and communicate. However, this ease of access has also led to growing concerns over illegal data acquisition, misuse, leakage, and the exchange of personal information. Privacy and data security have become increasingly critical issues.

Due to the rapid development of technology and the Internet of Things, devices such as portable health monitors are inherently becoming vulnerable to hacking. There are many ways that malicious third-party attacks can wreak havoc on unsuspecting personal data products. Developers of portable ECG acquisition devices must ensure security features are built into their products. As cybersecurity becomes a greater priority in healthcare, security must be a top design consideration. In addition, wearable ECG devices may present a series of safety hazards, such as inaccurate data and static electricity on the device, which must be addressed while keeping costs under control.

4 CONCLUSION

The heart is the foundation of human life, driving blood circulation and ensuring the body receives the oxygen and nutrients it needs to function properly. Heart health is closely related to life expectancy, and a healthy heart contributes to a long and healthy life. However, heart disease remains one of the leading causes of death worldwide.

With the rapid development of science and technology, wearable devices designed to collect ECG signals are continually being optimized and upgraded to better understand the real-time conditions of the heart and help maintain heart health. Today's wearable ECG devices are highly portable and are capable of accurately measuring ECG signals in time and sending them to a computer terminal. These innovations allow for a better understanding of the real-time heart conditions of patients and greatly improve the success rate of heart disease treatment.

As the global population ages and technology continues to advance, the incidence of cardiovascular disease is rising. It remains one of the leading causes of death. Real-time cardiac devices are now widely used to help prevent cardiac diseases in the early stages. However, conventional ECG surveillance devices have the disadvantages of being large in volume, expensive, and inconvenient to use. Portable ECG sensors, integrated with ECG monitors and other terminals, provide a practical solution so that the device can be used in high-risk patients in daily life. The increasing application of wearable devices for ECG signal collection is expected to become a widespread trend, which is likely to significantly reduce the risk of developing heart disease.

REFERENCES

Baig M. M., Gholamhosseini H. and Connolly M. J. (2013). *Medical & Biological Engineering & Computing*, **51**, 485

Belgacem N., Assous S. and Bereksi-Reguig F. (2011). *International Workshop on Systems, Signal Processing and their Applications, WOSSPA*

Fong E.-M. and Chung W.-Y. (2015). *Sensors*, **15**, 19237

Jarusriboonchai P. and Häkkilä J. (2019). *Proceedings of the 18th International Conference on Mobile and Ubiquitous Multimedia*

Khan M. A., Hashim M. J., Mustafa H., Baniyas M. Y., Suwaidi S. K. B. M. A., Alkatheeri R., Alblooshi F. M. K., Almatrooshi M. E. A. H., Alzaabi M. E. H., Darmaki R. S. A. and H. Lootah S. N. A. (2020). *Cureus* **2**

Motti V.G. and Caine K. (2014). *Proceedings of the Human Factors and Ergonomics Society Annual Meeting*, **58**,1820

Plesnik E., Malgina O., Tasic J. F., Zajc M. (2010). *Melecon 2010 - 2010 15th IEEE Mediterranean Electrotechnical Conference*

Wasimuddin M., Elleithy K., Abuzneid A., Faezipour M. and Abuzaghleh O. (2020). *IEEE Access*, **8**,177782

Wang K., Ma S., Feng J., Zhang W., Fan M. and Zhao D. (2012). *Procedia Engineering*, **29**, 3763

Zhang Q., Zahed C., Nathan V., Hall D. A. and Jafari R. (2015). *2015 IEEE Biomedical Circuits and Systems Conference (BioCAS)*

Biological Sciences and Environmental Health – Gao (Ed.)

Application of electrochemical ELISA in cancer detection

Yilei Zhao
West China School of Basic Medical Sciences & Forensic Medicine, Sichuan University, Chengdu, Sichuan, China

ABSTRACT: Currently, public health is a widespread concern in society, with over half of the global cancer mortality rate. However, there are currently few efficient approaches to improve the poor prevalence of cancer early diagnosis. The current mainstream detection method is enzyme-linked immunosorbent assay (ELISA) based on antibody-antigen immune response. It mainly observes the changes in the solution after enzymatic reactions occur. But this judgment will be influenced by the turbidity of the solution and the interference of its color. Electrochemical ELISA avoids this situation, as it can generate electrically active substances through electrical detection methods with high sensitivity, ease of use, and effectiveness. It is often used to identify various tumor biomarkers, including alpha-fetoprotein (AFP), carcinoembryonic antigen (CEA), horseradish peroxidase (HRP), etc. In addition, it can also be used for the clinical detection of serum tumor markers, which is crucial for the early identification and treatment of cancer. Therefore, this article explores the mechanism of electrochemical ELISA and its application in biomarker detection by collecting relevant data and analyzing references related to cutting-edge ELISA technologies.

1 INTRODUCTION

Cancer has recently emerged as a major global public health concern that threatens people's physical well-being. Most cancer-related deaths result from the metastasis of the primary tumor. The detection of these diseases is of great significance in terms of early diagnosis and following clinical treatment to improve the patient's survival rate (Zhou *et al.* 2022).

For the identification of cancer biomarkers, a variety of techniques have been developed, including chemiluminescence, radioimmunoassay, and enzyme-linked immunosorbent assay (ELISA). Nowadays, electrochemical ELISA is gaining more and more attention and is applied in cancer detection, as it has higher sensitivity, higher specificity wider detection range, and better efficiency compared with conventional ELISA biosensors.

Focused on electrochemical biosensors and ELISA, this review summarizes and outlines some literature about electrochemical ELISA, and will illustrate the mechanism and application of this biosensor in the detection of cancer and tumor.

This review can provide us a better insight into the determination of cancer and the application of ELISA and has referential significance in the effective evaluation of the diagnosis and treatment procedures of the disease.

DOI: 10.1201/9781003587590-38

2 ELECTROCHEMICAL ELISA

2.1 *Basic mechanism of ELISA*

Many methods, including chemiluminescence, radioimmunoassay, and ELISA, have been developed to identify cancer biomarkers. ELISA is the most widely applied enzyme immunoassay technology used for the detection of antigens and antibodies.

The antigen-antibody-specific response serves as the foundation for ELISA. An antigen (or antibody) needs to be adhered to the solid phase carrier's surface before the test. The test sample and the enzyme-labeled antigen (or antibody) are intended to interact with the antigen (or antibody) on the solid carrier throughout the testing process. The surplus material is removed after the development of antigen-antibody complexes, and the substrate is then added. Then the substrate is catalyzed by the enzyme and produces colored substances. By detecting the qualitative or quantitative of the amount of the colored substances in the sample, the content of the material to be tested in the sample can be determined (Huang and Ning 2022).

Direct ELISA, indirect ELISA, sandwich ELISA, and competitive ELISA are the four fundamental ELISA experiment types. The electrochemical ELISA technique most frequently employed is the sandwich-type test (Díaz-Fernández and Ferapontova 2023).

In Figure 1, the four distinct ELISA types are compared. In a direct ELISA, the antigen is first immobilized on the ELISA plate and is afterward directly detected by an antibody that has been enzyme-labeled. In an indirect ELISA, the antigen is immobilized on the ELISA plate, a detection antibody is added, adhering to the antigen only when necessary, and then a secondary antibody is added that has been enzyme-tagged, detecting the antigen and enabling the color to be developed using the substrate. In a sandwich ELISA, the analyte or sample is introduced first, followed by the detection antibody, which is immobilized in the ELISA plate. In a competitive ELISA assay, antigens or antibodies in the sample compete to bind a specific amount of enzyme-labeled antibody or antigen. The quantity of antigen in the sample has an inverse relationship with the output signal.

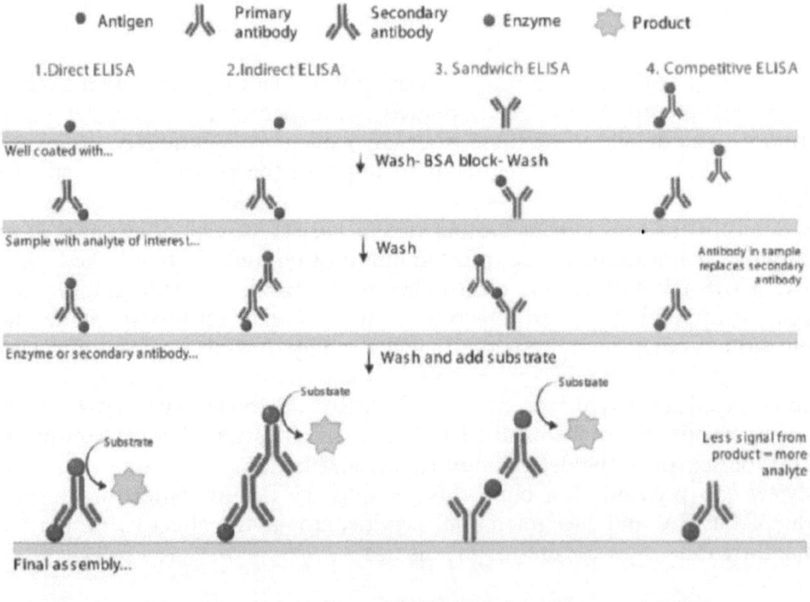

Figure 1. Lustration of four types of traditional ELISA (Ochoa-Ruiz *et al.* 2023).

2.2 *Electrochemical sandwich ELISA*

Electrochemical sandwich ELISA is recognized as one category of electrochemical immunosensors. The composition of the electrochemical sandwich ELISA mainly contains three parts (Arya and Estrela 2018). First, the surface of the sensor is coated with a recognition element, such as an antigen or antibody. The target analyte, which forms an antigen-antibody complex by preferentially binding to the recognition element, is the second layer. As a result of the binding processes, an electrochemical signal is created. The electrochemical signal tag is then bound by a secondary recognition molecule, and the signal is transduced and measured by the transducer. The concentration of the analyte can be determined by the signal's strength.

2.3 *Evolution and research progress*

Since the invention of ELISA in the 1960s, this detecting method has experienced rapid development and now become a frequently used immunoassay method in clinical diagnosis and scientific research.

Antibodies are the main recognition elements of conventional ELISA. In early research, mouse antibodies are widely applied. However, it is found in further studies that rabbit antibodies have better similarity to human antibodies, and goats can produce larger amounts of antibodies for experimental needs. So, antibodies from rabbits and goats have become comparatively new and more preferred recognition elements (Peng *et al.* 2022).

As for cancer detection, the concentration of tumor-related markers is below the detection range of ELISA (Xiong *et al.* 2012), so more sensitive electrochemical immunoassays based on ELISA are developed with signal amplification, and the possibility of automation (Arya and Estrela 2018).

3 APPLICATIONS IN CANCER DETECTION

Serum, urine, tissue, and other samples taken from tumor patients include biomarkers that can be used to identify tumors and cancers. Their existence indicates that there might be tumor cells in one's body, and their concentration is closely linked to the type, position, size, and malignancy degree of the tumor.

Electrochemical ELISA can be used for the detection of numerous biomarkers, such as Carbohydrate Antigen 125 (CA-125) related to ovarian cancer, CA-153 related to breast cancer, CA-199 related to gastrointestinal cancer, Human Chorionic Gonadotophin (HCG) related to trophoblastic tumor, and Vascular Endothelial Growth Factor (VEGF) which has predictive value about many other tumor and cancer (Jia *et al.* 2010).

3.1 *Detection of Alpha-Fetoprotein (AFP)*

The concentration of the glycoprotein alpha-fetoprotein (AFP) in adult serum is very low. The concentration of AFP, which is regarded as a significant tumor marker, can show if a patient develops a tumor or even cancer. Normal human blood AFP levels are typically modest, however, individuals with liver cancer may experience large increases in AFP levels (Laocharoensuk 2016).

For the detection of AFP, a sandwich-type electrochemical immunosensor was created (Figure 2). This sandwich immunosensor amplifies the signal and improves sensitivity by using multienzyme-antibody labeling on graphene sheets (Du *et al.* 2010). Primary AFP antibodies (Ab1) are attached to the electrode as a capture antibody, and HRP-labeled AFP (HRP-Ab2) is attached to CNSs as a detection antibody. AFP acts as the biomarker and is supposed to be captured between these two layers of antibodies.

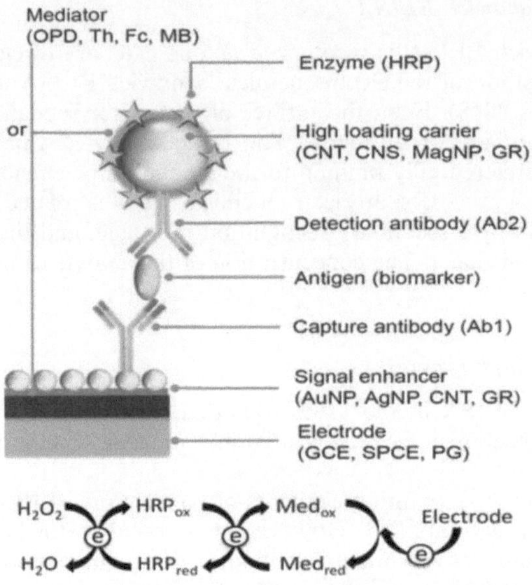

Figure 2. A sandwich-type electrochemical immunosensor for determination of AFP (Du *et al.* 2010).

Carboxylic acid–tethered polyaniline (PCOOH) is also applied in this kind of sandwich electrochemical biosensor for AFP detection. Compared with traditional Polyaniline (PANI), using PCOOH as an immobilization matrix provides a more intensive immobilization of biomolecules, higher reduction current, and faster charge transfer between electrode and PCOOH (Anbalagan and Sawant 2021). Higher amounts of antibodies are immobilized on the surface of the matrix as a result of the presence of several -COOH functional groups, which eventually improves the analytical performance of the biosensor (Anbalagan and Sawant 2021).

For the detection of alpha-fetoprotein (AFP), Wang *et al.* created a sensitive sandwich electrochemical immunosensor based on Co_3O_4 @ MnO_2-methionine and a screen printing technique. In the meanwhile, immunosensors were made using the pseudo-enzyme-linked immunosorbent assay. Differential pulse voltammetry (DPV), screen-printed carbon electrode (SPCE), and amino-functionalized Co_3O_4 @ MnO_2-Th are used as secondary markers, which can significantly enhance the electrochemical response signal and be useful for AFP detection. EIS (Electrochemical Impedance Spectroscopy) is used to verify if immunosensors were successfully manufactured. The immunosensor had a linear response to AFP, with a detection limit as low as 0.33 pg/mL and a range of 0.001 to 100 ng/mL. The immunosensor has remarkable repeatability and great stability (Wang *et al.* 2018).

To identify and track primary liver cancer, AFP has evolved into a particular clinical indicator. One of the crucial methods for diagnosing primary liver cancer is the detection of AFP levels.

3.2 *Detection of Carcinoembryonic Antigen (CEA)*

First discovered in fetal intestinal tissue and colon cancer, carcinoembryonic antigen (CEA) has minimal to no presence in healthy cells. Pancreatic cancer, gastric cancer, and medullary thyroid tumors are the three malignancies that typically have elevated levels of CEA, a non-specific tumor marker (Peng and Yu 2013), but most of the time the increasing CEA level is associated with colorectal cancer. In the clinical setting, quantitative analysis of CEA relies heavily on standard ELISA techniques, and recently electrochemical technology has also been combined with a common detection method (Laocharoensuk 2016).

An electrochemical immunosensor based on the principle of competitive immunoassay method was developed for CEA detection (Figure 3). Before the sample detection, standard CEA antigen is attached to the surface of nano- Fe_3O_4 modified carbon paste electrode (Fe_3O_4-CPE). The sample to be tested will be added to the solution with HRP-modified CEA antibody. After adding the solution to the electrode, the previous CEA antigen on the electrode and the CEA antigen in the sample will compete to bind with the antibody, and then the presence of the HRP-CEA antibody will be measured. This ELISA-based electrochemical immunosensor exhibits great selectivity, sensitivity, and reproducibility, making it a suitable and promising detection tool for CEA determination in clinical diagnosis (Tang and Xia 2008).

Except for the competitive type, sandwich-type electrochemical immunosensors are also widely applied. The sandwich-type immune complexes are formed by the primary antibody, HRP-labeled secondary antibody (Ab2) and the antigen to be detected between them (Tang and Xia 2008). Due to their superior biocompatibility and stable electrochemical capabilities, several conductive nanoparticles (NPs) have been employed to immobilize antibodies. The signal is amplified by these nanoparticles because they include significant amounts of HRP and CEA antibody that has been tagged with HRP. These characteristics, along with the multi-enzyme labeling strategy, increase the sensitivity of this technique to 100 times that of a standard ELISA, making the electrochemical sandwich ELISA suitable for detecting minute variations in the CEA concentration (Gan *et al.* 2011).

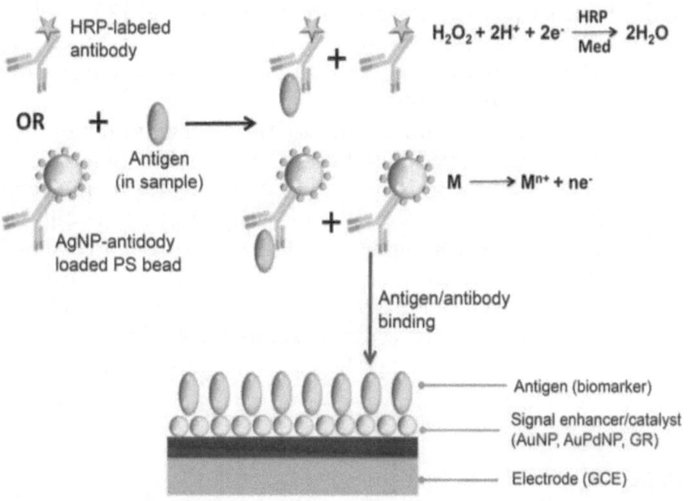

Figure 3. A competitive type electrochemical ELISA for determination of CEA (Tang and Xia 2008).

An unlabeled electrochemical immunosensor for detecting CEA in the human body was created by Jozghorbani *et al.* First, a platform for antibody binding is created on the partly reduced graphene oxide surface of the GC electrode. The electrode surface is coated with antibodies after the EDC/NHS junction activates the carboxyl group of rGO. Cyclic voltammetry and electrochemical impedance spectroscopy were used to examine the electrochemical behavior of electrodes treated with antibodies and the parameters of interactions between antibody and antigen immune complexes. According to research, the immune complex layer reduces the electrochemical current, a useful indicator for estimating the antigen concentration. With a detection limit of 0.05 ng/mL, the immunosensor has an excellent amperometric response to CEA in the concentration range of 0.1 to 5 ng/mL. The new approach was also tested for its ability to identify CEA in actual samples (human serum), and its outcomes were shown to be equivalent to the reference values acquired using ELISA (Jozghorbani *et al.* 2021).

3.3 *Detection of Horseradish peroxidase (HRP)*

One of the most popular labeling enzymes in the ELISA technique for cancer biomarkers is horseradish peroxidase (HRP), which is simple to extract, heat- and solvent-resistant, and seldom loses activity after interacting with antigen or antibody.

The potentiometric method for measuring catalase can also be applied to determine the activity of peroxidase. Immerse two platinum electrodes in a peroxide solution, and when a microcurrent of 2 microamps is input to the electrode, a stable starting voltage of 0.40 volts is presented. When peroxygenase is added, the voltage increases until it reaches the voltage generated by the release of oxygen from water. The slope (voltage difference/time difference) of this curve is proportional to the concentration of peroxygenase within the enzyme activity range of 0.01~1.0 units/milliliter. Due to the need for hydrogen donors to facilitate the catalytic function of peroxygenase, the selected donors, whether oxidized or reduced, are nonelectroactive compounds (such as pyrogallol) under the voltage used.

In an electrochemical ELISA, the main antibody first attaches to the antigen before being selectively bound by the secondary antibody that is HRP-conjugated. Hydrogen peroxide will then be used by HRP to oxidize substrates like hydroquinone (HQ), and the electroactive result will then provide an electrochemical signal that can be observed and measured. In the process, HQ will be oxidized to p-benzoquinone (BQ), and BQ will be turned back to HQ by the electrode, generating electrocatalytic signals (Díaz-Fernández and Ferapontova 2023). So, the use of HRP labels with HQ substrate can enhance the sensitivity of electrochemical ELISA for biomarker detection.

A second sensitive electrochemical immunoassay for assessing human tissue polypeptide antigen (TPA) has also been developed based on the HRP label. Since the visible signal of the direct antigen-antibody interaction is typically small, tagging biomolecules like HRP is frequently necessary for an electrochemical immunoassay to be successful. In this sandwich immunocomplex, HRP-anti-TPA conjugates are labeled using a Prussian blue-nanogold hybrid microsphere (AuPB), a label on an anti-TPA-functionalized electrode. The HRP may catalyze the reduction of hydrogen oxide and electrons may be effectively transferred from the electrode surface to the HRP's redox center (Li *et al.* 2014). The TPA concentration will subsequently be determined by measuring the cathodic current caused by the reduction process.

4 CONCLUSION

Compared with traditional tumor diagnosis tools, electrochemical ELISA has the advantages of high sensitivity, fast detection speed, low cost, wide detection range and convenient operation. Due to the use of electrochemical technology for testing, it has the advantage of providing faster response and field testing in undiluted or treated samples. On the other hand, electrochemical ELISA provides a powerful and rapid tool for sensitive and selective analysis of these biomarkers in human serum, which can specifically detect the low serum concentration required for clinical analysis. At the same time, it is also a good tool to detect a variety of biomarkers, and it is a new trend of tumor sensitive and specific detection. Therefore, this paper introduces the basic principle and development of ELISA, focusing on the application of electrochemical ELISA in tumor detection, aiming to achieve early diagnosis and effective treatment of tumors.

However, the electrochemical ELISA sensor still needs further improvement in the stability, service life and renewal difficulties of the sensitive membrane to meet the needs of practical analysis. In order to improve the storage life and stability of the system, more detailed studies are needed to understand the properties of biomolecules on flat substrates and nanomaterials. In order to better block the surface to prevent nonspecific binding, while maintaining the conductivity of the sensor surface to obtain higher electrochemical signal and better sensitivity, people need to conduct in-depth research. In addition, newer and better packaging methods need to be developed to store all the chemicals and reagents required in the multi-step ELISA processor, thereby automating the analysis and reducing human errors. With the development of science and technology, these problems will be solved, and the performance of electrochemical ELISA will be better optimized. These will also be widely used in clinical practice.

REFERENCES

Anbalagan A.C., Sawant S.N., (2021). *Microchim Acta* 188, 403.

Arya S.K. and Estrela P., (2018). *Sensors*, 18, 2010

Díaz-Fernández A. and Ferapontova E.E., (2023). *Anal Bioanal Chem* **415**, 3831.

Du D., Zou Z., Shin Y., Wang J., Wu H., Mark H., Liu J., Aksay A.I. and Lin Y., (2010). *Analytical Chemistry* 82, 7

Gan N., Jia L. and Zheng L., (2011). *International Journal of Molecular Sciences* **12**, 7410

Huang Y. and Ning L., (2022). *Today's Animal Husbandry and Veterinary Medicine* **38**, 5

Jia L., Zheng L., Wang Q. and Gan N., (2010). *International Journal of Laboratory Medicine* 31, **11**

Jozghorbani M., Fathi M., Kazemi S.H. and Alinejadian N., (2021). *Analytical Biochemistry* **613**

Laocharoensuk R., (2016). *Electroanalysis* **28**, 1716

Li Q., Loua F. and Tang D., (2014). *Anal. Methods* **6**, 3442

Ochoa-Ruiz A.G., Parra G., López-Espinoza D., Astudillo P., Galyamin D.N., Esquivel J.P. and Vallejo-Cardona A.A., (2023). *Electroanalysis* **35**, e202200053

Peng P., Liu C., Li Z., Xue Z., Mao P., Hu J., Xu F., Yao C. and You M., (2022). *TrAC* **152**, 116605

Peng W. and Yu G., (2013). *Chinese and Foreign Medicine Research* **11**, 21

Tang D. and Xia B., (2008). *Microchim Acta* **163**, 41.

Wang Y., Zhao G., Wang H., Cao W., Du B. and Wei Q., (2018). *Technology and Applications of Biosensors and Related Devices*

Xiong P., Gan N., Cao Y., Hu F., Li T. and Zheng L., (2012). *Materials* **5**, 12

Zhou C., Zhang K. and Li L., (2022). *Chemistry Bulletin* **85**, 1

Biological Sciences and Environmental Health – Gao (Ed.)

Applications of microfluidics in cancer prediction and detection

Dongrui Lv
School of Material Science and Engineering, Wuhan University of Technology, Wuhan, Hubei, China

ABSTRACT: Cancer detection and prediction are crucial for cancer diagnosis, development, and even treatment. Because of its great advantages of miniaturization, high throughput, and low sample dosage, microfluidics is very promising and developing rapidly in biomedical applications. At present, organ-on-chips built on microfluidic chips can be used to establish more realistic cancer models, which can largely reflect the physiological and pathological status of cancer. This provides an important reference for cancer diagnosis and drug development. Based on the microfluidic chip, a platform for isolating circulating tumor cells can be designed, and other biological detection technologies can be further used to detect circulating tumor cells. Efficient and effective isolation and detection of circulating tumor cells positively affect accurate and rapid early cancer diagnosis in individual patients. Based on this, this article introduces two typical methods for cancer prediction and detection using microfluidic technology, and then summarizes the application of microfluidic chips in different cancer cells, aiming to provide certain reference significance for the development of cancer prediction and detection in the future.

1 INTRODUCTION

Cancer is currently the world's most serious disease, it is one of the most important causes of death around the world, and it causes a huge economic burden of trillions of yuan worldwide (Bargahi *et al.* 2022). Therefore, fighting cancer is a goal of many biological and medical scientists, and the prediction, diagnosis, and monitoring of cancer are also crucial for the treatment of cancer (Xie *et al.* 2023). Today, methods like magnetic resonance imaging, positron emission tomography, and so on have been applied in the diagnosis and staging of cancer, radiotherapy, chemotherapy, and surgical removal are classic methods of treating cancer, but these methods expose patients to high doses of radiation and chemotherapy, and cancer has the potential to recur and the process is long and painful, with a significant negative effect on the patient's health, wealth and quality of life (Guo *et al.* 2021). Many patients are diagnosed with cancer only in the late stages, at which point only painful treatment and impending death await them. Therefore, in vitro, cancer prediction and diagnosis methods are required, which are sensitive and accurate enough to detect cancer at an early stage, and the demand for miniaturization and personalization is also growing. At present, some methods based on microfluidic technology can meet some of the above needs, so the application of microfluidics in cancer detection is very promising.

Microfluidic technology is the technique of precisely manipulating small amounts of fluids in microtubes (Zhou *et al.* 2022). Microfluidic chips are made of microtubes on a certain material to accurately control trace fluids, which can miniature biology, chemistry, and other laboratories into a few square centimeters of chips, so it is also called a lab-on-a-chip (Cheng *et al.* 2018). Since the establishment of microfluidic methods, the understanding of microfluidic flow behavior and methods to control them at the micrometer scale have

 DOI: 10.1201/9781003587590-39

evolved rapidly, and these advances have enabled the successful application of microfluidic technology in fields such as biological sciences, healthcare, and materials science (Battat *et al.* 2022). Microfluidic technology already provides developing countries with inexpensive and reliable basic diagnoses, such as pregnancy tests, sexually transmitted disease tests, and blood glucose real-time monitoring, which are portable, cheap, practical, concise, and can be utilized on a large scale (Battat *et al.* 2022). Linas M. *et al.* developed the in-drop method based on microfluidics for single-cell sequencing, which sets barcodes for individual cells before sequencing (Zilionis *et al.* 2017). Microfluidics has also promoted the discovery and verification of therapeutic methods, which can be used to screen therapeutic antibodies, and can also be made into organ-on-chips to verify drug toxicity and effectiveness, and cancer models are also designed for this purpose (Battat *et al.* 2022; Guo *et al.* 2021). Microfluidics has also been developed as a device to detect foodborne pathogenic bacteria and can also be used as food labels, promoting food safety. Microfluidics can also be used to build platforms for fine material production and chemical synthesis (Battat *et al.* 2022).

This article reviews two typical methods for cancer prediction and detection that can be built on microfluidic technology: establishing a cancer model on a microfluidic chip and isolating and detecting a cancer marker–circulating tumor cells (CTCs). Firstly, the shortcomings of animal models and traditional liquid biopsy are briefly introduced. Then the advantages and achievements of establishing cancer models on microfluidic chips and the separation and detection of CTCs using microfluidic technology are introduced, some applications of microfluidic chips in different cancer cells are explained, and finally, the advantages and disadvantages of microfluidic technology in cancer detection and the future development direction are summarized.

In this paper, it can provide a certain reference for the development of cancer prediction and detection in the future. Fast, convenient, and non-invasive means will provide important support for cancer diagnosis and personalized treatment and are of extraordinary significance for in-depth research on cancer.

2 ESTABLISHMENT OF CANCER MODELS

Preclinical cancer models can help medical scientists explore key molecular and cellular mechanisms of cancer (Guo *et al.* 2021). Traditional planar cancer cell culture cancer models, while convenient, do not reflect the complex tumor environment (Guo *et al.* 2021; Jihoon *et al.* 2019). Animal models are widely used in clinical experiments, but after all, animals cannot fully reflect the human environment, cannot accurately predict the reflection of cancer and drug effects, and the establishment of animal models is time-consuming and costly, requiring strict screening and culture (Guo *et al.* 2021). Therefore, the great potential of growing cancer cells on organ-on-a-chips to build 3D cancer models is gradually attracting attention.

Microfluidic technology enables cancer cells to simulate the cancer environment together with a variety of tissue cells and can achieve automated culture (Jihoon *et al.* 2019). After a period of development, many studies have fabricated and verified organ-on-a-chip cancer models. These models enable researchers to reproduce the multicellular architecture, tissue and tissue interface, and physical and biochemistry microenvironment of cancer growth within some physiological systems of the living human body (Alexandra *et al.* 2019). The materials used to make microfluidic devices are mostly oligomers such as Polydimethylsiloxane (PDMS) and polystyrene (PS) (Jihoon *et al.* 2019). These materials are generally manufactured into microfluidic chips by microprocessing such as mold injection, photolithography, and micro-engraving. Although these methods have high precision, most of them are complex and expensive (Alexandra *et al.* 2019; Jihoon *et al.* 2019). 3D printing has become an important method for cancer modeling on organ chips in recent years because of its streamlined operation and relatively low cost (Jihoon *et al.* 2019). Donald E. Ingber *et al.* developed a plastic array 3D spheroid culture platform using polystyrene as a raw material using an injection molding process and demonstrated the establishment of a tumor spheroid model. This platform provides robust and reproducible preclinical predictions and associated drug studies relevant to vascularized cancer research (Alexandra *et al.* 2019). Roger D. Kamm et al established a 3D model of vascularization in the microenvironment of human peritoneal and metastatic ovarian cancer on a microfluidic chip based on PDMS (Figure 1) (Lina *et al.* 2022). This model can be used to study the influence of some stromal cells and blood vessels on tumor cells to predict the behavior of this type of cancer.

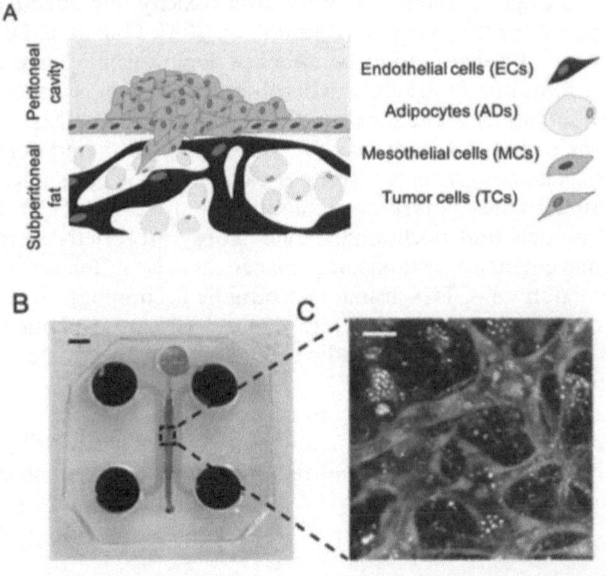

Figure 1. In vitro model of peritoneal microvascular networks: (a) Schematic illustration of the peritoneum, which is made up of an adipocyte-rich stroma, an overlaying mesothelial cell (MC) simple squamous membrane, and endothelial cell (EC) vessels. (b) Soft lithography was used to create a PDMS mold with patterned channels that were then adhered to a glass coverslip. A fibrin hydrogel and cells were present in the center gel area (green). Cell culture media was poured into the bottom channel and reservoir (blue), side channels and reservoirs (purple), and top channel and reservoir (orange). (c) A picture captured by confocal microscopy of the device's microvascular networks. (Lina *et al.* 2022).

It can be seen that preclinical or metastatic models based on organ chips can largely reproduce the physiological and pathological state of a specific cancer (Jihoon *et al.* 2019). So microfluidic chips can play a more far-reaching work in the discovery and detection of biomarkers and the sieving of anticancer drugs (Alexandra *et al.* 2019; Jihoon *et al.* 2019; Lina *et al.* 2022).

3 MICROFLUIDIC SEPARATION AND DETECTION OF CTCS

At present, tissue biopsy has important reference significance in the early diagnosis of cancer, but it involves the use of invasive surgical tools to remove part of the tumor tissue, and the resected tissue may not fully reflect the tumor status due to spatial and temporal heterogeneity, and liquid biopsy as an alternative diagnostic method has big latent capacity in early detection of cancer, therapy instruct, and relapse monitoring. Liquid biopsy targets include: circulating tumor cells (CTCs) which is the focus of this paper, extracellular vesicles (EVs) which also have a wide range of applications, circulating tumor DNA (ctDNA) which is also a useful target, various characteristic proteins, and other metabolites. These targets are formed from the tumor site and can be obtained from body fluids near tumors (Xie *et al.* 2023).

In a liquid biopsy, CTC is important for tumor prognosis evaluation, It enters the blood from primary and metastatic lesions, carries important features of cancer progression and metastasis, can provide important information for cancer detection, characterization, and monitoring, and only needs to routinely measure biomarkers in a little specimen from cancer patients, which helps push personalized medicine (Bargahi *et al.* 2022; Guo *et al.* 2021). However, the detection of CTCs is challenging due to the scarcity of CTCs in blood, their diversity in size, their size, and their ability to be easily damaged during recognition (Guo *et al.* 2021).

Research on microfluidic systems for the detection of CTCs has yielded some results. Separating CTCs can use physical methods based on size and affinity, and biological methods that introduce specific identifying elements (such as antibodies and aptamers) into the specimen (Xie *et al.* 2023). Manifested on microfluidic chips, physical methods are manifested as designing membranes of different sizes, applying different forces, channel design, using viscoelasticity, etc., and biological methods are designing nanoparticles containing antibodies or aptamers in microtubules (Xie *et al.* 2023). Zhang *et al.* deplete the leukocyte and platelet in a deterministic transverse displacement (DLD) structure, and then further remove the remaining leukocytes by an immunomagnetic purification device, complete the isolation of CTCs, on a second chip CTCs will be recognized by Alexa Fluor 568 rabbit anti-cytokeratin 7 antibody, while a third chip collects CTCs for further single-cell detection later (Xu *et al.* 2020). Jin *et al.* designed a cascaded microfluidic chip. The chip can segregate CTCs, and it has the advantages of high throughput and low cost, and the purity of the separated CTC is very high (Figure 2) (Lu *et al.* 2023). The chip contains two successive structures, one of the structures is a spiral structure that is used to isolate CTCs from whole blood based on size, and the other is a junction of a single cell array that is utilized to trap CTCs. Then, based on the microfluidic array of captured CTCs, immunofluorescence staining is used to realize biochemical characterization of single-molecule heterogeneity analysis, and a cell imaging analysis system is used to realize single-cell functional heterogeneity analysis (Lu *et al.* 2023).

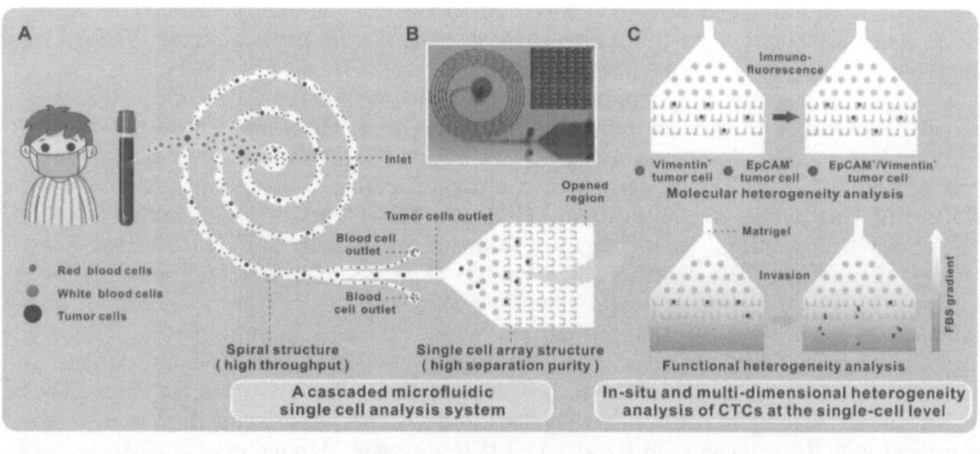

Figure 2. (A) Schematic diagram of the cascaded microfluidic chip. Helical structure and single-cell array are combined to isolate and capture CTCs. (B) Actual photo of the chip, filled with red ink to make it more clear to show the structure. (C) Schematic diagram of molecular heterogeneity analysis (Lu *et al.* 2023).

Various microfluidic technologies such as microfluidic peptide-based biosensors, microfluidic immune sensors, magnetic bead separation, nanostructure CTC capture design of microfluidic tubes have been tried for CTC separation, and biosensing techniques such as fluorescence colorimetry, chemiluminescence, electrochemistry, surface-enhanced Raman scattering (SERS) can be integrated on microfluidic chips, providing convenient and sensitive methods for CTC detection (Bargahi *et al.* 2022; Xie *et al.* 2023).

4 MICROFLUIDIC CHIPS FOR DIFFERENT CANCERS

There are many types of cancer, and microfluidics can be applied to different types of cancer through flexible design.

Breast cancer is a type of cancer in which microfluidic chips are more widely used. There are studies on co-culture tumor spheroids with human mammary ductal epithelial cells on microfluidic chips and breast fibroblasts to simulate the 3D organism structure and microenvironment of breast cancer, and various types of organ chips are designed to study the extravasation behavior and metastasis behavior of breast cancer in different organs (Alexandra *et al.* 2019; Guo *et al.* 2021). There are also combinations of size-based microfluidics with various biosensing methods to easily diagnose breast cancer through the detection of markers (Xie *et al.* 2023; Xu *et al.* 2020). Lung cancer, bowel cancer, liver cancer, ovarian cancer, gastric cancer, and other cancers have corresponding microfluidic models for studying their biological microenvironment and extravasation migration behavior, and researchers have also designed tumor microenvironment chips and human system chips to study a variety of different cancers with a certain behavior (Guo *et al.* 2021; Lina *et al.* 2022; Xu *et al.* 2020). Lung cancer, gastric cancer, colorectal cancer, and other commonly common malignant tumors can be diagnosed by the separation and detection of different CTCs, and the integration of detection into microfluidic chips can diagnose cancer at a relatively early stage (Bargahi *et al.* 2022; Xie *et al.* 2023; Xu *et al.* 2020). Some studies have also noted that glioblastoma, ovarian cancer, melanoma, and kidney cancer can also be diagnosed by microfluidic chips by detecting extracellular vesicles in the blood (Xie *et al.* 2023).

Hou *et al.* reported a microfluidic chip that is an acrylic acid-based multi-channel dual electric field (MDF) chip. The MDF chip offers eight combinations of electrical/chemical stimuli in a single test, considerably reducing the amount of time needed for the experiment while simultaneously increasing the precision of the findings. It was used to investigate how lung cancer cells responded to both chemical and electrical stimulation (Hou *et al.* 2015).

Carcinoembryonic antigen (CEA) and vascular endothelial growth factor (VEGF), two GC protein biomarkers, may be detected using a microfluidic device that Huang *et al.* created. The device has three sets of parallel channels, each with two response areas, allowing it to analyze several biomarkers in numerous samples at once. The 4-mercaptobenzoic acid (4-MBA) linked antibody functionalized gold nanosheets (GNS -) matrix may detect the presence of CEA and VEGF in the sample by causing a Raman frequency shift. As a result, the relationship between the concentrations of CEA and VEGF and the usual Raman frequency shift of 4-MBA is linear. According to the study's findings, the VEGF detection limit is 0.82 pg/mL and the CEA detection limit (LOD) of SERS microfluidic chips is as low as 0.38 pg/mL. The detection procedure requires only one step of sample addition, which eliminates non-specific adsorption brought on by several reactions and greatly enhances the simplicity and specificity of the detection. Additionally, blood samples from GC patients and healthy persons were analyzed. The results showed that SERS microfluidic chips may be used in the clinical setting for early diagnosis and GC prognosis, and they were in good agreement with the existing gold standard ELISA approach (Huang *et al.* 2023).

The presence of circulating tumor cells (CTC) in peripheral blood can be used to predict the prognosis and survival of cancer patients. Zhang *et al.* developed a microfluidic chip that includes a hexagonal array and a microtubule channel array, which can isolate and confirm individual circulating tumor cells. Through the analysis of clinical samples collected from 129 breast cancer patients and 50 healthy people, it was found that the chip could detect different immunophenotypes of circulating tumor cells in breast cancer patients, with high sensitivity (73.6%) and specificity (82.0%) (Zhang *et al.* 2021).

Nowadays, the vast majority of cancers that threaten human health can be diagnosed, monitored, and predicted by microfluidic technology, and the application of microfluidics in cancer continues to develop.

5 CONCLUSION

As a serious disease in the world, cancer is of great significance for its detection and prediction. At present, the diagnosis and treatment of cancer is very unfriendly to patients. Microfluidic chips have broad prospects in cancer detection and prediction due to their exceptional advantages such as high throughput, miniaturization, and designability. This paper introduces the advantages of establishing cancer models based on organ chips compared with traditional animal models, briefly describes the current status, some progress, and significance, introduces the advantages and development of using microfluidic technology to isolate and detect CTCs, and finally shows that microfluidics can be used for a variety of different cancers.

Although microfluidic technology has a very important positive impact on the diagnosis, treatment, and research of cancer, it still faces some problems and challenges. The biggest problem is that most microfluidic chips are only staying in the laboratory and have not been commercialized on a large scale, because microfluidic chips are still more complex in manufacturing and functionalization as a more sophisticated instrument, and their use currently requires the technical level of the operator. Microfluidic chips also lack usable standards. Many of the substrates of existing microfluidic chips are oligomers, which have a certain slow-release toxicity and may have an effect on sample cells.

In the future, microfluidic chips for cancer will gradually go out of the laboratory to benefit more cancer patients, which can realize the integration of production and research. Microfluidic chips should form a complete system with various other components, the structural functions of each part of the entire system, the connection of each part of the system, etc. should establish a unified standard, and at the same time can be connected to a cancer medical database that can be jointly built, providing a powerful and convenient means for cancer diagnosis and research.

REFERENCES

Alexandra S., Bryan A.H. and Donald E.I., (2019). *Nature Reviews Cancer* **19**, 2

Bargahi N., Ghasemali S., Jahandar-Lashaki S. and Nazari A., (2022). *Biological Procedures Online* **24**, 1

Battat S., David A.W. and George M.W., (2022). *Lab on a Chip* **22**, 3

Cheng Y., Chen Z. and Li J., (2018). *Applied Chemical Industry* **47**, 6

Guo Q., Zhang L., Liu J., Li Z., Li J., Zhou W., Wang H., Li J., Liu D., Yu X. and Zhang J., (2021). *Nanotheranostics* **5**, 1

Hou H.S., Chang H.F., Cheng J.Y., (2015). *J Vis Exp*

Huang Y., Liu Z., Qin X., Liu J., Yang Y. and Wei W., (2023). *Analyst* **148**

Jihoon K., Jungho A., Suryong K., Younggyun L., Jungseub L., Dohyun P. and Li J.N., (2019). *Lab on a Chip - Miniaturisation for Chemistry & Biology* **19**, 17

Lina I., Cynthia H., Giovanni S.O., Mark R.G. and Roger D.K., (2022). *Biomaterials* **288**

Lu Y., Yue S., Liang M., Wang T., Wang R., Chen Z. and Fang J., (2023). *Sensors and Actuators B: Chemical*

Xie Y., Xu X., Wang J., Lin J., Ren Y., Wu A., (2023). *Lab on a Chip* **23**, 13

Xu M., Zhao H., Chen J., Liu W., Li E., Wang Q. and Zhang L., (2020). *Cytometry* **97**

Zhang X., Lu X., Gao W., Wang Y., Jia C. and Cong H., (2021). *Translational Oncology* **14**, 1

Zhou Q., Guo M., Zheng Q. and Gao B., (2022). *Sci Sin Chim* **52**, 89

Zilionis R., Nainys J. and Veres A., (2017). *Nat Protoc* **12**, 44

Biological Sciences and Environmental Health – Gao (Ed.)
© 2025 the Author(s), ISBN: 978-1-032-96016-6

Orthotic treatment of adolescent idiopathic scoliosis

Ruixin Li
Clinical Medical College of Acupuncture Moxibustion and Rehabilitation, Guangzhou University of Chinese Medicine, Guangzhou, China

ABSTRACT: Nowadays, scoliosis, as a common disease, seriously jeopardizes the health of adolescents and children. Idiopathic scoliosis, which in turn accounts for 80% of scoliosis, is the most common type of scoliosis and is more common in adolescent girls. The physical characteristics of scoliosis are insidious and difficult to detect in the early stages of the disease, and by the time it is detected, it is often due to the development of significant symptoms. Therefore, it is necessary to study the pathogenesis of idiopathic scoliosis in adolescents and then apply effective treatments. Orthotic therapy is an important method of non-surgical treatment. It is an indispensable method and means of clinical treatment, as it promotes the healing of the lesion and achieves the purpose of preventing and correcting the deformity. This paper introduces the definition of adolescent scoliosis, pathogenesis, types of orthoses, role, treatment effect and other aspects of orthoses for adolescent idiopathic scoliosis.

1 INTRODUCTION

Adolescent idiopathic scoliosis (AIS) refers to scoliosis and rotational deformity of one or more segments of the spine in the absence of other organic diseases. AIS is the most common idiopathic spinal deformity, accounting for approximately 80% of all scolioses, and is most common in adolescents between 10 and 16 years of age (Negrini *et al.* 2018; Weinstein *et al.* 2008).

The spine is composed of 24 vertebrae, one sacrum and one coccyx, and is the central axis of the human body. The upper part of the spine supports the skull, and the lower part connects to the lower limbs. The intervertebral discs are connected to the cones, and they are tough and elastic, compressed when pressure is exerted and recovered when pressure is removed, which has a cushioning effect like an "elastic cushion" and allows the spine to move in all directions. The fibers of the anterior and posterior longitudinal ligaments and the intervertebral discs firmly connect the front and back of the vertebrae respectively, preventing the spine from over-extending or flexing forward. The intervertebral arches are connected by the ligamentum flavum, which restricts excessive forward flexion of the spine. The spinal canal, consisting of the foraminal connections of the vertebrae, holds and protects the spinal cord, nerves, blood vessels, and other tissues. When the position of the intervertebral disc changes, it may compress or damage the spinal cord, nerves or blood vessels, resulting in movement disorders (Bai and Li 2006). In the early stages of the disease, there may be no obvious symptoms, but as the disease progresses, symptoms such as low back pain and scoliosis deformity gradually appear, which in turn affects cardiac and pulmonary function, and ultimately leads to their failure. The cause of the disease is unclear. A Cobb's angle $>10°$ is diagnostic. So far, the treatment of AIS has been categorized into non-surgical and surgical treatments, and the International Scoliosis Research Society (SRS) recommends

 DOI: 10.1201/9781003587590-40

surgical treatment for severe scoliosis of 10°45° (Shi *et al.* 2023). This article is a review of the pathogenesis, diagnosis and evaluation of adolescent idiopathic scoliosis, types of orthoses and their therapeutic rationale, effects, advantages and disadvantages, and classic spinal orthoses.

2 DIAGNOSIS OF ADOLESCENT IDIOPATHIC SCOLIOSIS

Patients who are to be treated with orthoses first need to be examined and evaluated accordingly. Currently the commonly used clinical assessment methods are forward flexion test (Adams test) assessment and imaging assessment. Whole spine imaging, multislice CT (MSCT), and Mri are three widely used imaging methods.

2.1 *Total spine imaging*

Cobb measurement of the whole spine in the standing position is currently the gold standard for the diagnosis of scoliosis and is the most commonly used method for the diagnosis and evaluation of idiopathic scoliosis (Ng and Bettany-Saltikov 2017). Radiographs of the whole spine in the standing position were taken by a professional radiologist, and the orthopedic surgeon measured the scoliosis angle using the Cobb angle measurement method according to the results of the X-ray examination, and a Cobb angle of $\geq$ 10° was defined as positive, confirming the diagnosis of scoliosis (Spine Surgery Group of the Chinese Orthopaedic Association 2020).

2.2 *Multi-slice CT (MSCT) examination*

For atypical scoliosis, the spine, vertebral bodies, pedicles, spinal canal, and surrounding soft tissues need to be understood before surgery, which cannot be accurately detected and localized by X-ray, but MSCT reconstruction can accurately visualize the above mentioned structures, and detect abnormal changes that cannot be detected by X-ray. MSCT post-processing techniques include volume rendering imaging, surface shadow masking, multi-planar reconstruction, and curved surface reconstruction, through which cross-sectional, sagittal, and coronal impacts can be obtained, providing multidimensional observation for clinical diagnosis (Liu 2022).

2.3 *MRI examination*

Whole spine MRI has its own advantages in the detection of idiopathic scoliosis, such as no radiation, allowing the reconstruction of film information to be visualized and axial imaging to be accurately assessed (Liu 2022).

3 ORTHOTIC TREATMENT OF ADOLESCENT IDIOPATHIC SCOLIOSIS

3.1 *Orthotic treatment*

Orthotic device treatment is an important method of non-surgical treatment, which mainly plays the role of restricting spinal activities, so that the lesion joints are stabilized, local pain is reduced, vertebral body weight-bearing is reduced, and the healing of the lesion is promoted, so as to achieve the purpose of preventing and correcting deformity, and it is an indispensable method and means of clinical treatment (Zhao and Tian 2011)

3.2 *Four classic spinal orthoses*

3.2.1 *Boston brace*

Boston brace is the most widely used symmetrical thoracolumbosacral orthopedic brace in North America, which is required to be worn for more than 18h per day, and has a better effect on the correction of scoliosis vertebrae located in T8∼L2 (Karimi and Rabczuk 2019). At present, the Boston brace mainly adopts CAD/CAM technology, according to the patient's scanning data, the model material is processed and produced, and the pads in the brace are placed in the parietal vertebrae of scoliosis and underneath the lateral convexity, and the lateral window is opened to release the pressure, and the combination of CAD/CAM and finite element method in designing the brace can accurately correct the direction and position of force, and it has better effect on the correction of scoliosis (Gomez *et al.* 2016; Lu *et al.* 2020).

3.2.1 *Xenu orthosis*

The Xenu orthosis is an asymmetric brace for scoliosis with upper end vertebrae below T5 and Cobb angle of 25°∼45°, and the wearing time is 20∼23 h/d, which is the most widely used TLSO rigid brace in Europe (Rigo and Jelačić 2017). The three main types include the Rigo system Chêneau brace, the Chêneau light™ brace, and the Gensingen brace. The three modified Chêneau braces are based on the traditional Chêneau brace and follow the same principles, but each has its own characteristics. The Gensingen Brace Weiss (GBW), developed by Weiss in conjunction with a CAD/CAM system, is a further refinement of the chennu brace and is widely used in chennu braces because of its short fabrication time, ease of wear, and high level of comfort (Weiss 2010). The GBW is currently available in more than 35 different types of supports, ranging from athletic to pediatric torso models, and can be fine-tuned to fit a variety of patients. The Xenu brace has been shown to have good results in terms of Cobb's angle and the angle of rotation (AVR) of the parietal vertebrae (Lu *et al.* 2020).

3.2.3 *Milwaukee orthosis*

Milwaukee Scoliosis Orthosis: The Milwaukee Scoliosis Orthosis, consisting of an occipital brace, a laryngeal brace, a pelvic brace, anterior and posterior bars, and lateral pressure pads, is the earliest orthotic device used to correct scoliosis. It is characterized by longitudinal traction and lateral pressure when worn by the patient. It is mostly used for high level scoliosis (above T6), but the structure around the neck of this orthosis has greater limitations on the patient's daily life activities, and it is not aesthetically pleasing, which will bring psychological barriers to most adolescent female patients.

3.2.4 *Lyon scoliosis orthosis*

Lyon Scoliosis Orthosis: a combined orthosis, which consists of two pelvic fixation brackets and an underarm annular bracket connected by a metal bar in front and back, and the annular pressure pads in lumbar and thoracic vertebrae can be adjusted up and down according to the patient's needs. It can not only treat scoliosis, but can also be used as a fixed orthosis for postoperative immobilization of the thoracic and lumbar spine to support and stabilize the spine. Due to its adjustability and modifiability, it is extremely popular in Europe and the United States, and is suitable for thoracolumbar scoliosis deformity with a Cobb angle of 50° or less, and scoliosis of the middle and high thoracic segments, as well as immobilization of the thoracolumbar spine after surgery.

3.2.5 *33D-printed scoliosis orthoses 3D-printed orthoses are partial or partial orthoses*

3D printed orthoses are extracorporeal aids that are partially or fully fabricated by 3D printing technology and are used to modify the structure and function of the neuromuscular and skeletal systems.

Firstly, 3D scanning is used to take the mold instead of plaster bandage; after that, the software carries out computer-aided design, which is a great progress compared with the traditional production method, and 3D printing technology has a broad prospect in the field of scoliosis orthosis production. The 3D printed scoliosis orthosis is light in weight and beautiful in style, which has been widely used in clinic and achieved certain results.

3.2.6 *Effect evaluation*

After wearing the orthosis, it is not only to test it immediately, but also to follow up and test whether it is worn persistently and the effect of wearing. The evaluation of effect is based on the "Classification of scoliosis degree and rotation angle before and after using orthosis" as the evaluation standard, namely: Grade 0: Grade 0: Number of scoliosis $<10°$ and rotation angle < I degree; Grade I : Grade I: Scoliosis $10° \sim 20°$ and rotation I $\sim$ II degrees; Grade II: Number of degrees of lateral bending $21° \sim 35°$ and angle of rotation II $\sim$ III degrees; Grade III: Grade III: $36° \sim 45°$ of scoliosis and more than III degree of rotation. An improvement of more than 1 level is considered effective, a decrease in scoliosis without reaching 1 level is considered effective, and an increase in scoliosis is considered ineffective.

3.2.7 *The scoliosis orthosis must be worn continuously*

The continuity of wearing scoliosis orth osis is very important, which directly determines the effect of treatment.

The wearing time of the scoliosis orthosis can be gradually reduced as the condition improves, and the regression phenomenon caused by the withdrawal of the corrective force should be fully considered when the orthosis is completely removed. Usually, the orthosis should be worn until the age of maturity (5 degrees of the iliac spine Risser's sign on orthopantomogram), and the wearing time should be gradually reduced under the guidance of a professional rehabilitation doctor, and the orthosis should be taken X-ray regularly for review and observation of the changes of the scoliosis until the orthosis is completely taken off.

4 ADVANTAGES AND DISADVANTAGES OF ORTHOTIC TREATMENT AND OTHER TREATMENTS

Orthoses in scoliosis treatment can assist patients to maintain relatively correct position, reduce the weight of vertebral body, play a certain supportive role in stabilizing the disordered small joints, and play an important role in improving the trunk function of scoliosis patients. However, spinal stiffness and atrophy of paravertebral muscles easily caused by continuous wearing of orthoses (Lu 2012).

In addition to orthotic treatment, other non-surgical therapies are also widely used in the treatment of scoliosis, such as exercise therapy and electrical stimulation therapy.

5 CONCLUSION

Orthotic treatment is a very effective treatment for scoliosis, but the complications associated with orthotic treatment have been a barrier to its clinical application. The SOSORT guidelines suggest that orthotic treatment combined with scoliosis-specific exercise therapy is significantly more effective than a single treatment option, and that the specific exercise therapy can effectively avoid the complications associated with brace treatment, such as stiffness of the spine and loss of muscle strength, and can improve the efficacy of the orthotic treatment. It also improves orthotic efficacy. Orthotic treatment can also limit the growth of the patient's thorax, affecting the development of the heart and lungs in the thoracic cavity, which is contrary to the original purpose of the treatment and is also a defect of the orthosis.

At present, although the Xenu brace has the most advanced technology and design, it inevitably still has defects, and there are few studies and reports on this at home and abroad. The 3D printing technology can make the orthosis can solve part of the problem, but also lack of effective and unified product standards (Negrini *et al.* 2018). Now the scoliosis orthosis is generally worn for a long time, plus sports training time, the patient is almost 24 hours in the process of scoliosis treatment, coupled with the scoliosis orthosis in the appearance is not beautiful, the patient's mental health is very easy to be affected. Secondly, scoliosis braces are generally large in size and are not convenient to put on, and some patients even need the help of others to put them on. How to improve the appearance and size of scoliosis braces to make them more beautiful and compact while maintaining or even improving their therapeutic effects is a major focus of future practice research. In addition, combining the scoliosis orthosis with big data analysis, digital medicine, artificial intelligence and other advanced technologies to make the scoliosis orthosis have better therapeutic effect under the integrated use of multiple methods is also a future development direction for scoliosis treatment.

Adolescent idiopathic scoliosis mainly refers to the growth and development of adolescents in the period of scoliosis of unknown origin, when the condition is serious, it can affect the anatomical structure of the thorax, cardiopulmonary function to a certain extent, and there is also the possibility of spinal cord involvement, resulting in paraplegia. If it is not treated early and effectively, it will have a serious impact on the patient's quality of life, so orthotic treatment of scoliosis needs to be in the appropriate time period. The purpose of orthotic treatment is mainly to prevent further exacerbation of the curvature during the dangerous period of progression of the scoliosis curve until the patient becomes skeletally adult, with a view to minimizing the possibility of surgical treatment and reducing the trauma.

REFERENCES

Bai A. and Li S., (2006). *Journal of Nanjing Institute of Physical Education (Natural Science Edition)* **1**, 74.

Gomez J. A., Hresko M. T., and Glotzbecker M. P., (2016). *Journal of the American Academy of Orthopaedic Surgeons* **24**, 555.

Karimi M. T. and Rabczuk T., (2019). *The Journal of Spinal Cord Medicine* **43**, 824.

Li X., (2001). *Chinese Orthopaedic Surgery Miscellany* **8**, 184.

Liu M., (2022). *Journal of Molecular Imaging* **4**, 627.

Lu D., Wang C., Liu Z., Yang H., Wei H., Wang X., and Wang J., (2020). *Chinese Journal of Orthopaedics* **28**, 1215.

Lu Y., (2012). *Journal of Hebei Medical University* **33**, 566.

Negrini S., Donzelli S., Aulisa A. G., Czaprowski D., Schreiber S., de Mauroy J. C., Diers H., Grivas T. B., Knott P., Kotwicki T., Lebel A., Marti C., Maruyama T., O'Brien J., Price N., Parent E., Rigo M., Romano M., Stikeleather L., and Wynne J., (2018). *Scoliosis and Spinal Disorders* **13**.

Ng S.-Y. and Bettany-Saltikov J., (2017). *The Open Orthopaedics Journal* **11**, 1500.

Rigo M. and Jelačić M., (2017). *Scoliosis and Spinal Disorders* **12**.

Shi M., Ma Y., Ji W., and Wang X., (2023). *Orthopaedic Journal of China* **13**, 1189.

Spine Surgery Group of the Chinese Orthopaedic Association, *Chinese Journal of Orthopaedics* **23**, 1574 (2020).

Tao J., Hu J., and Zhao L., (2019). *Science and Technology Herald*, **37**, 87.

Weinstein S. L., Dolan L. A., Cheng J. C., Danielsson A., and Morcuende J. A., (2008). *The Lancet* **371**, 1527.

Weiss H.-R., (2010). *Scoliosis* **5**.

Zhang X. and Yang W., (2005). *China Clinical Rehabilitation* **9**, 118.

Zhao P. and Tian Q., (2011). *Medicine and Philosophy: Clinical Decision Forum Edition* **32**, 44.

Biological Sciences and Environmental Health – Gao (Ed.)

Fabric electrode materials for physiological signal monitoring

Qiqi Wang
School of Physics, Shandong University, Jinan, China

ABSTRACT: This paper introduces three distinct methods for integrating with textiles to monitor human physiological signals. These three methods can be applied in real-world scenarios, extending beyond laboratory or clinical environments, making them suitable for long-term use by both users and patients. Upon careful examination, it has been discovered that titanium metal holds significant potential for a wide range of applications in this context. By doping titanium with various metals and preparing it as dry electrodes, these methods offer the advantage of eliminating the need for ionic liquids or conductive gels, in contrast to traditional approaches. Alternatively, fabricating titanium into porous structures and combining it with silicon serves to prolong the lifespan of the electrodes, while also allowing for the removal of conductive gels, thereby expanding the range of applicable environments. Furthermore, the paper explores the use of different techniques for printing electrodes on textiles, achieving the objective of monitoring human physiological signals. To reduce impedance and enhance signal quality, methods such as uniformly applying ionic liquids or incorporating carbon nanotubes during fabrication are proposed. This paper provides an integrated overview of the preparation methods and parameter assessment techniques for these three materials.

1 INTRODUCTION

To record biological signals, electrodes for measuring bioelectric potentials are generally categorized into invasive electrodes, which penetrate the skin, and non-invasive electrodes, which do not breach the skin. The use of invasive electrodes necessitates skin penetration, rendering them unsuitable for prolonged continuous monitoring. Certainly, it is evident that invasive electrodes will induce wounds on the human body and may potentially trigger an inflammatory response (Lopes *et al.* 2021). Non-invasive electrodes are indeed conducive to long-term monitoring; however, they encounter numerous issues such as electrode corrosion leading to impedance escalation, integration with textiles, and alteration of physical and chemical properties due to stretching during washing, rendering them unusable (Fiedler 2014; Mihajlovic *et al.* 2015).

Electrodes can be divided into three types:

① Metal Electrodes: Metal electrodes are typically made of inert metals (such as silver/silver-chloride electrodes, platinum electrodes) and are used for measuring bioelectric signals, such as electroencephalograms (EEG), electrocardiograms, and electromyograms (EMG) (Chen *et al.* 2014).

② Conductive Gel Electrodes: Conductive gel electrodes have a layer of conductive gel applied to the electrode surface, aiming to enhance the quality of electrode-skin contact.

② Magneto-electrodes: Magneto-electrodes employ a magnetic field to measure biological signals, such as magnetoencephalograms (MEG). They do not directly contact the skin but instead measure the weak magnetic fields generated by the brain.

DOI: 10.1201/9781003587590-41

Clinical electrocardiogram monitoring is performed using wet electrodes with Ag/AgCl as the electrode material, with gel placed between skin and electrode. The principle behind this method involves measuring the electrochemical reactions at the electrode-electrolyte interface, primarily focusing on measuring resistive coupling outcomes. Additionally, the gel in wet electrodes moisturises the skin, reducing impedance (Geddes 1997). However, wet electrodes have significant drawbacks when measuring physiological signals from the human body, as they cannot be used outside of medical or laboratory settings.

Flexible textile dry electrodes have recently become a focal point of research. The aim is to transition the process of bio-monitoring to the use of non-invasive electrodes and even ensure comfort through integration with everyday clothing. Well-established electrode materials for monitoring electrocardiogram (ECG) include metals, intrinsically conductive polymers, and carbon-based materials.

In recent years, with the maturation of flexible printing or alloy thin-film technologies, physiological signal monitoring can exist outside laboratory or clinical settings.

2 TI-ME DOPED DRY ELECTRODES

2.1 *Dry electrodes*

Dry electrodes are a commonly used type of electrode in the measurement of biological signals. In contrast to traditional wet electrodes, dry electrodes do not require the use of conductive gel or liquid mediums, making them more convenient to use and maintain.

Dry electrodes typically exhibit higher impedance compared to wet electrodes, ranging from several kilohms to several megohms. In contrast, wet electrodes possess higher impedance, ranging from low kilohms to low megohms. According to existing research findings, combining metals with titanium to form alloys as monitoring electrodes for physiological signals can achieve results that are not inferior to traditional wet electrodes (Lopes *et al.* 2020).

2.1.1 *Advantage*

The advantages of dry electrodes include:

a) Convenience: They eliminate the need for conductive gel, reducing electrode preparation time and making installation and usage easier.
b) Comfort: Since they don't require contact with liquids, the risk of skin allergies is reduced.
c) Durability: Dry electrodes do not become ineffective due to the evaporation of conductive gel.
d) Portability: They are suitable for applications requiring movement or long-term monitoring, such as brain-computer interfaces and motion tracking.

2.1.2 *Conventional electrode materials*

The principle of dry electrodes involves using the surface material of the electrode to establish direct contact with the skin and acquire bioelectric signals. Dry electrodes employ specialized materials such as single metals, metal alloys, carbon nanotubes, polymers, and more.

In clinical and research applications, traditional typically employ silver chloride electrodes, often used with electrolyte gel. These allow them to function as reference electrodes, maintaining the necessary potential for the electrolytic process over time, while oxidation and reduction reactions occur at the anode and cathode, respectively. Non-polarizable electrodes generally exhibit low skin contact impedance that remains nearly frequency-independent, yielding more sensitive measurement results. As a result, they are often used in EMG, EEG, and ECG.

Dry electrodes typically exhibit higher contact impedance compared to traditional gel-based wet electrodes. However, with the use of electronic devices, dry electrodes can achieve signal-to-noise ratios comparable to gel electrodes, thereby ensuring similar performance level (Huigen *et al.* 2002).

2.2 *Reducing impedance*

Titanium is a biocompatible metal commonly utilized for biomedical implants, renowned for its low susceptibility to corrosion (Lopes *et al.* 2014). Furthermore, due to its high non-magnetic properties and minimal susceptibility to magnetic field interference, titanium continues to find widespread adoption, despite potential limitations, to mitigate potential harm associated with nuclear magnetic resonance imaging scans.

Using flexible and high modulus base materials can enhance electrode adaptability to body contours, improve comfort, and reduce the risk of skin contact allergies. However, balancing material elasticity and low impedance can currently be achieved through a method known as coating.

Coatings consist of conductive components, and can also be doped with conductive elements. Doped materials primarily include graphite, elastic substances with silver, or doped carbon nanotubes and nanofibers.

Commonly used materials for coating elasticity are Ag, Ag/AgCl, gold (Au), and titanium (Ti).

In order to efficiently incorporate dopants into electrode substrates flexibly and effectively, thin film technology based on flexible polymer substrates can be employed. Flexible polymer films provide a highly conductive pathway for biological signals while simultaneously preserving the polymer's elastic modulus and enhancing the film's surface mechanical elasticity.

Titanium is a material commonly employed in the field of medicine, and titanium-based alloys are increasingly used in various medical fields due to their excellent physical properties. Through multi-parameter investigation and comparison of titanium-based coatings, flexible polyurethane substrates are functionalized using different Ti-Me binary metal-intercalated films, incorporating metals. During this process, the addition of the metal "Me" into the titanium base forms intermetallic compounds, thus enhancing the well-known properties of titanium (Lopes *et al.* 2020).

2.3 *Electrochemical parameter assessment*

Rutherford Backscattering Spectroscopy was utilized to conduct a quantitative chemical composition analysis of Ti-Me films, followed by determining the crystal structure and phase distribution of titanium-metals (Ti-Me) films using X-ray diffractometry. These analyses facilitated the electrochemical parameter evaluation of Ti-Me dry electrodes.

2.4 *Analysis of the reasons for impedance reduction by Titanium*

When conducting electrical stimulation using neural electrodes, delivering a specific charge density of current is essential. For numerous microelectrode arrays, the contact area between actual neurons and electrodes is exceedingly small, leading to higher current density during transmission. When electrode current density is substantial, the overpotential exhibits a linear relationship with the logarithm of the current density, which can be represented using the Tafel equation:

$$\eta = a + b \cdot lg\ I \tag{1}$$

(The symbol η denotes the electrode's polarization potential, while I represents the polarization current density. The parameters 'a' and 'b' are associated with the material properties of the electrode, surface structure, and the effective electrode surface area.)

For implantable neural electrodes used in electrical stimulation, charge transfer efficiency diminishes over time due to the body's immune response. This necessitates higher charge injection densities to ensure sufficient stimulation of target neurons. However, excessive charge density may exacerbate electrode corrosion, especially when the electrode is corroded and its surface area reduced. Balancing current intensity with potential harm to the human body has been a persistent research challenge.

3 TEXTILE PRINTED ELECTRODES

3.1 *Review of existing research*

Mature textile electrodes are generally fashioned from 3D protruding carbon-based structures, each possessing a circular configuration with a diameter of 2 centimeters. Significant differences exist between flat electrodes made of carbon and 3D textile electrodes with protrusions. In experiments, printing coatings onto their surfaces containing carbon-conductive coating materials demonstrated excellent printing adaptability on the flat structure, regardless of the presence of ionic liquids. Furthermore, after printing, no significant cracks were observed in the coatings.

However, it should be noted that in experiments, conductive coating materials containing a high concentration of ionic liquid (7.5%) exhibited cracking when screen-printed onto carbon-containing flat textile substrates. Printing on prominent 3D textile substrates resulted in outright printing failures.

Rienzo *et al.* developed a vest with sensors. These textile sensors consist of two conductive fibers electrodes, positioned around the chest area for the purpose of monitoring cardiac arrhythmia events in patients (Rienzo *et al.* 2005). The novelty of this garment lies in utilizing the elasticity of the fabric to ensure contact between the electrodes and the body's skin, as opposed to using gel. Upon testing, the system demonstrated signal quality equivalent to that of traditional ECG devices.

Wattal *et al.* designed a T-shirt to motivate ECG and conducted testing on it (Wattal *et al.* 2018). The T-shirt was fabricated using a pyrrole polymerization process and featured two electrodes and connectors made of conductive Velcro. During manufacturing, the nylon hook-and-loop fasteners on it were rendered conductive, and elasticity was employed to ensure continuous contact between the fabric and the skin, enabling uninterrupted monitoring.

Conductive coating materials comprising PEDOT:PSS+PDMS (with or without CNTs) or containing appropriate concentrations of ionic liquids (for example, $\leq 5\%$) only exhibit printability on planar silver yarn textile substrates, without encountering mechanical cracking.

Furthermore, planar textile electrodes composed of silver yarn with carbon coatings present significantly higher impedance compared to planar textile electrodes with PEDOT: PSS coatings, reflecting results akin to prior research findings.

Ankhili *et al.* employed various PEDOT:PSS solutions to fabricate PEDOT:PSS-coated polyamide fabric electrodes (Ankhili 2019). Through experimentation, the quality of signal was assessed after 50 washing cycles. The findings indicate that, for the purpose of physiological signal monitoring, although there was a slight decline in signal quality, it still remained at an excellent level.

3.2 *Reducing impedance on textile printed electrodes*

Altering the conductivity of coating materials can reduce electrode impedance. Electrodes coated with PEDOT:PSS exhibit significantly higher impedance compared to dry textile electrodes coated with carbon-based materials. The addition of carbon nanotubes or ionic

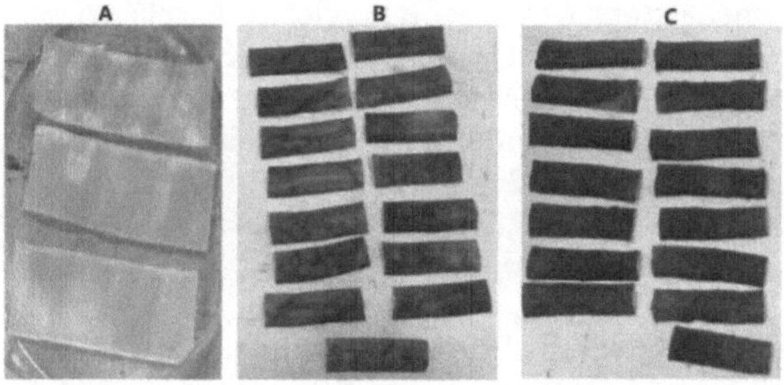

Figure 1. (A) Polyamide textile fabrics before immersion coating; (B) Polyamide textile electrodes coated by PEDOT:PSS (S1); (C) Polyamide textile electrodes coated by PEDOT:PSS (Ankhili 2019).

liquids can further reduce the impedance of PEDOT:PSS electrodes. Finally, the enhancement induced by CNTs may derive from suppressing the phase separation of PEDOT:PSS.

3.3 *Ensuring signal quality*

Because of the lack of adhesives on dry textile electrodes, it is necessary to exert the correct amount of pressure and enhance the quality of bioelectrical signals to ensure proper skin-electrode contact. During the evaluation of impedance in dry textile electrodes coated with different conductive materials, it was noted that silver yarn-based planar textile electrodes remained free from cracks. Pressure levels of 10 mmHg, 20 mmHg, and 30 mmHg were chosen, as they fall within the optimal pressure range for electrode compression applications. Researchers noted that the impedance of dry textile electrodes with different conductive coatings exhibited minimal sensitivity to pressure.

3.4 *Influence of other factors*

Current gel electrode research has shown that as the temperature decreases, both the resistive and capacitive aspects of the skin-electrode interface rised. Dry textile electrodes with a carbon-coated FS structure exhibit high impedance ($\sim$3000 Ω) and poor long-term stability (a $\sim$75% increase in impedance within 30 days).

Other properties of dry textile electrodes, for example, breathability, motion-induced artifacts, prolonged contact-induced skin irritation, warrant investigation. Furthermore, their actual performance under conditions of perspiration and stretching necessitates testing. Textile stretching and washing cycles, among other variables, also affect the performance of dry electrodes. Testing should encompass varying stretching, wear periods, and laundering frequencies across diverse applications (e.g., electrocardiography, electromyography, electroencephalography monitoring) and various textile shapes and uses (sleeves, vests, headbands, etc.). Presently, no comprehensive testing results have been researched or published

To ascertain optimal performance formulations for dry electrodes and suitable textile-material combinations, it is imperative to subject finished products to cycles of wear and tear using a range of laundering agents and methodologies, thus facilitating cyclic performance investigations.

4 PLICATION OF POROUS PLATINUM ELECTRODES IN IN-EAR MONITORING

To monitor human conditions, measurements can be taken using EEG or electromyography of muscle activity (Fiedler *et al.* 2017). Specifically, non-invasive methods like EEG can support insights into individuals' neural and physiological states (Grummett *et al.* 2015).

The EEG measurement approach involves electrode placement and preprocessing, requiring the attachment of numerous electrodes to the scalp. Such measurements must also be conducted in a clinical setting. Consequently, these measurements cannot be sustained over extended periods, necessitating alternative approaches for continuouly monitoring human physiological states (He *et al.* 2013).

4.1 *Principle*

Recent years have witnessed research efforts to measure auditory brain activity through ear-electroencephalography (ear-EEG) to overcome this limitation. Stefan Debener and colleagues conducted a study of monitoring EEG parameters using flexible printed electrodes applied onto thin films, combined with integration into smartphones. This device is worn on the ear and holds the potential for long-term monitoring in non-laboratory environments (Debener *et al.* 2015).

In addition, multiple electrodes are distributed on earplugs, which transmit cortical electrical signals through the ear canal and auricle. Porous silver chloride is frequently employed as an electrode material in such studies (Christensen *et al.* 2018). However, this material degrades over time and necessitates the use of conductive gel for measurements. Due to these drawbacks, porous silver chloride is unsuitable for long-term measurements (Greulich *et al.* 2009).

In Max Eickenscheidt's research, a comparison of the electrochemical properties of different materials was conducted, leading to the proposition of a platinum (Pt)-based electrode. This electrode significantly increases the active surface area while minimizing impedance in relevant frequency domains. Corrosion-resistant and biocompatible metals, such as gold, titanium, or platinum, are preferred choices for electrode surfaces. Platinum, due to its low ductility and absence of a native oxide layer like titanium, is generally regarded as the superior material. This research employed a galvanic co-deposition of Pt and copper (Cu), iteratively depositing both metals to create a highly porous Pt surface, releasing Cu after each cycle. The lower oxidation-reduction potential of copper compared to noble metals and its position above the hydrogen potential allows for controlled surface structuring of varying heights. The final product's electrode structure was tailored to techniques using laser cutting techniques to accommodate human physiological features.

4.2 *Fabrication techniques*

First, a 70 μm layer of silicone gel is spin-coated onto a flat substrate. Next, a pre-cured organic silicone layer will be laminated onto the gel layer, with a thickness of 25 μm, using metal foils of different materials (silver, platinum, MP35N chosen as controls in the experiment). Subsequently, laser cutting will be employed to obtain the predetermined dimensions of the electrodes. The organic silicone layer will cure and adhere to the metal structures during this process. The conductor traces are configured in a serpentine pattern to preserve the system's high flexibility (Figure 1A). A top coating of 10 μm poly (Figure 1B) was applied using a chemical vapor deposition system (Figure 1C). The active electrode sites on one end were exposed using prototype laser processing, while the other end was connected with a connector and isolated from the circuitry. Finally, the probes were released by laser cutting the outlines.

Once fabrication is complete, the electrode array is assembled with the connectors. Enamel-coated copper wires are spiral-welded onto the solder pads, and individual wires are soldered onto the header pins to establish separate connections for each electrode. Subsequently, residual substances or dust particles on the surface are removed using ethanol and deionized water. An electrochemical cleaning of the electrodes is performed by running 15 cycles within the range of -600 mV to +900 mV in a phosphate-buffered saline solution at a rate of 250 mV/s. The finalized electrodes are affixed onto acrylic resin molds created from

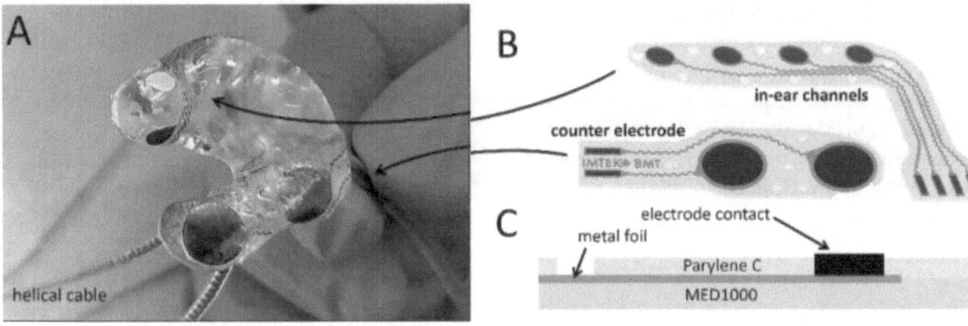

Figure 2. Image of the fully assembled Ear-EEG electrode with four electrodes in the ear (Eickenscheidt *et al.* 2020).

ear impressions of the test subjects. The electrodes are placed at the outer edge of the earpiece to enable measurements to penetrate as deeply into the ear canal as possible (Eickenscheidt *et al.* 2020).

4.3 *Electrodeposition*

Electrodeposition was carried out with the electrolyte placed within a nitrogen environment. Initially, nitrogen gas was bubbled through the solution remaining over 1200 seconds, followed by nitrogen purging across the electrolyte surface. The deposition was accomplished by utilizing a voltage of -500 mV versus SCE to the electrode on working for a duration of 9 seconds, after the solution had reached nitrogen saturation levels. The principle involved simultaneous deposition of Cu and Pt from the electrolyte. Experimental findings demonstrated that repeating this process 50 times facilitated the formation of Pt layers with thicknesses ranging from 5 to 20 μm.

Following deposition, copper was selectively dissolved for 4.5 seconds with a voltage of +700 mV vs. SCE, and repeated 50 times. To eliminate bubbles, continuous movement of a magnetic stirring bar was employed.

A direct current of 1 mA/cm2 of electrode surface area was applied for 15 seconds, utilizing a single Ag/AgCl reference electrode in a 3 moL potassium chloride solution to chloridize the silver electrode.

4.4 *Electrochemical electrode characterization*

Experiments conducted by Max Eickenscheidt *et al.* indicate that the access resistance is independent of electrode material or surface roughness and is solely related to the material's volume (Figures 2A, B). Using Solartron setup, a significant decrease in low-frequency impedance was observed on the surface after platinum-copper deposition, exhibiting purely resistive behavior above 1 Hz (Figures 2A). Comparable occurrences were noted in the chloride process of silver foils, albeit with a less marked decrease in impedance compared to the notable surface expansion observed in platinum.

Expanding the electrode surface area makes it possible to accurately record the bioelectric potentials associated with skin contact. In the experiments conducted by Max Eickenscheidt, two pairs of in-ear electrodes were fabricated for subjects to measure EEG signals. These electrodes were constructed using platinum-copper alloy and the conventional method employing silver chloride foil as materials.

The experimental findings revealed distinct differences in electrode performance. The power increase observed in that of the silver chloride electrodes from traditional method was

2.4±1.8μV^2, whereas the porous platinum electrodes exhibited a power increase of 4.5±3.7μV^2. This divergence underscores the contrasting capabilities of these electrodes. However, the power density of the silver electrodes exceeded that of the porous platinum electrodes by an order of magnitude as expected. Conversely, the platinum electrodes exhibited significantly lower signal variance.

The reference material MP35N, chosen for its biocompatibility, observed that there is a quicker rise in complex impedance compared to the smooth platinum foil., serving as a controlled benchmark.

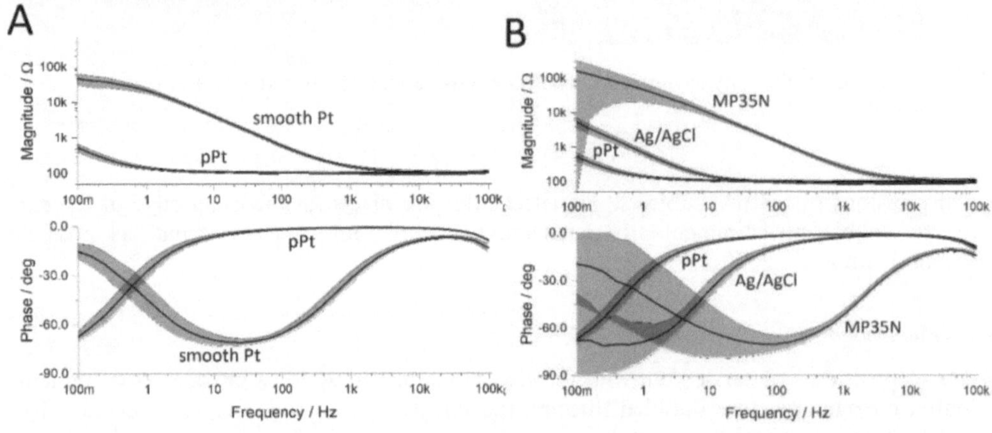

Figure 3. Electrochemical impedance measurement of different electrode materials (Eickenscheidt *et al.* 2020).

5 CONCLUSION

This paper examines three methods for wearable monitoring of human physiological signals. These methods involve incorporating metals into electrode materials during the manufacturing of dry electrodes, using carbon nanomaterials in the textile manufacturing process, and applying porous platinum electrodes in in-ear physiological monitoring.

5.1 *Ti-Me doped dry electrodes*

By incorporating Ti-Me metal films, it is possible to effectively decrease the electrode-skin contact surface's resistive impedance over prolonged monitoring periods. Experimental measurements demonstrate that Ti and Me content variations within the films are inversely proportional to the exposed surface area of Me on the target material. Concurrently, the sputtering of metal Me onto the films influences their chemical properties. Each Ti-Me system exhibits distinct structural characteristics, dependent on the composition of the Me dopant and its concentration within the film.

Three main structural zones have been identified as universally present in all prepared Ti-Me systems: (1) Ti-rich zone, representing films primarily composed of Ti; (2) intermetallic region, becoming prominent in films with pronounced Ti-Me intermetallic phase deposition; (3) Me-rich region, where the metal Me becomes the predominant contributor to the film's composition.

The results suggest that Ti-Me thin films can function as reliable bioelectric electrodes, exhibiting consistent and low impedance between the electrode and the skin and enduring and stable long-term contact.

5.2 *Textile printed electrodes*

Integrating electrodes with textiles for long-term monitoring presents more challenges than conventional electrode placement. Firstly, textiles are subjected to the effects of washing and stretching. Secondly, textiles cannot maintain constant contact pressure with the skin over extended periods, which can affect measurement outcomes. Lastly, physiological signals from the human body often fluctuate, and factors such as sweat and other contaminants can influence the measurement environment.

Experimental evidence has shown that using a conductive coating material composed of PEDOT: PSS+PDMS in conjunction with carbon nanotubes to embed electrodes into fabric effectively mitigates the impact of the aforementioned environmental factors.

5.3 *Plication of porous platinum electrodes*

Utilizing in-ear EEG measurement devices allows for EEG measurements outside laboratory or clinical environments, with measurement signals transmitted through the ear canal and auricle. Regarding electrode selection, it can be observed that porous platinum electrodes yield the most suitable experimental data. This is because, compared to other metals, platinum possesses excellent ductility, corrosion resistance, and electrical conductivity. Additionally, porous platinum offers a higher surface area within the same volume. An ideal surface structure can be achieved by electrodepositing platinum and copper together effectively reducing contact interface impedance and improving signal-to-noise ratio.

REFERENCES

Chen Y.H., Op De Beeck M., Vanderheyden L., Carrette E., Mihajlović V., Vanstreels K., Grundlehner B., Gadeyne S., Boon P., and van Hoof C., (2014). *Sensors-basel* **14(12)**, 23758–23780.

Christensen C.B., Harte J.M., Lunner T., and Kidmose P., (2018). *IEEE. Trans. Biomed. Eng.* **65(5)**, 1026–1034.

Debener S., Emkes R., De Vos M., and Bleichner M., (2015). *Sci. Rep* **5(1)**, 16743.

Di Rienzo M., Rizzo F., Parati G., Brambilla G., Ferratini M., Castiglioni P., (2005). *Conf Proc IEEE Eng Med Biol Soc* **2015**, 7167–7169.

Eickenscheidt M., Schäfer P., Baslan Y., Schwarz C., and Stieglitz T., (2020). *Sensors-basel* **20(11)**, 3176.

Fiedler L., Wostmann M., Graversen C., Brandmeyer A., Lunner T., and Obleser J., (2017). *J Neural Eng* **14 (3)**, 36020.

Geddes L.A., (1997). *Ann Biomed Eng* **25(1)**, 1–14.

Greulich C., Kittler S., Epple M., Muhr G., and Köller M., (2009). *Langenbeck Arch Surg* **394(3)**, 495–502

Grummett T.S., Leibbrandt R.E., Lewis T.W., DeLosAngeles D., Powers D.M.W., Willoughby J.O., Pope K. J., and Fitzgibbon S.P., (2015). *Physiol Meas* **36(7)**, 1469–1484.

H.J.J.D. and Fiedler P., (2014). *Acta Imeko*, **3**, 33–37.

He B., Coleman T., Genin G. M., Glover G., Hu X., Johnson N., Liu T., Makeig S., Sajda P., Ye K., (2013). *IEEE. Trans. Biomed. Eng.* **60(11)**, 2983–2992.

Huigen E., Peper A., and Grimbergen C.A., (2002). *Med Biol Eng Comput* **40(3)**, 332–338.

Lopes C., Fiedler P., Rodrigues M.S., Borges J., Bertollo M., Alves E., Barradas N.P., Comani S., Haueisen J., and Vaz F., (2021). *Sensors-basel* **21(23)**, 8143.

Lopes C., Fonseca P., Matamá T., Gomes A., Louro C., Paiva S., and Vaz F., (2014). *J Mater Sci Mater Med* **25(9)**, 2069–2081.

Lopes C., Gabor C., Cristea D., Costa R., Domingues R.P., Rodrigues M.S., Borges J., Alves E., Barradas N. P., Munteanu D., and Vaz F., (2020). *Appl. Surf. Sci.* **505**, 144617.

Mihajlovic V., Grundlehner B., Vullers R., and Penders J., (2015). *IEEE J Biomed Health* **19(1)**, 6–21.

T.X.C.C. and Ankhili A., (2019). *Sensors-basel* **19(2)**, 416.

Wattal S., Spear S. K., Imtiaz M. H., Sazonov E., (2018). *BSN* 54–57.

Chapter 5
Miscellaneous topics in medical research

Biological Sciences and Environmental Health – Gao (Ed.)

Emerging role of GCGR in diabetes

Yu Ji
Southwest Jiaotong University, China

ABSTRACT: Type 2 diabetes is a chronic metabolic disease characterized by elevated blood sugar levels in the body. It accounts for more than 90% of all diabetic cases and is increasingly prevalent with the age of patients becoming younger each year. The International Diabetes Federation estimates that the number of type 2 diabetes mellitus (T2DM) patients will increase to 629 million by 2045. GCGR, which belongs to a Class B G protein-coupled receptor (GPCR), usually binds to hormones that increase glucose concentrations in the body. By activating signaling pathways, it plays a crucial role in regulating the release of glucose in the liver. GCGR is also vital in triglyceride metabolism and maintaining glucose balance, making it a promising target for the pharmacological treatment of T2DM. Unlike Class A GPCRs such as the $\beta 2$ adrenergic receptor, GCGR has enormous cavities that act as ligand-binding pockets while extending 3 helical structures upward in helix 1, above the membrane, to form a stalk. The review explores the seven transmembrane helix domains of human GCGR and the model glucagon binding to GCGR to comprehend the molecular recognition of natural ligands by human GCGR. This review provides an overview of the GCGR's 7TM crystal structure, the binding model between glucagon and GCGR, and the regulation of lipid and glucose metabolism mediated by this binding.

1 INTRODUCTION

The G protein-coupled receptor (GPCR) is present in various tissues and organs in the human body and is anchored to the cell membrane by crossing it seven times. GCGR belongs to the Class B GPCR, the secretin receptor family (Siu *et al.* 2013). It consists of seven transmembrane helical domains, an N-terminus, a C-terminus, three extracellular loops, and three intracellular loops. Unlike Class A GPCRs, the larger cavity formed by the unique location of the extracellular tip is the main factor responsible for the ligand-specific binding of the GPCR (Pal *et al.* 2012). The extracellular domain of the N-terminus, which is globular and found in all Class B GCGR, is defined as a transmembrane domain with three disulfide bonds (IDF 2022). A thorough understanding of the structure of GCGR is of great significance to further study its regulatory mechanism and lays a theoretical foundation for the future research and development of biased ligand drugs.

It is estimated that more than 6.7 million people die from diabetes, with approximately 5.5 million suffering from type 2 diabetes mellitus (Cho *et al.* 2012). The primary causes of type 2 diabetes are improper lipid metabolism and hyperglycemia. GCGR binds to glucagon, which contains 29 amino acids and mediates signaling pathways related to glucose homeostasis, making it an ideal therapeutic target for type 2 diabetes mellitus (Bang and Choi 2015). Additionally, obesity is strongly linked to type 2 diabetes. As a member of GPCR, when linked with hormones, GCGR activates G proteins and stimulates the formation of cAMP, thereby promoting the breakdown of glycogen in liver cells. The physiological effects of glucagon are extensive, including its effect on lipid metabolism.

DOI: 10.1201/9781003587590-42

2 THE STRUCTURE OF GCGR

2.1 *β2 adrenergic receptor*

Secretin family receptors have unique structures that are different from those of Class A, so the seven transmembrane structures of *β*2 adrenergic receptors in Class A GCRR were first observed for subsequent comparison (Figure 1).

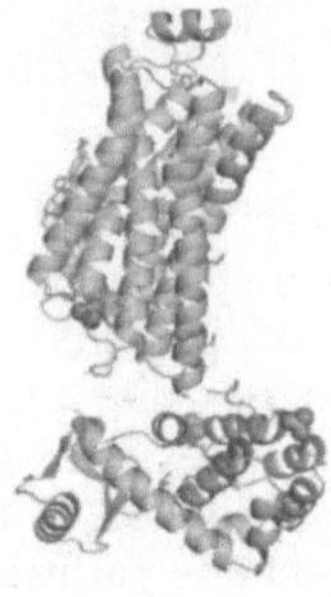

Figure 1. The 7TM structure of human *β*2AR (Wu *et al.* 2012).

The entire rhodopsin structure is distributed intracellularly and extracellularly and consists of seven transmembrane helices and three-ring regions. To stabilize the hydrocarbon skeleton located in the retina, hydrophobic residues in helix 5 and helix 6 form ligand-binding pockets. It is covalently bound to Lys296 of helix 7 (Siu *et al.* 2013). The D[E]RY motif on helix 3 is one of the frequent sequence motifs in rhodopsin-type GPCRs. It creates an ionic lock by forming a salt bridge in helix 6. This ionic lock is a feature of the GPCR's inactive conformation and has been proposed as a mechanism to prevent G protein binding at the cytoplasmic region. The NPXXY motif on helix 7 is another typical motif, believed to be crucial in GPCR activation, in contrast to the ionic lock, which maintains the inactive conformation. Although rhodopsin structure revealed the initial structural aspects of a GPCR, it was hypothesized that since rhodopsin has a covalently bonded ligand, the majority of other GPCRs, which interact with diffusible ligands with varied efficacies, would have different structural features (Wu *et al.* 2012).

2.2 *Extracellular side of GCGR*

Compared with most Class A GPCRs, GCGR has approximately 12 more residues in the extracellular loop (ECL1) (Figure 2).

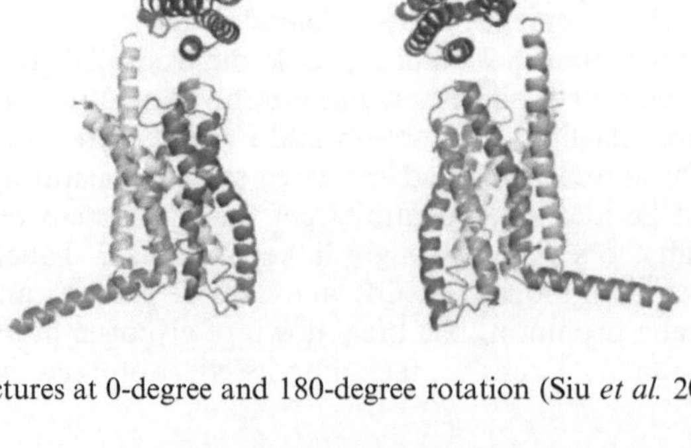

Figure 2. GCGR structures at 0-degree and 180-degree rotation (Siu *et al.* 2013).

The N-terminal end of helix 1 in GCGR is lengthier than that of GPCR because Lys136 to Glu126 form three additional helical turns, extending roughly 16 Å beyond the outer cell membrane (Siu *et al.* 2013). The stalk of GCGR, which determines how the extracellular domain is oriented in relation to the 7TM domain, may be important for glucagon binding (Figure 3).

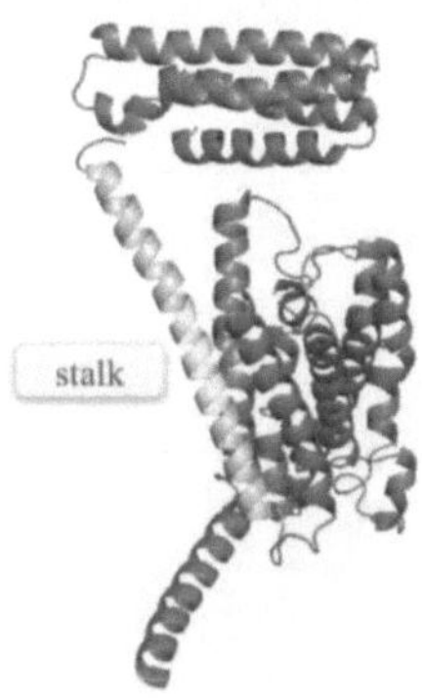

Figure 3. Stalk region in helix 1 of GCGR (Siu *et al.* 2013).

Compared with other GPCRs, the length between the extracellular (EC) tip is the greatest between helix 2 and 6, but this does not include kappa (κ-OR) and mu-opioid receptor (μ-OR). At the same time, the length between helix 3 and helix 7 is the largest (Katritch *et al.* 2013; Manglik *et al.* 2012). As can be seen from Figure 4, the ligand-binding pocket of GCGR is deeper and wider than the structure of rhodopsin-like receptors due to the arrangement of extracellular regions in the seven transmembrane structure.

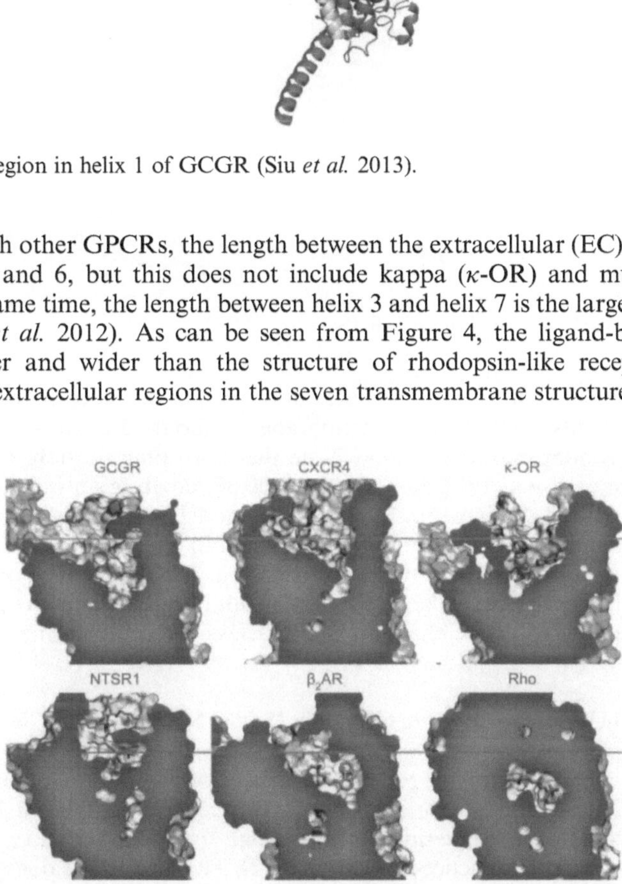

Figure 4. Ligand-binding pocket of GCGR compared with that of rhodopsin-like receptors (Siu *et al.* 2013).

2.3 *Intracellular side of GCGR*

With the exception of a significant inward displacement of helix 7's IC (intracellular) tip, the IC helical tips of GCGR and rhodopsin-like receptors are of similar length, though helix 7 of GCGR shows considerable intracellular movement. In rhodopsin-like receptors, the inward movement of the IC tip of helix 7 is a sign of receptor activation. However, the role of helix 7's intracellular region in GCGR remains unknown (Fredriksson *et al.* 2003). Proline kinks, which are a component in rhodopsin-like receptors, are absent from helix 7 of the receptor (Roberts *et al.* 2011). Conversely, Gly3937.50 on helix 7 of GCGR allows for bending the helix in this region. This glycine is part of the FQG7.50XXVXXXY7.57CF pattern found in helix 7 of the Class B receptors, including GCGR. The hydrophobic interactions between the Gly3937.50-induced bend and Phe1842.57 of helix 2 in GCGR stabilize the structure (Siu *et al.* 2013).

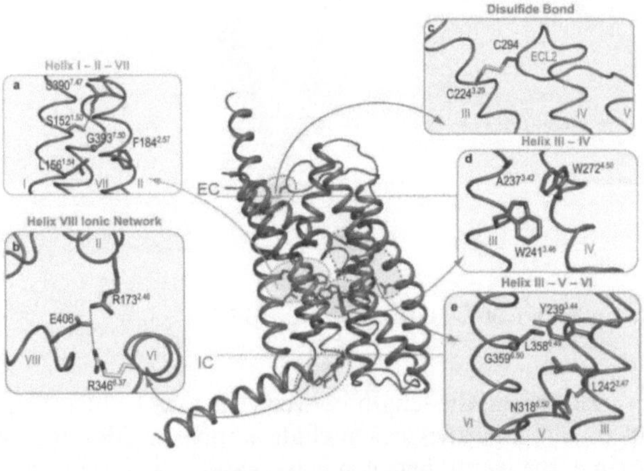

Figure 5. Ionic network of helix 8 in GCGR (Siu *et al.* 2013).

The IC helix 8 has 20 residues and is located at the end of the receptor's C-terminus in the GCGR structure. It tilts away from the membrane by about 25 degrees, which is the same location as in the rhodopsin-like receptor. Note that the filling illusion, Glu406 in helix 8 forms a salt bridge with Arg 1732.46 and Arg 3466.37, creating an interaction within this region of helices 2, 5, and 8 (Figure 5). By building a model, it has been shown that while the tilt of helix 8 has the potential for interactions that could alter its position, the Glu406 salt bridge can be retained and maintain this conformation. Due to the lack of significant conservation that exists in rhodopsin-like receptors, the salt bridges created by these residues are believed to represent a distinctive characteristic of Class B receptors (Siu *et al.* 2013).

3 THE STRUCTURE OF THE GCGR-GLUCAGON MODEL

As shown in Figure 6, in GCGR, the residues associated with glucagon binding form binding sites that include ECL1, ECL 2, and ECL 3, and six other transmembrane helical structures in addition to helix 6. At the same time, these binding sites penetrate deep into the pockets between seven transmembrane helices (Siu *et al.* 2013). The GCGR residues Arg201, Tyr202, Asp208, and Trp215 either interact with glucagon directly or stabilize the ECL1 conformation in the loop region (Figure 6). Additionally, residues Trp295 and Asn298 interact with glucagon in a direct manner. Although mutations in Glu290, Arg225, Lys286, Cys294 Asp218 (Prevost *et al.* 2010), and Cys224 (Koth *et al.* 2012; Prevost *et al.* 2010) also disrupt ligand binding, it is possible that these residues maintain the receptor's conformation with glucagon, but do not interact directly with the hormone. For instance, a disulfide bridge between Cys294 and Cys2243.29 and possible salt bridges between Lys286 and Glu290 and Asp218 and Arg225 stabilize ECL2 and ECL1, respectively. In addition,

Trp3045.36 stabilizes ECL2 between helix 5 and helix 6, while Arg378, which stabilizes ECL3, also affects the binding of GCGR to hormones. (Siu *et al.* 2013).

Depending on crystallography data and in agreement with the findings of mutant binding tests, the GCGR-glucagon model shown in Figure 6 is supported by these data (Koth *et al.* 2012; Prevost *et al.* 2010; Unger and Orci 1975).

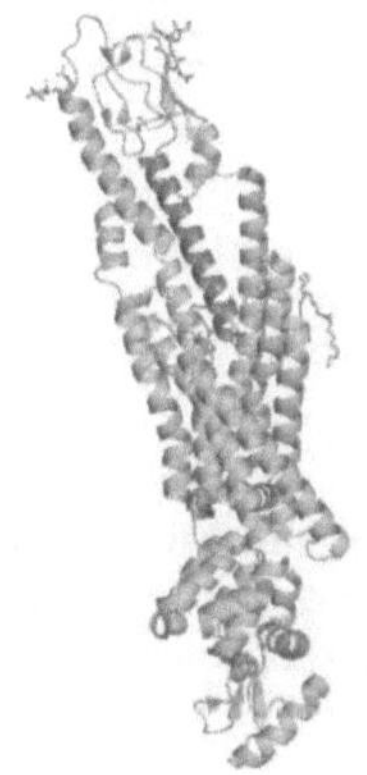

Figure 6. Seven transmembrane domains in GCGR and extracellular structural regions (green) bind to glucagon (blue) (Siu *et al.* 2013).

4 MECHANISM OF GCGR AND GLUCAGON IN DIABETES AND OBESITY

4.1 *Bihormonal regulation*

Diabetes is thought to be caused by the aberrant secretion of both glucagon and insulin, according to the bihormonal regulation theory (Unger 1976, 1978). Diabetes-related metabolic problems such as increased lipolysis, elevated proteolysis, and impaired glucose utilization are directly attributed to insulin shortage. In contrast, excessive glucagon directly promotes hepatic glycogenolysis, increased ketogenesis, decreased glycogen synthesis, and elevated gluconeogenesis (Muller *et al.* 1971; Unger 1976, 1978, 1981). When the insulin in the body is at a low level, blood sugar levels in diabetic patients rise significantly, causing endogenous hyperglycemia, while increased ketone levels lead to hyperketonemia. These conditions are a result of abnormal levels of glucagon in patients that promote gluconeogenesis, accelerate glycogen breakdown, and enhance ketone body production (Campbell and Drucker 2015). Hyperglycemia and glycosuria occur due to elevated glucagon levels in diabetic patients, despite largely constant insulin levels (Jia *et al.* 2022; Ramnanan *et al.* 2011).

4.2 *Mechanism between glucagon and GCGR*

One of the main roles of the signaling pathway mediated by GCGR and glucagon is to regulate glucose levels in the body (Elrick *et al.* 1958). Glucagon in the blood stimulates the breakdown of polysaccharides into simple sugars, thereby increasing the concentration of glucose in the liver (Reiband *et al.* 2015). As a result, glucagon helps regulate low blood sugar levels following insulin release (Jiang and Zhang 2003). The normal range of blood sugar in the human body is critically related to the balance of glucagon and insulin. Therefore, drugs targeting GCGR are promising for the treatment of T2DM. Inhibition of glycogen production and glycolysis, as well as stimulation of glycogenolysis and gluconeogenesis, contribute to the increase in liver glucose synthesis that occurs due to elevated glucagon secretion during hypoglycemia. Whether glycolysis is inhibited and gluconeogenesis is promoted, or glycogen synthesis and breakdown are affected, glucagon secretion and glucose synthesis in the liver are enhanced when the blood sugar levels are low (Habegger *et al.* 2010; Wewer *et al.* 2016). The binding of glucagon to GCGR activates Gs-coupled proteins. As a result, adenylate cyclase gets triggered, increasing the amount of cAMP by stimulating cAMP response element-binding protein and protein kinase A (Wewer *et al.* 2016).

CREB transcription induces G-6-Pase and PEP carboxykinase, both of which stimulate the conversion of non-sugar substances into glucose or glycogen. At the same time, PKA adds a phosphate group to the bifunctional enzyme and activates it. When PFK-2 is phosphorylated, it inhibits PFK-2 activity while activating FBPase2. Thus, glucagon decreases the amount of allosteric modulator while increasing the amount of lactacidogen, inhibiting the breakdown of glucose into pyruvate and promoting the conversion of non-sugar substances into monosaccharides (Janah *et al.* 2019). Additionally, PKA adds a phosphate group to pyruvate kinase, which increases the amount of fructose 1,6 bisphosphate and decreases the amount of pyruvate, resulting in decreased glycolysis. Most crucially, PKA causes the phosphorylase kinase to add a phosphate group, which promotes the conversion of glycogen to Cori ester. At the same time, PKA also causes glycogen synthetase to be phosphorylated and inhibited. The blue down arrow indicates the inhibitory GCGR signal, while the red up arrow indicates the stimulatory GCGR signal (Longuet *et al.* 2008).

4.3 *Glucagon and lipid metabolism*

As mentioned above, glucagon receptors are considered targets for hypoglycemic drugs of T2DM. Since the liver exhibits the highest levels of GCGR expression, it is recognized that glucagon primarily affects hepatocytes. Although adipocytes may express the glucagon receptor, it appears that only rats, not humans, appear to possess this capability. Therefore, hepatic signaling is likely the primary mechanism through which glucagon controls lipid metabolism. The following mechanisms might be involved: First, cAMP is activated when glucagon attaches to GCCR. And then cAMP builds up and activates the CREB protein (Longuet *et al.* 2008). Moreover, the effect of Carnitine O-palmitoyltransferase I(CPT-1) is enhanced, which may lead to an increase in the production of acylcarnitine, thereby activating β-oxidation and producing acetate (DiMarco and Hoppel 1975). Coenzyme A combines with acetic acid to form acetyl coenzyme A, which subsequently forms citrate. Citrate participates in the citric acid cycle and inhibits glycolysis. Hepatic glucagon signaling thus promotes citric acid cycle activation, slows glycolysis, and boosts fatty acid catabolism (Berglund *et al.* 2009).

Additionally, malonyl-CoA inhibits CPT-1, which reduces β-oxidation. As a result, the formation of triglycerides will be inhibited, and β-oxidation will increase as the malonyl-CoA quantity decreases. Malonyl-CoA will reduce β-oxidation in the body by blocking the normal action of CPT-1. Therefore, a decrease in malonyl-CoA content will inhibit the production of triglycerides and increase β-oxidation (Longuet *et al.* 2008).

Normally, triglycerides are stored in the form of free fatty acids. Eventually, very low-density lipoproteins (VLDLs) enter the next process. Glucagon reduces the production of VLDLs and de novo fatty acid synthesis. Finally, glucagon signaling might enhance the AMP/ATP ratio required for the activation of AMP-activated kinase. As a result, this activation leads to the transcription of genes associated with β-oxidation, including acetyl-CoA oxidase and CPT-1, through peroxisome proliferator-activated receptors.

5 CONCLUSION

The analysis of the details of GCGR 7TM structure, the binding of GCGR and hormone, and insulin provides a theoretical basis for the future design of ligands. At the same time, the summary of the mechanism of lipid metabolism and blood glucose regulation can effectively reduce drug side effects by selectively inhibiting the activation of specific effector proteins and promoting the development of T2DM drugs.

REFERENCES

Bang I. and Choi H.J., (2015). *Mol Cells*, 38, 105–111.

Berglund E.D., Lee-Young R.S., Lustig D.G., Lynes S.E., Donahue E.P., Camacho R.C., Meredith M.E., Magnuson M.A., Charron M.J., (2009). *J. Clin. Investig*, 119, 2412–22.

Campbell J.E., Drucker D.J., (2015). *Nat. Rev. Endocrinol*, 11, 329–38.

Cho Y., Merchant C.E. and Kieffer T.J., (2012). *Pharmacol Ther*, 135, 247–278.

DiMarco J.P. and Hoppel C.J., (1975). *Clin. Investig*, 55, 1237–44.

Elrick H., Witten T.A., Arai Y., (1958). *N. Engl. J. Med*, 258, 476–80.

Fredriksson R., Lagerstrom M.C., Lundin L.G., Schioth H.B., (2003). *Mol Pharmacol*, 63, 1256–72

Habegger K.M., Heppner K.M., Geary N., Bartness T.J., DiMarch R., Tschop M.H., (2010). *Nat. Rev. Endocrinol*, 6, 689–97.

International Diabetes Federation (IDF). IDF Diabetes Atlas, 10th ed. (2022), Available online at: https://diabetesatlas.org/

Janah L., Kjeldsen S., Galsgaard K.D., Winther-Sørensen M., Stojanovska E., Pedersen J., Knop F.K., Holst J.J., Wewer Albrechtsen N.J., (2019). *Int J Mol Sci*, 20, 3314.

Jia Y., Liu Y., Feng L., Sun S., Sun G., (2022). *Front Endocrinol (Lausanne)*, 13.

Jiang G. and Zhang B.B., (2003). *Am. J. Physiol. Endocrinol. Metab*, 284, 71–78

Katritch V., Cherezov V., Stevens R.C., (2013). *Annu Rev Pharmacol Toxicol*, 53, 531–556.

Koth C.M., Murray J.M., Mukund S., Madjidi A., Minn A., Clarke H.J., Wong T., Chiang V., Luis E. and Estevez A. (2012). *Proc Natl Acad Sci U S A*, 109, 14393–398.

Longuet C., Sinclair E.M., Maida A., Baggio L.L., Maziarz M., Charron M.J., Drucker D.J., (2008). *Cell Metab*, 8, 359–71.

Manglik A., Kruse A.C., Kobilka T.S., Thian F.S., Mathiesen J.M., Sunahara R.K., Pardo L., Weis W.I., Kobilka B.K. and Granier S., (2012). *Nature*, 485, 321–326.

Muller W.A., Faloona G.R. and Unger R.H., (1971). *J Clin Invest*, 50, 1992–9.

Pal K., Melcher K. and Xu H., (2012). *Acta Pharmacol Sin*, 33, 300–311.

Prevost M., Vertongen P., Raussens V., Roberts D.J., Cnudde J., Perret J. and Waelbroeck M., (2010). *J Biol Chem*, 285, 30951–58.

Ramnanan C.J., Edgerton D.S., Kraft G. and Cherrington A.D. (2011). *Diabetesobes Metab*, 13, 118–125.

Reiband H.K., Schmidt S., Ranjan A., Holst J.J., Madsbad S. and Norgaard K., (2015). *Diabetes Metab. Res. Rev*, 31, 672–79.

Roberts D.J., Vertongen P. and Waelbroeck M., (2011). *Peptides*, 32, 1593–99.

Siu F.Y., He M., de Graaf C., Han G.W., Yang D., Zhang Z., Zhou C., Xu Q., Wacker D., Joseph J.S., Liu W., Lau J., Cherezov V., Katritch V., Wang M.W. and Stevens R.C., (2013). *Nature*, 499, 444–449

Unger R.H. and Orci L., (1975). Lancet, 1, 14–16

Unger R.H. and Orci L., (1981). *N Engl J Med*, 304, 1575–80.

Unger R.H., (1976). *Diabetes*, 25, 136–51.

Unger R.H., (1978). *Metabolism*, 27, 1691–709.

Wewer Albrechtsen N.J., Kuhre R.E., Pedersen J., Knop F.K., Holst J.J., (2016). *Biomark. Med*, 10, 1141–51.

Wu H., Wacker D., Mileni M., Katritch V., Han G.W., Vardy E., Liu W., Thompson A.A., Huang X.P., Carroll F.I., Mascarella S.W., Westkaemper R.B., Mosier P.D., Roth B.L., Cherezov V., Stevens R.C., *Nature*, (2012). 485, 327–332.

Biological Sciences and Environmental Health – Gao (Ed.)

Bisphosphonates in the treatment of osteoporosis, drug holidays, and future perspectives

Yuhan Xu
Biological Sciences, University of Liverpool, Liverpool, United Kingdom of Great Britain and Northern Ireland

ABSTRACT: Osteoporosis is a frequently seen condition among individuals in the middle-aged and older population due to its extensive reach and substantial incidence. This ailment gives rise to fragility fractures and a range of consequences that significantly damage the quality of life experienced by affected patients. With the increasing aging population, osteoporosis has emerged as a prevalent metabolic bone disorder on a global scale, necessitating the development of safe and easily accessible therapeutic interventions. Complete reversal of osteoporosis is not currently achievable, necessitating long-term treatment for people with the illness to rebuild and sustain bone density and mitigate the risk of fractures. Bisphosphonates are extensively employed in the management of osteoporosis. Bisphosphonates, being counterparts of pyrophosphate, exert their effects on bone loss via suppressing osteoclastic activity. This article provides a comprehensive evaluation of the effectiveness and safety profiles of several bisphosphonates often employed in therapeutic interventions. Additionally, it examines the optimal duration of bisphosphonate administration and the potential implementation of drug holidays. Furthermore, it explores potential advancements that may expand the scope of bisphosphonate treatments in the future.

1 INTRODUCTION

Osteoporosis is a chronic and progressive skeletal disorder that mostly arises due to menopause and the natural process of aging. It is a significant contributor to disability and mortality among older individuals, and its prevalence is increasing worldwide as the global population ages. Osteoporosis does not have a direct impact on the process of bone production by osteoblasts. Instead, it disrupts both bone resorption and formation, resulting in a decrease in resorptive bone formation and ultimately leading to a decline in bone density (Gupta *et al.* 2018). As a result of the significant prevalence of osteoporosis and low bone mass, this condition is strongly correlated with a heightened susceptibility to fractures and falls, diminished physical and social capabilities, compromised quality of life, and, in severe instances, complications arising from localized fragility fractures. These fractures are particularly challenging to manage and contribute to elevated rates of mortality, disability, and healthcare expenditures (Rizzo *et al.* 2022). Annually, a staggering 8.9 million individuals worldwide experience fractures as a direct consequence of osteoporosis (Zhu and Song 2018). Primary osteoporosis is the prevailing form of osteoporosis, distinguished by heightened bone fragility and bone loss resulting from the activity of osteoclasts, degradation of bone structure, and bone loss associated with the natural aging process and diminished gonadal function, encompassing postmenopausal and senile osteoporosis. Given that osteoporosis is a condition that cannot be fully reversed, many therapeutic approaches are employed to manage and mitigate its effects. Several treatment approaches are employed for managing

 DOI: 10.1201/9781003587590-43

osteoporosis, including hormone replacement therapy, selective estrogen receptor modulators, bisphosphonates, fluoride, parathyroid hormone, and calcitonin (Gupta *et al.* 2018).

Bisphosphonates, one of the main treatments for osteoporosis, have been shown in clinical trials to reduce fractures in patients with osteoporosis and bone loss and are widely used to treat osteoporosis in postmenopausal women and older men (Compston 2020). Bisphosphonates are pyrophosphate analogues that reduce bone loss by inhibiting osteoclast recruitment and affecting osteoblast activity. Bisphosphonates used to treat osteoporosis include etidronate, alendronate, ibandronate, risedronate and zoledronic acid (Gupta *et al.* 2018).

Despite the widespread use of bisphosphonates in therapy and the large amount of research and data available, there is still a lack of concise and clear summaries of the different drugs and their advantages and disadvantages. This article provides an overview of the use of bisphosphonates in osteoporosis, including the efficacy of several common bisphosphonate drugs in osteoporosis, the safety of their use, and the directions in which bisphosphonate drug therapy may be refined in the future.

2 APPLICATION AND EFFICACY OF DIFFERENT BISPHOSPHONATES

2.1 *Alendronate*

Among the most widely used antiresorptive bisphosphonates, the most clinically used is alendronate, an oral bisphosphonate currently used in the treatment of various types of osteoporosis, which inhibits osteoclasts from destroying and digesting bone, thereby reducing osteoporosis symptoms. Bisphosphonates are the mainstay of osteoporosis treatment and should usually be used as the drug of choice because of their long history of use, safety and anti-fracture efficacy (Luz *et al.* 2017).

A total of 6,457 women diagnosed with osteoporosis were enrolled in a single trial. Among them, 2,023 had a history of vertebral fractures, whereas 4,434 did not. The osteoporotic female participants were administered a daily dosage of 5 mg of alendronate for a duration of 2 years. Subsequently, they were either given a daily dosage of 10 mg of alendronate or a placebo for the remaining duration of the trial. During a median follow-up period of 3.8 years, the administration of alendronate demonstrated efficacy in mitigating the likelihood of vertebral fractures among women diagnosed with osteoporosis, regardless of whether they had previously experienced a vertebral fracture (Rdn *et al.* 2018). In the context of osteoporosis in males, three clinical trials were conducted, wherein a daily dosage of 10 mg of alendronate was administered for durations of 1, 2, and 3 years, respectively. Two additional cohorts administered a weekly dosage of 70 mg of alendronate during a period of either 6 months or 1 year. The administration of alendronate demonstrated a notable enhancement in bone density at the lumbar spine in comparison to the administration of a placebo (Beaudart *et al.* 2023).

Furthermore, it has been observed that the continuous weekly oral administration of 70 mg of alendronate over a period of 12 months has proven to be efficacious in enhancing spinal bone density and alleviating back pain among individuals suffering from thalassaemic osteoporosis (Piriyakhuntorn *et al.* 2023). The therapeutic efficacy of alendronate is seen in both male and female patients, as well as in some subtypes of osteoporosis.

The administration of alendronate is generally well received and deemed safe, with occurrences of side effects being quite infrequent. Bisphosphonates have been found to be related with several adverse effects, including hypocalcemia, gastrointestinal side effects, osteonecrosis of the jaw, and atypical femur fractures (Piriyakhuntorn *et al.* 2023). Among the observed adverse effects, dyspepsia and epigastric discomfort exhibit a higher prevalence, manifesting in around 5% of those on alendronate treatment. Furthermore, it should be noted that prolonged adherence of alendronate oral tablets to the oesophageal wall has the potential to induce the formation of oesophageal ulcers (Radwan *et al.* 2018).

2.2 *Risedronate*

In the year 2000, risedronate received approval as the second bisphosphonate for the therapeutic management of osteoporosis (Luz *et al.* 2017). Risedronate, a bisphosphonate compound containing nitrogen, is employed for the purpose of enhancing bone strength and managing or preventing osteoporosis. As a result of its very brief half-life, this substance necessitates repeated administrations and has conventionally been offered in oral formulations designed for daily, weekly, or monthly consumption (Fazil *et al.* 2015).

In a study including 2,458 women under the age of 85 who had previously suffered a vertebral fracture, the administration of risedronate for a duration of 3 years resulted in a significant decrease in the occurrence of both vertebral and nonvertebral fractures. Specifically, the risk of experiencing vertebral fractures was decreased by 41%, while the likelihood of nonvertebral fractures was reduced by 39%. A comprehensive study involving a sample size of 5445 women diagnosed with osteoporosis and falling within the age range of 70 to 79 years revealed a significant decrease of 40% in the likelihood of experiencing a hip fracture over a period of 2 years, as observed during the follow-up period (Luz *et al.* 2017). Two clinical trials were conducted to compare the efficacy of risedronate with placebo in the treatment of osteoporosis in a sample of 600 male participants. The study conducted by Boonen *et al.* administered a weekly dose of 35 mg of risedronate or placebo, while the study conducted by Ringe *et al.* administered a daily dose of 5 mg of risedronate or placebo. Both trials had a duration of 2 years. The results of the study indicated that risedronate demonstrated favorable effects across all measured outcomes (Beaudart *et al.* 2023).

While certain studies have provided evidence regarding the therapeutic effectiveness of risedronate in individuals diagnosed with osteoporosis, there exists a study that examined the therapeutic efficacy and upper gastrointestinal tolerability of alendronate and risedronate. This particular study involved the allocation of 520 patients to receive alendronate 70 mg in the morning after fasting, while an additional 533 patients were assigned to risedronate 35 mg. The study evaluated changes in bone mineral density at the acetabulum, total hip, femoral neck, and lumbar spine after 6 and 12 months. It also examined the percentage of patients who experienced a predetermined change in bone mineral density at the acetabulum and lumbar spine after 12 months. Additionally, changes in biochemical markers of bone turnover were measured at 3, 6, and 12 months. Results The study found that alendronate had a considerably higher impact on bone density at all assessed sites, and there was no significant difference in the likelihood of cessation or gastrointestinal adverse effects (Rosen *et al.* 2004). The comparative analysis suggests that alendronate exhibits superior efficacy in enhancing bone density compared to risedronate, while maintaining a similar level of tolerability. Consequently, alendronate may be considered a more favorable therapeutic choice for managing osteoporosis, despite the potential adverse effects encountered by patients towards the conclusion of treatment.

2.3 *Ibandronate*

Ibandronate, which was granted approval in 2005 as a therapeutic option for osteoporosis, represents the most recent iteration, or third generation, of bisphosphonate medications. These treatments have demonstrated notable efficacy, minimal toxicity, convenient administration, and are accessible in both oral and intravenous formulations (Chen *et al.* 2020).

In a trial including a 3-year duration, a total of 2946 female individuals diagnosed with osteoporosis and aged between 55 and 80 years, who had experienced one or more cone fractures, were subjected to treatment with the administration of ibandronate. The findings of this study revealed a significant reduction in the likelihood of vertebral fractures by 62% (Luz *et al.* 2017). A separate investigation including a cohort of 132 males diagnosed with osteoporosis, who had undergone a one-year treatment regimen, was conducted to assess the efficacy of ibandronate at a dosage of 150mg per month in comparison to a placebo.

The results of this study demonstrated noteworthy enhancements in lumbar spine and total hip bone density within the ibandronate group, as opposed to the placebo group (Beaudart *et al.* 2023).

A study was undertaken in Japan to observe the effects of monthly intravenous ibandronate 1 mg treatment on bone mineral density, bone turnover indicators, and adverse events in a cohort of 887 female patients and 138 male patients. The participants were followed for a duration of 12 months. The study observed a substantial increase in bone mineral density at the lumbar spine, femoral neck, and whole hip after 12 months compared to the initial measurements. Additionally, all markers of bone turnover showed a significant decrease after the 12-month period. A total of 75 adverse events were documented, occurring in 54 of the patients. A total of four individuals experienced significant adverse effects, with one instance specifically involving osteonecrosis of the jaw. A total of 21 patients experienced acute phase reactions, with 50% of these reactions manifesting following the initial administration of ibandronate. According to the cited source (Takeuchi *et al.* 2018), there was a lack of unreported adverse occurrences. The findings of this study provide evidence supporting the favorable therapeutic effectiveness and safety profile of ibandronate.

Nevertheless, a prior investigation with a cohort of 2946 individuals diagnosed with osteoporosis and treated with ibandronate revealed that the administration of ibandronate did not demonstrate any significant reduction in the incidence of non-vertebral fractures, as indicated by the results of placebo-controlled studies (Luz *et al.* 2017). This observation suggests that the treatment efficacy of ibandronate may be limited to cone osteoporosis. It is conceivable that future investigations will be conducted to provide evidence or validate the potential of ibandronate in mitigating non-vertebral fractures.

2.4 *Zoledronic acid*

In 2007, the approval for the use of zoledronic acid, a bisphosphonate known for its superior antiresorptive efficacy, was granted for the treatment of osteoporosis. This particular medication exhibits the highest rate of bone retention when compared to alendronate, ebandronate, and etidronate, mostly attributed to its strong affinity for hydroxyapatite (Radwan *et al.* 2018).

A study was conducted to evaluate the efficacy of annual infusions of zoledronic acid over a period of three years in a sample of 7765 women aged 65-89 with osteoporosis and a vertebral fracture. The results indicated a significant reduction in the risk of vertebral, femoral, and nonvertebral fractures by 70%, 41%, and 25% respectively, over the follow-up period (Luz *et al.* 2017). In a separate investigation, it was determined that the administration of zoledronic acid by annual intravenous infusions proved to be efficacious in mitigating the likelihood of fractures occurring in the vertebrae, femur, and other nonvertebral regions among women between the ages of 65 and 89. In a separate study, a notable enhancement in lumbar spine bone density was observed among a cohort of 1,199 individuals who received an annual intravenous administration of 44 mg of zoledronic acid. A study conducted on a cohort of 21 males who had recently experienced hip fractures likewise shown noteworthy enhancements in both total hip bone mineral density and femoral neck bone mineral density (Beaudart *et al.* 2023). The paper also documented and compared the alterations in bone mineral density and serum bone turnover marker levels in the left forearm, lumbar spine, and left hip before and after therapy in 21 individuals from each of the two groups. The findings indicated that individuals who received zoledronic acid had a notable augmentation in bone mineral density across all measured locations as compared to the baseline period. No new fractures were observed in either group for the duration of the therapy period. The findings indicate that the administration of Zoledronic acid leads to a substantial enhancement in the blood markers of bone turnover among patients, resulting in a notable improvement in bone density and a reduction in the incidence of new fractures. Furthermore, the treatment demonstrates favorable safety and tolerability profiles (Feng *et al.* 2020).

Zoledronic acid is widely regarded as a safe pharmaceutical agent for the management of osteoporosis, with minimal occurrence of adverse effects. Acute temporary responses, specifically transient flu-like symptoms, have been documented in individuals with osteoporosis who are undergoing treatment with ZOL. The highest occurrence of this phenomenon is observed following the administration of the initial dose, and then diminishes with each consecutive dose (Radwan *et al.* 2018). A research investigation was conducted to evaluate the occurrence of adverse reactions among a group of patients receiving annual intravenous infusions of zoledronic acid. The study involved 50 female and 9 male patients, and utilized a questionnaire consisting of 7 items to assess the presence of such reactions. The findings revealed that 14 patients, accounting for 23.7% of the sample, reported experiencing mild adverse reactions subsequent to their initial infusion. These reactions included symptoms such as myalgia, arthralgia, flu-like syndrome, fever, headache, and pruritus (Dilek *et al.* 2017). The incidence of bisphosphonate-associated osteonecrosis of the jaw has been demonstrated in cases where large oncological dosages of zoledronic acid were administered, however the probability of its manifestation was found to be minimal. Cardiac arrhythmias may also be induced by the administration of zoledronic acid (Radwan *et al.* 2018).

3 DRUG HOLIDAY IN BISPHOSPHONATE THERAPY

The utilization of oral bisphosphonates has played a significant role in the global decline of osteoporotic fractures. The concept of a medication holiday is unique to osteoporosis, as it is the only chronic condition where this approach is considered. In contrast, other chronic diseases like hypertension, hypercholesterolemia, diabetes, and gout typically require constant therapy (Bandeira *et al.* 2020). In recent years, there has been a growing focus among medical professionals and individuals with regards to the detrimental consequences associated with prolonged utilization of bisphosphonates for the management of osteoporosis.

The underlying justification for drug holidays is to capitalize on the lingering anti-fracture properties of bisphosphonates, while discontinuing the ongoing buildup of the medication and potentially mitigating unfavorable occurrences. The extended utilization of bisphosphonates has been associated with infrequent although significant side consequences. The occurrence of osteonecrosis of the jaw is predominantly associated with the administration of high dosages of bisphosphonates. Additionally, there seems to be an elevated likelihood of atypical femur fractures after 3-5 years of bisphosphonate treatment. Additional risk factors for atypical femur fractures encompass Asian ethnicity, diabetes mellitus, rheumatoid arthritis, the utilization of glucocorticoids and proton pump inhibitors, as well as bone demineralization (Hayes *et al.* 2021). The current recommendations prioritize the implementation of drug holidays following a duration of 5 years for alendronate usage or 3 years for zoledronic acid usage, provided that the individual is assessed to have a low-risk status at the conclusion of these time frames (Bandeira *et al.* 2020).

Typically, the cessation of drug intake following prolonged bisphosphonate therapy, known as a medication holiday, does not result in a return to the pre-treatment level of fracture risk due to the continued anti-fracture effects of residual bisphosphonates, even while bone turnover markers remain suppressed. A retrospective cohort study was conducted to evaluate the fracture risk associated with a medication holiday in a population of 39,502 women aged 45 years or older who had been prescribed bisphosphonates for a duration exceeding 3 years for the management of osteoporosis. In a study comparing individuals who took a bisphosphonate holiday lasting over 12 months (11,497), those who used bisphosphonates continuously (17,123), and those who did not use bisphosphonates continuously (10,882), it was found that women on a bisphosphonate holiday exceeding 12 months did not exhibit a heightened risk of fragility fractures related to osteoporosis, hip fractures, or vertebral fractures (Bandeira *et al.* 2020). Previous studies have demonstrated that cessation of treatment with three oral bisphosphonates (ibandronate, alendronate, and risedronate) in postmenopausal women with osteoporosis resulted in an elevation of bone turnover markers and a reduction in hip bone mineral density. These post-treatment values remained below the initial baseline values prior to the commencement of treatment (Naylor *et al.* 2018).

While there is a prevailing consensus regarding the necessity of implementing a drug holiday after bisphosphonate therapy for patients with a low to moderate risk of fracture, the optimal duration and potential discontinuation of this drug holiday remain uncertain. Several authors have proposed that future investigations on the duration of drug holidays should take into account several parameters, such as the cumulative exposure to bisphosphonates prior to the holiday, the specific type of bisphosphonate medication administered, alterations in fracture risk factors, and the unique characteristics of individual patients (Hayes *et al.* 2021).

3.1 *Total bisphosphonate exposure*

The cumulative exposure impact of bisphosphonates manifests in their ability to adequately suppress osteoclasts and provide fracture protection, although this effect is observed only after a period of 6-12 months of consistent usage. The role of cumulative exposure on the anti-fracture effect after withdrawal should also be considered, as the presence of leftover bisphosphonates in bone during dosage is insufficient to eternally lower fracture risk. As an illustration, the in vivo effective dose following the cessation of alendronate therapy after a decade of treatment amounts to merely 25% of the dosage administered during the treatment period (Hayes *et al.* 2021).

3.2 *Bisphosphonates used before drug holidays*

Various bisphosphonates have varying levels of potency in inhibiting osteoclasts and differing affinities for hydroxyapatite. Zoledronic acid demonstrates the highest affinity for hydroxyapatite, while alendronate, ibandronate, and risedronate exhibit diminishing affinities in the aforementioned sequence. The diminished affinity of risedronate for hydroxyapatite could potentially impact the accumulation of bisphosphonates inside the skeletal system. Due to its potential for reduced accumulation and faster clearance from the body, risedronate may exhibit a more transient protective effect on fractures upon discontinuation of treatment. This is evident in a study comparing the physiological changes in patients undergoing a drug holiday, where the risedronate group demonstrated less inhibition on bone turnover markers compared to the alendronate and ibandronate groups (Naylor *et al.* 2018). It is evident that medication holidays following prolonged administration of risedronate should be of appropriate duration and necessitate additional extensive monitoring.

3.3 *Bone mineral density and fall risk*

The reevaluation of the suitability of an extended pharmaceutical holiday should primarily focus on the alterations in fracture risk factors. In cases where a patient exhibits an elevated susceptibility to falls, it may be deemed advisable to forego the pharmaceutical hiatus as a means of mitigating the potential for fractures resulting from falls. This course of action should be accompanied by the implementation of supplementary measures aimed at diminishing the occurrence of falls.

3.4 *Patient characteristics*

Multiple factors have been found to increase the risk of fracture in patients with osteoporosis who are undergoing treatment. These factors include patient adherence to treatment, sex (specifically female), body weight (particularly low body weight), and ethnicity (namely

Caucasian race) (Hayes *et al.* 2021). Nevertheless, there is a dearth of research investigating the impact of these attributes on the efficacy of medication getaways.

It is evident that there is potential for further refinement of reporting and data analysis pertaining to bisphosphonate medication holidays. Additionally, there is a need to examine the distinct characteristics of individual patients in relation to the aforementioned four aspects, and to compare them. This exploration aims to investigate the effects of various influences on bisphosphonate medication holidays and provide recommendations regarding suitable medication schedules for patients.

4 ADDITIONAL FUTURE DIRECTIONS FOR IMPROVEMENT

4.1 *Medication mode: Oral to topical administration*

Currently, the primary approach to the prevention and treatment of osteoporosis in clinical settings is around the utilization of systemic medications. However, systemic medicines are associated with several challenges, including limited bioavailability, delayed onset of therapeutic effects, and the potential for severe adverse reactions resulting from prolonged bisphosphonate administration. Furthermore, osteoporosis, being a chronic condition characterized by subtle symptoms, presents challenges in terms of patient awareness. Oral bisphosphonates have a higher propensity to induce irritation to the gastrointestinal tract. Prior to and following oral delivery, fasting is necessary. Additionally, it is important to maintain an upright position after medication administration. Failure to adhere to adequate administration methods can lead to gastrointestinal responses, and in severe cases, ulcerative esophagitis (Zhu and Song 2018). In the realm of clinical practice, it is frequently observed that oral bisphosphonate therapy exhibits a notable lack of compliance among patients, resulting in suboptimal adherence prior to the initiation of a medication holiday (Hayes *et al.* 2021). Several studies have proposed potential options and approaches for localized treatment. However, it is important to note that current methods such as local drug injection therapy and biologics are both costly and imperfect. Therefore, future research efforts should be focused on finding ways to prolong the effectiveness or even achieve controllable duration of localized treatment (Zhu and Song 2018). The integration of oral and topical medications has the potential to significantly enhance the efficacy of osteoporosis treatment and improve patient adherence.

4.2 *Eliminating side effects*

In conjunction with the aforementioned topical drugs, which aid in mitigating the adverse effects linked to bisphosphonates, dietary patterns and insufficient awareness regarding dietary practices also exert a significant influence on the onset of osteoporosis. Several scholarly papers have posited that the regular consumption of specific vegetables, adherence to a balanced diet, and the incorporation of herbal medicines may potentially mitigate the effects of osteoporosis (Gupta *et al.* 2018). Nevertheless, the utilization of plant-derived or other naturally occurring bioactive compounds for the treatment of osteoporosis has not yet been explored in clinical trials. Hence, it is recommended that the exploration of natural and plant-derived medicines be pursued as a means to mitigate the problems and adverse effects associated with chemical-pharmacological interventions.

5 CONCLUSION

In summary, bisphosphonates such as alendronate, ibandronate, risedronate, and zoledronic acid have demonstrated efficacy in the treatment of osteoporosis in both experimental and clinical contexts. The selection of a specific bisphosphonate should be guided by the physician, who must consider the patient's individual response to the drug and the occurrence of any adverse effects following administration and prolonged use. Following prolonged administration of a bisphosphonate, it is advisable to implement a drug holiday, which should be periodically evaluated, in order to mitigate the potential occurrence of infrequent adverse effects. The duration of the drug hiatus and the factors that impact it remain uncertain. One potential avenue for advancing bisphosphonate therapy involves modifying the drug's delivery method. Currently, oral administration is commonly employed, but it presents challenges in terms of low absorption rates and patient adherence. In contrast, topical administration offers a promising alternative, as it requires less frequent dosing and exhibits a higher rate of absorption. Furthermore, the implementation of dietary and lifestyle modifications, with the concurrent utilization of herbal remedies, has the potential to mitigate the adverse effects and complications associated with bisphosphonate therapy, thereby enhancing the management of osteoporosis.

REFERENCES

Bandeira F., Dantas W., Bilezikian J. P., (2020). *Arch Endocrin. Metab* **64**, 331.

Beaudart C., Céline Demonceau, Sabico S., Veronese N., Cooper C., Harvey N. C., Fuggle N. R., Bruyere O., René Rizzoli and Jean-Yves Reginster, (2023). *Aging. Clin. Exp. Res* **35**, 1789.

Chen C., Zhou S., Zhang W., Hou W., Xiang L., and Wu J., (2020). *Chinese J. Tissue Eng. Res.* **24**, 2625.

Compston J., (2020). *Bone* **136**, 115330.

Dilek B., Şahin E., Erdem D., Bulut D., Gülbahar S., (2017). *Turk. Osteoporoz. Derg* **23**, 21.

Fazil M., Hassan M. Q., Baboota S. and Ali J., (2015). *Drug Deliv* **23**, 2428.

Feng Y., Wu L., Kuerbanjiang Y. and Adina S., (2020). *Xinjiang Med.* J **50**, 787.

Gupta T., Das N., Imran S., (2018). *J. Diet. Suppl* **16**, 699.

Hayes K. N., Winter E. M., Cadarette S. M., Burden A. M., (2021). *J. Clin. Med* **10**, 1140.

Luz E., Bezerra M. C., Flávia A., Márcia S., Cristina S., Alva C. B., (2017). *Rev. Bras. Reumatol* **57**, 254.

Naylor K. E., Bradburn M., Paggiosi M. A., Gossiel F., Peel N. F. A., McCloskey E. V., Walsh J. S. and Eastell R., (2018). *Osteoporos. Int* **29**, 1407.

Piriyakhuntorn P., Tantiworawit A., Phimphilai M., Srichairatanakool S., Teeyasoontranon W., Rattanathammethee T., Hantrakool S., Chai-Adisaksopha C., Rattarittamrong E., Norasetthada L., Fanhchaksai K., Charoenkwan P., (2023). *Front. Endocrinol* **14**, 1178761.

Radwan I. A., Korany N. S., Ezzat B. A., (2018). *Case Rep. Cli. Med* **07**, 324.

Rizzo M., Tammaro G., Guarino A., Basso M., Cozzolino A., Mariconda M., (2022). *Orthop. Rev* **14**, 1.

Rosen C. J., Hochberg M. C., Bonnick S. L., McClung M., Miller P., Broy S., Kagan R., Chen E., Petruschke R. A., Thompson D. E. and de Papp A. E., (2004). *J. Bone Miner. Res* **20**, 141.

Takeuchi Y., Hashimoto J., Nishida Y., Chiemi Yamagiwa, Tamura T., Atsumi A., (2018). *Osteoporos. Sarcopenia* **4**, 22.

Zhu J. and Song C., (2018). *Chin. J. Osteoporos* **24**, 806.

Biological Sciences and Environmental Health – Gao (Ed.)

Gut hormonal responses to sucralose in healthy subjects

Jiaruo Hu
School of Chemical Engineering, University of Birmingham, Birmingham, UK

ABSTRACT: In the continuously evolving domain of food additives, sucralose, identified as a chlorinated derivative of sucrose in 1976, has risen to prominence. Its allure stems not only from its potent sweetening capabilities but also from its calorie-free nature, making it a favored choice among health-conscious consumers and the food industry alike. This research undertakes a meticulous examination of the physiological ramifications of sucralose consumption, specifically focusing on its potential interactions with pivotal intestinal hormones: GLP-1, GIP, and PYY in healthy human subjects. The data suggests that despite sucralose's ubiquity in modern diets, its influence on the secretion patterns of GLP-1, GIP, and PYY in healthy human participants appears minimal. Such findings have profound implications, particularly in the context of appetite regulation, nutrient absorption, and overall metabolic homeostasis. This research aims to empower consumers with evidence-based insights, fostering informed decision-making and promoting healthier, safer dietary choices in an era where food additives are omnipresent.

1 INTRODUCTION

Sucralose has become a prominent figure in the growing field of food additives. Originally discovered in 1976, this chlorinated derivative of sucrose has since gained widespread acceptance as a calorie-free artificial sweetener and is widely used in a range of food and beverage products (Grice and Goldsmith 2000). Although its sweetening ability has been well documented, the physiological effects of its consumption, particularly in relation to gut hormones, remain the subject of lively debate (Siddiqui *et al.* 2022).

Gut hormones are a complex series of peptides secreted by enteroendocrine cells in the gastrointestinal tract that play a key role in coordinating various physiological processes. These processes include appetite regulation, nutrient absorption and maintenance of metabolic homeostasis. Among these hormones, glucagon-like peptide-1 (GLP-1) is mainly involved in the regulation of insulin secretion and appetite suppression. Gastric inhibitory polypeptide (GIP), on the other hand, is mainly associated with insulin secretion and promotion of lipid storage. Peptide YY (PYY) is mainly involved in appetite suppression and regulation of gastric emptying rate. Given the intricate nature of these hormones, any foreign substance that interacts with them can have far-reaching effects. Sucralose, a widely used artificial sweetener, is hypothesised to interact with sweet taste receptors in the gut. This potential interaction raises pertinent questions about how sucralose modulates the secretion and function of these key gut hormones. Such interactions have important practical implications as they may influence appetite cues, determine nutrient intake patterns and alter overall metabolic trajectories. Understanding the interactions between sucralose and these hormones is therefore not only an academic issue, but is also critical for assessing the broader impact of sucralose consumption on human health. As people continue to add artificial sweeteners to diets, it is imperative to elucidate their potential physiological effects to ensure make informed dietary choices.

 DOI: 10.1201/9781003587590-44

The main purpose of this study is twofold. Firstly, it aims to provide food safety regulators and medical professionals with more accurate and comprehensive information on the physiological effects of sucralose. Such information will assist in the development of guidelines, recommendations and potential warnings related to sucralose-containing products. Second, by elucidating the complex interactions between sucralose and gut hormones, this research works to empower consumers to make healthier and safer food choices. In an era when dietary choices significantly impact health outcomes, understanding the potential impact of widely consumed additives such as sucralose is not only beneficial, but imperative.

2 SUCRALOSE

2.1 *Definition of sucralose*

Sucralose is a non-nutritive artificial sweetener synthesised by the selective substitution of chlorine atoms for three hydroxyl groups in the sucrose molecule. This chlorination process converts natural sugar compounds into highly effective sweeteners with a sweetness intensity approximately 600 times that of sucrose itself (Grice and Goldsmith 2000). A recent study by Dyab *et al.* demonstrated that unlike conventional sugar, sucralose is not metabolically broken down in the body and therefore sucralose in pomegranate juice successfully replaces sucrose, resulting in a reduction of the total carbohydrate content and the total number of calories without affecting the sensory properties (Dyab *et al.* 2021). Sucralose has been successfully substituted for sucralose in pomegranate juice. Sucralose is also highly stable at the high temperatures often used in the manufacturing of food, beverages and pharmaceuticals and therefore maintains the sweetness level of the product after cooking, baking and/or pasteurisation leading to the widespread use of sucralose in a variety of culinary applications.

2.2 *Safety of sucralose*

The safety of sucralose, a chlorinated derivative of sucrose, can be inferred from its molecular structure and physico-chemical properties. The molecular structure of sucralose is similar to that of other disaccharides and is highly water soluble and non-lipophilic due to the substitution of three hydroxyl groups by chlorine. It is not bioaccumulative. Also studies in animals have found that a large proportion of sucralose (about 85%) is not absorbed and is excreted by the body in feces (Sims *et al.* 2000). In humans, sucralose is neither a substrate for the gastrointestinal microbiota nor does it produce gastrointestinal side effects because large doses are not absorbed. Radiological studies surface no evidence of any protein binding production after sucralose administration. No relationship between plasma concentrations and the amount of sucralose ingested in humans was found in a 13-week human experiment with increased sucralose intake (Baird *et al.* 2000).

2.3 *Widespread use of sucralose in the food industry*

Increasing consumer awareness of climate change and sustainability is further driving the adoption of sucralose as a preferred sweetener, in keeping with trends arising from Fourth Industrial Revolution technologies (Hassoun *et al.* 2022). In addition to its role in reducing calorie content, sucralose's stability under various processing conditions makes it suitable for innovative applications such as nutrient encapsulation and delivery, edible coatings and fat substitutes. The shift towards natural ingredients in the food industry and the strategic avoidance of new food phobias have also contributed to the acceptance of sucralose. The growing awareness of health and wellness makes sucralose chemically stable, widely sustainable and the trend towards natural ingredients an attractive option for consumers who seek to reduce sugar consumption or manage their weight (Siddiqui *et al.* 2022).

3 INTESTINAL HORMONES

3.1 *Definition of glucagon*

Glucagon is a peptide hormone produced by alpha cells in the pancreas, specifically in the pancreatic islets. It maintains blood sugar levels by stimulating the liver to convert stored glycogen into glucose, which is then released into the bloodstream. This counter-regulatory mechanism is essential to prevent hypoglycaemia, especially during fasting or hypoglycaemia. Glucagon secretion is influenced by glucose concentration, amino acids and other hormones. Almaça *et al.* revealed that human β-cells produce and secrete serotonin, which inhibits glucagon secretion from α-cells by decreasing cyclic AMP (cAMP) levels (Almaça *et al.* 2016). The biological function of glucagon is not limited to glucose regulation. It has been found to interact with other hormones, such as growth hormone-releasing peptide, which directly stimulates glucagon secretion from pancreatic α-cells (Chuang *et al.* 2011).

3.2 *Definition of PYY*

PYY is an intestinal-derived hormone secreted primarily by enteroendocrine L cells located in the distal intestine that acts as a satiety signal, reduces food intake and regulates energy homeostasis (Kerem and Lawson 2021), PYY is secreted into the bloodstream primarily after a meal, hence the name 'postprandial' (Alhussain *et al.* 2016). once released, PYY acts as an anorexic factor, i.e., suppresses hunger. This is achieved by signalling a satiety or fullness state to the brain, thus ensuring that people do not consume more food than necessary (Alhussain *et al.* 2016). the complex interplay between PYY, appetite control and the regulation of energy metabolism attests to its important role in ensuring energy balance in the body (Yoshikawa 2011). This balance is essential for maintaining optimal health and preventing diseases such as obesity.

3.3 *Definition of GIP*

GIP is an important incretin hormone that is synthesised and secreted mainly by specialised endocrine cells located within the intestinal mucosa (Deacon and Ahrén 2011). The secretion of GIP is subject to a complex regulation that is mainly triggered by ingested nutrients. Notably, macronutrients such as carbohydrates, fats and proteins are potent stimulators of its release (Deacon and Ahrén 2011). Mechanistically, the main physiological action of GIP is to promote insulin secretion from pancreatic β-cells in a glucose-dependent manner. This action ensures that postprandial glucose concentrations are carefully regulated and maintained within physiological ranges (Kim and Lee 2010). In addition to its role in glucose homeostasis, GIP has been shown to regulate a variety of cell signalling pathways. Of particular importance is its interaction with the Akt/protein kinase B pathway, which plays a key role in ensuring the survival, proliferation and optimal function of pancreatic β-cells (Widenmaier *et al.* 2009). The dynamics of GIP, including its secretion and action, have been observed in the broader context of health and disease in pathological conditions such as type 2 diabetes mellitus (T2DM). In the setting of T2DM, the delicate balance between insulin secretion and peripheral insulin sensitivity is disturbed, thus increasing the importance of the regulatory role of GIP.

4 RESPONSE OF SUCRALOSE TO INTESTINAL HORMONES

4.1 *Response of sucralose to GLP-1*

In the study conducted by Ma *et al.* seven healthy individuals participated in the experiment. These participants underwent an intragastric infusion under four different conditions.

Specifically, these conditions included sucrose dissolved in water, two different concentrations of sucralose (sucralose) in saline, and saline itself. It is worth noting that the sucrose used for the infusion was labelled with ^{13}C acetate. As demonstrated in Figure 1, sucralose does not affect GLP-1 when injected intragastrically in humans, regardless of whether the concentration is matched to sucrose (0.4 mM) or higher (4 mM) (Ma *et al.* 2009). In contrast, rodent model studies have shown that sucralose stimulates GLP-1 production in mice through activation of sweet taste receptors on enteroendocrine cells. However, human trials have contradicted this, suggesting that intragastric administration of sucralose does not stimulate GLP-1 secretion and does not reduce the rate of gastric emptying (Olsson *et al.* 2006).

In a controlled experimental setting involving healthy participants, it was observed that a single oral dose of sucralose, ranging from 48 mg to 52 mg, did not produce any significant effect on the response to GLP-1. glucose load (Pepino *et al.* 2013). This finding suggests that sucralose may not interfere with physiological mechanisms controlling glucose homeostasis in healthy individuals in this specific dose range.

Another study conducted by Lertrit *et al.* suggested that chronic sucralose exposure in healthy populations may have effects on glucose metabolism and GLP-1 secretion (Lertrit *et al.* 2018). Specifically, their findings showed that oral administration of 200 mg sucralose per day for four weeks resulted in decreased systemic and hepatic insulin sensitivity. This was evidenced by a diminished insulin response, reduced insulin sensitivity and a significant increase in the area under the curve of active GLP-1.

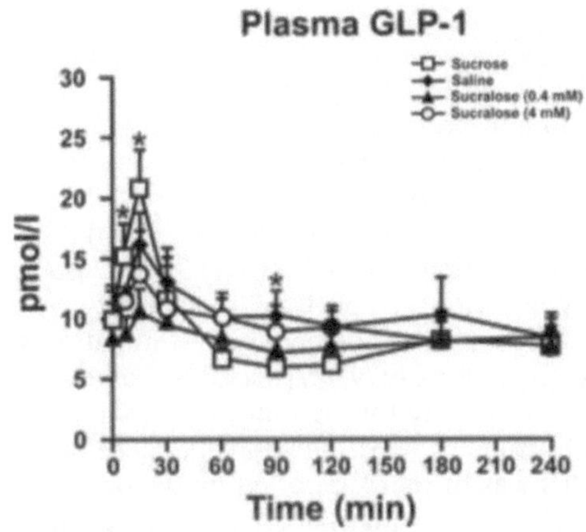

Figure 1. The effects of sucralose on GLP-1 (Ma *et al.* 2009).

4.2 *Response of sucralose to GIP*

In a comprehensive study led by Ma et al, researchers scrutinised the potential effects of sucralose on GIP secretion in healthy human subjects (Ma *et al.* 2009). As shown in Figure 2 they administered sucralose intragastrically at two different concentrations (i.e., 0.4 mM and 4 mM). Their results showed that this administration did not result in any significant changes in GIP secretion, suggesting that sucralose may not affect the physiological release of this specific peptide in these concentration ranges.

In a parallel study focusing on oral intake of sucralose, it was observed that mean plasma GIP concentrations were generally elevated following sucralose ingestion compared to water alone. However, it is worth noting that this elevation was minimal and the difference was not considered significant from a statistical point of view ($P=0.08$) (Pepino *et al.* 2013). This suggests that although there may be a tendency for GIP levels to increase following sucralose ingestion, the magnitude of this change is not sufficient to be clinically or biologically significant.

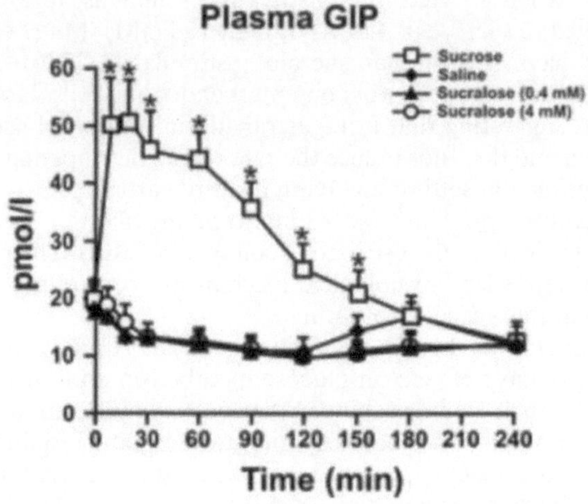

Figure 2. The potential effects of sucralose on GIP secretion in healthy human subjects (Ma *et al.* 2009).

4.3 *Response of sucralose to PYY*

In a well-designed study conducted by Ford *et al.* eight young volunteers, consisting primarily of females (n=7) and one male participant, were recruited for the survey. These participants were characterised by normal weight and overall health status and were aged between 22 and 27 years. The test solution consisted of 1.50 ml of plain water as a control.2. Sucralose solution at a concentration of 0.083% (w/v).3. Glucose polymer solution fortified with sucralose, specifically consisting of 50% maltodextrin (w/v) and 0.083% sucralose.4. Modified Sham-Feeding (MSF) protocol, where oral stimulation was provided by an oral stimulus at a concentration of 0.083% (w/v). /v) sucralose solution was provided. Systematic measurements were taken periodically throughout the experiment to assess appetite ratings and PYY levels. The final results showed that oral sucralose did not cause any significant increase in PYY levels. This was further supported by the observation that the incremental area under the curve (iAUC) of the plasma PYY concentration over a 120-min period remained consistent across all four treatment groups. This suggests that under the conditions of the present study, sucralose intake does not modulate PYY secretion in a manner that may affect appetite in healthy young people (Ford *et al.* 2011).

5 CONCLUSION

The physiological effects of artificial sweeteners (especially sucralose) on gastrointestinal hormone secretion have become a focus of attention during the ongoing evolution of dietary composition. The complex dance of gastrointestinal hormones comprising key peptides such as GLP-1, GIP and PYY plays a key role in numerous physiological processes such as appetite regulation, nutrient absorption and metabolic homeostasis.

These findings highlight that despite its widespread use as a calorie-free sweetener, sucralose has minimal impact on the secretion of these key gut hormones in healthy individuals. Specifically, the secretion and function of GLP-1, a hormone inextricably linked to insulin secretion and appetite suppression, was largely unaffected by acute ingestion of sucralose, even at higher dose ranges. This observation is particularly noteworthy given the critical role of GLP-1 in glucose homeostasis and its potential impact on metabolic health. Similarly, GIP, another important incretin hormone associated with insulin secretion and lipid storage, showed no significant changes in its secretion pattern after sucralose administration. This suggests that sucralose largely did not interfere with the physiological mechanisms of GIP release, thus reinforcing its inertia in incretin regulation. Furthermore, the regulation of PYY, a hormone closely related to appetite suppression and gastric emptying rate, remained consistent across sucralose intake. The absence of significant changes in PYY levels after sucralose intake emphasises the neutral position of sweeteners in appetite regulation and overall metabolic regulation.

In conclusion, the physiological profile of gastrointestinal hormone secretion in healthy individuals appears to be largely undisturbed by sucralose intake. These findings provide a foundation for understanding the broader effects of sucralose in the diet and emphasise the importance of continued research in this area. As the consumption of artificial sweeteners continues to rise, it is imperative to understand their subtle effects on human health and ensure that consumers are equipped with the knowledge to make informed dietary choices.

REFERENCES

Alhussain M. H., Macdonald I. A. and Taylor M. A., (2016). *Am J Clin Nutr*, **104(1)**, 21–32.

Almaça J., Molina J., Menegaz D., Pronin A. N., Tamayo A., Slepak V., Berggren P. O. and Caicedo A., (2016). *Cell Rep*, **17(12)**, 3281–3291.

Baird I. M., Shephard N. W., Merritt R. J. and Hildick-Smith G., (2000). *Food Chem Toxicol*, **38**, 123–129.

Chuang J. C., Sakata I., Kohno D., Perello M., Osborne-Lawrence S., Repa J. J. and Zigman J. M., (2011). *Mol Endocrinol*, **25(9)**, 1600–1611.

Deacon C. F. and Ahrén B., (2011). *Rev Diabet Stud*, **8(3)**, 293.

Dyab A., El-Tukhy H. M., Ghazal G. A., Mahmoud M. H. and Abolila R. M., (2021). *Egyptian Journal of Food Science*, **49(2)**, 239–248.

Ford H. E., Peters V., Martin N. M., Sleeth M. L., Ghatei M. A., Frost G. S. and Bloom S. R., (2011). *Eur J Clin Nutr*, **65(4)**, 508–513.

Grice H. and Goldsmith L., (2000). *Food Chem Toxicol*, **38**, 1–6.

Hassoun A., Cropotova J., Trif M., Rusu A. V., Bobiş O., Nayik G. A., Jagdale Y. D., Saeed Afzaal F. and Mostashari P. M., (2022). *Front Nutr*, **9**, 972154.

Kerem L. and Lawson E. A., (2021). *Int J Mol Sci*, **22(14)**, 7737.

Kim M. H. and Lee M. K., (2010). *Korean Diabetes J*, **34(1)**, 2–9.

Lertrit A., Srimachai S., Saetung S., Chanprasertyothin S., Chailurkit L., Areevut C., Katekao P., Ongphiphadhanakul B. and Sriphrapradang C., (2018). *Nutrition*, **55**, 125–130.

Ma J., Bellon M.,Wishart J. M., Young R., Blackshaw L. A, Jones K. L., Horowitz M. and Rayner C. K., (2009). *Am J Physiol Gastrointest Liver Physiol*, **296(4)**, G735–G739.

Olsson C., Chen B. N., Jones S., Chataway T. K., Costa M. and Brookes S. J. H., (2006). *J Comp Neurol*, **496 (6)**, 787–801.

Pepino M. Y., Tiemann C. D., Patterson B. W., Wice B. M. and Klein S., (2013). *Diabetes Care*, **36(9)**, 2530–2535.

Siddiqui S. A., Zannou O., Karim I., Kasmiati, Awad N. M. H., Gołaszewski J., Heinz V. and Smetana S., (2022). *Sustainability*, **14(16)**, 10391.

Sims J., Roberts A., Daniel J. W. and Renwick A. G., (2000). *Food Chem Toxicol*, **38**, 115–121.

Widenmaier S. B., Sampaio A. V., Underhill T. M. and McIntosh C. H. S., (2009). *J Biol Chem*, **284(16)**, 10764–10773.

Yoshikawa T., (2011). *Update on Mechanisms of Hormone Action-Focus on Metabolism, Growth and Reproduction* (IntechOpen).

Biological Sciences and Environmental Health – Gao (Ed.)
© 2025 the Author(s), ISBN: 978-1-032-96016-6

Malnutrition problems caused by vitamin deficiency in African countries

Yixuan Sun
Windermere Preparatory School, Windermere, Florida, USA

ABSTRACT: Malnutrition, a global health issue, is particularly prevalent in many African nations, resulting from inadequate nutrient consumption, frequent infections, socio-economic challenges, lack of nutrition education, and political instability. This paper discusses the malnutrition problems in African countries, focusing on protein and vitamin deficiencies and the holistic approach necessary for addressing the issue. Malnutrition manifests as Protein-Energy Malnutrition (PEM) and micronutrient deficiencies, affecting primarily children under five and expectant mothers. Factors contributing to malnutrition include poverty, lack of education, cultural beliefs, and environmental factors. The impact of malnutrition on health and development includes stunted growth, cognitive impairment, decreased work efficiency, and economic consequences. Current strategies to address malnutrition involve government policies, international assistance, and community-based approaches but face challenges such as corruption, insufficient funding, and coordination deficits. Proposed solutions include enhancing food availability through agricultural development, food fortification, distribution of supplements, education and awareness programs, partnerships with NGOs and international organizations, and robust monitoring and evaluation. In conclusion, addressing malnutrition in Africa requires a multifaceted approach involving improved agricultural practices, education, international collaborations, and continuous program evaluation.

1 INTRODUCTION

Malnutrition is a condition that develops from poor diets or eating habits which need to provide more or more of one or more nutrients. Nutrients are substances found in food essential for an organism's survival, reproduction, and growth (Sawe and Keino 2022). The macronutrients are building blocks of a person's diet and are usually consumed in large amounts as they provide energy to the body. Minerals and vitamins are called micronutrients as they are consumed and required in small quantities but perform a vital role in the body for a long time. Vitamin deficiency means the body is not getting enough of these essential micronutrients to function effectively. Vitamins are indispensable in ensuring health and vitality. They facilitate critical bodily functions, including energy generation, immune system operations, blood coagulation, and other essential processes. As a result, a dearth of any particular vitamin can manifest in various health issues, ranging from mild symptoms like fatigue to severe conditions like scurvy or rickets (Oldewage-Theron and Grobler 2021).

Malnutrition is a widespread and pressing global health issue, with a particularly significant presence in many African nations. This multifaceted problem does not stem from a single cause but from myriad interrelated factors. One of the primary reasons is inadequate nutrient consumption. Many individuals in these regions need access to a balanced diet, leading to deficiencies in essential vitamins and minerals (Finlay and Darnton-Hill 2001). Additionally, frequent infections, often due to limited access to clean water and proper sanitation,

 DOI: 10.1201/9781003587590-45

exacerbate the situation by weakening the immune system and reducing the body's ability to absorb nutrients. Beyond these immediate causes, there are other foundational determinants, including socio-economic challenges, lack of education about proper nutrition, and even political instability, which can disrupt food supply chains. Addressing malnutrition, therefore, requires a holistic approach that considers all these underlying factors (Zuma and Modi 2022). This paper discusses malnutrition problems caused by deficiencies in protein and vitamin deficiency in African countries and the holistic approach necessary for addressing the issue.

2 TYPES OF MALNUTRITION PREVALENT IN AFRICAN COUNTRIES

Across the African continent, malnutrition presents itself in multiple guises.

2.1 *Protein-Energy Malnutrition (PEM)*

PEM is the most fatal form of malnutrition. Protein-Energy Malnutrition (PEM) is a severe health concern primarily impacting children under five. This condition is characterized by a marked deficiency in calories and protein, essential for growth and development (Sifri *et al.* 2002). There are two primary manifestations of PEM: Kwashiorkor and Marasmus. Kwashiorkor arises primarily from a deficiency in protein intake, leading to symptoms like swelling, liver enlargement, and skin disorders.

On the other hand, Marasmus results from a severe caloric deficiency, causing extreme thinness and muscle wasting (Jones *et al.* 2018). Children suffering from PEM often exhibit a range of concerning symptoms. These include stunted growth, which can have long-term implications for their physical development. Their immune systems are also compromised, making them more susceptible to infections and diseases. Additionally, cognitive setbacks are expected, with affected children facing challenges in learning and memory. Addressing PEM is crucial, as it can impact a child's health and future potential.

2.2 *Micronutrient deficiencies*

Often referred to as "hidden hunger," micronutrient deficiencies might not be as overt as PEM but are equally harmful (Sondo *et al.* 2021). This is because although they are only required in small quantities, the impact of micronutrients on the body's health is crucial. Any deficiencies might cause severe and life-threatening conditions. These micronutrients participate in several bodily functions, including producing hormones, enzymes, and other bodily messengers essential for average growth and development. Commonly observed deficiencies encompass iron, iodine, vitamin A, and zinc. Such deficiencies can precipitate conditions like anemia, blindness, cognitive impairment, and heightened infection vulnerability (Ssentongo *et al.* 2021).

2.3 *Demographics most affected*

Although malnutrition can afflict individuals across all age brackets, children below five years and expectant mothers remain the most susceptible. In Africa, rural inhabitants, refugees, and internally displaced individuals confront elevated risks, primarily due to constrained access to nutritious sustenance and medical care (Schoeman *et al.* 2020).

3 ANALYSIS OF MALNUTRITION PROBLEMS IN AFRICAN COUNTRIES

3.1 *Factors contributing to malnutrition*

Africa has had to grapple with much more regarding the malnutrition burden; Africa accounts for 30% of malnourished children worldwide. Studies established that countries in

West and East Africa bear the most significant burden of malnutrition globally (Obasohan *et al.* 2020). With undernutrition as the prevalent form of malnutrition, several factors underpin the rampant malnutrition observed in Africa.

3.1.1 *Poverty and economic constraints*

Poverty is the primary factor for malnutrition across Africa as it influences the people's ability to access adequate food, quality healthcare, education, and sanitation (Raut *et al.* 2018). Financially strained families often grapple with procuring nutritious sustenance, culminating in diets devoid of essential vitamins and minerals.

3.1.2 *Lack of education*

The vicious cycle of poverty increases due to poor education, as most families cannot access quality formal education. This does not only impair civilization and the family's ability to have a successful future but also to live a healthy life. As a result, the absence of nutritional awareness can culminate in suboptimal dietary selections, even when resources are accessible (Zeba *et al.* 2014).

3.1.3 *Cultural beliefs*

Certain cultural norms and practices can inadvertently intensify malnutrition (Lusamba-Dikassa 2019). For instance, some communities might allocate more food to male members or harbor reservations against consuming specific nutrient-rich edibles. Meanwhile, certain nutritious foods have been restricted to a particular gender or age group, thus impairing nutrition.

3.1.4 *Environmental factors*

Environmental adversities like droughts and floods can disrupt agricultural yields, leading to food shortages and escalating malnutrition (Figure 1) (Jonah *et al.* 2018). Food shortages from environmental catastrophes have adversely affected the continent as most of its population relies on agriculture as its significant socio-economic activity. Also referred to as food insecurity, unfavorable weather patterns have interrupted Africa's food supply, especially among low-income families relying on farms for food.

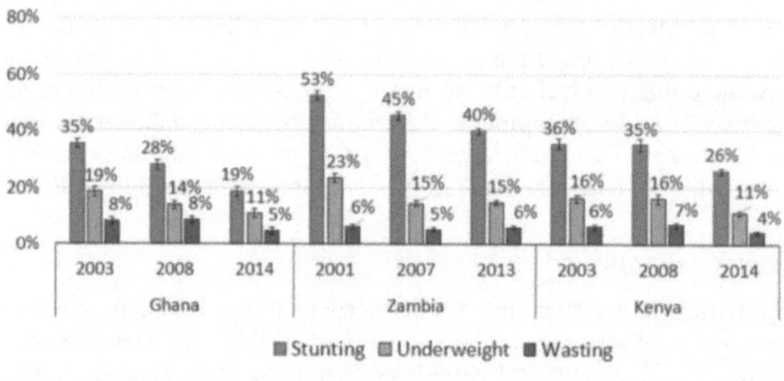

Figure 1. Levels of malnutrition in Ghana, Kenya, and Zambia (Jonah *et al.* 2018).

3.2 *Impact on health and development*

3.2.1 *Child growth and development*

Malnourished children frequently exhibit stunted physical growth, cognitive lags, and diminished immune responses, rendering them more prone to illnesses (Prioreschi *et al.* 2017). The deficiency in certain micro and macro nutrients impairs a child's growth and development in several ways. This includes delayed motor skills and physical growth, decreased intellectual capacity, poor social skills, and behavioral problems.

3.2.2 *Impact on ADULT Health*

In adults, malnutrition can diminish work efficiency, heightened disease susceptibility, and complications during gestation (Alem *et al.* 2023). This is because the body lacks the necessary nutrients to sustain itself. As a result, the body begins breaking down or using some of its tissues and shutting down some essential functions, thus decreasing work efficiency.

3.2.3 *Economic consequences*

Malnutrition can stymie a nation's economic ascent (Herrador *et al.* 2014). A workforce plagued by malnutrition is inherently less productive, and the financial burden of addressing malnutrition-linked ailments can strain healthcare infrastructures. Besides, an unhealthy population is unproductive, thus impairing economic growth.

3.3 *Regional variations in malnutrition*

Disparities in malnutrition rates are evident across African nations and regions (Ahmed *et al.* 2016). Climatic conditions, political stability, and infrastructural robustness can shape these variations. With favorable climatic conditions, political stability, and a well-developed infrastructural system, parts of African regions enjoy economic growth, decreased poverty, food security, and improved health outcomes.

4 CURRENT STRATEGIES FOR MALNUTRITION

4.1 *Government policies and interventions*

Numerous African governments have rolled out policies and initiatives to counteract malnutrition, encompassing measures like school meal programs and public health drives (Delange and West 2003). This strategy immediately addresses malnutrition by ensuring families and children can access nutritious food. This was particularly important during the COVID-19 pandemic and other natural disasters such as droughts, conflicts, and violence. However, this strategy needs to provide a long-term solution to the malnutrition problem in Africa.

4.2 *International assistance*

Global entities like UNICEF and the World Food Programme extend aid, which includes food distribution endeavors and nutritional education initiatives (Aguiar *et al.* 2020). International aid from these global international entities is an intervention or a short-term solution to the malnutrition problem in Africa. This is because the initiatives are primarily targeted toward areas or regions worst affected or at the highest risk of experiencing malnutrition.

4.3 *Community-based approaches*

Grassroots movements, frequently spearheaded by local NGOs, emphasize community farming projects, nutritional education, and indigenous solutions to combat malnutrition (Gernand *et al.* 2016). These long-term solutions focus on alleviating Africa's malnutrition problem by empowering local communities. These community-based programs ensure that communities know and know the available solutions, such as drought-resistant food crops, improved farming techniques, and alternative nutritious food sources.

4.4 *Successes and failures of current strategies*

While specific strategies have curtailed malnutrition rates, corruption, insufficient funding, and coordination deficits can impede their efficacy (Bain *et al.* 2013). As a result, the problem of malnutrition continues to persist despite the development and implementation of various strategies. Corruption due to poor leadership at the national level leads to poor implementation of the developed programs or initiatives. The misappropriation of funds allocated for short-term interventions such as school feeding programs has derailed and impaired the approach's effectiveness. Additionally, inadequate funding due to corruption from poor leadership has influenced how the strategies are implemented. Also, since the different programs have different objectives and are applied across different regions in Africa, the inefficiency of the programs due to poor coordination is bound to be a problem.

5 SOLUTIONS AND RECOMMENDATIONS

Despite developing and implementing several strategic interventions to address malnutrition among African communities, the problem persists. This could be attributed to several factors, including poor agricultural practices (Hwang *et al.* 2012). Figure 2 below shows the different sources of staple foods in West and East Africa.

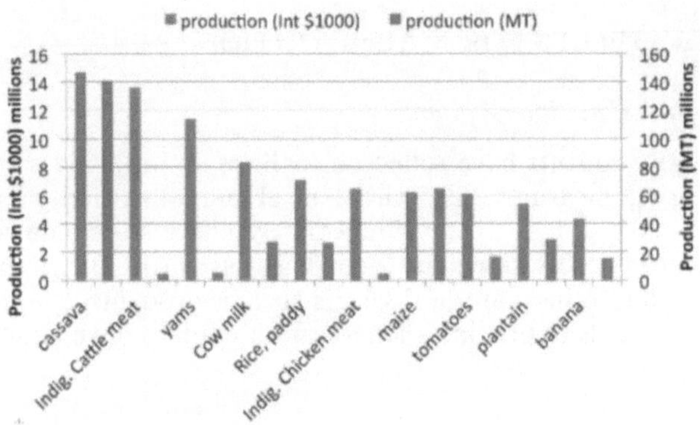

Figure 2. The highest valued and produced foods in West and East Africa. Data from FAO STAT (2015).

5.1 *Enhancing food availability*

This means developing programs and initiatives to help Africa achieve sustainable and equitable socio-economic growth. This is because malnutrition impairs growth and development among children and economic growth due to poor education, decreased intellectual ability, and poor work efficiency, thus the vicious cycle of poverty (Mukisa and Shumba 2023). However, enhancing food availability would improve nutrition and thus address poverty to some extent.

5.1.1 *Agricultural development*

Championing sustainable agricultural practices can bolster food production, ensuring a consistent supply of nutritious edibles (Aryeetey and Covic 2020). This is particularly important since most African families rely on agriculture and farming for food. Agricultural developments mean introducing modern and sustainable farming techniques, such as the growth of climate-resistant crops using environmentally friendly farming techniques.

5.1.2 *Food fortification*

Enriching staple foods with vital vitamins and minerals can address specific micronutrient shortfalls (Oldewage-Theron 2021). This solution involves educating the communities on alternative nutritious food sources and accompaniments from well-known staple foods. For instance, since maize, rice, and cassava are stable foods across several communities, other alternatives such as millet, sorghum, and wheat could be combined with other foods such as beans, peas, and green grams, among others, and introduced to these communities.

5.1.3 *Distribution of supplements*

Administering vitamin and mineral supplements can swiftly rectify deficiencies, especially among high-risk demographics (Cloete and Idsardi 2013). This involves the provision of diet supplements through food distribution programs such as school feeding initiatives. This is an effective intervention in helping those worst affected or at the highest risk of experiencing malnutrition.

5.2 *Education and awareness*

This approach mainly involves empowering the communities to adopt alternative techniques, food sources, or dietary habits to restore health and alleviate malnutrition.

5.2.1 *Community education programs*

Imparting nutritional knowledge within communities can foster improved dietary decisions (Delisle *et al.* 2021). This involves conducting campaigns on diet and nutrition to educate and empower the community. The education programs conducted through campaigns would focus on equipping the public, more so mothers, with appropriate knowledge on diets and nutrition that promote optimum growth and development.

5.3 *Training for healthcare providers*

Equipping healthcare professionals with the skills to identify and manage malnutrition can enhance patient outcomes (Caleyachetty *et al.* 2022). This means training and educating healthcare professionals on malnutrition through seminars, workshops, and webinars. Equipping healthcare professionals with appropriate knowledge helps develop early intervention plans among malnourished families and communities. This approach would help decrease the fatalities or consequences of malnutrition.

5.4 *Partnerships and collaborations*

Collaboratively working with one another through partnerships with international agencies, such as UNICEF and WFP, would help develop and implement effective strategies to eradicate malnutrition in Africa.

5.4.1 *Working with NGOs*

Collaborative endeavors with NGOs can harness their expertise and resources to address malnutrition (Tirivangasi 2018). Locally based organizations or government agencies could provide insights into the types and causes of malnutrition within the community, which would be addressed using the NGOs' resources. This approach would ensure that resources are allocated and managed appropriately according to the severity of the problem, thus enhancing its effectiveness through improved coordination. This would be achieved through the partnership of NGOs with other agencies in addressing malnutrition.

5.4.2 *Collaborating with international organizations*

Partnerships with international organizations can offer financial support, specialized knowledge, and logistical assistance (Onyeak *et al.* 2021). One of the challenges in addressing malnutrition in Africa was inadequate funding, which can be addressed through partnerships with international organizations. This means that national governments should collaborate with international organizations such as the WFP and UNICEF to develop and implement effective food programs that address malnutrition across the continent.

5.5 *Monitoring and evaluation*

This approach aims to enhance accountability and transparency during the development and implementation of various programs (Delisle and Faber 2021). This step also assesses the program's effectiveness in addressing malnutrition in Africa.

5.5.1 *Developing robust data collection*

Accurate data capturing malnutrition rates and causative factors can guide impactful interventions (Haradhan 2022). This involves using appropriate tools to collect relevant data on the severity and situation of malnutrition across different regions. Accurate data would provide insights into the prevalence of malnutrition and the effectiveness of the interventions.

5.5.2 *Continuous evaluation of programs*

Periodic assessments of malnutrition-focused initiatives ensure they achieve their objectives and facilitate necessary adjustments. This involves collecting relevant data and information on the different implemented programs and assessing their effectiveness in achieving the desired outcomes (Olanbiwoninu *et al.* 2023). These continuous evaluations promote accountability and highlight the factors that need improvements to enhance the program's effectiveness.

6 CONCLUSION

In conclusion, although the past few decades have witnessed extensive economic growth globally, including some of the poorest countries in Africa, millions are still locked in the vicious cycle of hunger and poverty. This means some parents cannot feed their children or families nutritious food, causing malnutrition. Malnutrition due to the deficiency of essential micronutrients has several irreversible effects, such as stunted growth and development among children and poor productivity among adults. The adults cannot work effectively and earn a living as poor diets have decreased their body energy levels, thus the inability to earn a living or escape the cycle of poverty. Poor education among African communities, especially among women, is a major causative factor of malnutrition across the continent. Without knowing what diet or foods provide the essential nutrients the body requires, most families or communities continue consuming what they are used to, hence the deficiencies. Long-term solutions to the problem of malnutrition across the continent include enhancing the availability of foods by changing the existing agricultural practices, partnerships, and collaborations with international agencies, as well as effective monitoring and evaluating the effectiveness of the proposed strategies.

REFERENCES

Aguiar M., Andronis L., Pallan M., Högler W. and Frew E., (2020). *Public Health Nutr.* **23**,1165–1172.
Ahmed F., Prendiville N. and Narayan A., (2016). *J Nutr Sci.* **5**, e46.

Alem A. Z, Yeshaw Y., Liyew A.M. and Z. T, (2023). *BMC Public Health.* **23**, 1479.
Aryeetey R. and Covic N. (2020). *Food Nutr Bull.* **41**, 380–396.
Bain L. E., Awah P.K., Geraldine N., Kindong N. P, Sigal Y., Bernard N. and Tanjeko A. T., (2013). *Pan Afr Med* J. **15**, 120.
Caleyachetty R., Kumar N. S. and Bekele H., (2022). *Med Rxiv Preprint.* 367.
Cloete P.C. and Idsardi E. F., (2013). *Agroecol. Sustain. Food Syst.* **37**, 902.
Delange F. and West K. P., (2003). *Nestle Nutr. Inst. Workshop Ser.* **52.**
Delisle H. and Faber M., (2021). *Public Health Nutr.* **24**, 3577–3580 .
Delisle H., Faber M. and Revault P., (2021). *Public Health Nutr.* **24**, 3577–3580.
Egal, W. (2021). Oldewage-Theron, *South Afr J Clin Nutr.* **33**, 142–143.
Finlay D. and Darnton-Hill I., (2001). *Food Nutr Bull* **22,** 469.
Gernand A.D., Schulze K. J., Stewart C. P., West JR K. P. and Christan P., (2016) *Nat. Rev. Endocrinol.* **12**, 274–89.
Haradhan M., *JEDEP.* **11**, 24–34 (2022).
Herrador Z., Sordo L., Gadisa E., Gadisa E., Buñoet A., Gómez-Rioja R., Iturzaeta J. M., Armas L. F .D., Benito A., Aseffa A., Moreno J., Cañavate C. and Custodio E., (2014). *PLoS One.* **9**, e112858.
Hwang C., Mahadevan V. and Ross. U., (2012). *Inflamm Bowel Dis.* **18**, 1961–81.
Jonah C.M. P., Sambu W.C. and May J. D, (2018). *Arch Public Health* **76**, 77.
Jones K. D. J., Hachmeister C. U, Khasira M., L. Cox, Schoenmakers I., Munyi C., Nassir H. S., Hünten-Kirsch B., Prentice A. and Berkley J. A., (2018). *Matern Child Nutr.* **14**, e12452.
Lusamba-Dikassa P.S., Nsue-Milang D. and Okello D., (2019). *AJFAND* **12.**
Mukisa G.W. and Shumba T.W.A. (2023). *Lourens Nutr Health,* **2023**, 02601060231185815 (2023).
Obasohan P.E., Walters S. J., Jacques R. and Khatab K., (2020). *Int J Environ Res Public Health* **17**, 8782.
Olanbiwoninu, Greppi A. and Awotundun T., (2023). *Food Biosci.* **55**, 102996.
Oldewage-Theron W. and Grobler C., *Curr Dev Nutr* **7**, 172.
Onyeaka H., Agbugba I. and Ekwebelem O. C., (2021). *Eur. J. Nutr.* **13**, 104.
Prioreschi, Wrottesley S., Draper C. E., Tomaz S. A., Cooket C. J., Watson E. D., Van Poppel M. N. M., Said-Mohamed R., Norris S. A, Lambert E. V. and Micklesfield L. K., (2017). *Glob Health Action.* **10**, 1301085 (2017).
Raut M.K, JReddy J.C. and Bera K D., (2018). *IJCMPH* **6**, 395–411.
Sawe C. and S. Keino, *Curr Dev Nutr* **6**, 171 (2022).
Schoeman J., Kellerman I.M. and Rogers P.C., (2023). *Pediatr Hematol Oncol* 1–14
Sifri Z., Darnton-Hill D. I., Baker S. K, Ag Bendech M., Baker S. K. and Aguayo V. M., (2002). *AJFAND. Dev.* **2**, 78.
Sondo P., Tahita M.C., Rouamba T., erra K. D, Kaboré B, Compaoré C. S, Ouédraogo F., Rouamba E., Ilboudo H., Bambara E. A., Nana M., Sawadogo E. Y., Sorgho H, Somé A. M., Valéa I., Dahal P., Traoré M., Tinto C. and Tinto H., (2021). *Trials* **22**, 360.
Ssentongo P., Ba D.M., Ssentongo A.E., Fronterre C., Whalen A., Yang Y., Ericson J. E. and Chinchilli V. M. (2021). *PLoS One* **16**, e0250138.
Tirivangasi H. M., (2018). *Jamba.* **10**, 468.
Zeba A.N., Delisle H.F. and Renier G., (2014). *J Nutr Sci.* **3**, e50.
Zuma M. and Modi U. A., (2022). *AJFAND* **22**, 19230.

Biological Sciences and Environmental Health – Gao (Ed.)
© 2025 the Author(s), ISBN: 978-1-032-96016-6

Deficient nutrition intake and overtraining in female CrossFit athletes

Yumeng He
Rabun Gap Nacoochee School, Rabun Gap, USA

ABSTRACT: CrossFit training aims to improve overall health and physical conditioning, making it a popular activity across different age groups and genders. Its adaptable nature allows people of various fitness levels to join and benefit from the workouts. However, a concerning trend of deficient nutrition intake and excessive training has been observed among female CrossFit athletes. This study analyzes the macronutrient intake of this group, focusing on their dietary patterns and exercise intensity. Training load was assessed through a comparison with biomarkers and recovery status. A deficiency in carbohydrates, particularly in relation to the 4:3:3 macronutrient ratio of carbohydrate, fat, and protein diet, was found to be a primary problem. The lack of attention toward increased micronutrient needs in dietary intake, combined with overburden from inappropriate training intensity, results in poor recovery from elevated hormone levels and inflammatory and oxidative damage. This can result in a higher risk of stress fracture and infection, reduced muscle adaptation, and impaired performance. Addressing the increased micronutrient requirements in general, and specifically for women, shall be considered. Supportive educational programs could improve the overall condition of this popular sport.

1 INTRODUCTION

CrossFit is a high-intensity, interval training program that combines a variety of aerobic and anaerobic exercises. Workouts typically include cardiovascular activities such as biking, running, and rowing, along with resistance activities such as deadlifts and squats. The goal of this comprehensive functional training is to improve overall health and physical attributes, including strength, endurance, agility, flexibility, and balance. With its easy accessibility to local gyms and adaptive training plans suited to people of various fitness levels, CrossFit has gained increasing popularity in recent years.

While pursuing a lean body shape and better performance, female CrossFit athletes engage in extremely high-intensity training at a high-frequency level. However, the dietary intake recommended by the official training guide struggles to meet even basic macronutrient requirements. Furthermore, the elevated micronutrient needs essential for women, especially for post-exercise recovery, are not addressed at all. As more individuals take up CrossFit, it is crucial to understand the balance between training intensity and nutritional needs to ensure healthy and safe training.

This paper aims to explore the phenomenon of unbalanced nutrition intake and overtraining in female CrossFit athletes. By assessing the macronutrient status of female CrossFitters, the study highlights potential flaws in the dietary structure recommended on the official CrossFit website.

DOI: 10.1201/9781003587590-46

2 DIETARY PATTERN

The CrossFit Level 1 Training Guide (2020) recommends the zone diet to athletes, introducing it as a performance-maximizing and disease-minimizing meal plan. The guide summarizes the diet principle of consuming "meat and vegetables, nuts and seeds, some fruit, little starch, and no sugar." The diet assigned the macronutrients into blocks, where 1 block of protein equals 7g of protein, 1 block of carbohydrate equals 9g of carbohydrate, and 1 block of fat equals 3g of fat. To follow this meal plan, individuals are advised to consume the same number of blocks of each nutrient per meal.

2.1 *Carbohydrate*

When the zone diet is followed accurately, the energy provided by carbs, fat, and protein is in the ratio of 4:3:3. However, according to the 2020–2025 Dietary Guidelines for Americans, individuals of all sexes over the age of two should gain 45%–65% of their daily calorie intake from carbohydrates (US Department of Agriculture and US Department of Health and Human Services 2020). The diet is 5% off the lower limit recommended by the Acceptable Macronutrients Distribution Range (AMDR).

The carbohydrate insufficiency in the diet becomes even more apparent when considering the exercise level of CrossFit athletes. Daily training of CrossFit athletes focuses on both resistance and endurance capacity, activating a mix of anaerobic and aerobic metabolic pathways. Carbohydrates serve as the primary energy source for both systems. During resistance training that requires short bursts of explosive power (such as pull-ups), ATP is rapidly produced from glucose in the blood without the presence of oxygen. Due to limited ATP production and accumulation of lactate in muscle, this anaerobic pathway is inefficient and only lasts less than two minutes. Endurance training, which lasts longer than two minutes, also depends heavily on carbohydrates as the primary fuel source. In this case, glucose is broken down into two pyruvate molecules, which enter the citric acid cycle and eventually produce over 30 ATP molecules in the electron transport chain with the presence of oxygen. This aerobic pathway dominates much of CrossFit training.

Either the anaerobic or aerobic metabolism utilizes glucose from blood or muscle glycogen stored as the primary fuel source. A typical CrossFit workout incorporates both fueling systems, thus drastically increasing the rate of glucose depletion in the body. To support this, the International Society of Sports Nutrition recommends consuming 5–8 g of carbohydrates (CHO) per kilogram of body mass to maintain adequate glycogen levels before, during, and after exercise (Kerksick *et al.* 2018). A study carried out by Capistrano *et al.* (2022) discovered an average carbohydrate intake of 4.5 g/kg body mass among Brazilian female CrossFit athletes. Similarly, Gogojewicz *et al.* (2020) reported an even lower average carbohydrate intake of 3.9 g/kg body mass. The data points to a significant carbohydrate and overall energy deficit among female CrossFit athletes.

Adequate carbohydrates replenish the depleted glycogen stored in muscle through glycogenesis. Without sufficient carbohydrates, the body resorts to using muscle protein for fuel, hindering muscle growth and resulting in the loss of lean muscle mass. The energy deficit would also exacerbate fatigue, increase perceived exertion and heart rate, and elevate the risk of injury.

Carbohydrates are also a major source of dietary fiber. A low-carb diet usually correlates with inadequate fiber intake, leading to constipation and other bowel disorders.

Post-exercise cravings for sweets are common, especially among women, which can be alleviated with carbohydrate consumption, providing satiety and stabilizing appetite. Cutting staple foods and sweets from the diet increases the risk of binge eating and may lead to eating disorders. The psychological stress associated with measuring and eating an accurate amount, similarly, puts athletes at risk of depression and elevated cortisol levels.

2.2 *Fat*

Fat can only be utilized as a fuel in the aerobic pathway. The fatty acids and triglycerides stored in the body undergo beta-oxidation to produce acetyl-CoA, which then generates ATP through the citric acid cycle and electron transport chain. As the main form of stored energy in the body, each gram of fat would generate four times more ATP compared to carbohydrates. At the same time, however, the oxygen requirement for the process is also four times higher, making fat a primary fuel source for long-duration, low-intensity activities such as walking and golfing.

Generally, the percentage of fuel from fat decreases as exercise intensity increases, although this percentage can be elevated through training. Endurance athletes are commonly trained to improve efficient fat oxidation. Relying more on stored fat for energy allows them to spare muscle glycogen use and potentially sustain longer durations of exercise. In high-intensity CrossFit training, the percentage of fuel from fat remains low, typically ranging from 10%–40%. For CrossFitters, intentionally training for higher fat oxidation would not have a significant impact on performance, as fat cannot support the high power output that carbohydrates provide.

The USDA recommends that male and female adults consume 20%–35% of their daily calorie needs from lipids. Based on this guideline, the 30% fat suggested in the Zone Diet falls within the safe range. However, the CrossFit Level 1 Training Guide (2020) emphasizes on the benefits of fats and recommends elite CrossFitters to double or triple their fat intake to optimize performance while maintaining leanness. According to the blocks set by zone parameter, a meal composed of X blocks of carbohydrate, X blocks of protein, and 3X blocks of fat would result in 56% of the energy coming from fat.

2.2.1 *High-fat diets*

Limited human research has been conducted on the effects of the Zone Diet on the performance of athletes. To explore the potential benefits and drawbacks of the Zone Diet, studies on some of the more popular high-fat diets are often referenced. The ketogenic diet is one such highly praised weight-loss diet. The diet is composed of extremely low carbohydrate (<20g/day), moderate protein (20%–25%), and high fat (70%–80%) (Kerksick *et al.* 2018). Without sufficient carbohydrate intake, the low blood glucose level triggers the release of glucagon, a hormone that promotes gluconeogenesis, i.e., the production of glucose from other substrates. In this case, fatty acids stored in adipose cells are released and transformed into acetyl-CoA to produce ATP. However, the huge backup of acetyl-CoA flushing into the citric acid cycle slows the cycle down, causing acetyl-CoA to unite in pairs and form ketones. After three to five days of extremely low carbohydrate intake, the body enters ketosis, where the brain begins to metabolize ketones to preserve lean body mass.

The effects of high-fat low-carb diets on athletic performance are under debate. A recent study examining the effect of four weeks of ketogenic diet on CrossFit athletes found a significant decrease in VO2peak in female participants after intervention (Durkalec-Michalski *et al.* 2021). However, contradictory observations from similar studies have also been reported. Overall, diets based on the existing knowledge, no significant ergogenic benefit can be guaranteed by consuming high-fat low-carb diets (Kerksick *et al.* 2018).

2.2.2 *Risk factors*

High-fat content usually indicates a high intake of saturated fat and high cholesterol intake, which can lead to increased levels of LDL cholesterol in the body (Kephart *et al.* 2018). LDL cholesterol that cannot be absorbed by cells remains in the blood, where it could eventually kill the macrophages. Over time, dead macrophages accumulate in the blood vessel wall as cholesterol plaques that could eventually block blood flow or break off to cause a heart attack. Other potential fat-induced risks were observed in a study where rats were fed a 40%–60% fat diet (Wali *et al.* 2020). This resulted in elevated levels of obesity, blood glucose, blood insulin, and blood fat, as well as insulin resistance, in the group after intervention. These biomarkers are associated with an increased risk of cardiovascular and chronic diseases.

2.3 *Protein*

Adequate protein intake is essential for preserving lean muscle mass. For athletes, sufficient protein is even more important to ensure positive nitrogen balance, efficient muscle synthesis, and recovery. The AMDR recommends adult females consume 10%–35% of their daily calorie intake from protein (US Department of Agriculture and US Department of Health and Human Services 2020). Proper implementation of the Zone Diet would provide 30% energy from protein, which is a reasonable amount.

The International Society of Sports Nutrition has specific recommendations regarding the protein intake of athletes (Kerksick *et al.* 2018). Depending on the intensity of daily training, a protein intake ranging from 1.4–1.8g/kg/day is considered appropriate, which is about double the Recommended Dietary Allowance (RDA) for normal adults.

3 OVERTRAINING AND INCREASED NUTRITIONAL NEEDS

Elite athletes striving for improvements often push themselves to achieve higher training capacities. A training plan designed with a reasonable distribution of different training intensities and adequate recovery methods is usually more effective in improving performance.

3.1 *Training intensity*

Higher training intensity is associated with greater improvements in performance. Indications of training intensity include heart rate, blood lactate, VO2max, and perceived exertion (Rosenblat *et al.* 2019). Endurance athletes such as cross-country runners and rowers usually train in the low-intensity range. CrossFitters, on the other hand, are usually trained in high intensity, combining long-duration aerobic and maximum power anaerobic exercises.

Heart rate is a straightforward measurement of the training intensity. A general sports watch categorizes heart rate during exercise into five zones, with Z1 referring to rest state and Z5 referring to very high intensity. During a typical CrossFit training session, it is not uncommon for athletes' heart rate to stay above 170 beats per minute (Schlegel 2020), which lies in Z5 of the heart rate zone. Spending too much time in this extremely high-intensity zone can overload cardiovascular muscles and require a longer recovery period. Moreover, CrossFit training tends to induce a significant increase in blood lactate concentration and a high rate of perceived exertion (Schlegel 2020). When combined, these biomarkers indicate a high potential risk of overtraining in CrossFitters.

3.2 *Poor recovery and increased nutritional needs*

The CrossFit Level 1 Training Guide (2020) recommends training for five to six days per week. Although this is considered a reasonable frequency for moderate exercises, it does not offer CrossFitters enough time to fully recover from the high-intensity Z5 training. The negative effects of poor recovery are reflected in multiple aspects.

3.2.1 *Glycogen replenishment*

Impairment of performance occurs under inadequate recovery, despite the higher training capacity. An intense training of over an hour depletes the glycogen stored in the body.

Glycogenesis, which replenishes muscles and liver glycogen, proceeds during the recovery period and typically takes 20–24 hours. For CrossFit athletes training twice a day, inadequate glycogen would be produced during the short recovery window. This leads to fatigue, increased perceived effort, and decreased maximal workload during training sessions. Incorporating appropriate pre-workout and post-workout meals may help strengthen performance. Optimal food choices include simple sugars that can be consumed and utilized efficiently.

3.2.2 *Rehydration*

Proper fluid replenishment after training is significant for restoring homeostasis and controlling heart rate recovery time. Depending on the level of exercise, 4–24 hours are needed to rehydrate from the fluid and electrolytes lost. Efficient rehydration should address the significant sodium and potassium lost through sweating. Incorporating electrolytes in the rehydration strategy aids recovery by increasing fluid retention and decreasing urine production.

3.2.3 *Cortisol*

Inadequate recovery and insufficient caloric intake fail to address elevated hormone levels after training (Gogojewicz *et al.* 2020). CrossFit has been monitored to induce acute elevation of cortisol levels in both males and females (Schlegel 2020). Elevated cortisol levels put the body into an alert state, breaking down muscle glycogen as ready energy. Other negative consequences include poor sleep quantity and quality, slower digestion, increased heart rate, rising blood glucose level, and increased rate of fat storage.

3.2.4 *Calcium and vitamin D*

Low body mass index, overtraining, and menstrual dysfunction put female CrossFitters at higher risk of stress fractures. Many athletes only give six weeks for these microdamages to fully repair. At the same time, a significant percentage of the female population struggles to meet the RDA for calcium. For women under 30 who are still depositing bone calcium, not consuming enough calcium increases the risk of osteoporosis in the later stages of life. Female athletes are particularly susceptible to low bone mineral density due to low calcium and vitamin D intake and low energy availability (Kerksick *et al.* 2018). Therefore, adequate consumption of calcium from diet or supplements is essential.

3.2.5 *Iron*

Iron deficiency is another prolonged issue among female athletes due to its low bioavailability and higher needs. Iron is essential for oxygen transportation throughout the body and the production of hemoglobin and red blood cells. Intense exercise stimulates expansion in plasma volume, causing iron turnover in tissues with the increased red blood cell mass. Iron loss from sweating, hemoglobin synthesis, and gastrointestinal bleeding is also more significant in athletes (Ponorac *et al.* 2020). Moreover, exercise-induced inflammation is associated with elevated hepcidin levels, which can limit iron absorption (Badenhorst *et al.* 2021). Together, these factors contribute to iron deficiency in athletes, eventually leading to impaired aerobic capacity, faster onset of fatigue, and an impaired menstrual cycle. Incorporating iron-rich foods, such as red meat, and ensuring adequate vitamin C intake or moderate iron supplements would be ideal for proper recovery (Badenhorst *et al.* 2021).

3.2.6 *Antioxidant, immune, and inflammatory systems*

Significantly higher oxygen uptake during strenuous exercise stimulates the production of reactive oxygen species (ROS), also known as free radicals. The accumulation of ROS could overwhelm the antioxidant defense system and lead to oxidative stress (Mastaloudis *et al.* 2001). In non-athletes, a normal level of dietary antioxidants can scavenge free radicals and eliminate the damage. For CrossFitters engaged in extremely high-intensity training, a faster turnover of these antioxidants has been observed (Mastaloudis *et al.* 2001). This indicates that increasing the intake of dietary antioxidants, primarily vitamin E, vitamin C, carotenoids, selenium, and zinc, may be beneficial for CrossFitters to reduce oxidative damage.

While moderate exercise has been shown to boost immunity, studies indicate that the risk of infection and inflammation likely increases as exercise workload exceeds the recommended level (Simpson *et al.* 2020). In terms of inflammation, high-frequency heavy training stresses joints and elevates high-sensitive C-reactive protein levels, which may not adequately recover over time. Poor recovery, combined with low energy availability in female endurance athletes, can impair immune system functions. Other environmental factors, such as traveling for competitions and disrupted sleep schedules, can also contribute to weakened immunity. To maintain healthy immune functions, athletes should ensure adequate dietary intake of vitamin C, B6, zinc, copper, and anti-inflammatory foods.

4 DRIVING FACTORS AND POTENTIAL RISKS

As CrossFit becomes more popular and more grand games are held, elite athletes push themselves harder to stay competitive and make a name in the meets. Besides pressure from competitors, Dimuzio suggests that an altered perception of body image may underlie the discrepancy between the energy intake and training intensity of the female CrossFitters (Dimuzio 2019).

CrossFit claims itself as an adaptive training program suitable for all sexes and age groups, encouraging shared training space and minimal distinction between male and female athletes. However, this has led to the perception that the muscular ripped physiques of male CrossFitters set the same body shape expectations for female athletes (Dimuzio 2019). As a result, female CrossFitters often implement greater workloads and stricter diets to build larger muscles and achieve low body fat, similar to male athletes.

However, female athletes are more susceptible to training addiction and eating disorders, often driven by internal psychological factors. The accurate measurements of food intake and workout capacity can give athletes a sense of control over their bodies as a function. Perfectionism drives them to continually implement stricter diets and harder training to achieve progress (Dimuzio 2019). This mindset fails to address the biological differences and heightens the risks of overtraining and low energy availability.

5 CONCLUSION

As the official handbook for new CrossFitters, the *Level 1 Training Guide* has a significant impact on shaping the training routines of the athletes. Therefore, it should exercise greater caution in its dietary recommendations to ensure they align with national nutrition guidelines. Additionally, the effects of intense exercise on bodily functions, hormone levels, and micronutrient needs should be included to help athletes manage potential effects. At the same time, attention should be given to the elevated micronutrient requirements, both in general and for specific sex groups. It is also worth noting that when suggesting supplements, proper doses and bioavailability should be clearly addressed.

In conclusion, balancing nutrition and training is an area often overlooked by CrossFitters and many other athletes. Correctly identifying and addressing nutritional deficiencies, such as inadequate carbohydrate intake, is closely associated with improved performance outcomes. Neglecting elevated micronutrient needs further exaggerates the physiological impacts induced by intense exercise and poor recovery. Female CrossFitters, in particular, are highly susceptible to these issues under the influences of multiple external and internal factors. Thus, more well-developed supportive educational programs are necessary to improve the overall well-being of participants in this growing sport.

REFERENCES

Badenhorst C. E., Goto K., O'Brien W. J. and Sims S., (2021). *J Sports Sci*, **39**, 1565

Capistrano Jr, V. L. M., Gonçalves Y. T., Costa E. E., Caetano M. L., Naves A., Cordeiro B., Teixeira D. C., Loureiro L. L. and Leandro Ribeiro de Souza M., (2022). *IJKSS*, **10**, 55

CrossFit Level 1 Training Guide, (2020). http://library.crossfit.com/free/pdf/CFJ_English_Level1_TrainingGuide.pd

Dimuzio N., (2019). *Open Access Theses & Dissertations*, **2019**, 2847

Durkalec-Michalski K., Nowaczyk P. M., Główka N., Ziobrowskav A. and Podgórski T., (2021). *Nutrients*, **13**, 864

Gogojewicz A., Śliwicka E. and Durkalec-Michalski K., (2022). *Int J Environ Res Public Health*, **17**, 4772

Kephart W., Pledge C., Roberson P., Mumford P., Romero M., Mobley C., Martin J., Young K., R. Lowery R., Wilson J., Huggins K. and Roberts M., (2018). *Sports (Basel)*, **6**, 1

Kerksick C. M., Wilborn C. D., Roberts M. D., Smith-Ryan A., Kleiner S. M., Jäger R., Collins R., Cooke M., Davis J. N., Galvan E., Greenwood M., Lowery L. M., Wildman R., Antonio J. and Kreider R. B., (2018). *J Int Soc Sports Nutr.*, **15**, 38

Mastaloudis A., Leonard S. W. and Traber M. G., (2001). *Free Radic Biol Med*, **31**, 911

Ponorac N., Popović M., Karaba-Jakovljević D., Bajić Z., Scanlan A., Stojanović E. and Radovanović D., (2020). *Int J Sport Nutr Exerc Metab*, **30**, 48

Rosenblat M. A., Perrotta A. S. and Vicenzino B., (2019). *J Strength Cond Res.*, **33**, 3491

Schlegel P., (2020). *J Sports Sci Med*, **19**, 670

Simpson R. J., Campbell J. P., Gleeson M., Krüger K., Nieman D. C., Pyne D. B., Turner J. E. and Walsh N. P., (2020). *Exerc Immunol Rev*, **26**, 8

U.S. Department of Agriculture and U.S. Department of Health and Human Services, (2020). *Dietary Guidelines for Americans, 2020-2025, 9th Edition*

Wali J. A., Jarzebska N., Raubenheimer D., Simpson S. J., Rodionov R. N. and O'Sullivan J. F., (2020). *Nutrients*, **12**, 1505

Biological Sciences and Environmental Health – Gao (Ed.)

Correlation between chronic constipation and sacral perineural (Tarlov) cyst growth

Haijun Li
Department of Neurosurgery, Tianjin Medical University General Hospital, Tianjin, China

ABSTRACT: Objective: To explore the relationship between chronic constipation and the growth of sacral perineural (Tarlov) cysts.

Methods: This retrospective cohort study included image data from GE Healthcare Picture Archiving and Communication Systems (PACS) and symptom information from the Patient Assessment of Constipation Symptoms (PAC-SYM) score. Subjects were patients with radiologically diagnosed sacral perineural cysts, with examinations conducted more than once across time. The primary outcome was the relationship between constipation and the growth of sacral perineural cysts, measured by odds ratio (OR) and correlation coefficient (R).

Results: The study involved 40 consecutive patients. Of them, 11 (27.5%; 3 males and 8 females) showed growing cysts, and another 11 (27.5%; 2 males and 9 females) had constipation problems. Constant chronic constipation was associated with a higher likelihood of cyst growing (controlling for sex and age, P = .003, OR = 5.800). Cyst number (P = .025, P = 2.646), constipation duration (P = .037, OR = 1.035), and average defecation time (ADT, P = .049, OR=1.277, CI=1.002-1.628) also correlated with growing cysts. Among patients with both growing cysts and chronic constipation, ADT showed a correlation with size change per month (SCPM).

Conclusions: Chronic constipation strongly correlated with the growth of sacral perineural cysts, especially in those with long-term constipation.

1 INTRODUCTION

In 1938, Dr. Tarlov was the first to describe the cysts that developed in the perineurial space between the endoneurial (pial) and the perineurial (arachnoid) sheaths, now known as Tarlov cysts (TCs) (Tarlov 1938). In previous studies, these cysts were initially considered dilatations of the nerve root sleeves (Hulens *et al.* 2022). The global prevalence of TCs is about 4.27%, with frequent occurrence in the sacral and coccygeal roots (Klepinowski *et al.* 2021). TCs are more common in women (7.01%) than in men (4.05%) (Klepinowski *et al.* 2021). While most TCs are considered asymptomatic, the proportion believed to cause clinical symptoms has risen from 1% in 1994 to 15.59% now, potentially due to increased awareness among clinical researchers (Klepinowski *et al.* 2021). However, the majority of symptomatic TCs should be differentially diagnosed from other spinal lesions (Hulens *et al.* 2019).

Symptoms of TCs may be related to their locations, adjacency, number, and size, with presentation depending on the compression of the nerve roots (Fletcher-Sandersjoo *et al.* 2019). In most cases, TCs are found in the sacral spinal ganglia, with the most common location being the spinal roots in the sacral level 2 (S2) segment (about 46.7%) (Sharma *et al.* 2019). About 42.6% of patients suffer from more than one cyst (Klepinowski *et al.* 2021).

DOI: 10.1201/9781003587590-47

Consequently, symptoms of TCs vary and may include low back pain, perineal pain, coccygodynia, sciatica, sensory deficits, bowel/bladder dysfunction, and other uncommon symptoms (Langdown *et al.* 2005).

A widely accepted theory is the ball-valve mechanism, where cerebrospinal fluid (CSF) enters the cyst into the perineurial (subarachnoid) space and is unable to efflux through the same path (Tarlov 1970). The hydrostatic and pulsatile forces of CSF lead to the development of the cyst (Yang *et al.* 2020). Yang et al. proposed that cysts grow when symptoms deteriorate, or new symptoms, such as orthostatic or positional headaches, arise (Yang *et al.* 2020). Besides, the Valsalva maneuver can increase CSF pressure remarkably within the first 20 seconds (Zhang *et al.* 2014). Defecation is a typical and representative condition that triggers a Valsalva maneuver in daily life, and chronic constipation (CC) prolongs defecation time (Pstras *et al.* 2016). However, TC pathogenesis and its development remain unclear. Based on the above, this study will investigate the relationship between TCs and CC.

2 MATERIAL AND METHODS

2.1 *Subject*

The study reviewed magnetic resonance imaging (MRI) reports with radiological diagnosis of sacral perineural cysts in Tianjin Medical University General Hospital between 2015 and 2021 (the available time span in the hospital's electronic record system). Patients who had undergone MRI examinations more than once (with an interval of at least 1 month) in the imaging database across time were considered in the study. Furthermore, the patients' images explicitly covered the lumbosacral region, with cysts present in more than one plane. Patients who underwent surgical treatment during the examination interval were excluded, as their data would not reflect the natural growth of TCs. To minimize recall bias, all eligible patients were included in the PACS. A total of 46 subjects met the eligibility criteria and were considered for inclusion in the study. Regardless of symptoms, these patients required repetitive or enhanced MRI scans for various reasons, such as persistent or recurrent back/low back pain, spine-related lower limb pain or sensory changes, trauma, multiple abdominal or pelvic examinations without spinal pathology, repeated tumor re-examinations, and issues in the lumbar vertebral areas.

2.2 *Cyst measurement and constipation evaluation*

All patients were examined in the supine position. Almost all images obtained from the Picture Archiving and Communication Systems (PACS) were not purposely aimed at sacral perineural cysts. Therefore, to ensure the consistency of the measurement results, this study could only measure the diameters of their TCs in the sagittal view in most instances. The professional imaging technicians located their acquisition planes at the same anatomical level and with a consistent slice thickness (3 mm). The MRI results of some patients indicated cyst growth in the same plane (Figure 1). The study calculated the diameters along two axes from the first to the subsequent examinations: the craniocaudal line (CL, the longest diameter along the spinal cord) and the anteroposterior line (AL, the longest diameter perpendicular to CL) (Figure 2).

The interval time (IT) was defined as the time period in months from the first to the last acquisition. The study defined Li as the sum of the initial-time diameters of both axes; Lf as the sum of final (latest)-time diameters of both axes; and (Lf-Li)/IT as size changes per month (SCPM). The study also measured CL and AL size changes separately. Additionally, the dimensions of the cysts were averaged over two types of imaging: T2-weighted imaging (T2WI) and fat suppression T2WI.

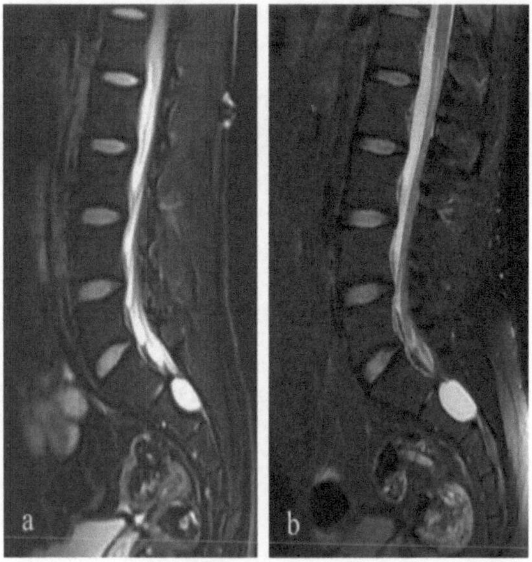

Figure 1. MRI of Tarlov cyst changes. (a) The first image of an MRI examination. (b) The last image of an MRI examination. Picture credit: Original.

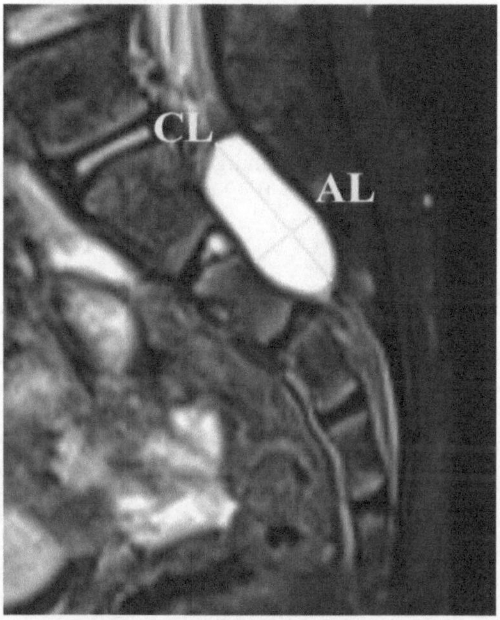

Figure 2. Schematic diagram of the measurement. (Picture credit: Original).

Rome IV criteria were introduced as the diagnostic criteria of chronic constipation, including functional constipation and irritable bowel syndrome with predominant constipation (Drossman and Hasler 2016). The study utilized the Patient Assessment of Constipation Symptom Questionnaire (PAC-SYM), a standard questionnaire to identify and evaluate CC, as the central part of the assessment of the average degree of symptoms in the past few years (Bellini *et al.* 2017). The study also added the average defecation time (ADT) in minutes and constipation duration in months, as key factors in cyst growth. The questionnaires were administered by professional physicians. To control researcher bias, the study did not separate the patients into different cohorts until after data analysis was completed.

2.3 *Statistical analysis*

The study used SPSS (Version 26.0) to record and analyze data. Logistic regression analysis was used to verify the correlation with cyst growth, including factors such as age, sex, number of cysts, CC, ADT, and constipation duration. In the group of patients with both cyst growth and CC, the bivariate correlation method was used to examine the relationship between the degree of size change (CL, AL, and SCPM) and variables like cyst number, PAC-SYM scores, ADT, and constipation duration. Data are presented as mean ± standard deviation (range), and a P-value <.05 was set as the threshold for statistical significance.

3 RESULTS

3.1 *General results*

Of the 46 consecutive patients, six were excluded because of unavailable contact details. The remaining 40 patients, including 7 males and 33 females with a mean age of 60.83±14.81 (7-82) years, had 65 cysts in total (1.62±1.13 cysts per patient). Among these patients, 11 patients (27.5; 3 males and 8 females) belonged to the cyst growing group (CGG), and 6 of them were considered CC (Table 1). Of all 40 patients, 11 patients (27.5%; 2 males and 9 females) had constipation problems. The mean of the interval between the first and the last examination was 19.43 ± 16.24 (2-60) months, without significant difference between CGG and non-CGG groups (15.10 ± 14.80 months [range: 3–51] versus 21.07 ± 16.71 months [range 2–60], P = .23). The average cyst-size changes in the CGG group were 1.59 ± 1.01 mm (range -.40–3.00 mm) in the CL and 1.22 ± 0.79 mm (.10-2.60) mm in the AL.

Table 1. 11 Patients observed with Tarlov cyst growth.

Group	Age	Sex	Number of cysts	First-time size CC×AL (mm)	Last-time size CC×AL (mm)	Interval time (month)	PAC-SYM Score	Average defecation time (minutes)	Constipation duration (months)
Normal	78	Female	1	9.2×10.4	10.5×11.9	14	0	5	0
	43	Male	2	11.3×9.5	13.7×10.4	51	0	5	0
	72	Female	2	11.5×4.6	14.5×7.0	3	0	5	0
	60	Female	1	36.5×19,9	36.2×22.7	13	0	5	0
	68	Female	1	9.5×5.0	10.9×5.8	4	0	5	0
Constipation	76	Female	1	8.7×6.6	9.2×8.3	3	20	15	50
	39	Female	3	21.6×30.2	24.6×31.6	9	8	10	60
	79	Male	5	6.6×5.6	8.6×6.0	14	6	10	36
	69	Female	5	10.7×8.4	12.4×10.1	15	7	10	48
	47	Male	5	7.0×5.4	8.5×6.4	34	8	10	60
	7	Female	1	32.2×22.4	34.0×23.7	6	6	10	40

CC = chronic constipation; AL, anteroposterior line; PAC-SYM = patient assessment of constipation symptoms.

3.2 *Statistical results*

Logistic regression analysis, controlling the variables of sex and age, indicated that CC (P = .003, OR = 5.800, CI = 1.185–28.385), number of cysts (P = .025, OR = 2.646, CI = 1.133–6.178), constipation duration (P = .037, OR = 1.035, CI = 1.002-1.068), and ADT (P = .049, OR = 1.277, CI = 1.002–1.628) significantly correlated with cyst growth. However, sex (P=.325, OR = .427, CI = .078–2.325), age (P = .458, OR = .983, CI = .939–1.029), and PAC-SYM score (P = .110, OR = 1.123, CI = .974–1.296) did not (Figure 3). Furthermore, in the group of patients with both growing cysts and CC, only ADT showed a significant correlation with SCPM per month (R = .843, P = .033).

3.3 *Cases*

A 7-year-old girl took part in the study with the consent and help of her parents. She was the only underage participant. The primary symptom was uracratia, which caused her to unconsciously urinate and experience stress urinary incontinence. The size of the cyst grew from 30.1 ×28.4mm before 12 months to 33.3 × 29.2 mm at diagnosis. The patient also experienced difficult defecation, lasting around 30 minutes and characterized by weakness. The patient did not experience pain or numbness. The patient underwent percutaneous cyst aspiration under local anesthesia, as there were no surgical contraindications. The patient's symptoms of urinary incontinence were significantly improved on the first postoperative day, and she was able to control urination autonomously. However, the symptoms recurred seven days later. The patient subsequently underwent cyst surgery, and the symptoms did not reappear within one year of follow-up after treatment.

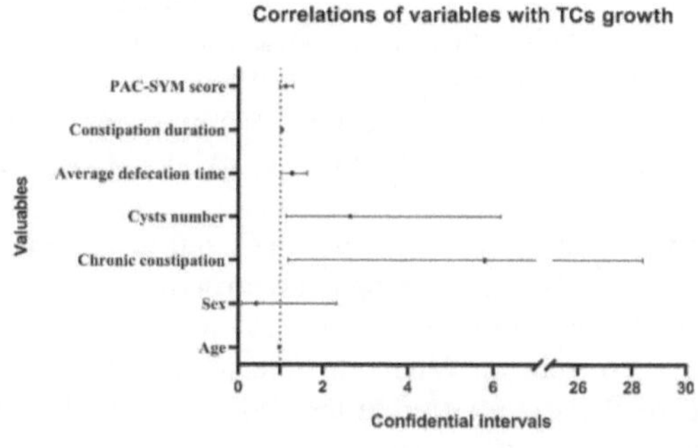

Figure 3. Result of main binary logistic regression showing odds ratios and confidence intervals. Picture credit: Original.

Of all patients, two showed a decrease in cyst size. One patient's cyst reduced from 15.5 × 9.1 to 14.1 × 9.4 mm, and the other patient's from 5.9 × 4.3 to 4.3 × 4.3 mm. Neither of these patients experienced constipation and none reported worsening of their constipation symptoms, which remained stable.

4 DISCUSSION

4.1 *Characteristics of distribution*

Previous research has found that the prevalence of TCs is significantly higher in women compared to men, with women having almost twice the prevalence. The study also observed a higher number of female patients, consistent with previous findings. However, the statistical analysis did not indicate a significant association between TC growth and gender. Men and women exhibit many physical differences, such as tissue structure, metabolic rate, and internal environment, which could affect the prevalence of TCs. However, currently there are no studies to explain the difference in the prevalence of TCs between men and women, nor do they discuss the lack of difference in disease progression between genders.

4.2 *Correlation between chronic constipation and Tarlov cyst growth*

This study focuses on the relationship between TC growth and chronic constipation, with the statistical results showing that the two affected each other. On the one hand, the function of the sphincter is mainly controlled by the sacral 2 to sacral 4 nerves, which are also the nerves commonly involved in cysts, including the pelvic visceral nerves that control the intestinal, bladder, and sexual functions. When the cyst grows, it can affect or compress the related conduction nerve, causing dysuria and difficult defecation. When TCs involves the nerves innervating the anal muscles, the function of the corresponding nerves may be weakened, resulting in sphincter dysfunction, such as uncoordinated or weak muscle contraction (Shimauchi-Ohtaki *et al.* 2022). This can lead to symptoms such as a prolonged defecation process, laborious defecation, and persistent defecation, which is in line with the disease symptoms and diagnostic conditions of chronic constipation.

However, chronic constipation is multifactorial, and it cannot be completely attributed to neurological dysfunction. A comprehensive evaluation was conducted to analyze the clinical symptoms of chronic constipation, including the duration of the condition, stool characteristics, rectal signs, and abdominal symptoms. The PAC-SYM questionnaire was also used for assessment. Regardless of the cause of constipation, patients tend to perform the Valsalva maneuver during defecation, which can significantly increase the CSF pressure within 20 seconds (Neville and Egan 2005). This rise in pressure leads to an increase in the extracapsular CSF pressure of TCs, which can cause the pressure outside the cyst to drive CSF into the cyst. After the pressure equalizes inside and outside the cyst, the surface tension of the cyst increases. This repeated force provides dynamic conditions for cyst growth, in accord with the pain associated with symptomatic sacral nerve root cysts when performing the Valsalva maneuver.

There is a potential connection between CC and TC that could lead to a feedback loop in disease development. If TCs invade the motor nerves related to the anorectum, the patient may experience functional chronic constipation due to motility issues, which can persist for a long time and be challenging to relieve. When chronic constipation continues, the increase in CSF pressure during forced defecation can cause CSF to enter the saccular cavity of TCs, increasing the intra-cystic pressure and providing repeated and long-term impetus for the growth of TC. This creates a harmful cycle that can only be broken by therapeutic interventions when symptoms become unbearable or new ones develop. Therefore, controlling difficult defecation symptoms and reducing the duration of defecation may help slow the growth of the cyst compared to ignoring these symptoms.

Research shows a strong link between CC and cyst growth. When defecation time is prolonged, the pressure of CSF increases significantly, enhancing TC growth. This means that patients who take too long to defecate are more likely to experience faster cyst growth. The growth of TCs is not related to the PAC-SYM score but is connected to the duration of chronic constipation. This implies that repeated and prolonged constipation is the key factor in the growth of TCs. Unfortunately, CC is often overlooked by patients and clinicians, providing an opportunity for the mutual causal relationship between the growth of TCs and chronic constipation to continue unnoticed.

While the Valsalva maneuver can manifest in various ways, patients with TCs often experience difficulty with defecation. The study focuses on chronic and long-term symptoms accompanying TCs, which can include chronic constipation. However, chronic constipation can be easily overlooked by both patients and clinicians in clinical diagnosis and treatment and may become a long-term influencing factor in the progression of TCs (Hulens *et al.* 2019). Multiple factors influence the development of cysts, leading to growth, stabilization, or shrinkage. This study discusses one possible factor that may contribute to TC growth.

4.3 *Other factors*

Previous research has shown that having multiple TCs is a common occurrence. In this study, however, the average number of cysts found per patient was 1.62 ± 1.13. The regression analysis revealed a statistically significant relationship between the growth of TC and the number of cysts. This suggests that having multiple sacral nerve cysts may be a risk factor for the growth of TC. Patients with this condition may have a predisposition to developing cysts, with a higher likelihood of cyst growth. This susceptibility may be due to congenital defects in tissue structures or organs that provide the conditions for the formation and growth of sacral nerve root cysts.

4.4 *Limitations*

The number and the type of patients were limited due to geographic restrictions and the constraints of COVID-19, resulting in a wide confidence interval. The PACS records of the medical centers only date back to 2015, limiting the research scope to that timeframe. At the time of study design and conduct, no suitable and standard measurement method were available.

5 CONCLUSIONS

Chronic constipation and TC growth may be correlated, especially in patients with long-term constipation problems. For TC patients who present with constipation, assistance with defecation might help manage the condition. Future studies should include larger sample sizes to reduce the bias inherent in retrospective studies. Additionally, more precise and standard measurement methods should be used to calibrate the results.

ACKNOWLEDGMENT

Dr. Shiwei Li assisted with the statistical analysis. This work was supported by the Tianjin Municipal Health Commission (Grant ZC20175).

REFERENCES

Bellini M., Usai-Satta P., Bove A., Bocchini R., Galeazzi F., Battaglia E., Alduini P., Buscarini E., Bassotti G. and ChroCoDiTe Study Group A., (2017). Chronic constipation diagnosis and treatment evaluation: the "CHRO.CO.DI.T.E." study, *BMC Gastroenterol* **17**(1), 11.

Drossman D. A. and Hasler W. L., (2016). Rome IV-functional GI disorders: Disorders of gut-brain interaction, *Gastroenterology* **150**(6), 1257–61.

Fletcher-Sandersjoo A., Mirza S., Burstrom G., Pedersen K., Kuntze Soderqvist A., Grane P., Fagerlund M., Edstrom E. and Elmi-Terander A., (2019). Management of perineural (Tarlov) cysts: a population-based cohort study and algorithm for the selection of surgical candidates, *Acta Neurochir* **161**(9), 1909–1915.

Hulens M., Bruyninckx F., Thal D. R., Rasschaert R., Bervoets C. and Dankaerts W., (2022). Large- and small-fiber neuropathy in patients with Tarlov Cysts, *J Pain Res* 15, 193–202.

Hulens M., Rasschaert R., Bruyninckx F., Dankaerts W., Stalmans I., De Mulder P. and Vansant G., (2019). Symptomatic Tarlov cysts are often overlooked: ten reasons why-a narrative review, *Eur. Spine J.* **28**(10), 2237–2248.

Klepinowski T., Orbik W. and Sagan L., (2021). Global incidence of spinal perineural Tarlov's cysts and their morphological characteristics: a meta-analysis of 13,266 subjects, *Surg Radiol Anat* **43**(6), 855–863.
Langdown A. J., Grundy J. R. and Birch N. C., (2005). The clinical relevance of Tarlov cysts, *J. Spinal Disord. Tech.* **18**(1), 29–33.
Neville L. and Egan R. A., (2005). Frequency and amplitude of elevation of cerebrospinal fluid resting pressure by the Valsalva maneuver, *Can J Ophthalmol* **40**(6), 775–7.
Pstras L., Thomaseth K., Waniewski J., Balzani I. and Bellavere F., (2016). The Valsalva manoeuvre: physiology and clinical examples, *Acta Physiol (Oxf)* **217**(2), 103–19.
Sharma M., SirDeshpande P., Ugiliweneza B., Dietz N. and Boakye M., (2019). A systematic comparative outcome analysis of surgical versus percutaneous techniques in the management of symptomatic sacral perineural (Tarlov) cysts: a meta-analysis, *J. Neurosurg. Spine* **30**(5), 1–12.
Shimauchi-Ohtaki H., Honda F., Nakamura S. and Yoshimoto Y., (2022). Severe constipation due to sacral perineural cysts in a pediatrics patient: A case report, *Surg. Neurol. Intl.* 13, 317.
Tarlov I. M., (1938). Perineurial cysts of the spinal nerve roots, *Arch. Neurol.* **40**(6), 1067–1074.
Tarlov I. M., (1970). Spinal perineurial and meningeal cysts, *J Neurol Neurosurg Psychiatry* 33(6), 833–43.
Yang A. I., Rinehart C. D., McShane B. J., Hitti F. L. and Welch W. C., (2020). Growth of Lumbosacral Perineural (Tarlov) Cysts: A Natural History Analysis, *Neurosurgery* **86**(1), 88–92.
Zhang Z., Wang X., Jonas J. B., Wang H., Zhang X., Peng X., Ritch R., Tian G., Yang D., Li L., Li J. and Wang N., (2014). Valsalva manoeuver, intra-ocular pressure, cerebrospinal fluid pressure, optic disc topography: Beijing intracranial and intra-ocular pressure study, *Acta Ophthalmologica* **92**(6), e475–e480.

Biological Sciences and Environmental Health – Gao (Ed.)
© 2025 the Author(s), ISBN: 978-1-032-96016-6

Five hallmarks and different theories for aging

Haonian Zhou
Biology Department, Geogia State University, Atlanta, USA

ABSTRACT: Aging, a phenomenon that has intrigued humanity for centuries, remains a topic of intense scientific investigation. This paper presents a comprehensive review of key aspects surrounding the aging process, with a focus on the molecular hallmarks and mechanisms underlying this complex phenomenon. The discussion centers around five primary hallmarks of aging: DNA instability, telomere attrition, loss of proteostasis, epigenetic alterations and mitochondrial dysfunction. Each hallmark is examined in detail, highlighting its contribution to the overall aging process. Additionally, the paper delves into the diverse theories surrounding aging, including debates about the circumventability of aging and contrasting viewpoints that emphasize aging's natural occurrence driven by thermodynamics. Furthermore, the paper explores the three mechanisms of aging observed in vertebrates: rapid senescence, gradual senescence, and negligible senescence, elucidating how different species experience aging-related changes. By presenting a comprehensive synthesis of current knowledge, this paper aims to enhance our comprehension of the aging process. and its potential implications for future therapeutic interventions, ultimately contributing to the enhancement of human health span.

1 INTRODUCTION

Aging is a pervasive process, manifesting sequentially throughout the body, with the timing and order varying among individuals. One of the most prevalent and conspicuous signs of aging is the narrowing of blood vessels throughout the body, resulting in inadequate blood supply to organs. This, in turn, leads to a decline or weakening of organ functionality. Specifically, significant atherosclerotic changes in cardiovascular vessels can culminate in myocardial infarctions and strokes. As aging progresses, there's a widespread decline in immune function, leading to decreased resistance to infections. A minimal invasion by pathogens can result in severe infections, especially in organs such as the lungs. Hormonal reductions in the aging process leads to muscle atrophy, osteoporosis, increased susceptibility to falls, and fractures. Aging brains experience a reduction in cell numbers and intercellular connections, leading to diminished memory capacity and, in severe cases, degenerative mental disorders like dementia. The onset of memory loss and cognitive decline become increasingly common. Furthermore, aging is characterized by increased errors in genetic replication, transcription, and translation. The cumulative effect of these errors, coupled with a reduced immune response's error-correcting ability, substantially elevates the risk of cancer, among other diseases (Li *et al.* 2021). In addition, scientists have also identified other characteristics of aging, including DNA damage, telomere shortening, epigenetic changes, and so on. However, until the last century, a unified understanding of the core features of aging had not yet been established.

In order to coupe with that, scientists have worked for centuries to overcome. In 20th century, several features of aging have been identified including Instabilities in DNA,

DOI: 10.1201/9781003587590-48

telomere attrition, epigenetic alterations, loss of proteostasis, deregulated nutrient sensing, mitochondrial dysfunction, cellular senescence, stem cell exhaustion, and altered intercellular communication (López-Otín *et al.* 2013). All of them are considered the core characteristics of aging and received unanimous recognition. Three supplementary hallmarks been identified later: impaired macroautophagy, persistent inflammation, and microbial dysbiosis (López-Otín *et al.* 2023). Recent studies have validated and expanded on the significance of each of these markers. However, these hallmarks have not been definitively elucidated, potentially limited by the constraints of the data or technological advancements. Additionally, as research on aging progresses, there is a need to incorporate a broader spectrum of findings. Thus, it is timely to consolidate the literature and re-evaluate the various features of aging and their underlying mechanisms.

In this article, five traits of aging are chosen, including DNA damage, telomere attrition, epigenetic alterations, loss of proteostasis, and mitochondrial dysfunction. Those characteristics all take place inside the cell, which are the most basic elements for aging. Besides, more researches have been done on such area recently and have made great progress. By researching these characteristics, it grants a deeper understanding of the aging process for the general populace and also paves the way for potential therapeutic interventions in the future. Additionally, Integrated methods are anticipated to provide detailed insights into the mechanisms behind aging characteristics and foster future interventions to enhance human health span.

2 DNA INSTABILITY

Genomic instability delineates the propensity of the genome to accrue mutations, encompassing heritable alterations in the DNA sequence, such as base substitutions, insertions, deletions, copy number variations, chromosomal aberrations, or retrotransposition events. Broadly construed, genomic instability also signifies instances wherein DNA's intrinsic characteristics undergo chemical modifications, often referred to as DNA damage, thereby modulating the DNA's structural and functional attributes. This category of DNA damage incorporates spontaneous deamination, hydrolysis, and an array of chemical perturbations including, but not limited to, diverse strand breaks, nicks, gaps, a basic site, adduct formations, and both inter-strand and intra-strand DNA-protein crosslinks, alongside other nuanced chemical modifications. Such damage poses challenges to the precise replication, regimented transcription, and secure storage of genetic information (Vijg and Suh 2013).

In the trajectory of standard senescence, DNA incurs damage extensively, attributed to a gamut of exogenous and endogenous genotoxic agents. Estimates suggest that an active mammalian cell may experience up to 105 instances of DNA damage daily. Albeit a significant proportion of these damages are effectively ameliorated, certain elusive damages persist either due to late or incorrect reparative mechanisms or a complete lack thereof. As temporal progression ensues, the inexorable accumulation of DNA damage epitomizes genomic instability as a quintessential hallmark of aging.

DNA harm is pivotal in the onset of several illnesses, notably cancer. Mutations from this damage can upset the usual cell growth and division controls, resulting in unchecked cell growth and potential tumor genesis. Moreover, DNA damage can lead to genetic irregularities, a characteristic often seen in cancerous cells, facilitating additional mutations and the advancement of tumors. There's also a complex interplay between DNA damage, its repair mechanisms, and the immune system. Such damage can initiate immune reactions, causing persistent inflammation, a prevalent trait in aging and many diseases associated with age. This continuous inflammation can intensify DNA damage and accelerate tissue breakdown.

3 TELOMERE ATTRITION

Telomeres represent the termini of chromosomes, characterized by repetitive non-coding DNA sequences. They function as protective caps, safeguarding chromosomal integrity from deleterious events, analogous to the aglets on shoelaces that prevent fraying. With each cellular division, telomeres undergo attrition, and once they reach a critically reduced length, the cell enters a state of replicative senescence. Historically, telomere length has been postulated as a pivotal biomarker for human aging and associated pathologies (Vaiserman and Krasnienkov 2021).

The activation of telomere-dependent DNA Damage Response (tDDR) results in the formation of telomere-induced DNA damage foci (TIF) or telomere-associated DDR foci (TAF), serving as significant indicators of cellular senescence. In tissues with active cell division, telomeres undergo attrition over successive cell cycles. When their length becomes critically shortened, they no longer effectively interact with shelterin proteins. This triggers the cellular machinery to perceive them as exposed DNA ends, setting off the DNA Damage Response (DDR) pathway. In tissues with limited cell division (such as cardiomyocytes, adipocytes, neurons, osteocytes, and osteoblasts), telomere dysfunction can result from irreparable DNA lesions inherent to the telomeres. In both scenarios, continuous activation of DDR leads to chronic senescence characterized by cell growth arrest and the emergence of the Senescence-Associated Secretory Phenotype (SASP). The SASP involves the secretion of various pro-inflammatory cytokines, which are not only stimulated by DDR but also contribute to the further activation of DDR and the formation of TAF through autocrine and paracrine mechanisms (Casagrande and Hau 2019).

Various health issues, including lung diseases, skeletal problems, cardiovascular disorders, neurodegenerative conditions, metabolic disorders, kidney diseases, and fertility decline, are linked to aging. In these ailments, dysfunctional telomeres and accumulated cellular senescence play crucial causal roles. Shortened telomeres are closely associated with lung diseases like idiopathic pulmonary fibrosis. Cardiovascular disease risks correlate with telomere shortening. Neurodegenerative disorders and age-related macular degeneration have connections to aging markers. Additionally, skeletal issues, renal problems, and fertility decline are also influenced by telomere damage. Research indicates complex relationships between cellular senescence and these health issues, but deteriorating telomere function seems to play a pivotal role, influencing the progression of these related conditions (Rossiello *et al.* 2022).

4 EPIGENETIC ALTERATIONS

Epigenetics means changes in phenotype or gene expression caused by mechanisms (encompassing DNA methylation, histone modifications, and non-coding RNA (NcRNA) regulation) beyond DNA sequence variations. These changes usually caused by a combination of random events or other environmental factors, which play pivotal roles in gene expression control. DNA methylation involves adding a methyl group to cytosine nucleotides, influencing gene expression by recruiting repressive proteins or blocking transcription factor binding. Histone modifications like acetylation and methylation impact gene regulation and chromatin structure. NcRNAs, such as microRNAs (miRNAs), control gene expression by degrading mRNA or inhibiting translation. In aging, distinct epigenetic changes occur. DNA methylation patterns shift, with decreased methylation in heterochromatin and increased methylation in CpG islands near promoters. Histone modifications change, affecting chromatin structure and gene expression. RNA changes include reduced mRNA methylation and altered miRNA expression, both influencing gene regulation. These epigenetic changes have implications for aging-related processes, exemplified by epigenetic clocks like the Horvath clock estimating physiological age and predicting lifespan (Gonzalo 2010).

Epigenetics affects cellular aging, as well as age-related diseases like cancer, diabetes, atherosclerosis and Alzheimer's disease. Genes involved in these processes are subject to epigenetic modifications that contribute to disease development. In summary, epigenetics plays a significant role in influencing aging and age-related diseases through modifications that impact gene expression and cellular processes.

5 LOSS OF PROTEOSTASIS

In cells, proteins play various critical roles, including enzyme catalysis, cell signaling, and structural support. With aging, many biochemical processes within cells may undergo changes, affecting the balance of protein synthesis, degradation, and regulation. This can lead to the over-accumulation or reduction of certain proteins and the dysregulation of functional proteins.

Aging is characterized by disturbances in crucial cellular functions. Intrinsically disordered proteins (IDPs) and regions (IDRs) are unique in that they don't have a fixed structure, making them versatile connectors in signaling pathways, which might have an impact on processes related to aging. We gathered a dataset comprising 1,702 proteins associated with aging. Approximately 36% of these are IDPs/IDRs, a figure slightly below the general percentage of disorder content in the human proteome, which is around 40%. Upon assessing this aging-related proteome through Gene Ontology, it was observed that about one-third of the aging processes have a high concentration of IDPs/IDRs, particularly in genome regulation. IDPs/IDRs also feature prominently across various levels of aging-centric signaling pathways, emphasizing their role in the aging "structure-function spectrum." An analysis of the protein interaction network showcased IDPs associated with several key aging characteristics (Labbadia and Morimoto 2015).

Clusters enriched with IDPs have high likelihoods of liquid-liquid phase separation (LLPS), "nuclear" localization, and DNA-associated functions. These are linked to aging hallmarks like genomic instability, telomere attrition, epigenetic changes, and stem cell depletion. Intrinsic disorder, LLPS, and aggregation tendencies might indicate pathogenic proteins. Overall, IDPs/IDRs significantly impact aging-related processes, notably in DNA regulation. Aggregation of IDPs, leading to functional loss and toxicity, can be detrimental to cells. Analyzing aging structurally and identifying vulnerable proteins enhance our understanding of aging's molecular mechanisms, offering new avenues to slow down the process.

Protein imbalance during the aging process is a complicated phenomenon that may arise from various factors, including genetic factors, environmental influences, and changes in cellular regulatory mechanisms. This imbalance could have significant implications for cellular and organismal health. For instance, the reduction of certain functional proteins may hinder cells from effectively performing specific physiological processes, potentially affecting the function of tissues and organs. Besides, the abnormal accumulation of proteins can lead to aberrant cellular activities and may even be associated with the development of certain diseases, like neurodegenerative disorders and tumors. Yet the specific mechanisms and consequences require further research for better understanding.

6 MITOCHONDRIAL DYSFUNCTION

Mitochondrial dysfunction stands at the forefront of factors influencing the aging process. It notably affects cell operations and plays a significant role in the age-related physiological alterations. As individuals age, mitochondrial DNA experiences an uptick in mutations due to increased oxidative stress and weakening repair capabilities. These mutations hinder the smooth operation of the electron transport chain, which in turn cuts down the production of

ATP, compromising the energy needed for vital cellular activities. Moreover, malfunctioning mitochondria emit higher levels of reactive oxygen species (ROS), leading to oxidative harm to cellular structures. Such oxidative stress can induce apoptosis and accelerate cell aging, feeding into a wide array of age-associated characteristics. Additionally, with decreased mitophagy efficiency, which usually handles the removal of damaged mitochondria, cells end up harboring more of these faulty powerhouses. This, coupled with a hindered mitochondrial biogenesis, further obstructs the replacement of these damaged units (Lidsky *et al.* 2022).

The consequences of mitochondrial dysfunction are especially notable in energy-demanding tissues like the brain and muscles, contributing to the gradual decline in their functional capacities during aging. Beyond cellular consequences, dysfunctional mitochondria also play a significant role in the emergence and development of age-related diseases, including neurodegenerative disorders, cardiovascular ailments, diabetes, and cancer. In essence, addressing mitochondrial dysfunction is a crucial avenue for comprehending the intricacies of aging and developing interventions to promote healthier aging trajectories and mitigate age-associated diseases.

7 DIFFERENT VIEWS ON AGING

7.1 *Aging might be circumventable*

The reason for aging is still debatable nowadays. Recent propositions suggest that senescence might be circumventable, implying that under ideal circumstances, a form of perpetual existence might be feasible. At its core, when positioned in an optimal environment, comparing to hydra and bacteria, "Immortality" is an inherent attribute of life. After the emergence of mechanisms of death, the duration of life for the vast majority of multicellular organisms is actually adjustable – it's a variable that can be changed. The length of life for a particular species is not an inherent constant; rather, it's a result of natural selection and competition. When competition and the environment change, life tends to adapt in the direction most favorable for competition by altering this variable. In essence, the duration of life for complex organisms is not only controllable but also adaptable to environmental changes through adjustments in its length. All of these mechanisms are merely means of competition (Guo *et al.* 2023).

7.1.1 *Aging is not a disease and cannot be circumventable*

Distinct from diseases, aging is characterized by the following attributes: It manifests in all multicellular organisms upon reaching adulthood; It is present across all species; It becomes evident only post-reproductive maturation within each species; It is observed in all organisms isolated by humans from their natural environments, even those that may have been exempt from aging for nearly a millennium; It manifests in both animate and inanimate entities; It shares a universal molecular origin across all matter, namely thermodynamic instability. No known disease exhibits these six concurrent characteristics. More importantly, the indispensable and sufficient stochastic events leading to aging are the loss of functional molecules and the accumulation of dysfunctional molecules. Thermodynamic instability is the driving force behind the loss and accumulation of these molecules. In other words, the underlying cause of aging is rooted in the Second Law of Thermodynamics and the increasing entropy associated with growth (Gladyshev 2013).

7.1.2 *Aging in vertebrates has revealed three distinct mechanisms*

Other theories go in depth of aging theories and show more details and differences for aging. The study of aging in vertebrates has revealed three distinct mechanisms of aging: rapid senescence, gradual senescence, and negligible senescence. Rapid senescence is characterized by a swift decline in physiological functions and health, leading to a significant increase in mortality rates as organisms age. An example of rapid senescence can be observed in some species of mice, where their health deteriorates rapidly as they age, resulting in a shortened lifespan. On the other hand, gradual senescence involves a more moderate decline in physiological functions and health over time. Organisms with gradual senescence experience incremental changes in reproductive capabilities and overall vitality as they age. Dogs, for instance, exhibit gradual senescence, with a relatively consistent rate of decline in health and a gradual increase in mortality rates as they reach older ages. Negligible senescence is a unique mechanism observed in certain species, where there is minimal deterioration in physiological functions and health with age. These organisms maintain reproductive capabilities and vitality well into advanced ages. The naked mole-rat is a prime example of negligible senescence, as it shows little to no signs of aging, retains its reproductive abilities even at 30 years of age, and is rarely susceptible to age-related diseases like cancer. These three aging mechanisms reflect the diversity of ways in which organisms experience changes in health, reproductive capabilities, and mortality rates over their lifetimes (Buffenstein 2008).

It's evident that there are currently many disagreements among scholars regarding the understanding of aging. With the increasing number of discoveries, the previous assertion that aging is irreversible seems to be less reliable, and new perspectives on the relationship between aging and death have emerged. Even the previously summarized characteristics of aging are merely superficial and fail to explain the essence of aging. The journey to uncover the essence and mechanisms of aging is, at least for now, a challenging and lengthy path.

8 CONCLUSION

In conclusion, the exploration of aging is a multidimensional journey that intertwines scientific discovery with philosophical contemplation. People have delved into the intricate hallmarks of aging, shedding light on the molecular intricacies that drive the gradual decline of physiological functions. The hallmarks, encompassing DNA instability, telomere attrition, epigenetic alterations, loss of proteostasis, and mitochondrial dysfunction, collectively paint a comprehensive portrait of the aging process. These molecular changes not only affect individual cells but also reverberate through organs and systems, culminating in the visible signs of aging and increased susceptibility to age-related diseases.

The discourse on the theories of aging has provided contrasting viewpoints, reflecting the depth of uncertainty surrounding this phenomenon. The intriguing proposition of circumventability has sparked hope for potential interventions that could extend human lifespans significantly. Conversely, the perspective rooted in thermodynamics reminds us that aging is an inherent consequence of existence, shaped by the inexorable march of entropy.By discussing the three mechanisms of aging observed in vertebrates—rapid senescence, gradual senescence, and negligible senescence, remarkable diversity in the aging experiences of different species has been showned. Such insights not only enrich our understanding of aging but also underscore the complexity of aging-related processes, sparking avenues for future research and interventions.

However, there are several limitations in this study. Firstly, the characteristics of aging extend beyond the five listed in this paper. Many recent studies, including factors such as lipid droplets and immune system collapse, have not been addressed. Secondly, these identified features may not be the fundamental causes of aging; they might not delve into the underlying mechanisms of aging but rather remain on the surface as observed phenomena. Additionally, the various perspectives on aging have not been comprehensively summarized. The paper briefly touches upon the reversibility and irreversibility of aging, as well as the three types of aging. In reality, there is a wide range of viewpoints on aging; some argue that aging is a result of evolution, while others propose the existence of a control switch for aging within the human body. These divergent opinions have not yet converged into a unified consensus and have not been incorporated into this paper.

In the future, a deeper understanding of the characteristics of aging may offer more comprehensive biological explanations for longevity-enhancing measures, such as calorie restriction, cold exposure, and other measures. Additionally, these identified aging features can serve as targets for the development of specific drugs, such as protein-degrading agents or activators of telomerase activity, with potential clinical implications. Moreover, unraveling the mechanisms of aging can help dispel uncertainties and guide researchers in the field of aging toward new directions.

REFERENCES

Buffenstein R. (2008). *J Comp Physiol B*, 178**(4),** 439–445.

Casagrande S., Hau M. (2019). *Biol Lett. Mar* 29;15**(3):**20180885.

Gladyshev V. N. (2013). *Trends Genet*, 29**(9),** 506–512.

Gonzalo S. (2010). *J Appl Physiol (1985)*. Aug;109**(2)**:586-97

Guo Y., Guan T., Shafiq K., Yu Q., Jiao X., Na D., Li M. and Zhang G., (2023). *J. Kong. Ageing Res Rev*, **88,** 101955.

Labbadia J. and Morimoto R. I. (2015). *Annu Rev Biochem*, **84,** 435–464.

Li Z., Zhang Z., Ren Y., Wang Y., Fang J., Yue H., Ma S. and Guan F. (2021). *Biogerontology*, 22**(2),** 165–187.

Lidsky P. V., Yuan J., Rulison J. M. and Andino-Pavlovsky R. (2022). *Biochemistry (Mosc)*, 87**(12),** 1413–1445.

López-Otín C., Blasco M. A., Partridge L., Serrano M. and Kroemer G. (2013). *Cell*, 153**(6),** 1194–1217.

López-Otín C., Blasco M. A., Partridge L., Serrano M. and Kroemer G. (2023). *Cell*, **186(2),** 243–278.

Rossiello F., Jurk D., Passos J. F. and d'Adda di Fagagna F. (2022). *Nat Cell Biol*, **24**, 135–147.

Vaiserman A. and Krasnienkov D. (2021). *Front Genet*, **11**, 630186.

Vijg J. and Suh Y. (2013). *Annu Rev Physiol*, **75**, 645–668.

Biological Sciences and Environmental Health – Gao (Ed.)

Correlation analysis of neurodegenerative diseases – Alzheimer's disease and Parkinson's disease

ZiJun Zhou
Undergraduate Biology Program at Stony Brook University, NY, USA

ABSTRACT: Neurodegenerative disorders affect a large number of people globally, particularly represented by Alzheimer's disease and Parkinson's disease. Alzheimer's disease is considered to be the fourth leading cause of death worldwide, and its impact is mainly concentrated in the older age group of 65 years and above. Parkinson's disease, on the other hand, is another neurodegenerative disorder whose prevalence in this category is second only to that of AD. Each of these two diseases exhibits unique pathophysiological mechanisms and clinical manifestations, thus leading to separate therapeutic strategies. Nonetheless, they exhibit significant similarities in several aspects including pathogenesis, clinical manifestations and targeted drug designs. The purpose of this article is to provide insight into the similarities and differences between Alzheimer's disease and Parkinson's disease in terms of their cytopathophysiology, clinical features, and potential common treatment options, therefore seeking to further understand the molecular mechanisms and screening potential targets for specific therapies in neurodegenerative diseases.

1 INTRODUCTION

The currently recognized pathogenesis of Alzheimer's disease (AD) encompasses neuronal apoptosis, gene mutations, and a variety of biochemical and cell biological responses associated with them. At the pathological level, deposition of β-amyloid (Aβ), neurofibrillary tangles due to excessive and aberrant phosphorylation of tau proteins, and neurodegenerative phenomena are considered as the core pathogenic mechanisms of AD. Of particular note, the accumulation of pathologic tau protein has emerged as a key hallmark of AD.

Environmental factors such as MPTP, genes, and age may trigger Parkinson's disease (PD), but the abnormal folding of α-synuclein (aSyn) and its accumulation in Lewy bodies are considered to be the main etiological factor. αSyn triggers a significant decrease in dopamine, which, together with excessive oxidation of dopamine free radical metabolism, leads to oxidative stress and mitochondrial dysfunction in cells, which ultimately induces the clinical symptoms of PD. According to statistics, the incidence of the disease is significantly higher in men than in women. In the early stages of the disease, patients often experience decreased sense of smell and gastrointestinal dysfunction. As the disease progresses, patients may also exhibit clinical symptoms such as 4-6 Hz tremor, postural instability, rapid eye movements, depression and constipation.

Interestingly, although AD and PD differ significantly in etiology and clinical manifestations, they do share some similar pathologic features. Specifically, both AD and PD are associated with PMD, and both Tau and aSyn are considered to be typical representatives of PMD (Soto 2012). In addition, prion disease, the most talked about PMD, exhibits similar characteristics and mechanisms in both Tau and α-syn. On the other hand, the two diseases

DOI: 10.1201/9781003587590-49

differ in clinical features and therapeutic approaches, but similarities still exist. Therefore, this paper will delve into the correlation between AD and PD.

2 PATHOGENESIS CORRELATION OF AD AND PD

2.1 *Structural and functions of Tau protein*

Tau proteins are associated with microproteins in living cells, a major constituent form of microtubule-associated proteins (MAPs). Microtubules, as the main cytoskeletal component of eukaryotic cells, are commonly found in plant and animal cells and play a role in maintaining cellular morphology and structural stability. Structurally, the primary sequence of Tau protein can be divided into two major regions, N-terminal and C-terminal. Compared with the C-terminal, the N-terminal sequence variation of tau is more significant. In tau proteins, the occurrence of threonine and alanine residues within the N-terminal domain is non-random, being densely populated in specific regions. Tau proteins are characterized as intrinsically disordered proteins (IDPs), exhibiting complex long-range intramolecular interactions and lacking a defined secondary structure (Avila *et al.* 2016).

In terms of structural and functional diversity, Tau proteins can be further categorized into six different isoforms with amino acid lengths ranging from 352 to 441 amino acids. These isoforms can be separated by polyacrylamide gel electrophoresis in the presence of sodium dodecyl sulfate (SDS-PAGE) and have molecular weights ranging from 45 to 65 kDa. These isoforms are distinguished by the incorporation of either three repeat regions (3R) or four repeat regions (4R) within their C-terminal domain, whereas the N-terminus may be free of insertion, have one or two insertion fragments (29 or 58 amino acids, respectively). Different isoforms may perform specific functions in different physiological environments or contexts.

The phosphorylation status of Tau proteins is directly related to their binding stability to microtubules. One of the most extended Tau isoforms features 441 putative serine (Ser) or threonine (Thr) phosphorylation sites. A majority of the kinases implicated in Tau protein phosphorylation are members of the proline-directed protein kinase (PDPK) family, encompassing enzymes such as mitogen-activated protein kinase (MAPK). Phosphorylation of Tau proteins leads to dissociation from microtubules and consequent damage to microtubule structure, which in the long term leads to loss of neuronal function and has been linked to the development of a variety of neurodegenerative disorders (e.g., AD and frontal lobe degeneration).

2.2 *Structural and functions of aSyn*

α-synuclein, primarily composed of a sequence of 140 amino acids, exhibits a predicted molecular weight of 14,460.16 Da and is characterized by an isoelectric point of 4.67 (Mor *et al.* 2016). aSyn sequence consists of three functionally defined structural domains. The amino-terminal structural domain (N-terminal, residues 1-60) can be regarded as the region where genetic or familial mutational factors are located (Appel-Cresswell *et al.* 2013). The central structural domain (residues 61-95) tends to form a beta-folded lamellar structure, which may be associated with key pathological mechanisms of the disease. The carboxy-terminal structural domain (C-terminal, spanning residues 96-140) is enriched with proline and acidic residues. These residues are hallmarks of intrinsically disordered proteins that not only display significant conformational disorder but are also prone to phosphorylation and other post-translational modifications. The propensity of these residues to induce turns and perturb the regularity of secondary protein structures alludes to the absence of a well-defined secondary structure in this domain (Mor *et al.* 2016). Conversely, the N-terminal region (encompassing amino acids 1-60) is distinguished by its unique and highly conserved truncated tandem repeats. Central to these repeats is a consensus motif: KT(A)KE(Q)G(Q)V and K(M)T(A)K(R)E(Q)G(Q)V(A), with KTKEGV standing out as the prototypical sequence associated with synaptic proteins (Jakes, Spillantini and Goedert 1994).

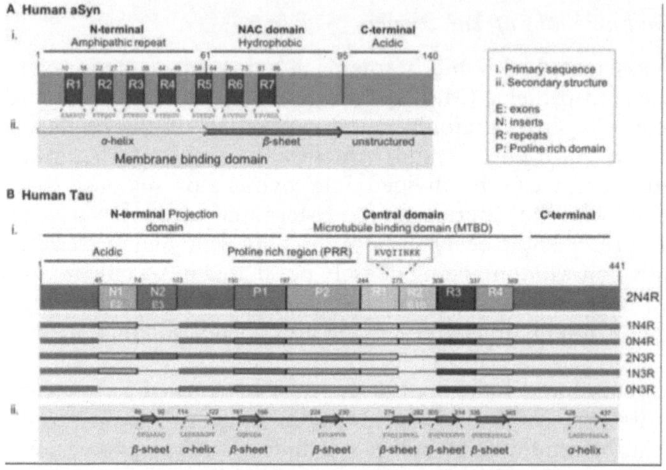

Figure 1. Structure of Tau and aSyn proteins (Vasili *et al.* 2019).

2.3 *Pathogenic role of Tau and aSyn*

2.3.1 *Characteristics of prions*

As mentioned previously, specifically, both AD and PD are associated *with* protein misfolding disorder (PMD), and both Tau and aSyn are considered to be representative factors of PMD (1). The article would like to provide an overview of the transmission pathways of AD and PD (mainly with aSyn and Tau) as well as attempt to understand the relationship with prions.

In delving into the mechanisms of protein infectious diseases, prion research has demonstrated that they are distinct from traditional infectious agents (e.g., bacteria and viruses), but still possess key attributes of infectious agents. Specifically, they are able to proliferate exponentially in suitable hosts, are capable of inter-individual transmission, can be titrated for infectivity by bioassay, show resistance to bioclearance mechanisms, penetrate biofilm barriers, and undergo structural changes to form so-called "mutant" strains, whose propagation is constrained by species-specific process of transmission is further constrained by the species barrier. Considering the striking similarities in pathogenesis between transmissible spongiform encephalopathies (TSEs) and other PMDs and prions, we have come to realize that proteins also have the ability to act as infectious agents to spread disease (Soto 2012).

2.3.2 *Characterization and transmission of Tau proteins*

Tau proteins show many similarities to prions in their mechanisms of transmission, and they are capable of spreading by multiple routes. It is important to note that the transmission of Tau proteins does not depend solely on spatial proximity, but is closely related to the pathway of synaptic connectivity. Further studies revealed that the concentration of Tau protein in the nucleus was significantly increased in the presence of P301SBE. To verify this finding, we compared P301SBE with PBS and other controls. The experimental results indeed showed that Tau proteins were significantly increased in the nuclei of mice receiving

P301SBE injection. Further experimental analyses suggested that these accumulated Tau proteins were taken up by the cells and transported along the axons either in a paracrine or retrograde manner. In particular, the increase of Tau protein in the nuclei of cells in the hippocampal region was particularly pronounced, suggesting a pattern of Tau protein propagation within the axon (Ahmed *et al.* 2014).

Under physiologically normal conditions, Tau proteins provide the necessary stability for microtubules, thereby safeguarding the structural integrity of microtubules within the cell. However, overexpression or aberrant aggregation of Tau proteins may lead to impairment of their function in stabilizing microtubules, resulting in potential damage to nerve cells. Similar to the abnormally folded proteins in prions, Tau proteins exhibit seeding effects, in which their six isoforms undergo structural changes in certain pathological environments (Soto 2012), leading to the formation of exogenous Tau pffs. When these Tau pffs are taken up by neuronal cells, they act as seeds, triggering abnormal folding and aggregation of endogenous Tau proteins. Intriguingly, even if only a small amount of exogenous Tau pffs are ingested, they are effective in inducing large amounts of Tau protein aggregation within the cell to form structures similar to those of NFT. This seeding effect is thought to be a central mechanism of protein aggregation in a variety of neurodegenerative diseases. Tau protein aggregation induced by pffs may reduce the concentration of soluble Tau, which in turn impairs its normal stabilizing effect on microtubules. In addition, the cellular uptake of Tau pffs, especially via WGA (wheat germ agglutinin)-mediated uptake, further corroborates the mechanism of cell-to-cell propagation of Tau proteins in neurodegenerative diseases (Guo and Lee 2011).

2.3.3 *Characterization and propagation of aSyn proteins*

PD is represented as a neuromyasthenia gravis PMD in which the accumulation of aSyn protein is widely recognized as a central pathological feature of this disease. Interestingly, the mechanism of aSyn protein propagation shows remarkable similarity to the way certain prion proteins propagate from cell to cell.

In order to investigate the transmissibility of aSyn proteins from primary cells to transplanted cells in detail, we used Alexa-Fluor-488-labeled aSyn medium to incubate mouse cortical neuronal stem cells (MCNSCs) in our experiments. The results showed that after 24 hours of incubation, 47% of GFP-positive MCNSCs exhibited punctate cytoplasmic accumulation associated with human aSyn. By 4 weeks, this percentage increased to 15%, and some cells even generated dense aSyn inclusion bodies within the cytoplasm (Desplats *et al.* 2009).

This pattern of cell-to-cell spread of aSyn resembles the behavior of prions in some respects. Under certain conditions, misfolding of the aSyn protein seems to induce similar misfolding of its neighboring homologous proteins, which is similar to the self-replicating mode of the prion protein. More importantly, aSyn aggregation and formation of inclusion bodies in neuronal cells are hallmarks of neurodegenerative diseases, whereas the prion protein exhibits a similar structure in infected neuronal cells.

We further found that the cell-to-cell spread of the aSyn protein does not appear to depend on direct contact between cells, which echoes the mode of spread of some prions. Recipient cells take up extracellular aSyn aggregates by an endosome mechanism and subsequently transport them to the lysosome for catabolism via the endoplasmic reticulum pathway. When the lysosomal function of the receptor cell is inhibited, the delivered aSyn gradually accumulates intracellularly, implying that diminished lysosomal function may be associated with increased aSyn. It has been shown that lysosomal enzyme activity decreases progressively with age and that mutations in certain lysosomal enzyme genes are associated with a range of inherited neurodegenerative diseases. In addition, overexpression of α-synuclein may be an important factor contributing to the rapid propagation of the aSyn protein we observed.

3 CLINICAL PROBLEMS OF AD AND PD AND THEIR CORRELATION

3.1 *Clinical problem of AD*

AD is the most common type of dementia, which is mainly characterized by a progressive impairment of brain function, leading to sustained cognitive decline. From a clinical point of view, dementia manifests itself as a marked deterioration of the cognitive and functional state previously achieved by the individual, to the extent that it affects his or her daily functioning. Although natural cognitive decline is inevitable with age, e.g., older adults may perform worse than younger adults in terms of mental processing speed, simple reaction time, choice reaction time, and perceptual time, this is not associated with significant brain function impairment.

Risk factors for AD include cardiovascular problems such as bleeding, vascular disease, blocked blood vessels, and infarction; and lifestyle and health conditions such as hypertension, type 2 diabetes, obesity, depression, and ongoing stress. Although family history and brain injuries have been associated with the onset of AD, the age factor remains the predominant risk factor. Typically, clinical symptoms of AD are not common until the age of 50, which is considered a late-onset disease. Initial symptoms are mainly impaired short-term memory and difficulty in remembering new information, while long term memory and implicit memory are relatively maintained. In addition, patients may have mild difficulties with temporal or spatial orientation, such as judging time and finding their way, and may experience mild behavioral or personality changes.

Cognitive decline worsens further in patients with moderate AD, leading to additional functional deficits such as muscle rigidity and motor delays that make them more dependent on others. The patient's ability to grasp information decreases dramatically, executive function and logical reasoning are significantly impaired, disorientation is lost, and he or she may begin to fail to recognize loved ones.

In severe or advanced stages, patients may experience hallucinations and optical illusions, a complete loss of cognitive abilities, and a dramatic decline in language skills, only being able to produce simple phrases or words. Due to the deterioration of their physical functions, they are completely dependent on others for care and may experience symptoms such as incontinence (Tarawneh and Holtzman 2012).

The primary method of diagnosing AD is by evaluating the patient's cognitive status and considering a combination of the potential factors listed above.

3.2 *Clinical problems of PD*

James Parkinson published an academic paper describing the neurological disorder that bears his name in the early 1800s. He meticulously described the clinical symptoms of patients with the disease, including involuntary tremors, muscle weakness, rigidity, and a tendency to transition from a slow pace to running in walking. Parkinson emphasized that despite the impairment of bodily functions, the senses and intellect were not affected. He originally referred to the disease as "shaking paralysis," but today's knowledge suggests that PD is not really a paralysis, but rather a motor dysfunction.

The pathology of PD is characterized by a decrease in nigrostriatal neurons, which is manifested by depigmentation, neuronal death, and glial cell proliferation. Although PD can present at all ages, its high prevalence is around 60 years of age, and the risk of developing the disease gradually increases with age, with a lifetime prevalence of about 2%. Most PD symptoms appear gradually and may initially be an imperceptible resting tremor. However, some patients may first experience bradykinesia, and some may never develop a tremor. Early symptoms of PD are associated with reduced levels of dopamine in the nigrostriatal pathway, but as the disease progresses, some symptoms may not respond to conventional dopamine therapy.

In addition to motor symptoms, patients with PD often experience non-motor symptoms such as fatigue, depression, anxiety, sleep disturbances, and autonomic dysfunction, which includes cardiovascular system and gastrointestinal problems. In addition, about 40% of patients may experience sensory symptoms such as pain, numbness or tingling. As the disease progresses, cognitive impairment and even dementia may also occur, especially in older patients (Fahn 2003).

Diagnosing PD relies heavily on its clinical presentation and assessment of responsiveness to dopamine therapy. Despite the use of advanced diagnostic tools, such as PET, the error rate in clinical diagnosis may remain high in the early stages of the disease, even in specialized centers. By rigorously applying established clinical diagnostic criteria, we can improve the diagnostic accuracy of PD.

4 THERAPEUTIC OPTIONS FOR AD AND PD

Alzheimer's Disease (AD) and Parkinson's Disease (PD) are classified under neurodegenerative disorders. PD predominantly arises from the diminution of dopaminergic neurotransmitters, leading to dopamine replacement therapy becoming the cornerstone of its clinical management. Various dopaminergic agents are employed in this realm, with levodopa (L-DOPA) being the most efficacious. Levodopa is typically co-administered with peripheral decarboxylase inhibitors to circumvent peripheral dopamine synthesis. Beyond its metabolic breakdown by aromatic amino acid decarboxylases, levodopa undergoes enzymatic conversion by catechol-O-methyltransferase (COMT), forming 3-O-methyldopa. By inhibiting COMT, the plasma longevity of levodopa can be extended, thereby amplifying its therapeutic efficacy without intensifying its peak concentrations. Nevertheless, empirical evidence underscores that roughly 60% of individuals diagnosed with PD experience motor complications, often termed the "wear-off" phenomena, after five years of sustained levodopa administration. Notably, patients younger than 60 tend to manifest these complications quickly (Fahn 2003).

At the same time, PD is not just a motor disorder; it also involves cognitive decline. When it comes to the treatment of Parkinson's disease dementia (PDD), the therapeutic strategy may be similar to that of AD.

4.1 *Pharmaceutical approaches for AD and PD*

4.1.1 *Cholinesterase inhibitors*

Donepezil, exhibiting an IC50 value of 5.7 nM, is the second FDA-approved therapeutic for Alzheimer's Disease (AD). It is recognized for its safety profile and is a recommended therapeutic intervention for AD-afflicted patients. The pharmacodynamic properties of donepezil derive from its interaction with the aromatic active site of acetylcholinesterase (AChE) and the peripheral anionic site (PAS). Specifically, its benzylpiperidine and indanone structural moieties interface with the canyon bottom anionic subsite of Trp 84 and the peripheral site of Trp 279 of the enzyme, respectively. The compound boasts notable in vitro AChE inhibitory prowess, exhibiting an extraordinary selectivity for AChE over butyrylcholinesterase (BuChE), displaying a potency 3200-fold greater against the former. A comprehensive randomized, double-blinded study indicated that patients with moderate-to-severe AD, previously on a ten mg/d regimen of donepezil IR, showed statistically meaningful enhancements in 10 out of the 23 pre-established primary endpoints when treated with two mg/d of donepezil in comparison to one mg/d dosage. However, even as cognitive metrics on the SIB displayed improvements, no pronounced effects were discerned beyond a ten mg/d dosage in the comprehensive functional evaluations using the CIBIC+. This evidence intimates that therapy remains beneficial for even late-stage AD patients (Farlow *et al.* 2010). Regarding Parkinson's disease-associated dementia (PDD), the scarcity of investigative studies implies a data deficit in affirming donepezil's therapeutic efficacy, underscoring the necessity for additional research.

4.1.2 *N-methyl-D-aspartate (NMDA) receptor antagonists*

Glutamate-mediated neurotoxicity is gradually gaining acceptance in the etiology of AD. The central hypothesis is that glutamate receptors of the NMDA type undergo excessive sustained activation rather than transient peak activation. This sustained mild activation may lead to neuronal damage under chronicity. Furthermore, damage during learning may not only stem from direct neuronal damage, but may also be related to sustained activation of NMDA receptors (Danysz and Parsons 2003). As a noncompetitive antagonist of NMDA receptors, memantine has been shown to have symptomatic therapeutic effects in diseases such as AD and vascular dementia, and may have a role in the treatment of PDD (Danysz *et al.* 2000). In addition, memantine may have neuroprotective effects against glutamate toxicity. Memantine is approved for the symptomatic treatment of moderate to severe AD and has been associated with a moderate improvement in the clinical course of AD. Its beneficial effects have been demonstrated in several clinical trials, albeit with smaller improvements, in cognition, mood, behavior, and daily functioning in patients with moderate to severe AD. Its effect in mild to moderate AD is unclear. The efficacy and safety of memantine has been demonstrated in placebo-controlled trials in moderate-to-severe AD and may be enhanced in combination with the aforementioned donepezil and other cholinesterase inhibitors. The utility of memantine in the treatment of PDD still requires further study.

4.2 *Non-pharmacological treatment*

We have explored in depth the pharmacologic treatment strategies for AD and PD. However, in addition to pharmacologic interventions, AD and PD share a range of common strategies in the area of non-pharmacologic treatments. For AD, biological therapies, such as photobiomodulation (PBM), have been shown to exert neuroprotective effects and present significant potential benefits in slowing the progression of AD. In addition, modulation of gut microbes has been widely recognized as promising as a therapeutic tool; restoration of gut microbial homeostasis may be beneficial in slowing the symptomatic manifestations of AD (Huynh *et al.* 2022). In the case of PD, on the other hand, given that the core symptom is impairment of motor function, therapeutic strategies tend to be more focused on the restoration of motor function. However, Parkinson's disease with dementia (PDD) is also a problem that cannot be ignored. Given that the focus of this paper is to explore the relevance of AD to PD in terms of non-pharmacologic treatment, we will next explore in detail the cross-cutting strategies of these two disorders in the non-pharmacologic realm.

4.2.1 *Cognitive interventions*

Within the domain of neurology, cognitive interventions are categorized into three primary paradigms. Firstly, Cognitive Stimulation (CS) emphasizes the repetitive execution of standardized tasks crafted to enhance specific cognitive functions. Secondly, Cognitive Training (CT) follows a similar methodology, focusing on rigorous training through standardized exercises targeting particular cognitive domains. Lastly, Cognitive Rehabilitation (CR) adopts a patient-centric methodology, initiating from an identified cognitive impairment and subsequently formulating personalized strategies to facilitate the patient in achieving the desired cognitive tasks or functions (Huntley *et al.* 2015). Current literature indicates a paucity of robust evidence supporting the efficacy of cognitive training. Notably, some trial findings suggest that prevalent standardized outcome measures might need to encapsulate such interventions' potential benefits comprehensively (Bahar-Fuchs *et al.* 2013). A recent meta-analysis, resonating with a Cochrane review, underscored the lack of substantial evidence supporting CT's efficacy in dementia. Furthermore, combinatorial approaches integrating CT and CS have yet to enhance holistic cognitive performance significantly. However, a salient observation is the therapeutic potential of CS, particularly in ameliorating AD symptoms (Huntley *et al.* 2015). Shifting the lens to Parkinson's Disease (PD), a study encompassing 45 patients illustrated the potential of a four-week CT regimen, with participants demonstrating enhanced performance across multiple cognitive metrics, including processing speed and executive functions (París *et al.* 2011). This suggests the potential applicability of cognitive interventions across both AD and PD spectra. Nonetheless, the scientific community acknowledges the need for extensive research to corroborate these preliminary findings.

4.2.2 *Exercise interventions*

The importance of exercise as a means of disease prevention has been widely recognized. However, in the case of AD, which has long been positioned primarily as a disease of cognitive impairment, exercise therapy has not been sufficiently emphasized in its management strategy. However, a systematic analysis of studies indicates that exercise actually positively affects the rate of cognitive deterioration in AD patients. A meta-analysis further revealed that exercise interventions can indeed produce positive benefits on overall cognitive function. Nonetheless, more high-quality, rigorous randomized controlled trials are needed to definitively determine the effects of exercise in delaying cognitive decline in AD (Farina *et al.* 2014). Notably, quantitative physical activity (PA) has been shown to reduce the risk of developing AD. According to the study, physical activity was significantly associated with survival in patients with AD: there was a gradual downward trend in the risk of death as the reported amount of physical activity increased. Correspondingly, median survival data show that people who engage in some kind of physical activity have a life expectancy of about 5.5 years longer than those who are physically inactive, while those who are physically active at a high intensity have a life expectancy of up to about 8 years (Scarmeas *et al.* 2011).

In the case of PD, since it has traditionally been viewed as a major movement disorder, treatment strategies have mostly focused on motor symptoms. However, nowadays, the impact of PD on cognitive function is also widely accepted. Although in the past there was a clear definition between cognition and motor function, it is now recognized that the loss of motor function in PD actually involves a wide range of impaired cognitive abilities, and the impairment of these abilities in turn affects the daily life of the patient. Research findings have shown that physical training does help with PD symptoms. For example, while rehabilitative exercise may not have shown significant improvements in executive function or attention in PD, aerobic training did produce positive results. In addition, although memory function did not significantly improve with exercise therapy alone, a growing number of integrated strategies, such as the combination of physical activity and cognitive training, have now yielded promising preliminary results for memory improvement (Pupíková and Rektorová 2020). Another study also confirmed that a weekly treatment program combining computer-assisted cognitive training with physical rehabilitation had particularly significant and long-lasting improvements in verbal fluency and situational verbal memory (Disbrow *et al.* 2012).

5 CONCLUSION

Alzheimer's disease (AD) and Parkinson's disease (PD) present some surprising commonalities in neuropathology and clinical manifestations. When comparing the neurobiology of the two in detail, a series of similar patterns are observed from molecular to cellular to overall clinical manifestations. For example, at the molecular level, the characteristic proteins of AD and PD, Tau and aSyn, exhibit similarities at the structural level, where they are both predominantly primary structures with no apparent secondary structure but also functionally exhibit prion-like propagation properties. Such proteins undergo misfolding, which leads to similar alterations in homologous proteins, a pattern that closely resembles the self-replication and propagation mechanism of prion proteins. Clinically, AD and PD also have a significant cross-presentation. For example, while AD patients primarily demonstrate cognitive dysfunction, many also have somatic symptoms; conversely, PD patients have a degree of cognitive impairment (e.g., Parkinson's dementia (PDD)), although they have predominantly motor symptoms.

Furthermore, regarding treatment strategies, AD and PD share certain potential treatments and strategies. Nonetheless, we must be cautious because these similarities are mainly based on current observational and experimental data. There are still substantial areas to be mined and explored in the interrelationships and intersections between AD and PD, especially in cell signaling mechanisms and therapeutic options. However, current evidence suggests that there are certain common mechanisms and interactions between the two.

REFERENCES

Ahmed Z. et al., (2014). *Acta Neuropathologica,* 127, 667–683.
Appel-Cresswell S. et al., (2013). *Movement disorders,* 28(6), 811–813.
Avila J. et al., (2016). *Frontiers in aging neuroscience,* 8(262).
Bahar-Fuchs A., Clare L., and Woods B., (2013). *Cochrane database of systematic reviews,* 6.
Danysz W. and Parsons C. G., (2003). *International journal of geriatric psychiatry,* 18, S1, S23–S32.
Danysz W., Parsons C. G., Mobius H. J., Stoffler A., and Quack G., (2000). *Neurotox Res,* 2, 2–3, 85–97.
Desplats P. et al., (2009). *Proceedings of the National Academy of Sciences,* 106, 31, 13010–13015.
Disbrow E. et al., (2012). *Brain research,* 1452, 151–164.
Fahn S., (2003). *Annals of the New York Academy of Sciences,* 991, 1, 1–14.
Farina N., Rusted J., and Tabet N., (2014). *International Psychogeriatrics,* 26, 1, 9–18.
Farlow M. R. et al., (2010). *Clinical therapeutics,* 32, 7, 1234–1251 .
Guo J. L. and Lee V. M., (2011). *J Biol Chem,* 286(17) 15317–31
Huntley J., Gould R., Liu K., Smith M., and Howard R., (2015). *BMJ open,* 5, 4, p. e005247.
Huynh Q.-S., Elangovan S., and Holsinger R. D., (2002). *International Journal of Molecular Sciences,* 23, 19, p. 11037.
Jakes R., Spillantini M. G., and Goedert M., (1994). *FEBS letters,* 345(1), 27–32.
Mor D. E., Ugras S. E., Daniels M. J., and Ischiropoulos H., (2016). *Neurobiology of disease,* 88. 66–74.
París A. P. et al., (2011). *Movement Disorders,* 26, 7, 1251–1258.
Pupíková M. and Rektorová I., (2020). *Journal of Neural Transmission,* 127, 5, 799–820.
Scarmeas N. et al., (2011). 19, 5, 471–481.
Soto C., (2012). *Cell,* 149(5), 968–977.
Tarawneh R. and Holtzman D. M., (2012). *Cold Spring Harb Perspect Med,* 2, 5, p. a006148.
Vasili E., Dominguez-Meijide A., and Outeiro T. F., (2019). *Frontiers in molecular neuroscience,* 12, 107.

Biological Sciences and Environmental Health – Gao (Ed.)

Modeling and forecasting Covid-19 deaths in the United States

Tianyi Feng
Zhejiang University, Hangzhou, PR China

ABSTRACT: The spread of COVID-19 has made it a pandemic, causing tremendous damage to daily life, both directly and indirectly. The goal of this study is to use ARIMA modeling to assist the government and health departments to better respond to the virus by analyzing trends in deaths from previous COVID outbreaks in the United States and to predict future COVID-19 deaths. In this study, the seasonal autoregressive integrated moving average (SARIMA) model was used to analyze the COVID-19 death data, which was based on the number of COVID-19 deaths from January 2020 to July 2023. Through the necessary steps of constructing the SARIMA model, such as smoothness test, parameter identification, model test, etc., the study successfully constructed the SARIMA model of (2,1,3)(1,0,0)52, which can be well applied to COVID-19 ground data. Compared with the ARMR model, this model better handles the specificity of seasonality in the data and can better predict the number of COVID-19 deaths in the future, which is more consistent with the trend of deaths in reality. The idea of modeling has important implications for public health. If models can be constructed to accurately predict COVID-19 deaths, health departments and policymakers can provide valuable insights to develop proactive data-driven strategies. This includes resource allocation, hospital preparedness, and timely implementation of interventions to mitigate the public health impact of a pandemic.

1 INTRODUCTION

Since the outbreak in early January 2020, Covid-19 rapidly disseminated throughout the United States. COVID-19 has been responsible for more than 88 million cases and 1 million deaths across the United States (Centers for Disease Control and Prevention 2019). COVID-19 has had a tremendous impact on the US society, economy, and healthcare (Regan *et al.* 2021). As of August 2023, the United States experienced at least five relatively large waves: the first around March 2020–April 2020, followed by the second on July 2020, the third around November 2020–January 2021, the fourth on August 2021–September 2021, and the final around January 2022. Covid-19 leads to substantial disruptions not only in daily life and the economy but also imposes immense pressures on the healthcare infrastructure.

The spread of COVID-19 is characterized by its complexity and rapid transmission, making traditional epidemiological models challenging to apply accurately. As a result, there is a growing need for advanced predictive modeling techniques that can capture the nuances of Covid-19 trends. One such approach is the use of the auto-regressive integrated moving average (ARIMA) model, renowned for its ability to analyze time series data and forecast future values (Jiang *et al.* 2020).

ARIMA is a time-series auto-regressive technique that calculates future short-term predictions by analyzing time series of historical data (Box *et al.* 2015). The ARIMA model has been widely used in areas including stock markets, economic indicators, industrial output, and weather forecasting. Of course, it is also quite commonly used for disease trend

DOI: 10.1201/9781003587590-50

prediction, especially during the past COVID-19 outbreak. The ARIMA model is particularly effective in capturing the temporal trends and patterns in COVID-19 data. By analyzing historical data points over time, the ARIMA model can identify underlying patterns, seasonal variations, and potential future trajectories of COVID-19. This enables policymakers to anticipate surges in COVID-19 cases, plan resource allocation, and implement appropriate public health interventions. Many researchers have made predictions about COVID-19 infection, deaths, hospitalizations, and other data based on the ARIMA model.

At the beginning of the COVID-19 outbreak, Benvenuto *et al.* (2020) used available data to predict future infection and mortality rates. Tandon *et al.* (2020) also used the ARIMA model to predict the number of infections in India in 2020. Similarly, Chintalapudi *et al.* (2020) built a model using ARIMA to forecast the number of infections and recoveries from COVID-19 in Italy for May 2020. These studies illustrated that in the case of COVID-19, ARIMA models could provide forecasts for various key metrics such as infection rates, hospitalizations, and deaths. These predictions help the government estimate the potential strain on healthcare facilities due to COVID-19 and guide the formulation of strategies to curb the spread of COVID-19. For instance, if the model predicts an upcoming spike in hospitalizations, authorities can proactively arrange for additional beds, medical supplies, and staff to ensure sufficient capacity to handle patients.

Moreover, ARIMA models contribute to informed decision-making by allowing officials to assess the impact of different policy measures related to COVID-19. By simulating different scenarios and observing their potential outcomes, policymakers can choose the most effective strategies to contain the spread of COVID-19 while minimizing social and economic disruptions caused by COVID-19.

Although many researchers have used ARIMA models to predict various kinds of data related to COVID-19, such as deaths, infected cases, hospitalizations, vaccinations, and so on since the early days of the COVID-19 outbreak, at the same time, some researchers have suggested that simple ARIMA models cannot solve the problem in the context of a nonlinear relationship in most cases, especially since the actual problem is often dynamic and complex (Papastefanopoulos *et al.* 2020). This leads to a significant limitation in the accuracy and usability of the ARIMA model in many cases, i.e., the model is unable to take into account and deal with situations where nonlinear relationships are likely to be present in time series data (Zhu and Wei 2013). However, this is not to suggest that research based on ARIMA models on time series problems such as the COVID-19 correlation is meaningless. In fact, the prediction results based on the ARIMA model are in many cases quite similar to the trend of the actual results, with only a certain gap in accuracy, which depends precisely on the dataset used for the training of the model and the parameters of the model chosen by the researcher. Therefore, using accuracy metrics to select the most appropriate model has become the preferred approach taken by many researchers to test their models. However, it is important to note that the values predicted by the model do not have to be exactly the same as the actual values over the same period of time but only have to keep the gap within a reasonable interval (Holshue *et al.* 2020). It is important to recognize that while ARIMA models offer a powerful predictive tool, they are not immune to limitations. Variability in data quality, the impact of external factors, and the evolving nature of the pandemic can all influence the model's performance. Nonetheless, the application of ARIMA models to predict COVID-19 data holds great promise in assisting authorities to make data-driven decisions that can effectively mitigate the impact of the pandemic on public health and society as a whole.

The goal of this study is to find the model with the best prediction results by comparing the models under different parameters. The accuracy of the predictions can be checked by comparing them with newly published data, and some parameters can be adjusted to improve the model based on the comparison results. Regarding the period of the model's prediction, the study aims to be able to accurately predict the data from one day to one week in the future and the trend of the epidemic over a longer period of time, for example, one month.

2 METHODS

2.1 *Data sources*

The study obtained data on the number of COVID-19 deaths and hospitalizations from the Centers for Disease Control and Prevention website and the number of COVID-19 infections from the Our World in Data website. The data on deaths covers the period from January 11, 2020, to July 15, 2023; data on hospitalizations spans from August 8, 2020, to July 8, 2023; and data on infections is from 4 January 2020 to 20 May 2023. All of the data is recorded at weekly intervals.

2.2 *Introduction of SARIMA model*

ARIMA model consists of three components, usually denoted by ARIMA(p, d, q):

Autoregression (AR(p)) is used to express the interconnectedness between the current values of the model and the observations of the past periods.

$$y_t = c + \varphi_1 y_{t-1} + \varphi_2 y_{t-2} + \cdots + \varphi_P y_{t-p} + \varepsilon_t \tag{1}$$

Where $\varphi_1, \ldots, \varphi_P$ are autoregressive coefficients, ε_t represent white noise, c is constant term (Liu *et al.* 2022).

The integral (I(d)) indicates that the time series is differenced. By differencing, a non-stationary series can be converted into a stationary series.

$$\Delta^d x_t = \Delta x_t - \Delta x_{t-1} \tag{2}$$

where Δ is the difference operator.

The moving average (MA(q)) represents a time series model, where the current value is expressed as a linear regression of the prediction errors (or residuals) from a number of points in time in the past.

$$y_t = c + \varepsilon_t + \theta_1 \varepsilon_{t-1} + \theta_2 \varepsilon_{t-2} + \cdots + \theta_q \varepsilon_{t-q} \tag{3}$$

Where $\theta_1, \ldots, \theta_q$ are moving average coefficients and $\varepsilon_{t-1}, \ldots, \varepsilon_{t-q}$ represent forecast errors. ε_t and c are white noise and constant terms, respectively.

The SARIMA model is generally expressed as SARIMA(p, d, q)(P, D, Q)s.

The expression of the SARIMA model is as follows:

$$\Phi_P(B^s)\varphi(B)\nabla_s^D \nabla^d x_t = \Theta_Q(B^s)\theta(B)\omega_t \tag{4}$$

where x_t is the nonstationary time series; ω_t is the white process. $\Phi_P(B^s)$; and $\Theta_Q(B^s)$ represent the autoregressive and moving average of the seasonal component; ∇_s^D and ∇^d indicate the differencing components and trend components; $\boldsymbol{B}$ is the backshift operator. The autoregressive and moving average process of the trend component are represented by polynomials $\varphi(B)$ and $\theta(B)$ (Liu *et al.* 2022).

2.3 *SARIMA model establishment process*

The data we use have evolved over time, reflecting the developmental changes in COVID-19 over time. Therefore, they can be considered as time series data. The SARIMA model establishment process involves several stages.

2.3.1 *Stationarity check*

Before building the SARIMA model, it is necessary to assess the stationarity of the time series data. One common method to test for stationarity is the Augmented Dickey-Fuller

(ADF) test. The ADF test helps determine if the time series exhibits a unit root, which would indicate non-stationarity. If the ADF test results show that the time series is stationary, it provides a solid foundation for proceeding with SARIMA model construction. In contrast, if the time series is found to be non-stationary, appropriate transformations, such as differencing, can be applied to achieve stationarity before building the model.

2.3.2 *Model identification*

The autocorrelation coefficient (ACF) and partial autocorrelation coefficient (PACF) plots are examined to identify the SARIMA model. The ACF helps determine the seasonal component, while the PACF provides insights into the autoregressive and moving average components. Based on these plots, potential values for seasonal and non-seasonal orders are selected.

2.3.3 *Model testing*

If the SARIMA model is specified, it needs validation. This involves testing the model's residuals for randomness and normality. The QQ-plot is used to visually assess the residuals' normality against a standard normal distribution. Additionally, statistical tests, such as the residual normality test, can be employed to check if the residuals follow a normal distribution.

2.3.4 *Model estimation and validation*

Once the orders are determined, the SARIMA model can be estimated and validated using historical data. Model performance is assessed using various evaluation metrics, and adjustments may be made to improve the model's accuracy.

3 RESULTS AND DISCUSSION

3.1 *Time series trend analysis*

Figure 1 shows the time series trend graph of the number of COVID-19 deaths. From Figure 1, it can be seen that the change in the number of deaths generally displays a horizontal change pattern, with significant fluctuations from 2020 onward, yet remaining within a stable range. The time series of the number of COVID-19 deaths appears to exhibit stationary behavior, although further testing is necessary.

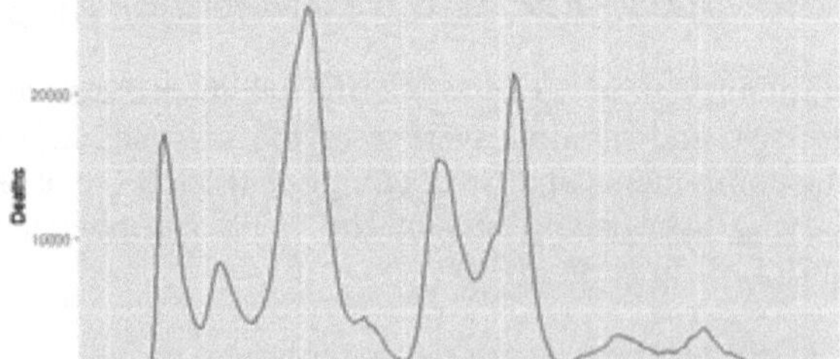

Figure 1. Time series trend of COVID-19 death cases (Picture credit: Original).

Figure 2 displays a scatterplot matrix of the correlation between the number of COVID-19 deaths and the number of deaths lagged 1 to 4 periods. The figure reveals a significant positive correlation between the number of COVID-19 deaths and the number of COVID-19 deaths lagging from period 1 to 4. This suggests a possible autocorrelation in the time series.

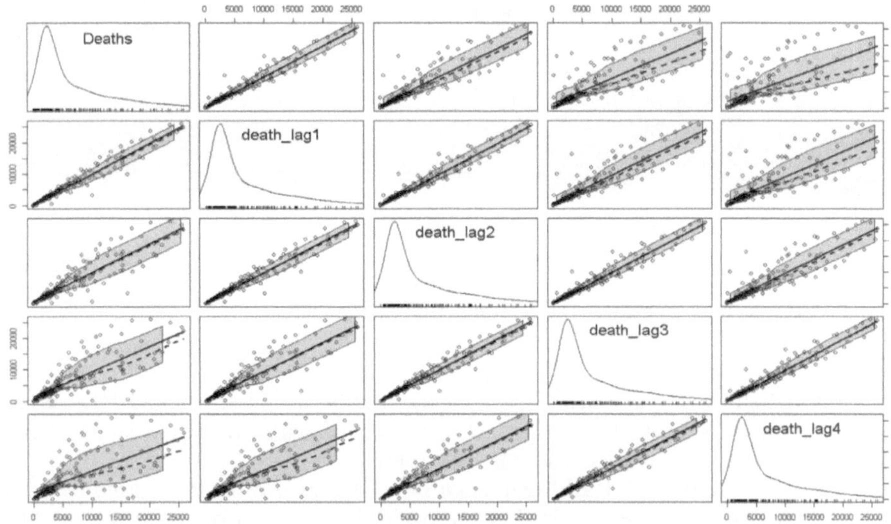

Figure 2. Scatterplot matrix for COVID-19 death case (Picture credit: Original).

3.2 *Time series stationarity test*

The ADF method was used to test the stationarity of the number of deaths.

Table 1. ADF test results of death cases.

Variable	lag	T value	P value	Conclusion
Case	5	-3.8199	0.01948	Steady

Table 1 presents the ADF test results for the original series of the number of COVID-19 deaths; the t-value in the test results is -3.8199; and it has a P-value of 0.01948, which is less than 0.05, so the time series of the number of deaths of the COVID-19 is a stationary time series at the 0.05 level of significance.

3.3 *Model order determination*

As a stationary time series is a prerequisite for establishing an ARMA model, we can proceed with constructing an ARMA model to predict the time series. The next step involves utilizing the ACF and PACF to determine the order of the model.

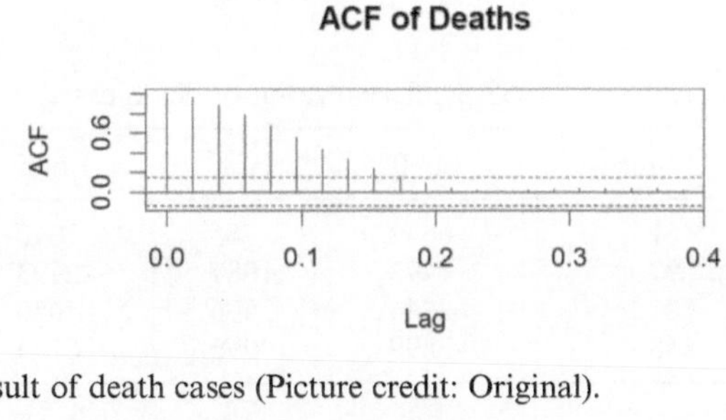

Figure 3. ACF test result of death cases (Picture credit: Original).

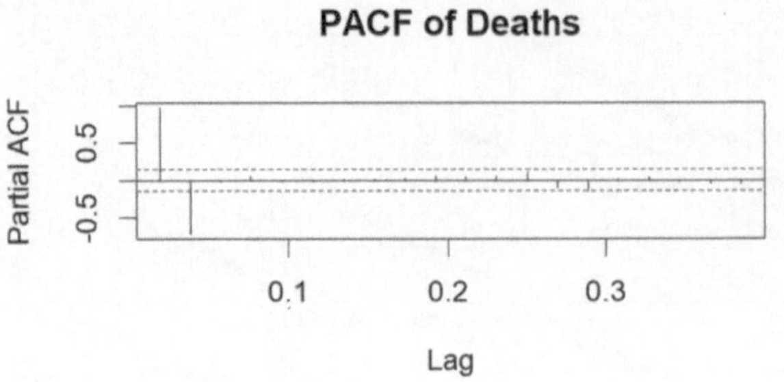

Figure 4. PACF test result of death cases (Picture credit: Original).

Figures 3 and 4 show the ACF and PACF of the number of deaths in COVID-19, and it can be seen that the ACF of the time series of the number of deaths decreases slowly from the first period, so there is an obvious "trailing" phenomenon.

The PACF of the number of deaths exhibits a rapid decrease from the second period and reaches the vicinity of twice the standard deviation in the third period, indicating a distinct second-order "truncated tail" phenomenon.

Therefore, from the plots of ACF and PACF, we get the model parameters as p = 2, q= 0, leading to the ARMA (2, 0) model.

Based on these results, we can determine the parameters p, d, q, and s for the SARIMA model, where p = 2, d = 0, q = 0, and s = 52. In this case, we calculate the optimal *P*, *D*, *Q* values, resulting in the optimal SARIMA model $(2,0,0)(1,1,0)_{52}$. The corresponding AIC and BIC values are 2170.77 and 2182.3, respectively.

The SARIMA$(2,0,0)(1,1,0)_{52}$ model is an extension of ARMA(2,0) with the addition of a seasonal component. The parameters p = 2, d = 0, and q = 0 represent the non-seasonal part, indicating the use of second-order autoregression, zeroth-order differencing, and zeroth-order moving average. The parameter P = 1 represents the seasonal autoregression, utilizing data from the previous 1 seasonal cycle. Parameters D = 1 and Q = 0 indicate that the model performs first-order seasonal differencing to remove seasonal effects, but does not have a seasonal moving average term. At the same time, the auto.arima function was used to search for the best model, which led to the result $(2,1,3)(1,0,0)_{52}$. The corresponding AIC and BIC values are 2844.53 and 2866.99, respectively.

Based solely on the AIC and BIC values, we cannot make a judgment on the results of the model selection. We need to adjust the model based on its predictions with the smallest AIC and BIC values, and therefore the parameter values that are most consistent with the model.

3.4 *Predicted outcome*

Using the above two SARIMA models with different parameters, we derived their predictions for the number of COVID-19 deaths in the next four weeks.

Table 2. Model (2,1,3)(1,0,0)52 prediction result of death cases.

Time	Forecast	Lo80	Hi80	Lo95	Hi95
2023.7.22	51	-6633	765	-1040	1143
2023.7.29	97	-1793	1987	-2793	2988
2023.8.05	281	-2944	3506	-4650	5213
2023.8.12	548	-3899	4996	-6254	7350

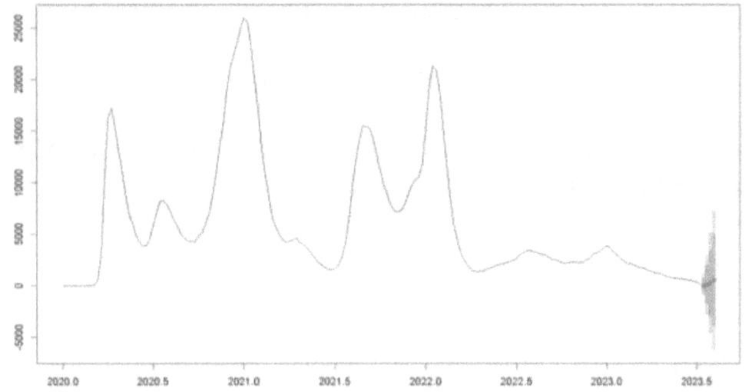

Figure 5. Model (2,1,3)(1,0,0)52 prediction result of death cases (Picture credit: Original).

From the above graphs, it can be seen that the number of deaths predicted by the model (2,1,3)(1,0,0)52 for the next four weeks is 51, 97, 281, and 548. The prediction result shows an upward trend.

Table 3. Model (2,0,0)(1,1,0)52 prediction result of death cases.

Time	Forecast	Lo80	Hi80	Lo95	Hi95
2023.7.22	261	-794	1315	-1352	1874
2023.7.29	527	-1677	2731	-2844	3898
2023.8.05	1107	-2318	4532	-4132	6345
2023.8.12	1979	-2645	6603	-5092	9051

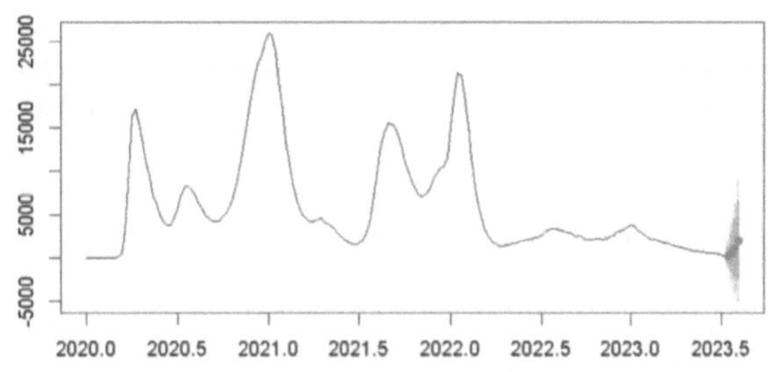

Figure 6. Model (2,0,0)(1,1,0)52 prediction result of death cases (Picture credit: Original).

The results of the predictions made through Model B were 261, 527, 1107, and 1979, which is consistent with the trend of the data predicted through Model A, showing an upward trend. This indicates that the two models are predicting in the right direction but with differences in accuracy. Therefore, the accuracy and validity of the models need to be further tested to select and optimize the models. The following sections discuss the relevant steps in this regard.

3.5 *Model comparison and checking*

3.5.1 *Error metrics testing*

Comparing SARIMA model predictions using MSE, ASE, and RMSE is essential for assessing forecast accuracy. These metrics measure prediction errors as follows:

- Mean squared error (MSE) averages squared errors, with lower values indicating better accuracy.
- Absolute squared error (ASE) captures absolute errors, highlighting closeness to actual values.
- Root mean squared error (RMSE), the square root of MSE, provides an interpretable measure that penalizes larger errors.

Table 4. Results of error metrics.

	Model $(2,1,3)(1,0,0)_{52}$			
Metrics	7.22	7.29	8.5	8.12
MSE	215097.4	178556.2	122384.8	15356.7
ASE	463.8	422.6	349.8	123.9
RMSE	463.8	422.6	349.8	123.9
	Model $(2,0,0)(1,1,0)_{52}$			
Metrics	7.22	7.29	8.5	8.12
MSE	64647.4	47.0	226488	1708894
ASE	254.3	6.857	475.9	1307.2
RMSE	254.3	6.857	475.9	1307.2

By comparing these metrics, we can determine which SARIMA model delivers more accurate and consistent forecasts, aiding in model selection for time series analysis.

So far, we have four weeks of actual death data from publicly available sources: 515 on July 22, 520 on July 29, 631 on August 5, and 672 on August 12. Calculations have yielded the results presented in Table 4.

From Table 4, it is evident that the model $(2,1,3)(1,0,0)_{52}$ has smaller error indicators – MSE, ASE, and RMSE – for the prediction results in the latter two weeks, indicating that the prediction results are more accurate. Whereas the model $(2,0,0)(1,1,0)_{52}$ shows better prediction results in the short term (the first two weeks) with smaller error indicators.

3.5.2 *Residual analysis*

Figures 7 and 8 show the QQ plot of the model residuals.

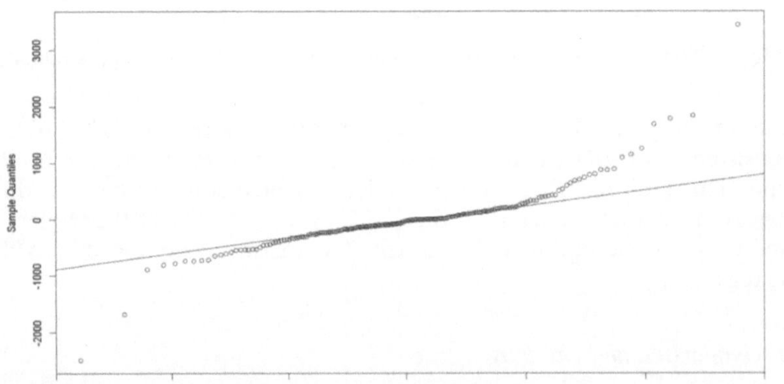

Figure 7. QQ plot of residuals for SARIMA model (2,1,3)(1,0,0)52.

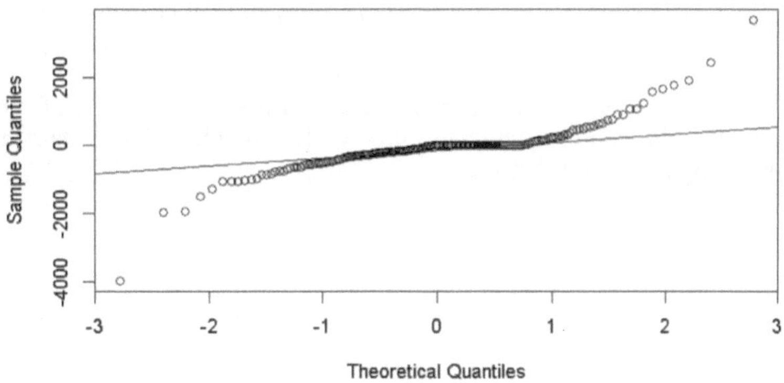

Figure 8. QQ plot of residuals for the SARIMA model (2,0,0)(1,1,0)52 (Picture credit: Original).

By analyzing the QQ plots of the residuals, we observe that the residuals of the model $(2,1,3)(1,0,0)_{52}$ coincide with the 45-degree line in the middle region, although the deviate at both ends, indicating that the residuals are close to the normal distribution to a certain extent, with a certain degree of stochasticity, and that the model extracts sufficient information. In contrast, the QQ plot results for the residuals of the model $(2,0,0)(1,1,0)_{52}$ were less successful, with more points deviating from the line at both ends.

From Figure 9, the histogram of residuals for the model $(2,1,3)(1,0,0)_{52}$ further confirms their proximity to a normal distribution, providing additional evidence of the model's effectiveness in capturing the underlying patterns. In contrast, the residual normality test results for the model $(2,0,0)(1,1,0)_{52}$ are not as strong as those for the model $(2,1,3)(1,0,0)_{52}$, but they still exhibit an overall trend of normal distribution.

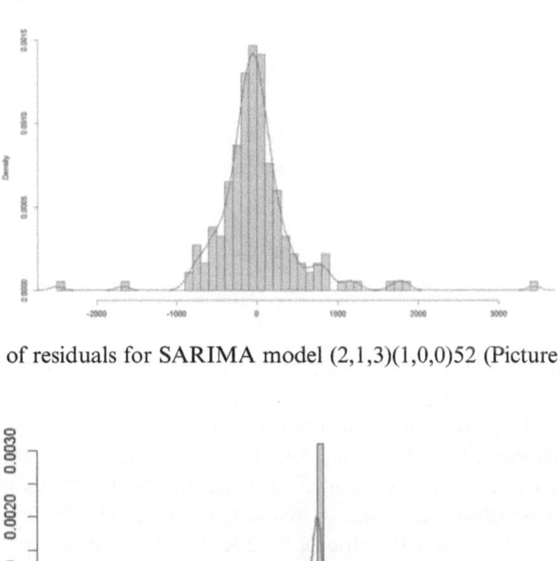

Figure 9. Histogram of residuals for SARIMA model (2,1,3)(1,0,0)52 (Picture credit: Original).

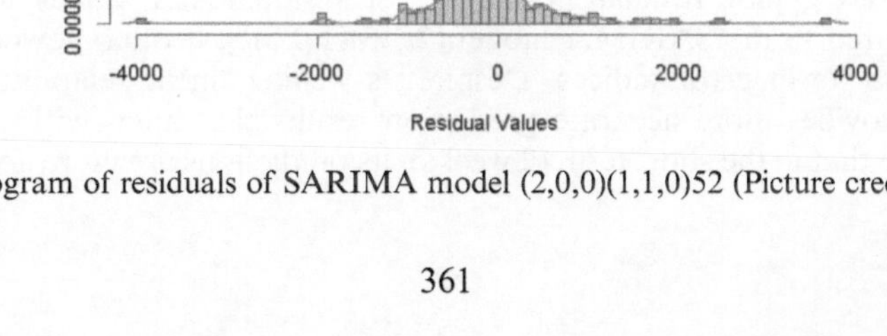

Figure 10. Histogram of residuals of SARIMA model (2,0,0)(1,1,0)52 (Picture credit: Original).

As can be seen from Figure 11, for the SARIMA model $(2,1,3)(1,0,0)_{52}$, only the ACF at order 0 exceeds the confidence interval. Since the ACF at order 0 represents the variance of the residual series, its impact on the residual ACF test is minimal. In all other cases, the ACF values do not exceed the confidence interval, indicating that the outcome of the ACF test strongly suggests the absence of significant autocorrelation. This affirms that the residuals conform to the properties of white noise.

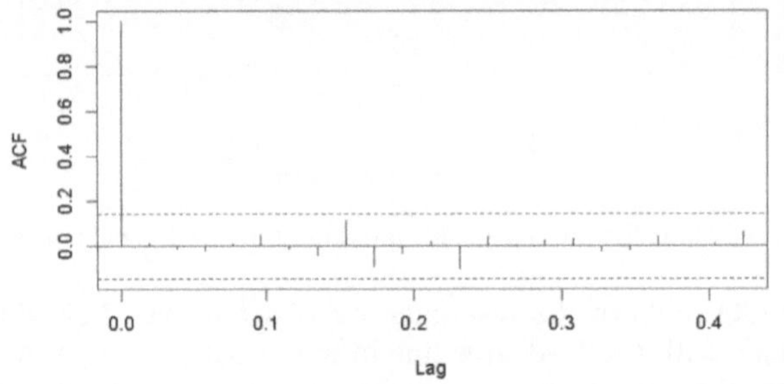

Figure 11. ACF test results of residuals for model (2,1,3)(1,0,0)52 (Picture credit: Original).

In the model $(2,0,0)(1,1,0)_{52}$, there are still ACFs exceeding the confidence interval in the subsequent orders, indicating the presence of autocorrelation in the model to some extent.

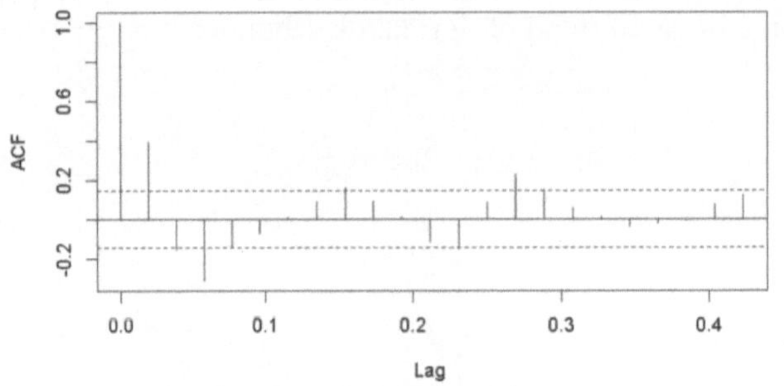

Figure 12. ACF test results of residuals for model (2,0,0)(1,1,0)52 (Picture credit: Original).

To further authenticate the model's efficacy, a Ljung-Box test was conducted as the subsequent step. This statistical test is utilized to assess the overall randomness and independence of the residuals, a pivotal characteristic of a well-behaved SARIMA model. Remarkably, in the model $(2,1,3)(1,0,0)_{52}$, the Ljung-Box test returned a high p-value of 0.9878, indicating the absence of serial correlation within the residuals and confirming their adherence to white noise characteristics. However, in contrast, the Ljung-box test for the model $(2,0,0)(1,1,0)_{52}$ resulted in a P-value of 8.753e-11, suggesting that the test is not white noise and indicating the presence of autocorrelation in the model.

In summary, the test results indicate that while the SARIMA model $(2,0,0)(1,1,0)_{52}$ is not optimal in terms of QQ plot, residual normality test, residual ACF values, and Ljung-BOX test results compared to the SARIMA model $(2,1,3)(1,0,0)_{52}$, it offers lower AIC and BIC values, along with lower error indices. Despite its weaker linear relationship, the model $(2,0,0)(1,1,0)_{52}$ provides more accurate prediction results that align with our needs. It is interesting to note that in the short term (2 weeks), its predictions are more accurate, whereas model $(2,1,3)(1,0,0)_{52}$ significantly underestimates the number of deaths during this period. Thus, despite its accurate predictions in the long term, the model's shortcomings make it less meaningful. Ultimately, we conclude that the model $(2,0,0)(1,1,0)_{52}$ is the best choice.

4 CONCLUSION

In this study, we successfully constructed a SARIMA model for predicting future COVID-19 deaths based on data from January 2020 to July 2023. After careful adjustment and comparison of model parameters, we identified the optimal combination $(2, 0, 0)\ (1, 1, 0)_{52}$, which yields the lowest AIC value (2170.77) and BIC value (2182.3). This preferred model was selected for its excellent performance in fitting historical data and forecasting future trends.

The construction of this SARIMA model represents an in-depth analysis of time series data, fully considering the effects of seasonality and trends. By predicting the number of COVID-19 deaths, people are able to better understand the trend of the epidemic. This would enable the health departments and the government to develop more effective prevention and control strategies.

Future research will focus on two main areas to further optimize the SARIMA model. First, we plan to introduce external factors to construct the ARIMAX model, which will make our model more capable of taking into account the effects of external factors on the time series and improve forecasting accuracy. Second, we can also try to explore the application of time series cross-validation to more comprehensively assess the performance of the model. It is believed that these efforts will help to continuously improve our model to ensure that it still provides reliable forecasting capabilities amid changing data patterns.

REFERENCES

Benvenuto D., Giovanetti M., Vassallo L., Angeletti S., Ciccozzi M., (2020). *Data Brief.*, 105340

Box G. E., Jenkins G. M., Reinsel G. C., Ljung G. M., (2015). *John Wiley & Sons.*

Centers for Disease Control and Prevention, What you need to know about variants. Cent. Dis. Control Prevent. 2023, https://www. cdc.gov/coronavirus/2019-ncov/variants/about variants.html.

Chintalapudi N., Battineni G., Amenta F., (2020). *J Micro. Imm.*, 396–403

Holshue M. L., et al. (2020). *J. Med*, **382**, 929–936

Jiang F., Zhao Z., Shao X., (2020). *J. Econo.*, **39**

Liu J., Zhao Z., Zhong Y., Zhao C., Zhang G., (2022). *Energy Reports*, 1360–1367

Papastefanopoulos V., Linardatos P., Kotsiantis S., (2020). *Appl Sci.*, **10(11)**, 3880

Regan D. O., Jackson M. L., Young A. H., Rosenzweig I., (2021). *Nat Sci Sleep*, **13**, 2053–2064

Tandon H., Ranjan P., Chakraborty T., Suhag V., (2020). *The Arixb.*

Zhu B., Wei Y., (2013). *Omega*, **41(3)**, 517–524

Biological Sciences and Environmental Health – Gao (Ed.)
© 2025 the Author(s), ISBN: 978-1-032-96016-6

Pharmacology and therapeutic applications of monoclonal antibodies

Yichen Zhou
Suzhou Foreign Language School Sciences, Suzhou, China

Zhenqi Zhou
Beijing New Oriental Foreign School at Yangzhou, Yangzhou, China

ABSTRACT: Monoclonal antibodies (mAbs), a category of drugs with approximately eighty approved variants, have surged in popularity. Recent years have witnessed a growing number of these antibodies gaining approval, expanding their use beyond oncology and infectious diseases. While mAbs are more complex than small molecules, they offer distinct advantages, such as high specificity, fewer side effects, and prolonged effectiveness. This review explores the impact of structural characteristics on monoclonal antibody properties, their benefits in treating specific diseases, and the contrast with small molecule drugs in terms of administration routes and accessibility. Understanding these facets can enhance our grasp of mAbs, reduce drug interactions, and improve oral bioavailability. However, further clinical development is essential to fully exploit their potential. Continued efforts in comprehending and utilizing mAbs are crucial, promising to broaden their application in medicine and enhance therapeutic outcomes.

1 INTRODUCTION

For a significant portion of history, drug research primarily focused on synthetic chemical pharmaceuticals. This involved studying the principles governing their impact on the human body, which eventually evolved into a distinct field known as pharmacokinetics. Pharmacokinetics encompasses the mechanisms governing the absorption, effects, and metabolism of small molecule drugs within the human body. Small molecule drugs undergo extensive experimentation before receiving marketing approval to mitigate potential adverse effects. Consequently, they often lack the precision to specifically target desired molecules, potentially leading to unintended consequences.mAbs are seen as option of curing diseases refractory to conventional immunosuppressive treatments, moreover, they may slow disease progression and prevent severe complications compared with traditional drugs, and can also improve patients' quality of life.

In recent decades, mAbs have emerged as a prominent player in the pharmaceutical market. This success can be largely attributed to advancements in molecular biology and immunology, which have enabled the production of mAbs from a clone of the same B-cell. This process yields monospecific antibodies, enhancing their therapeutic effectiveness. In contrast to naturally produced polyclonal antibodies, which may have a higher affinity, the presence of both neutralizing and non-neutralizing antibodies with varying affinities makes them less advantageous than mAbs, which offer homogeneity. This limitation restricts their suitability for therapeutic applications.

Muromonab-CD3 became the first monoclonal antibody to receive approval for use in 1986. However, it was generated from mice, leading to severe allergic reactions and reduced half-life in subsequent human treatments, as humans produce human anti-murine antibodies.

 DOI: 10.1201/9781003587590-51

Over the past thirty years, there has been an average of more than three marketing-approved mAbs per year. With the expanded application of mAbs for therapeutic purposes, their targets have broadened to include not only cytokines but also membrane-bound targets.

The production of mAbs was considered unattainable until the introduction of the hybridoma technique in 1975, for which the Nobel Prize was awarded. This technique involved fusing myeloma cells with lymphocytes to generate a continuous supply of B cells. These cells were then employed to select the most potent and high-affinity antibodies, which had previously been obtained from splenocytes of animals (Singh *et al.* 2018).

This review delves into the structural characteristics and classification of mAbs, accompanied by a brief historical overview. It also explains the therapeutic applications and markets of these antibodies, as well as regulatory oversight. Several examples will illustrate why mAbs have a lower marketing approval rate than small molecule drugs. Furthermore, the review will evaluate the differences between mAbs and small molecules, specifically examining their pharmacokinetic and pharmacodynamic properties, mode of administration, and metabolism. Technical terminology will be clarified upon first use. Additional variations, including drug accessibility and the therapeutic mechanism of infectious diseases, will also be addressed.

2 STRUCTURE AND FUNCTIONAL FEATURES OF ANTIBODIES

The fundamental constituent of human antibodies is immunoglobulin, a molecule consisting of two identical light chains and two identical heavy chains, which come together to create a Y-shaped structure. Each light chain is connected to a heavy chain through a disulfide bond. Antibodies are categorized based on the heavy chain isoforms they contain, giving rise to five distinct classes: IgA, IgD, IgE, IgG, and IgM. These classes encompass the heavy chain isoforms α, δ, ε, γ, and μ, which exist in varying proportions within the circulatory system and serve disparate roles. Notably, IgG is the most prevalent class found in the bloodstream. Additionally, each antibody class is further subdivided into multiple subclasses. During the 1950s, experiments involving the hydrolysis of antibodies yielded the revelation of fragments with diverse sizes. Among these fragments, certain ones demonstrated the ability to bind to antigens and were subsequently termed "Fab" fragments. Conversely, some fragments exhibited a propensity to readily crystallize, earning them the designation of "Fc fragments" (Kuroda and Tsumoto 2023). These distinctive characteristics were progressively elucidated through subsequent research endeavors. Each light or heavy chain is endowed with both variable and constant 55approximately 110 amino acid residues. Notably, both light and heavy chains exhibit this uniformity in their composition. Within an antibody molecule, two distinct chain variable regions collectively constitute the antigen-binding regions, which are denoted as "Fabs." It is noteworthy that within the same antibody molecule, both antigen-binding regions have the capacity to interact with the same antigen. The direct connection of the antigen-binding region to the hinge region imparts a remarkable degree of flexibility to the antibody structure. As shown in Figure 1, the Fab regions within an immunoglobulin are established through the fusion of VL and CL domains from the light chains with VH and CH1 domains from the heavy chains. This particular pairing of VL and VH domains culminates in the formation of the binding site responsible for antigen interaction. The two β-sheets, constructed from β-strands in the order of ↓C'' ↑C' ↓C ↑F ↓B, closely associate to give rise to a barrel-like structure. This structural arrangement aligns the connecting loops, thus creating the antigen-binding site. Concurrently, the CH1 and CL domains securely adhere to one another in an almost perpendicular orientation, capitalizing on the complementary surfaces of the opposing ↓A ↑B ↓E ↑D β-sheet. The constant region found in the two heavy chains constitutes the crystallizable fragment, a region capable of binding to receptor molecules, thereby initiating immune system responses. These responses encompass activities such as antibody-dependent cell-mediated cytotoxicity (ADCC) and complement-dependent cytotoxicity (CDC). Due to variations in the effects of different antibody subtypes on host cells hosting the receptor molecules, certain subtypes are extensively employed in the treatment of specific diseases (Chiu *et al.* 2019). For instance, IgG1 is employed in cancer therapy due to its capacity to induce lysis in the cells it binds to. Rituximab, for example, primarily employs the CDC mechanism to trigger apoptosis in tumor cells. In the process, it also incorporates a segment of the ADCC mechanism.

The engineering of the Fc region has assumed significant importance owing to its role in modulating the immune system and the effector functions of immune cells, including macrophages, monocytes, lymphocytes, and others.

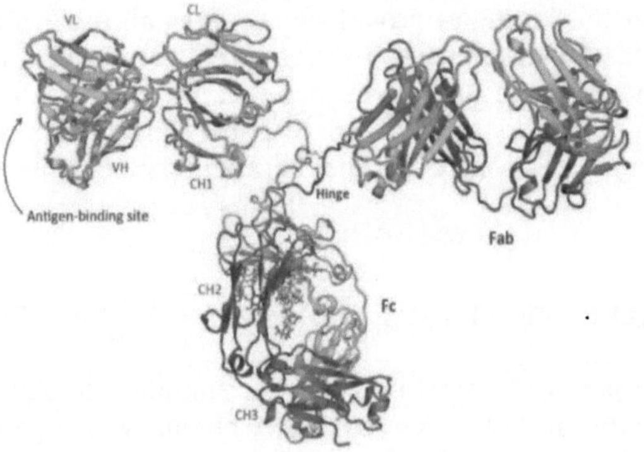

Figure 1. The structure of CAR. Light chains are represented in green, heavy chains in cyan and blue, glycan structures are shown as orange sticks, and interchain disulfides are illustrated in yellow sticks (Chiu *et al.* 2019).

3 THERAPEUTIC APPLICATIONS OF MARKETED MABS

mAbs are highly specific antibodies produced by B lymphocytes in response to a particular antigen epitope. After over three decades of research, mAbs have evolved towards miniaturization and multifunctionality. This evolution has given rise to various innovative forms, including humanized monoclonal antibody drugs, antibody conjugate drugs, bispecific antibodies, antibody fusion proteins, small molecule antibodies, and other novel antibody derivatives (Behl *et al.* 2023). These advancements have significantly expanded the therapeutic options for malignant tumors and autoimmune diseases (Mansouur *et al.* 2023; Schafer *et al.* 2023).

3.1 *Immune-mediated diseases*

In autoimmune disorders, a key hallmark is the activation of autoreactive CD4+ lymphocytes within peripheral lymph nodes. This activation occurs as naive T cells engage with antigen-presenting cells (APCs) and B cells. mAbs employ various mechanisms to address autoimmune disorders, such as blocking and depleting T cells and/or B cells, inhibiting the interaction between T cells and APCs, preventing the recruitment of T and B cells, halting T cell differentiation or activation, and suppressing the production of pro-inflammatory cytokines (Sofía and McGonigle 2019).

mAbs have demonstrated their effectiveness in rheumatoid arthritis treatment for over a decade. Additionally, they have proven to be efficacious in managing a range of other conditions, including psoriatic arthritis, Crohn's disease, ulcerative colitis, psoriasis, and ankylosing spondylitis (Schafer *et al.* 2023).

3.2 *Oncology*

The first category targets antigens expressed by tumor cells, either in a specific manner, as seen with Her2-neu in breast cancer and other carcinomas, or in conjunction with normal cells, such as differentiation antigens like CD20, CD52, CD19, and others (Sofía and McGonigle 2019). The aim of these antibodies is to induce tumor cell death, either by promoting apoptosis, neutralizing the effects of growth factors, or triggering host-effector mechanisms like complement activation or the elimination of tumor cells by macrophages or NK cells through their interaction with cellular IgG receptors (Fcg receptors - FcgR) (Beh *et al.* 2023; Sofía and McGonigle 2019).

The second category centers on addressing the stromal reactions surrounding the tumor. Within this category, a prominent example is mAbs that neutralize V-EGF, a factor derived from tumors that promotes neo-angiogenesis—an essential requirement for the tumor's oxygen and nutrient supply.

The third category focuses on boosting immune responses against tumors, and mAbs can also be employed for the targeted delivery of radioisotopes to cancer cells. For instance, Ibritumab tiuxetan (Zevalin), a monoclonal antibody labeled with either Yttrium 90 or Indium 111, is utilized in the management of non-Hodgkin's lymphoma (Sofía and McGonigle 2019). Furthermore, some mAbs target the tumor microenvironment, aiming to inhibit angiogenesis and other processes. Nevertheless, therapeutic vaccinations remain modestly effective in the context of progressing malignancies. Tumors employ various strategies to evade the immune system, one of which involves inducing regulatory lymphocytes with immunosuppressive properties (Sofía and McGonigle 2019). These regulatory lymphocytes, often referred to as suppressors, display specific markers (CD25, CTLA-4, PD1) that mAbs can target to inhibit or eliminate these cells, thereby bolstering the immune response against the tumor (Sofía and McGonigle 2019). Principal targets for immune-checkpoint inhibitors include Programmed Cell Death Protein 1 (PD1)/PD1 Ligand 1 (PDL1) and the immune-checkpoint molecule CTLA4, both of which play pivotal roles in regulatory mechanisms associated with tumor immune evasion (Sofía and McGonigle 2019).

4 PHARMACOLOGY OF MABS VERSUS SMALL MOLECULE DRUGS

There exist several notable distinctions between small molecule drugs and mAbs, with the most apparent being their size. mAbs typically have a size of around 150 kDa, whereas small molecule medications have a much lower molecular weight, approximately 700 Da. Due to this considerable difference in size, mAbs are primarily suited for targeting extracellular components, as they are unable to access intracellular targets effectively. Furthermore, because of their larger size, the distribution of mAbs within tissues occurs at a slower pace when compared to small molecules. Notably, mAbs are incapable of traversing the blood-brain barrier.

Another crucial difference lies in their production methods. Small molecule drugs are synthesized through chemical processes, whereas mAbs are generated by cells, often through biotechnological methods.

4.1 *Pharmacodynamics*

mAbs are known for their high affinity for their intended target, which reduces the likelihood of off-target effects (Behl *et al.* 2023). Conversely, small molecules may have compound-related effects and can interact with various expected and unexpected targets.

Antibody-drug conjugates (ADCs) are a notable application where highly cytotoxic small molecules, referred to as payloads, are chemically linked to mAbs using specialized linkers

(Sofía and McGonigle 2019). ADCs offer the advantage of providing sustained and selective cytotoxic drug delivery to tumors, expanding the therapeutic window compared to using cytotoxic agents alone (Sofía and McGonigle 2019). This makes ADCs a valuable tool in targeted cancer therapy.

An example of an ADC is Trastuzumab. Trastuzumab targets the human epidermal growth factor receptor 2 (HER2), a transmembrane receptor tyrosine kinase involved in cell proliferation, differentiation, and survival. In cases of endometrial cancer with overexpressed HER2, which often carries a poor prognosis, is aggressive, and is resistant to conventional treatments, Trastuzumab has shown promise (Behl *et al.* 2023; Mao *et al.* 2023).

Currently, Trastuzumab is the first-line therapy for metastatic breast cancer with HER2/neu overexpression, demonstrating its efficacy as a humanized monoclonal antibody (Mao *et al.* 2023). Recent research has also indicated that HER2-targeted treatments, including Trastuzumab, can be beneficial when combined with chemotherapy for HER2-positive endometrial cancer. Trastuzumab maintenance therapy is utilized in the management of advanced-stage HER2-positive uterine serous carcinoma, often administered alongside adjuvant platinum-based chemotherapy and concurrent Trastuzumab treatment. In certain situations, consolidation therapy involving tumor-directed radiation may also be contemplated (Mao *et al.* 2023). Ibritumab tiux- etan (Zevalin) is an example of monoclonal antibody used for the selective delivery of radioisotopes to cancer cells.

Zevalin is labeled with Yttrium 90 or Indium 111, used for treatment of non-Hodgkin's lymphoma. Some other monoclonal antibodies are target on the microenvironment of tumors, and act as inhibition of angiogenesis.

4.2 *Pharmacokinetics*

In terms of administration, oral delivery of mAbs is generally ineffective due to their large molecular size and poor membrane permeability, resulting in low bioavailability (usually $\leq 1\%$). Consequently, the most commonly used routes of administration for mAbs are intravenous, subcutaneous, and intramuscular. Subcutaneous injections are often preferred over intramuscular injections due to the potential for muscle tissue damage associated with the latter. Intramuscular injections can lead to a quicker peak concentration of the medication in the bloodstream compared to subcutaneous injections (Castelli *et al.* 2019).

mAbs typically exhibit a prolonged half-life in the bloodstream, typically ranging from 11 to 30 days in the human body, as compared to small molecule drugs (Castelli *et al.* 2019). However, ongoing research aims to further extend the half-life of mAbs, with the goal of providing patients with extended protection while reducing the frequency of administrations (Castelli *et al.* 2019; Ecker, Jones and Levine 2015).

Unlike small molecule drugs, the majority of mAbs cannot be filtered by the kidneys and eliminated through urine owing to their substantial size. which are typically metabolized by renal enzymes. Instead, mAbs are primarily eliminated from the body through bile or renal excretion.

Regarding medication risk, the primary concern lies in the use of mAbs for autoimmune conditions, including thyroid disorders and lupus-like syndromes. Comprehensive assessment of immunogenicity during drug development, testing on patients with varying sensitivities and immune functions, and stringent risk assessments for potential harm are essential practices. Additionally, technical term abbreviations should be clarified when first introduced to ensure clear understanding (Mao *et al.* 2023).

The presence of mAbs in the circulatory system, coupled with their high volume, can impede their ability to effectively reach the target tissue. A common solution is to use antibody fragments to improve targeting or enhance the antibody's affinity for the binding site while improving its hydrophilic properties.

5 CONCLUSION

mAbs are highly specific antibodies produced by B lymphocytes in response to specific antigenic epitopes. Over the past three decades, significant advancements have been made in the development of mAbs, leading to miniaturization and multifunctionality in this field. Consequently, a range of therapeutic options has emerged, including humanized monoclonal antibody drugs, antibody conjugate drugs, bispecific antibodies, antibody fusion proteins, small molecule antibodies, and novel antibody variants. These innovations have expanded treatment options for various conditions, including malignant tumors and autoimmune diseases.

In the realm of oncology, mAbs have made remarkable strides, with different antibody subtypes exhibiting varying effects on cells bearing the receptor molecule. Certain subtypes, such as IgG1, are widely utilized in cancer therapy due to their ability to induce cell lysis. For example, Rituximab primarily employs the CDC mechanism to induce tumor cell apoptosis while also involving the ADCC mechanism.

The market demand for mAbs has grown significantly in recent years, owing to their versatility in treating various diseases, including autoimmune disorders, cancer, and infectious diseases. mAbs possess characteristics like high specificity, multifunctionality, flexibility due to the direct antigen-binding region attachment to the hinge region, high target affinity, and a reduced likelihood of off-target effects. Moreover, Fc fusion proteins, ADCs, and bispecific mAbs have further diversified the avenues for monoclonal antibody development. It is anticipated that the market for mAbs will continue to expand exponentially in the future.

In the process of monoclonal antibody drug development, comprehensive analysis of immunogenicity and immune function among patients with varying sensitivities is crucial. Additionally, ongoing research focuses on understanding the side effects of mAbs and finding effective solutions. Given that monoclonal antibody drugs often remain in the human body for extended periods with a long half-life, ensuring patient safety and protection over the long term is essential. Addressing the challenge of mAbs' presence in the circulatory system and their potential to hinder target tissue will be crucial for optimizing the pharmacodynamic properties of mAbs and minimizing side effects in the future.

AUTHORS CONTRIBUTION

All the authors contributed equally and their names were listed in alphabetical order.

REFERENCES

Behl A., Wani Z. A., Nath Das N., Parmar V. S., Len C., Malhotra S. and Chhillar A.K. (2023). *Crit Rev Oncol Hemat*, **183**, 103915

Castelli, M. S., McGonigle, P., and Hornby, P. J. (2019). *Pharmacol Res Perspect*, **76**, 10.

Chiu M. L., Goulet D. R., Teplyakov A. and Gilliland G. L. (2019). Antibody structure and function: The basis for engineering therapeutics. *Antibodies*, **8**, 1.

Ecker D. M., Jones S. D. and Levine H. L. (2015). The therapeutic monoclonal antibody market. *MAbs.*, **71**, 6

Kuroda D., Tsumoto K. (2023). Structural classification of CDR-H3 in single-domain VHH antibodies. *Methods Mol Biol.*, **2522**, 3.

Mansouur I., Murugapandian S., Tanriover B. and Thajudeen B. (2023). *Mayo Clin. Proc.*, **7**, 276.

Mao S., Sravines D., Zarei S., Viswanathan A. and Fader A. (2023). *Gynecol. Oncol*, **49**, 101250.

Schafer C., Young D., Singh H., Jayakrishnan R., Banerjee S., Song Y., Dobi A., Petrovics G., Srivastava S., Srivastava S., Sesterhenn I. A., Chesnut G. T. and Tan S. (2023). *Journal of Immunological Methods*, **518**, 113493

Singh S., Kumar N. K., Dwiwedi P., Charan J, Kaur R., Preeti. Sidhu and Chugh V. K., (2018). *Curr. Clin. Pharmacol.*, **13**, 85

Sofia Castelli M., McGonigle P. and Hornby P.J. (2019). *Pharmacol*, **7**, 535.

Biological Sciences and Environmental Health – Gao (Ed.)
© 2025 the Author(s), ISBN: 978-1-032-96016-6

Effect of medical nutrition on gestational diabetes mellitus

Yingze Gao
Nursery Faculty, Sun Yat-sen University, Guangzhou, China

Shangbo Liu
College of Health and Rehabilitation, Chengdu University of Traditional Chinese Medicine, Chengdu, China

Ziyang Mu
Camford Royal School, Beijing, China

Siwei Yang
College of Pharmacy, Shenyang Pharmaceutical University, Shenyang, China

ABSTRACT: Gestational diabetes mellitus (GDM) presents dangers to both maternal and fetal well-being. The effectiveness of management depends on medical nutrition therapy. This study emphasizes on four major challenges, namely weight management during pregnancy, lack of exercise, inadequate nutritional knowledge, and suboptimal dietary patterns. Gestational diabetes mellitus patients often have difficulty with weight gain, making it crucial for them to maintain a balanced diet and ensure adequate nutrient intake for optimal blood sugar regulation. Simultaneously, consistent physical activity improves insulin sensitivity, thereby supporting glucose management. Moreover, a comprehensive understanding of nutrition is crucial. Pregnant women must distinguish beneficial foods, craft balanced diets, and steer clear of high-sugar and fatty items. Personalized nutritional guidance can serve as a bridge to fill knowledge gaps and facilitate the adjustment of dietary habits. A crucial aspect in enhancing the effectiveness of medical nutrition therapy for GDM involves the comprehensive management of weight, physical activity, and nutritional education.

1 INTRODUCTION

Gestational diabetes mellitus (GDM) is a common endocrine complication during pregnancy, and its prevalence has been increasing globally in recent years (Huang *et al.* 2022; Zhang and Gong 2021). It has been reported that patients with GDM account for 1% to 14% of the total number of pregnant women. GMD can cause macrosomia, premature delivery, neonatal respiratory distress syndrome, etc. It will affect the long-term tissue and organ development of newborns (Wang 2020; Zhang 2020). Without timely and effective treatment, it is easy to cause near and long-term complications with the continuous progression of the disease, which will bring great harm to mother and child, and should be paid enough attention to. Common nutritional problems of pregnant women with gestational diabetes include difficulty in weight management, lack of exercise, lack of accurate knowledge about nutrition and unreasonable diet structure (Huang *et al.* 2023). Lack of exercise will easily lead to the decrease of insulin utilization, and thus diabetes will more easily occur.

 DOI: 10.1201/9781003587590-52

Clinically, gestational diabetes mellitus is mostly treated by conventional treatment: insulin therapy, routine care, diet care and routine exercise for gestational diabetes mellitus patients (Metzger 2008). However, based on the therapeutic effect, it cannot meet the existing therapeutic requirements, and blood sugar fluctuations may still occur in clinical practice (Liu *et al.* 2020).

As a non-invasive, safe and effective means, medical nutrition therapy (MNT) has good universality and operability, and should be widely used in the management of gestational diabetes mellitus. Nutritional therapy by adjusting the total energy of the diet, diet structure and meal distribution ratio, is conducive to blood sugar control, help maintain the ideal weight and prevent malnutrition, diabetes and its complications prevention, treatment, self-management and education is an important part of the MNT way to optimize the diet structure of pregnant women, adjust the nutritional intake and provide appropriate exercise guidance (Huang *et al.* 2023). To a certain extent , the enhancement of the nutritional status among pregnant women diagnosed with gestational diabetes can be effectively achieved. Weight management is one of the most basic medical nutritional treatment means, so this paper reviews the improvement effect of medical nutritional treatment on the common nutritional problems of pregnant women with gestational diabetes.

2 COMMON NUTRITIONAL PROBLEMS IN PREGNANT WOMEN WITH GESTATIONAL DIABETES MELLITUS (GDM)

GDM is a common complication during pregnancy where women experience impaired sugar metabolism and abnormal levels of glucose, leading to diabetes. Pregnant women with GDM have prolonged periods of high blood sugar levels if not properly controlled, which can result in excessive blood sugar levels (Hughes *et al.* 2022). Prolonged high blood sugar levels can increase health risks for both the mother and the fetus, such as macrosomia, premature birth, and fetal developmental abnormalities.

2.1 *Influences of unreasonable diet structure on blood sugar control*

An unreasonable diet structure in pregnant women with GDM can negatively affect disease control. Pregnant women with poor dietary habits have a higher incidence of GDM, which is an independent risk factor (OR = 1.931 95% CI: 1.056-3.531, $P<0.001$). In order to mitigate the potential development of gestational diabetes mellitus (GDM), it is imperative to proactively monitor and intervene at an early stage (Hughes *et al.* 2022). Excessive consumption of high-sugar and high-fat foods, as well as an imbalanced diet structure, can lead to blood sugar fluctuations and nutritional imbalances. By adjusting the diet structure, properly selecting and proportioning food types, avoiding excessive intake of simple sugars and saturated fats, and scientifically controlling energy intake, individualized nutritional guidance should be given based on different pre-pregnancy BMI of pregnant women. The energy coefficient should be determined according to the pre-pregnancy BMI, with a BMI of 25kg/m^2 having an energy coefficient between 25-30. In general, the daily total energy intake during pregnancy should not be lower than 1500kcal (Rasmussen and Yaktine 2009).

2.2 *The impact of difficulties in weight management on blood sugar control*

Insufficient weight gain during pregnancy (odds ratio [OR] =1.485, 95% confidence interval [CI]: 1.164-1.893, $P = 0.001$) and being overweight before pregnancy (OR = 1.634, 95% CI: 1.241-2.151, $P < 0.001$) are identified as autonomous risk factors associated with the development of gestational diabetes mellitus (GDM) (Langer 2005). Weight management in pregnant women primarily includes two stages: pre-pregnancy BMI control and weight gain during pregnancy. (1) According to the WHO classification criteria, pre-pregnancy BMI can be divided into four categories: underweight (<18.5 kg/m^2), normal (18.5-<25.0 kg/m^2), overweight (25.0-<30.0 kg/m^2), and obese ($\geq$ 30.0 kg/m^2) (Langer 2005). (2) Based on the recommended appropriate weight gain during pregnancy in 2009 by the Institute of Medicine (IOM), weight gain during pregnancy can be classified as follows: underweight, normal, overweight, and obese women are advised to gain 12.5-18.0 kg, 11.5-16.0 kg, 7.0-11.5 kg, and 5.0-9.0 kg, respectively (Meng *et al.* 2022). Excessive weight gain during pregnancy is particularly evident in China, with pregnant women typically gaining 5.6-7.8% of their pre-pregnancy weight (Li 2019). Without appropriate weight management, this may even increase to 9.8%. Additionally, excessive weight gain can affect the insulin resistance level in pregnant women, further complicating blood sugar control.

2.3 *The impact of a lack of exercise on blood sugar control*

Pregnant women with gestational diabetes who remain sedentary or lack physical activity for long periods may experience reduced muscle utilization of insulin and impaired blood sugar regulation. This can lead to unstable blood sugar levels and high blood sugar occurrences. Moderate physical activity helps improve insulin sensitivity, promote effective insulin utilization, lower blood sugar levels, and prevent or control the occurrence of gestational diabetes. In one study, 387 pregnant women from routine obstetrics and gynecology outpatient visits were divided into observation and control groups. Both groups received routine prenatal care interventions: distribution of a self-developed GDM health education booklet - "Caring for Life, Avoiding GDM," and GDM-specific lectures covering four topics: ①GDM pathogenesis and its effects on mother and baby; ②GDM diagnosis and prevention; ③exercise and physical activity during pregnancy; ④psychological adjustment of exercise during pregnancy. The observation group received additional exercise interventions: ①assessment of the pregnant women's fitness levels, development of personalized exercise guidance, and establishment of follow-up records; ②individual or group counseling sessions after each lecture, answering specific and common questions, and then conducting group discussions lasting 30-40 minutes, focusing on strengthening confidence in exercise during pregnancy and sharing experiences in exercise management; ③telephone follow-ups on achieved exercise goals and any discomfort or adverse effects after exercise, encouraging pregnant women to record their daily exercise in a journal for self-monitoring; ④providing education to the pregnant women's partners and family members to ensure adequate emotional support and confidence in exercise. The findings of the study indicate that the observation group exhibited higher exercise self-efficacy scores and overall satisfaction compared to the control group ($P<0.01$). The prevalence of gestational diabetes mellitus (GDM) in the observation group was found to be significantly lower (6.19% or 12 out of 194) when compared to the control group (19.17% or 37 out of 193) ($P<0.01$). Hence, exercise interventions have demonstrated efficacy in mitigating the occurrence of gestational diabetes (Li 2019).

2.4 *The impact of lack of accurate nutrition knowledge on gestational diabetes blood sugar control*

Insufficient understanding of nutrition may potentially exert an adverse influence on the regulation of blood sugar levels among expectant mothers. Pregnant women with gestational diabetes often lack precise nutrition knowledge and may not understand their nutritional needs or the effects of their dietary habits on blood sugar control. In this situation, pregnant women may choose to consume high-sugar and high-fat foods, leading to an imbalanced diet structure. Additionally, cognitive biases, lack of care, and lack of scientific guidance may further influence blood sugar control. This can result in blood sugar fluctuations and nutritional imbalances, further affecting the control of gestational diabetes. A survey was conducted on a sample of 98 patients diagnosed with gestational diabetes who were admitted between April 2020 and October 2022. The participants were randomly assigned to either a control group or an observation group, with each group consisting of 49 cases. The control group received regular nursing care and underwent regular physical examinations, while the observation group received additional health education on top of regular nursing care. The results showed that the observation group had higher levels of satisfaction with nursing care, disease awareness, and self-care ability than the control group ($P<0.05$). The observation group also had lower rates of postpartum complications and neonatal complications compared to the control group ($P<0.05$). The implementation of health education for gestational diabetes patients had a positive effect, effectively improving their disease awareness, self-care abilities, and reducing the occurrence of adverse pregnancy outcomes. This, in turn, increased patient satisfaction with nursing care, ensured delivery safety, and better maintained the health of both mother and baby (Xia *et al.* 2023).

3 THE ASSOCIATION BETWEEN BLOOD GLUCOSE LEVELS IN PREGNANT WOMEN WITH GDM AND MNT

Gestational diabetes mellitus (GDM) poses a significant challenge to maternal health, primarily due to an imbalance in sugar metabolism in pregnant women, leading to unstable blood glucose levels. A study conducted on 531 Chinese pregnant women revealed that 192 of them were diagnosed with GDM. Furthermore, there were notable differences in the prevalence of GDM across various regions, emphasizing the importance of focusing on gestational diabetes in the prevention and control strategies for maternal diseases in China. Gestational diabetes mellitus (GDM) not only brings blood sugar fluctuations and related complications to pregnant women but also poses potential risks to the health of the fetus, such as inducing newborn macrosomia and long-term malnutrition. A comparative analysis was conducted on a cohort of 135 pregnant women diagnosed with gestational diabetes mellitus (GDM) who received diet and exercise management, and 105 pregnant women who received routine care without any specific interventions. The findings of this study revealed a notable reduction in the occurrence of pregnancy complications, including gestational hypertension, polyhydramnios,postpartum hemorrhage, and macrosomia, among the group of women who received diet and exercise management in comparison to those who received routine care alone. In the management of GDM, Medical Nutrition Therapy (MNT) has been proven to be an effective method. MNT relies on scientific dietary planning and appropriate exercise, aiming to prevent excessive weight gain in pregnant women, provide nutritional education for GDM patients, achieve optimal blood sugar control, maintain weight stability, and ensure the health of both mother and baby.

3.1 *MNT controls blood sugar levels by planning a reasonable dietary structure*

Diet is a crucial factor affecting blood sugar levels. By adjusting the dietary structure, reasonably allocating food types and proportions, and avoiding excessive intake of simple sugars and saturated fats, it helps control blood sugar levels and maintain nutritional balance. MNT will develop a personalized diet plan based on the physical condition of pregnant women, including weight, activity level, and blood sugar control. The proposed plan aims to delineate the recommended daily energy intake for pregnant women, as well as the appropriate proportions of protein, carbohydrates, and fats. Experiments have shown that the diet of GDM pregnant women should mainly consist of low-sugar, high-fiber foods to control the rise in blood sugar (American Diabetes Association 2018).

A clinical study, included 207 pregnant women with abnormal glucose metabolism (Yan 2020). After implementing individualized weight management and dietary control interventions for 73 GDM pregnant women, although the fasting blood glucose (FBG) and glycated hemoglobin (HbA1c) levels of GDM pregnant women were significantly higher than those of normal pregnant women, the blood sugar of these 73 pregnant women gradually came under control through MNT intervention, especially in the late pregnancy when placental hormone secretion increased. Furthermore, the present study examined the mean fluctuations in blood glucose levels among pregnant individuals within the preceding 8-12 weeks, utilizing HbA1c as a metric. The findings revealed that pregnant individuals diagnosed with gestational diabetes mellitus (GDM) exhibited higher HbA1c levels during the middle and late stages of pregnancy compared to those without GDM. However, the management of glycemic control in pregnant women with gestational diabetes mellitus (GDM) was notably more effective in the intervention group compared to the control group. This proves that MNT not only helps pregnant women change their dietary structure, but after reasonable dietary control, their blood sugar control status has significantly improved.

It is advisable to provide pregnant patients with a diverse diet of plant-based grains and to avoid excessive intake of risky factors in the diet, such as offal, sweets, meat, and potatoes. The nutritional requirements of pregnant women increase during pregnancy, and a good condition of the mother is beneficial for the healthy growth of the fetus, preventing the occurrence of future diseases such as obesity and type 2 diabetes.

3.2 *MNT controls blood sugar levels by managing weight*

Gestational diabetes mellitus (GDM) presents a significantly increased risk in overweight or obese pregnant women, with a likelihood 2.32 to 6.21 times higher than that of women with normal weight, and a GDM incidence rate as high as 12.8% (Macdonald *et al.* 2017). Associated with this is the fact that pregnant women with a higher body mass index (BMI) are more prone to complications during pregnancy, such as gestational hypertension, difficult delivery, cesarean section, and excessive weight gain (Artal *et al.* 2010; Shao *et al.* 2019). In this context, excessive weight gain has a negative impact on insulin sensitivity, thereby reducing blood sugar regulation. Medical Nutritional Therapy (MNT) provides personalized diet plans and appropriate exercise guidance for GDM pregnant women, not only effectively controlling weight gain but also improving insulin sensitivity and reducing blood sugar levels, thus reducing the risk of complications in pregnancy and diabetes. These complications include retinopathy, kidney disease, and cardiovascular disease. According to the "2022 China Guidelines for the Diagnosis and Treatment of Gestational Diabetes" and the "American Diabetes Association Guidelines for the Diagnosis and Treatment of Gestational Diabetes", empirical research has shown that MNT has demonstrated significant positive effects on weight management in GDM pregnant women, providing a healthier pregnancy experience for expectant mothers.

3.3 *MNT assists in blood sugar management through personalized exercise plans*

Exercise is an effective strategy for improving blood sugar management in diabetes patients and is crucial for managing blood sugar in GDM pregnant women. Exercise helps enhance the body's sensitivity to insulin and promotes the effective use of insulin. This can lower blood sugar levels and also prevent or control the occurrence of GDM. Research shows that implementing individualized medical nutrition therapy combined with exercise intervention in GDM patients can effectively lower blood sugar and blood pressure levels, and improve maternal and infant outcomes.

A randomized, single-blind, controlled trial was conducted to investigate the effects of a specific intervention on 92 patients diagnosed with gestational diabetes mellitus (GDM) who possessed a doctoral degree. The participants were randomly assigned to either a control group or an observation group, with each group consisting of 46 cases. The control group was administered conventional treatment, whereas the observation group implemented personalized medical nutrition therapy in conjunction with exercise therapy, following the same regimen as the control group.

For fasting blood glucose (FPG), the control group measured at 6.18 mmol/L, while the observation group was at 6.24 mmol/L (P=0.390). After treatment, the control group's level was 5.43mmol/L, with the observation group significantly dropping to 4.66 mmol/L ($P<0.001$).

In terms of 2-hour postprandial blood glucose (2hPG), the control group was 9.36mmol/L, and the observation group was 9.42mmol/L (P=0.826). Post-treatment, the control group measured at 8.29 mmol/L, with the observation group significantly reducing to 6.77 mmol/L ($P<0.001$).

Regarding systolic blood pressure (SBP), the control group was 146.94 mmHg, and the observation group was 147.38 mmHg (P=0.791). After treatment, the control group was 133.66mmHg, and the observation group was 118.07 mmHg ($P<0.001$).

For diastolic blood pressure (DBP), the control group was 107.53 mmHg, and the observation group was 108.11 mmHg (P=0.437). Post-treatment, the control group was 99.39 mmHg, and the observation group was 88.48 mmHg ($P<0.001$).

In brief, the group under observation exhibited noteworthy enhancements in fasting plasma glucose (FPG), 2-hour postprandial glucose (2hPG), systolic blood pressure (SBP), diastolic blood pressure (DBP), and other relevant indicators of blood glucose and blood pressure in comparison to the control group. Furthermore, the frequency of unfavorable outcomes in pregnant women and newborns within the observation group was shown to be reduced compared to the control group, with statistical significance ($P<0.05$) (Zhang *et al.* 2022).

MNT will design a suitable exercise plan based on the pregnant woman's physical condition and exercise habits. When choosing exercise, the intensity should be considered, as excessive exercise can pose unnecessary risks to the fetus and lead to pregnancy accidents. For pregnant women at 10 weeks of gestation, exercises with moderate to low intensity, such as walking, jogging, and swimming, are recommended. It is suggested to exercise for at least 30 minutes each time, with a frequency of 3-5 times per week (Liu *et al.* 2020).

MNT will also guide pregnant women on how to monitor the impact of exercise on blood sugar levels, and adjust the intensity and duration of exercise accordingly. This plays a significant role in preventing exercise-induced hypoglycemia and maximizing the effectiveness of exercise. Many pregnant women are confused about how to monitor blood sugar and interpret the results of blood glucose measurements. Healthcare professionals who provide MNT can offer assistance in order to achieve cooperation and obtain more accurate assessments and utilization of the results (ElSayed 2023).

3.4 *MNT controls blood glucose levels through nutritional education for pregnant women*

Nutritional education can help GDM (Gestational Diabetes Mellitus) pregnant women better understand their nutritional needs and the impact of diet on blood sugar control, thereby guiding them to make healthier food choices. In addition to the traditional management model of outpatient visits and regular follow-ups, there are also specialized practices, family support, and management based on internet platforms for the management of pregnant women with diabetes. This allows for continuous monitoring and supervision of their diet, exercise, and blood sugar levels. By establishing specialized obstetrics and diabetes clinics, enhancing family support, and utilizing platforms such as WeChat groups and online monitoring software, the educational and supervisory effects are strengthened. The specific content of nutritional education includes the pathophysiological mechanism of diabetes, the impact of food on blood sugar, how to read food nutrition labels, and how to plan a diet, among other aspects (Dyson *et al.* 2018). Research has shown that GDM pregnant women who receive nutritional education can significantly improve their blood sugar control and achieve more favorable pregnancy outcomes (Hoseth and Pediatr 2000).

4 CONCLUSION

Gestational diabetes mellitus (GDM) is a common clinical disease, which is mainly characterized by abnormal glucose metabolism in pregnant women during pregnancy, among which the common health problems of pregnant women such as unreasonable diet structures, weight management difficulties, lack of exercise and lack of accurate knowledge about nutrition have great correlation with gestational diabetes mellitus. Medical nutrition therapy (MNT), as a non-drug treatment, intervenes in the common health problems of pregnant women, such as weight management difficulties, lack of exercise, lack of accurate knowledge about nutrition and unreasonable diet structure, through reasonable diet planning, appropriate exercise, nutrition education and other ways. Metformin (MNT) has demonstrated efficacy in enhancing blood sugar regulation in pregnant women, promoting weight stability, enhancing quality of life, and offering a safe and effective therapeutic option for this population. However, the implementation of MNT requires the professional nutrition knowledge of medical staffs, as well as the active cooperation and continuous self - management of pregnant women. Therefore, for the treatment of gestational diabetes, in addition to drug treatment, nutrition education should be strengthened to improve the nutritional knowledge level of pregnant women and guide pregnant women to establish a healthy lifestyle in order to achieve the best MNT treatment effect.

AUTHORS CONTRIBUTION

All the authors contributed equally and their names were listed in alphabetical order.

REFERENCES

American Diabetes Association. (2018). *Diabetes Care.*

Artal R., Lockwood C. J. and Brown H. L. (2010). *Obstet Gynecol.* 115(**1**): 152–155.

Dyson P. A., Twenefour D. and Breen C. (2018). *Diabet Med.* 35(**5**): 541–547.

ElSayed N. A. (2023). *Diabetes Care.* 46(1): S267–S278,.

Hoseth E. (2000). *J Pediatr. Endocrinol Metab.* 13(**7**): 831–838.

Huang M., Dou Z. Y. and Zhong B. (2023). *Wisdom of Health.* 9(**08**): 153–158.

Huang X. M., Zha B. B. and Zhang M. N. (2022). *J Clin Endocrinol Metab.* 107(**1**): 192–204.

Hughes M. M., Black R. E. and Katz J. *Matern Chin J Dis Control Prev.* 26(**9**): 1015, (2022).

Langer O. (2005). *American Journal of Obstetrics and Gynecology.*

Li. R. *Medical Higher Vocational Education and Modern Nursing.* (2019). 2(**01**): 60–62.

Liao X. (2022). *Frontiers in Surgery.* 9.

Liu M., Xu W. and Wu K. (2020). *Henan Med Research.* 29(**35**): 6572–6574.

Macdonald S. C., Bodnár L. M. and Himmes K. P. (2017). Epidimiology. 28(**3**): 419.

Meng Y., Qu Y. and Zhan Y. (2022). *Chinese Journal of Disease Control.* 26(**09**): 1011–1016.

Metzger B.E. (2008). *Diabetes.*

Rasmussen K. M. and Yaktine A.L., (2009). Institute of Medicine (US) and National Research Council (US) Committee to Reexamine IOM Pregnancy Weight Guidelines. Weight Gain During Pregnancy: Reexamining the Guidelines. Washington (DC): National Academies Press (US).

Shao Y., He G., Wu P. (2019). *China Maternal and Child Health Care.* 34(**1**): 171–174.

Wang S. (2020). *New World Diabetes Mellitus.* 23(**19**): 48–49.

Xia L., Song X. and Qu X. (2023). *Practical Obstetrics and Gynecology Electronic Journal.* 10(01): 124–126.

Yan W.Y. (2020). *Chinese Journal of Social Medicine.* (**06**): 633–636.

Zhang H. (2020). *Chinese Journal of Health and Nutrition.* 30(**17**): 334–335

Zhang Q., Chen H., Lin L. (2022). *Diabetes in the New World.* (**17**): 52–55+59.

Zhang X., Gong Y.H. and Dellacorte K. (2021). *Clin Nutr.* 40(**5**): 2791–2799.

Biological Sciences and Environmental Health – Gao (Ed.)

Circadian rhythm: Implications for cardiovascular diseases

Weilun Chen
Faculty of Medicine, Macau University of Science and Technology, Macau, China

ABSTRACT: The human body has physiological processes that follow approximately 24-hour cycles, which are influenced by light and dark. These cycles are known as circadian rhythms. Circadian rhythms can be disrupted by factors such as jet lag, poor sleep habits, or shift work, which have been proven to affect the risk of cardiovascular diseases (CVDs). CVDs encompass a range of conditions impacting the heart and blood vessels, including diseases such as coronary heart disease, hypertension, and atherosclerosis. They are the leading cause of death worldwide and are linked to modern lifestyles involving irregular sleep schedules and excessive periods of wakefulness. The circadian system affects various cardiovascular processes, including blood pressure, cardiac rhythm, and endothelial function, through hormonal regulation of the hypothalamus-pituitary-adrenal axis and sympathetic nervous system. Disruptions in the circadian rhythm cause perturbations in these hormonal and physiological functions. There is accumulating evidence from both epidemiological and animal research showing that disruption of circadian rhythms is linked to an increased risk of CVD risk factors, including hypertension, hyperlipidemia, glucose intolerance, and inflammatory markers. Some animal studies also indicate that changes in core clock genes within the cardiovascular system can lead to pathologies such as arrhythmias, endothelial dysfunction, and accelerated atherosclerosis.

1 INTRODUCTION

Circadian rhythms are the natural endogenous cycles of the human body that regulate sleep cycle, metabolism, and other functions controlled by a set of genes, known as clock genes, which interact with each other and with environmental cues (Tahara and Shibata 2016). Circadian rhythms have cycles that last around 24 hours and can be found in behavior, physiology, or metabolism. When daily rhythms are disrupted by the environment, negative health effects follow, both in animal models and in clinical studies.

The circadian rhythm is the natural cycle of the human body that regulates various biological functions, including lipid metabolism that occurs in the liver. Lipid metabolism involves the synthesis, breakdown, storage, and transport of lipids, such as cholesterol and triglycerides (Gao *et al.* 2020). Situated in the hypothalamus, the suprachiasmatic nucleus (SCN) serves as the circadian governor, producing and harmonizing 24-hour periodicities via modulation of endogenous molecular oscillators. The SCN then receives input from light-sensitive retinal ganglion cells (RGCs) and sends output to various brain regions and hormonal systems. Circadian rhythms also affect the peripheral clocks in different tissues and organs (Rabinovich-Nikitin *et al.* 2019). It influences several aspects of metabolism, including nutrient absorption, energy expenditure, and hormone production. When the circadian rhythm is disrupted by factors, such as jet lag, shift work, or a high-fat diet, the liver may lose its ability to properly regulate lipid metabolism. This can lead to abnormal levels of cholesterol and triglycerides in the blood, which can increase the risk of cardiovascular diseases (CVDs), such as hyperlipidemia and atherosclerosis. Disruptions to the circadian rhythm from shift work or irregular sleep schedules can have detrimental effects on

DOI: 10.1201/9781003587590-53

metabolism. Individuals with irregular sleep patterns or disrupted circadian rhythms are more prone to metabolic disorders and CVDs. The mechanisms underlying the interactions between circadian rhythms and CVDs are complex and multifactorial, involving molecular, cellular, and systemic pathways.

CVDs, a term encompassing heart and blood vessel problems, are influenced by both circadian rhythms and metabolism (Rabinovich-Nikitin *et al.* 2019). Due to their position as the leading cause of death internationally, CVDs represent an important public health problem. An estimation, done by the World Health Organization (WHO), shows that according to recent data, CVD caused 17.9 million deaths in 2019, comprising 32% of total global mortality. Heart attack and stroke alone contributed to 85% of CVD-related fatalities. CVDs are also associated with high economic and social costs, as they affect people's quality of life, productivity, and healthcare expenditures.

The circadian system strongly influences cardiovascular health and the risk of related diseases. However, associations between disruptions to circadian rhythms and cardiovascular outcomes require further elucidation. Therefore, this systematic review aims to summarize past research by examining the link between circadian rhythms and cardiovascular health, evaluating current knowledge on how circadian disruptions may influence cardiovascular function and disease risk, and identifying evidence gaps and limitations of prior work to inform future research directions. A deeper insight into the interplay between circadian clocks and cardiovascular physiology may uncover avenues for preventive or interventional approaches. This systematic review strives to offer an encompassing analysis of available evidence to guide new explorations in this significant domain.

2 CIRCADIAN RHYTHMS AND CARDIOVASCULAR DISEASES

2.1 *Regulation effects of circadian rhythms on cardiovascular and metabolic functions*

Circadian oscillations are centrally controlled by the SCN in the hypothalamus (Brancaccio *et al.* 2014). SCN neurons use a variety of neurotransmitters to control their oscillations, and rhythmic neuronal firing influences downstream brain structures. An intrinsic feedback loop of core clock genes and proteins exists within the cells of almost every peripheral tissue. This molecular clockwork is regulated post-transcriptionally and post-translationally (Tahara and Shibata 2016). Self-sustained daily rhythmicity in the SCN arises from an interdependent interplay between the transcriptional and translational tiers of gene expression regulation conserved across cell types, which is the biological basis for circadian oscillation. Even when isolated in vitro, many tissues continue to exhibit circadian oscillations. Rhythmic body temperature, food intake, and hormones are some of the mechanisms by which the SCN controls these peripheral oscillators. Transcription factors, unfavorable regulators, and other molecules make up the molecular oscillator.

The circadian rhythm results from multiple overlapping feedback cycles that activate or repress levels of core clock genes over time, mainly including the interactions between CLOCK:BMAL1, PER:CRY, and Rev-Erbα/β:RORα/β genes and proteins. The body's natural circadian rhythm plays a role in numerous cardiovascular functions through time-of-day fluctuations in gene expression. Processes such as blood pressure, heart rate, cardiac output, vascular dynamics, endothelial health, platelet activity, and thrombosis are all subject to circadian regulation via transcriptionally mediated changes in downstream proteins integral to these systems over 24-hour cycles. The molecular clock synchronizes expression of genes responsible for diverse cardiovascular parameters, maintaining an internal temporal order across bodily processes and physiology (Rabinovich-Nikitin *et al.* 2019).

The mutation in Bmal1 also causes insulin resistance (IR) and obesity by affecting several mechanisms that involve the following:

- **Glucose metabolism impairment:** Bmal1 normally affects downstream targets; the circadian system modulates concentrations of proteins mediating glucose metabolism activities such as glucokinase, glucose transporter 4, and insulin receptor substrate 1. These genes are regulated by Bmal1 in a circadian manner to match glucose availability and demand. The mutation in Bmal1 disrupts this regulation and impairs glucose uptake and utilization.
- **Energy imbalance:** Bmal1 normally regulates the process involving the expression of genes that are associated with appetites, satiety, and thermogenesis, as well as lipid metabolisms, such as leptin, neuropeptide Y, uncoupling protein 1, and lipoprotein lipase. The mutation in Bmal1 disturbs this regulation and alters energy intake and expenditure.

The downstream genes that are regulated by the circadian rhythm include genes that are involved in vascular tone, inflammation, oxidative stress, coagulation, fibrinolysis, angiogenesis, and energy metabolism. Several genes involved in endothelial dysfunction include endothelin-1 (ET-1), nitric oxide synthase (NOS), cyclooxygenase-2 (COX-2), plasminogen activator inhibitor-1 (PAI-1), vascular endothelial growth factor (VEGF), and peroxisome proliferator-activated receptor gamma coactivator 1-alpha (PGC-1α) (Chen and Yang 2015). These genes exhibit diurnal variations in their expression or activity, which in turn affect the functions of the cardiovascular system in a time-dependent manner.

The circadian rhythm has a significant impact on the occurrence and severity of CVDs and related events, including myocardial infarction, ischemia-reperfusion injury, heart failure, arrhythmias, and sudden cardiac arrest. These diseases or events tend to occur more frequently and severely in certain time periods of the day, especially in the early morning. This may be related to the circadian regulation of cell death processes that are involved in cardiac injury and remodeling. Cell death is an important pathological mechanism of CVDs, and it has various types, such as apoptosis, necrosis, autophagy, etc. Cell death is affected by the circadian rhythm, which shows different sensitivity and protection in different time periods (Rabinovich-Nikitin *et al.* 2019).

2.2 *CVDs associated with circadian disruption*

Circadian disruption, or the disturbance of the natural 24-hour rhythm of biological processes, can increase the risk of developing CVDs by affecting various physiological and metabolic factors. For example, many people who have irregular schedules or travel across time zones may experience circadian disruption, which means their internal clock is out of sync with the external environment. This can have serious consequences for their cardiovascular health, as studies have shown. In a survey conducted as part of the US National Health and Nutrition Survey, approximately 4,000 flight attendants were found to have a higher risk of developing sleep disorders, depression, anxiety, and fatigue compared to the general population (Logan and McClung 2019) Depression has been linked to an increased risk of CVDs, which include heart attack and stroke (Meng *et al.* 2020). Insomnia can impair the function of the blood vessels and increase blood pressure, which can lead to CVDs. Therefore, these findings suggest that circadian disruption and sleep disorders can increase the risk of CVDs and other health problems. To circumvent or mitigate the ill effects of circadian disruption, it is important to establish a consistent sleep-wake rhythm and minimize light exposure at night.

2.2.1 *Hypertension*

Hypertension, defined as persistently high blood pressure, augments the risk for cardiovascular illnesses and cerebrovascular events. A recent animal study showed that test subjects, in this case, mice, with a mutation in the clock gene Bmal1 developed hypertension, IR, and obesity, suggesting that circadian clock disruption can lead to metabolic disorders that cause hypertension. As a key part of the circadian clockwork, gene Bmal1 influences the expression of numerous genes associated with metabolism, blood pressure, and inflammation (Lecarpentier *et al.* 2020; Smolensky *et al.* 2016). The mutation in Bmal1 affects several mechanisms that contribute to hypertension, such as follows:

- **RAAS dysregulation:** Hemodynamic and fluid homeostasis are largely governed by the renin-angiotensin-aldosterone system (RAAS). Bmal1 normally inhibits RAAS during the day and activates it at night. The mutation in Bmal1 abolishes this circadian regulation and results in a chronic elevation of RAAS components, such as angiotensin II, aldosterone, and renin.
- **Nitric oxide deficiency:** Under the regulation of Bmal1, endothelial nitric oxide synthase (eNOS) facilitates vessel relaxation and contributes to the lowering of blood pressure by synthesizing nitric oxide (NO). The mutation in Bmal1 reduces the expression and activity of eNOS and lowers NO levels.
- **Inflammation enhancement:** Under normal circumstances, Bmal1 helps regulate inflammation by suppressing cytokines with pro-inflammatory properties, such as interleukin-6 (IL-6) and tumor necrosis factor-alpha (TNF-α), and activating genes with anti-inflammatory properties, including heme oxygenase-1 (HO-1) and peroxisome proliferator-activated receptor gamma (PPARγ). However, a mutation in Bmal1 reverses this effect and increases inflammation.

The circadian regulation of blood pressure is mediated by several mechanisms, such as the sympathetic nervous system, the RAAS system, the natriuretic peptide system, and the vasopressin system. These mechanisms are influenced by the circadian rhythm at different levels, such as gene expression, hormone secretion, receptor sensitivity, and signal transduction (Rabinovich-Nikitin *et al.* 2019). The circadian regulation of heart rate is mainly dependent on the autonomic nervous system, which shows a rhythmic pattern of sympathetic and parasympathetic activity. Circadian patterning of cardiac contractility corresponds with daily fluctuations in calcium handling gene expression or activity, including sarcoplasmic reticulum calcium ATPase, phospholamban, and ryanodine receptor 2. The circadian regulation of hemodynamics is influenced by the balance between vasoconstriction and vasodilation, which is determined by the expression or activity of genes that are involved in vascular tone, such as ET-1, NOS, COX-2, and angiotensin II receptor 1. The circadian regulation of endothelial function is affected by the expression or activity of genes that are involved in processes that are related to inflammation and oxidative stress, including NO production, and angiogenesis, such as COX-2, NOS, VEGF, and nuclear factor kappa B (NF-κB). The circadian regulation of platelet aggregation and thrombus formation is influenced by the expression or activity of genes that are involved in coagulation and fibrinolysis, such as PAI-1, tissue factor, thrombin receptor (PAR), and von Willebrand factor (vWF).

2.2.2 *Coronary heart disease*

Coronary heart disease (CHD) develops as plaque accumulates in the coronary arteries, which are crucial for delivering oxygenated blood to the cardiac muscle. Insufficient blood flow and oxygen to the cardiac muscle can cause issues such as chest pain (angina) or heart attack. A heart attack transpires when a plaque buildup completely blocks an artery, preventing blood from flowing to part of the cardiac muscle. The process of plaque buildup, which is known as atherosclerosis, is the underlying condition and most common cause of CHD.

2.2.3 *Atherosclerosis*

Atherosclerosis is a condition that impacts the arteries, which carry oxygen and nutrients from the heart throughout the body. Atherosclerosis occurs when plaque, a substance made of fat, cholesterol, and other substances, deposits within the inner lining of the arteries, narrows the arteries, and reduces blood flow. Sometimes, plaque can also rupture and cause blood clots that can block the arteries completely. Atherosclerosis can result in serious complications such as myocardial infarction, cerebrovascular accident, peripheral arterial diseases, and renal dysfunction, depending on the arteries affected. Clock genes, such as Per2, are essential components of this system and are expressed in various tissues, including the liver and the blood vessels. Dysregulation of clock genes can lead to circadian disruption and affect the pathogenesis and advancement of CVDs, encompassing conditions like atherosclerosis.

One of the primary contributing factors associated with atherosclerosis is hyperlipidemia, which manifests as elevated levels of cholesterol and triglycerides in the bloodstream. Research found that mice with a mutation in Per2 exhibited elevated cholesterol and triglyceride levels compared to healthy mice, suggesting that Per2 exerts a substantial influence on regulating hepatic lipid metabolism (Turek *et al.* 2005). Moreover, circadian rhythms can be disturbed by various liver diseases, such as hepatic steatosis, biliary stasis, hepatitis, cirrhosis, and hepatocellular carcinoma, which can impair the functions of the liver and cause lipid disorders. These diseases can also worsen the condition of the liver by disrupting its own circadian rhythms (Tahara and Shibata 2016). Therefore, clock genes play crucial roles in maintaining regular metabolic processes and preventing CVDs.

2.2.4 *Indirect influences of circadian disruption*

Another risk factor for CVDs is inflammation, which is an immune response to tissue damage or contamination. However, inflammation can also contribute to atherosclerosis. The circadian rhythm system governs the modulation and functionality of numerous genes and proteins implicated in the processes of inflammation and atherosclerosis. These include peroxisome proliferator-activated receptor gamma (PPARγ), liver X receptor (LXR), sterol regulatory element-binding protein (SREBP), nuclear factor kappa B (NF-κB), chemokines, adhesion molecules, scavenger receptors, and inflammasomes (McAlpine and Swirski 2016; Song *et al.* 2022). These factors influence the synthesis, transport, and uptake of lipids; the production and release of inflammatory signaling molecules; and the behavior/function of immune effector cells such as macrophages, neutrophils, and T cells. These cells infiltrate the arterial wall and participate in plaque formation and instability.

Circadian disruption, caused by factors such as artificial light exposure, shift work, or jet lag, can impair the function of the SCN, the master clock that synchronizes the peripheral clocks in different tissues. This could lead to a disruption of the normal rhythm of the factors involved in inflammation and atherosclerosis and then lead to hyperlipidemia, oxidative stress, endothelial dysfunction, plaque formation, and plaque rupture. Circadian disruption can also induce pyroptosis, a type of inflammatory cell death that involves the activation of Gasdermin D by caspase-1 or caspase-11 (Song *et al.* 2022). Pyroptosis promotes the discharge of pro-inflammatory cytokines such as interleukin-1 beta (IL-1β) and interleukin-18 (IL-18), as well as damage signals including high-mobility group box 1 (HMGB1) and ATP. These molecules can further amplify the inflammatory response and aggravate atherosclerosis.

Furthermore, the circadian rhythm influences other aspects of cardiovascular parameters such as blood pressure, heart rate, and vascular tone, followed by daily patterns regulated by the SCN. Disruptions to this natural circadian rhythm from shift work, irregular sleep, or jet lag have been linked to higher risks of atherosclerosis and coronary artery disease. Such disruptions can cause imbalances in hormone levels, inflammation, oxidative stress, and lipid metabolism – all of which promote the development and progression of fatty plaques in the arteries (Song *et al.* 2022).

Specifically, the circadian rhythm controls enzymes involved in lipid processing. Interrupting this rhythm leads to abnormal lipid levels, including elevated LDL cholesterol levels and reduced HDL cholesterol levels. A higher LDL level is a major risk factor for atherosclerosis (Stone *et al.* 2023).

Blood pressure naturally dips at night and rises in the morning due to circadian influence. But rhythm disruptions can produce abnormal patterns like constant high nocturnal pressure. This sustained elevation promotes atherosclerosis development and worsening. The circadian rhythm also regulates platelet activity and blood clotting involved in thrombosis. Disruptions enhance pro-clotting and raise thrombosis risk. Additionally, plaque stability varies over the day's circadian cycle, with vulnerable plaques more prone to rupture at specific times (Stone *et al.* 2023).

Circadian disruption can impair the function of the endothelium. Endothelial dysfunction can lead to atherosclerosis, which is the buildup of plaque in the arteries that can cause heart attacks or strokes. A study found that healthy young adults who were exposed to bright light at night for 8 hours had reduced endothelial function and increased blood pressure compared with those who slept in darkness (Chellappa *et al.* 2019).

Circadian disruption can also alter the secretion and action of hormones that regulate blood pressure, glucose metabolism, and inflammation. For example, cortisol, which is normally highest in the morning and lowest at night, can be disrupted by circadian misalignment, resulting in elevated levels at night and reduced levels in the morning. This can increase the risk of hypertension, insulin resistance, and inflammation, which are all risk factors for coronary diseases (Fishbein *et al.* 2021).

3 HEALTHY CIRCADIAN RHYTHM—AN EFFECTIVE APPROACH TO PREVENT CVDS

To sum up, maintaining a healthy circadian rhythm is important for people, no matter whether people with CVDs and metabolic disorders or not, as these conditions can affect or be affected by the body's circadian rhythm. To stay in a healthy circadian rhythm, maintain a regular sleep-wake schedule, and avoid staying up too late or sleeping too much would help to synchronize the internal rhythm with the external light-dark cycle and improve the sleep quality and quantity (Xie *et al.* 2019). Avoid exposure to bright light at night, especially blue light from electronic devices, as this can suppress melatonin secretion and delay your circadian phase (Xie *et al.* 2019). Get enough exposure to natural sunlight during the day, especially in the morning, as this can enhance melatonin production at night and advance your circadian phase (Xie *et al.* 2019). Avoid caffeine, alcohol, nicotine, and other stimulants or depressants that can interfere with your sleep quality and circadian rhythm.

4 IDENTIFICATION OF PROBLEMS AND LIMITATIONS IN THIS FIELD

The molecular mechanisms that govern circadian rhythms involve intricate processes at the cellular and molecular levels, and their regulation of cardiovascular function is still not completely understood. More basic research is required to fully elucidate the interactions between biological clock genes, transcription factors, metabolic pathways, and the cardiovascular system.

Emerging research has demonstrated that molecular clock components are expressed not just in the SCN but also in peripheral tissues, including the heart and blood vessels (Allada and Bass 2021). Local circadian oscillators in cardiovascular tissues appear to control daily variations in cardiac contractility, heart rate, blood pressure, and vascular tone. Disruption of peripheral circadian clocks has been linked to cardiovascular pathology. However, the mechanisms by which clock genes regulate cardiovascular function are still not fully understood.

In addition, transcriptional factors and metabolic pathways that mediate crosstalk between the molecular clock and cardiovascular physiology need further exploration (Allada and Bass 2021). For example, how do circadian clock proteins interact with transcriptional regulators of cardiac and vascular genes? How do circadian oscillations in metabolic pathways like gluconeogenesis, and lipid metabolism influence cardiovascular health? Understanding these interactions at the molecular level could provide novel targets for chronotherapeutic approaches to treating cardiovascular diseases.

More comprehensive basic research using multidisciplinary techniques is still required to map out the molecular circuits connecting the circadian clockwork to cardiovascular pathways. Unraveling these complex regulatory networks will provide important insights into the circadian control of cardiovascular homeostasis and mechanisms underlying dysregulation leading to cardiometabolic diseases.

5 CONCLUSION

Circadian rhythms refer to the 24-hour cycles in the human body that regulate functions such as sleep, metabolism, blood pressure, heart rate, and more. They are influenced by factors within the body, such as clock genes, nerves, and hormones, as well as external environmental factors. Disturbances in circadian rhythms from issues such as shift work or irregular sleep can increase the risk of CVDs.

The molecular mechanisms behind circadian rhythms involve feedback loops among clock genes and proteins. Key players are the CLOCK:BMAL1, PER:CRY, and Rev-Erbα/β: RORα/β systems, which regulate downstream genes related to processes in the cardiovascular system. These downstream genes control things such as vascular tone, inflammation, oxidative stress, coagulation, and metabolism.

CVDs encompass conditions of the heart and blood vessels and are a leading global cause of death. Circadian rhythm disruptions can elevate CVD risk by impacting physiological and metabolic factors. For example, issues with blood pressure, cholesterol, triglycerides, inflammation, oxidative stress, endothelial function, atherosclerosis, and more have all been tied to circadian rhythm.

To prevent CVDs, maintaining a healthy circadian rhythm is important. This involves keeping a regular sleep-wake cycle, limiting late-night light and blue light exposure, and avoiding substances such as caffeine, alcohol, and nicotine that interfere with sleep quality and rhythms. Adjusting medication timing to biorhythms may also boost effectiveness and reduce side effects.

The knowledge of the circadian regulation of cardiovascular functions may provide novel insights for optimizing therapeutic strategies and improving cardiovascular outcomes. For example, chronotherapy, which is the adjustment of drug administration or intervention timing according to the circadian rhythm, may enhance drug efficacy and reduce adverse effects. Additionally, preserving a regular circadian rhythm or sleep pattern can lower the likelihood of cardiovascular events and support cardiac restoration.

REFERENCES

Allada R. and Bass J., M. D. (2021). *The New England Journal of Medicine*, 384(**6**), 550–561.

Brancaccio M., Enoki R., Mazuski C. N., Jones J., Evans J. A. and Azzi A. (2014). *Journal of Neuroscience*, **34** (46) 15192–15199.

Cardiovascular diseases (CVDs) (who.int)

Chellappa S. L., Vujovic N., Williams J. S. and Scheer F. A. L. (2019). *Trends in Endocrinology and Metabolism: TEM*, **30**(10), 767–779.

Chen L.H. and Yang G.R. (2015). *Front. Pharmacol.*, **01** April.

Fishbein A. B., Knutson K. L. and Zee P. C. (2021). *J.C. Invest.* 131(**19**):e148286.

Gao W., Shu Y., Ye J. and Pan X. (2020). *Shijie Huaren Xiaohua Zazhi*, **28**(20), 1025–1035

Lecarpentier Y., Schussler O., Hébert J. L. and Vallée A. (2020). *Curr Hypertens Rep* **22**, 50.

Logan R. W. and McClung C.A., (2019). *Nat Rev Neurosci* **20**, 49–65.

McAlpine C. S. and Swirski F. K. (2016). *Circulation Research*, **119**(1), 131–141.

Meng R. W., Yu C. Q. and Liu N. (2020). *JAMA Netw Open*. Feb 5;**3**(**2**):e1921043.

Rabinovich-Nikitin I., Lieberman B., Martino T. A. and Kirshenbaum L. A. (2019). *Circulation*, **139**(7), 965–980.

Smolensky M. H., Ohayon M. M. and Roth T. (2016). *Chronobiol Int.* **33**(8):1101–19.

Song D., Li M., Yu X., Wang Y. Q., Fan J. Y., Yang W., Yang L. M. and Li H. (2022). *Front. Cell Dev. Biol.*,

Stone P. H., Libby P. and Boden W. E. (2023). *JAMA Cardiology*, **8**(2), 192–201.

Tahara Y. and Shibata S. (2016). *Nature Reviews Gastroenterology & Hepatology*, **13**, 217–226

Turek F.W., Joshu C., Kohsaka A., Lin E., Ivanova G., Mcdearmon E., Laposky A., Losee-Olson S., Easton A., Jensen D. R., Eckel R. H., Takahashi J. S. and Bass J. (2005). *Science*. May 13; **308**(5724):1043–5.

Xie Y., Tang Q., Chen G., Xie M., Yu S., Zhao J. and Chen L. (2019). *Frontiers in Physiology*, **10**, 682.

Biological Sciences and Environmental Health – Gao (Ed.)
© 2025 the Author(s), ISBN: 978-1-032-96016-6

A review on immunoenhancement technology based on non-drug-loaded nanoparticles

Yi Jiang
Biology and Medical Engineering Department, Beihang University, Beijing, China

ABSTRACT: Infectious diseases and cancer are significant health concerns globally. Infectious diseases, caused by microorganisms like viruses and bacteria, spread from person to person and can lead to pandemics. Prevention involves vaccination, hygiene, and medications. Cancer, characterized by abnormal cell growth, results from genetic factors, environmental exposures, and lifestyle choices. Early detection through screenings like mammography and colonoscopy improves outcomes. Both diseases challenge healthcare systems. Advances in medicine, including immunotherapy, offer hope. Public health efforts and early intervention are vital in reducing their global impact. Non-drug-loaded nanoparticles (NDLNPs) have drawn public notice as promising tools for immunoenhancement, leveraging their unique properties to modulate immune responses. This comprehensive review explores the definition, components, properties, and advantages of NDLNPs in the context of immunotherapy. The applications of NDLNPs in infectious disease and cancer immunotherapy are elaborated, highlighting their potential in disrupting viral structures, harnessing photothermal effects, augmenting the immune system, and serving as vaccine adjuvants.

1 INTRODUCTION

The twenty-first century has seen several epidemics of infectious diseases. We have had several pandemics since the turn of the century, including SARS, Ebola, SARS-Cov-2, and others that have severely harmed our civilization (Baker *et al.* 2022). At the same time, medical technology aimed at enhancing the immune system is also developing rapidly, making great contributions to mankind's victory over these infectious diseases.

Additionally, cancer is becoming a serious global public health concern on an increasingly global scale (Siegel *et al* 2023). Cancer is a major cause of mortality in China, placing a heavy strain on families and society (Feng *et al.* 2019). Therefore, it is urgent to find effective treatments. Immunotherapy is a rapidly growing field in cancer treatment aiming to stimulate the function of the autoimmune system to detect and eliminate cancer cells. Conventional cancer therapies like radiation and chemotherapy target both malignant and healthy cells, which has serious negative effects. Immunotherapy, on the other hand, targets cancer cells only and spares healthy cells. Immunotherapy has proven to be extremely successful in treating a variety of malignancies (Esfahani *et al.* 2020). A rising number of people are interested in using nanoparticles for cancer treatment. Nanoparticles are tiny in size. They can be manufactured to have certain characteristics like specific tiny volume, surface charge state and surface chemistry property. They have a size range of 1 to 100 nanometers. These characteristics can be changed to best transport medications, genes, or antigens to the intended cells (Khan *et al.* 2019). Non-drug-loaded nanoparticles (NDLNPs) have emerged as a novel avenue in immunoenhancement, capitalizing on their distinct properties for

 DOI: 10.1201/9781003587590-54

modulating immune responses. In contrast to conventional drug-loaded nanoparticles, NDLNPs possess inherent immunomodulatory capabilities that make them attractive candidates for various immunotherapy strategies. This review aims to comprehensively elucidate the definition, components, properties, and advantages of NDLNPs in the context of immunotherapy. The multifaceted mechanisms by which NDLNPs boost immune responses are explored, along with their applications in infectious disease and cancer immunotherapy. The versatility and potential of NDLNPs to revolutionize the field of immunoenhancement were discussed.

2 BRIEFING OF NON-DRUG-LOADED NANOPARTICLES DESIGNED FOR IMMUNOENHANCEMENT

Non-drug-loaded nanoparticles (NDLNPs) have recently emerged as a novel approach for immunoenhancement, leveraging their distinctive properties to modulate the immune system's responses. This section aims to provide an overall view of NDLNPs, focusing on their definition, components, properties, and the advantages they bring to immunoenhancement strategies.

2.1 *Basic principle of NDLNPs*

NDLNPs refer to nanoparticles that are devoid of conventional drug payloads but possess intrinsic immunomodulatory properties. These nanoparticles are typically composed of biocompatible materials such as lipids, polymers, metals, or ceramics. The core components of NDLNPs may include targeting ligands, adjuvants, and functional coatings, which collectively contribute to their immunoenhancing capabilities.

NDLNPs exhibit a range of properties that are crucial for their immunomodulatory effects. These properties include size, surface charge, shape, and surface functionalization (Sarkar and Mukhopadhyay 2021 & Zhu *et al.* 2021). The nanoscale size of NDLNPs enables their interaction with immune cells, promoting enhanced cellular uptake and antigen presentation. Surface charge and functionalization further dictate their interactions with immune receptors and molecular pathways.

2.2 *Involution and advantages*

2.2.1 *Mechanisms of immunoenhancement based on NDLNPs*

Nanotechnology used for adjuvant immunotherapy has undergone an iterative process and is constantly evolving. Through a number of pathways, including the stimulation of antigen-presenting cells (APCs), alteration of cytokine profiles, and improvement of T cell responses, NDLNPs exercise their immunostimulatory effects (Akkın, Varan and Bilensoy, 2021). NDLNPs are effective adjuvants that can accelerate dendritic cell maturation and the subsequent start of adaptive immune responses. Recently, researchers discovered that NDLNPs might affect immune checkpoint pathways, enhancing the body's response to tumours (Yan *et al.* 2019).

2.2.2 *Advantages of NDLNPs in immunotherapy*

NDLNPs offer several distinct advantages in the context of immunotherapy. Their ability to selectively target immune cells and tissues allows for precise immune modulation (Gao *et al.* 2021). Furthermore, the absence of drug payloads reduces the potential for off-target effects and systemic toxicity (Liu *et al.* 2021). NDLNPs can be engineered to encapsulate specific antigens or nucleic acids, thereby enabling tailored immune responses for vaccination or cancer immunotherapy. The biocompatibility and versatility of NDLNPs make them attractive candidates for combination therapies and personalized treatment strategies (Fu *et al.* 2022 & Wang *et al.* 2021).

3 NON-DRUG-LOADED NANOPARTICLES IN INFECTIOUS DISEASE IMMUNOTHERAPY

Non-drug-loaded nanoparticles (NDLNPs), whose special qualities include a high specific surface and catalytic activity, have drawn a lot of attention in the field of infectious disease immunotherapy, even though the majority of nanoparticle research over the last few decades has focused on drug delivery. These characteristics give potential possibilities in viral destructions, harnessing photothermal effect and immune system augment, making NDLNPs attractive in infectious diseases' immunotherapy nowadays, opening up new opportunities in this field.

3.1 *NDLNPs for disrupting viral structures*

Certain metal nanoparticles exhibit intrinsic viral affinity. For instance, copper nanoparticles may breakdown viral capsids whereas gold nanoparticles have shown the potential to destroy the outer coat of several coronaviruses (Jeremiah *et al.* 2020). Silver nanoparticles, due to their strong affinity for sulphur-containing amino acids in viruses, non-specifically bind to viral proteins, causing cellular dysfunction. This disruption in viral structure contributes to viral neutralization. Mechanistic insights reveal the potential of metal NDLNPs in thwarting viral infections (Cai *et al.* 2020).

3.2 *NDLNPs for harnessing the photothermal effect*

Non-drug-loaded nanoparticles possess a unique potential in harnessing the photothermal effect. By incorporating specific antibodies onto these nanoparticles which could be combined with target delivery techniques to achieve localized virus killing effect. For instance, under near-infrared light exposure, these nanoparticles undergo plasmon resonance, converting light energy into localized heat. This thermal energy can inflict damage to viruses, as demonstrated by recent research using semiconductor nanoparticles that effectively neutralized SARS-CoV-2. The utilization of NDLNPs in photothermal therapy emerges as a promising avenue in infectious disease immunotherapy.

3.3 *Augmenting the immune system with NDLNPs*

In addition to their physical interactions, certain NDLNPs possess immunostimulatory properties. These nanoparticles have the capacity to activate important immune cells including dendritic cells and macrophages, which are necessary for effective immunological responses. Notably, the capacity of amantadine-assembled nano stimulators (AAS) to activate the RLR signaling pathway, resulting in dendritic cell and T helper cell maturation, has been studied. This immune activation culminates in potent antibody responses by B cells. NDLNPs thus serve as promising candidates for boosting the immune system against infectious agents (Zhang *et al.* 2022).

4 NON-DRUG-LOADED NANOPARTICLES IN CANCER IMMUNOTHERAPY

In addition to its use in the study of infectious illnesses, nanoparticles have revolutionized the treatment of tumor immunotherapy. These immunotherapies exploit the similar properties of nanoparticles. In addition to being also used for drug delivery and vaccine delivery, increasing interests have been developed on nanoparticles that carry no drug. Rapid-developing advances of immunotherapy based on NDLDPs offer several innovative combined approaches, including photothermal therapy, photodynamic immunotherapy, electrical stimulation therapy and so on.

4.1 *NDLNP-enhanced photodynamic therapy (PDT) and photothermal therapy (PTT) immunotherapy*

Photothermal and photodynamic therapies can induce various antitumor effects, including immune responses (Siegel *et al.* 2017). As a result of the considerable tumor cell death brought on by these therapies, immune effector cells may be redistributed and activated, cytokines may be produced and released, and memory T lymphocytes may undergo metamorphosis (Ray *et al.* 2018). Immune checkpoint blockade treatment can help these immune responses even more. Unlike conventional antitumor therapies like radiation therapy and chemotherapy, which have a lower degree of specificity and can be harmful over time, nanoparticle-based phototherapies, such as photothermal therapy (PTT) is a cutting-edge option for cancer treatment, as well as photodynamic therapy (PDT) (Takaki *et al.* 2017). NDLNPs have the potential to function as photothermal conversion agents in PTT, converting light energy into heat to destroy cancer cells. The intravenous injection of NDLNPs can also be adjusted with targeting molecules to achieve tumor-specific death. Additionally, NDLNPs can be designed to self-enrich oxygen, which is beneficial for enhancing the PDT effect and overcoming chemoresistance. Overall, NDLNPs can improve the efficacy and specificity of PTT and PDT, making them promising treatment options for cancer (Chen *et al.* 2019).

4.2 *NDLNP-enhanced radiotherapy*

NDLNPs can regulate the immune-suppressive microenvironment of tumor and stimulate the potent immunological responses of tumor debris following radiation-induced ICD (immunogenic cell death), according to research, which can improve the immune response to cancer cells during radiotherapy. The NDLNPs used in the study contained the TLR7 agonist R836, which can activate dendritic cells and promote the progress of presenting antigens of tumors to T cells. This can lead to the establishment of a systemic immune response that targets cancer cells, providing long-term immunological memory protection against cancer recurrence (Wei *et al.* 2018).

4.3 *NDLNP-enhanced chemotherapy*

New findings present the development of combined chemotherapy for brain cancer treatment. The study demonstrates that electrical stimulation based on NDLNPs, when used synergistically with a sub-toxic concentration of temozolomide (an oral chemotherapy medication used in the chemical treatment of specific types of brain tumors), increases sensitivity to chemotherapy treatment and has remarkable anticancer effects (Genchi *et al.* 2016). The study's findings offer new perspectives on nano treatment and may be beneficial for the home therapy of brain tumors and neurological illnesses. NDLNPs used for electrical stimulation have several advantages over traditional therapies for glioblastoma multiforme, including their ability in crossing the blood-brain barrier, targeting cancer cells, and giving far-reaching electric stimulation. The study shows that glioblastoma cells' chemosensitivity is increased when nanoparticles are added to remote electric stimulation. The synergistic approach dramatically reduces the quantity of cancer cells and the metabolic activity of glioblastoma cultures. It does this by combining chemical therapy with chemotherapeutic medication, physical therapy with remote electric stimulation, and both (Zhao *et al.* 2015). According to these results, electric nanoparticles can effectively increase a cell's permeability to immunological and therapeutic substances. This can reduce the need for high-dose, toxic injections, which are otherwise harmful to the body over time but are essential for cancer therapy.

4.4 *NDLNP-enhanced electrical stimulation therapy*

Electrical stimulation therapy has become a viable cancer treatment option because of its capacity to balance the immune system and improve immunotherapy's effectiveness. But the use of electrical stimulation alone has limitations in terms of its effectiveness and safety, for those continuous treatments relied on electrotherapy devices requires a significant investment of time and money. Also, the requirement for patients to wear electrodes on their scalp could lead to discomfort. To overcome these limitations, researchers have explored the combination of electrical stimulation with nanoparticles in recent years. Nano pulse electrical stimulation (NPS), which employs electrical pulses with a duration of only a couple of nanoseconds long to produce gaps in the cell membranes of cancer cells, is one of the most promising nanoparticle-enhanced electrical stimulation treatments. (Das *et al.* 2020). Another fascinating approach involves using biodegradable nanofiber scaffolds as electrical stimulators. These scaffolds have the ability to operate independently, remotely, and with nanoparticles to increase their effectiveness (Huang *et al.* 2022).

5 NDLNPS AS VACCINE ADJUVANTS

Non-drug-loaded nanoparticles have garnered significant attention in the field of vaccine development as potential adjuvants. Chemicals known as adjuvants are added to vaccines in some cases. This kind of substances could enhance the body's immune response to antigens. They work by activating and directing the immune system's response, leading to a stronger and longer-lasting immune reaction. In the context of vaccines, NDLNPs offer several advantages as adjuvants.

5.1 *Immune stimulation*

Non-drug-loaded nanoparticles can be designed to stimulate the immune system by acting as adjuvants. Adjuvants are chemicals that enhance the immune system's reaction to antigens. These nanoparticles can imitate pathogens or danger signals, which can activate immune cells and trigger a strong immune response against cancer cells. Aside from this, NDLNPs can also enhance the vaccine's stimulation to prevent cancer by being intricately engineered to serve as potent carriers for tumor antigens or fragments of tumor cells. The key to triggering a strong immune response lies in these painstakingly crafted nanoparticles, which deliver these antigens to essential immune cells such as dendritic cells. For example, NDLNPs-based antigen presentation platforms offer multifaceted advantages. They facilitate improved antigen presentation and T-helper cell activation by increasing not only the absorption of antigens by antigen-presenting cells (APCs), but also optimizing their volume to fall within the range suitable for effective APC uptake. Additionally, complement may effectively opsonize bigger NDLNPs, which facilitates attachment to the surface of follicular dendritic cells (FDCs) and extends the time that the NDLNPs remain inside lymph follicles. This extended presence in the lymphatic system enhances antigen presentation to B-cells, thus contributing to a more potent immune response (Gu *et al.* 2021). Furthermore, NDLNPs displaying multiple antigens excel in facilitating B-cell activation through the effective crosslinking of multiple B-cell receptors. In a groundbreaking development, protein platforms based on NDLNPs have enabled the presentation of self-antigens, typically dispersed and challenging to target. This innovative approach effectively disrupts self-tolerance mechanisms, triggering a robust immune response. As a result, protein platforms using

NDLNPs hold enormous promise for the creation of cancer vaccines by making tumor-associated antigens more visible.

5.2 *Targeted delivery*

Targeting certain immune cells or tumor microenvironments is possible with NDLNP design. A variety of compounds can be delivered to particular parts of the body by combining therapeutic medicines with nanoparticles that have distinctive physicochemical and biological characteristics and structuring their paths for effective targeting (Jahan *et al.* 2017). This targeted delivery ensures that immune-stimulating agents or antigens are delivered precisely where they are needed, enhancing their effectiveness while minimizing potential side effects (Wu *et al.* 2018).

5.3 *Modulation of immune suppression*

The microenvironment of tumor cells often creates an immune-suppressive environment that can limit the effectiveness of immunotherapy. Immune suppression can be brought on by a variety of factors, such as certain types of macrophages related to tumor, suppressor cells, and some specific T cells. A significant obstacle to the development of successful cancer immunotherapy is immune suppression. NDLNPs can be designed to counteract this immunosuppression by delivering immune-activating signals locally to the tumor microenvironment. This strategy can overcome immune suppression by transforming suppressive cells into immuno-stimulating ones.

6 CHALLENGES AND FUTURE PROSPECTS

The exploration of immunoenhancement technology through the use of NDLNPs holds great promise within the realm of biomedical research. However, this burgeoning field is not without its challenges and uncertainties, which demand careful consideration and strategic planning for future advancements. In this section, we will delve into the current challenges while envisioning the prospects of immunoenhancement technology using NDLNPs.

One of the paramount concerns in harnessing the potential of functional nanoparticles lies in ensuring their biocompatibility and safety. The possibility of unintended immune responses, cytotoxicity, and unforeseen long-term effects necessitates a thorough assessment and the development of robust risk mitigation strategies. Introducing nanoparticles into immune system carries the risk of triggering immune reactions, potentially compromising their effectiveness, or leading to adverse events. Hence, comprehending and effectively managing the immunogenicity of functional nanoparticles is imperative for their successful translation into clinical applications. Precisely targeting immune cells and tissues with functional nanoparticles remains a formidable challenge that demands advancements in targeting ligands, surface modifications, and innovative delivery strategies. Surmounting the biological barriers that hinder efficient nanoparticle accumulation at desired sites remains an ongoing pursuit. Determining optimal dosing regimens and administration routes for functional nanoparticles in immunoenhancement applications is a complex endeavor. Striking a delicate balance between therapeutic efficacy, minimization of side effects, and ensuring patient compliance requires meticulous optimization.

Functional nanoparticles have the potential to revolutionize immunotherapy by enabling personalized approaches tailored to individual patient profiles. Furthermore, the integration of functional nanoparticles with established immunotherapies, such as checkpoint inhibitors and vaccines, holds the potential for synergistic effects and enhanced treatment outcomes. The field is ripe for the development of rational combination strategies that could redefine the landscape of immunotherapy. Moreover, the convergence of immunoenhancement and drug delivery opens the door to innovative strategies for precise and controlled immune modulation. Functional nanoparticles can serve as carriers for immune-modulating agents, optimizing their pharmacokinetics and bioavailability, thereby enhancing treatment efficacy.

Incorporating bioinformatics, computational modeling, and data-driven approaches can provide invaluable insights into nanoparticle-immune interactions. These approaches can guide the design of nanoparticles with specific immunomodulatory effects, paving the way for more targeted and effective interventions in the future.

7 CONCLUSION

Non-drug-loaded nanoparticles represent a cutting-edge approach in immunoenhancement, leveraging their intrinsic properties to modulate immune responses. This review has provided a comprehensive overview of NDLNPs, covering their definition, components, properties, and advantages in immunotherapy. NDLNPs demonstrate remarkable potential in diverse applications, including infectious disease and cancer immunotherapy. Their ability to disrupt viral structures, harness photothermal effects, augment the immune system, and serve as vaccine adjuvants underscores their significance in precision immunomodulation. NDLNPs offer the advantages of targeted immune modulation, reduced off-target effects, and tailored immune responses. As ongoing research continues to unravel the intricacies of NDLNPs' immunoenhancing mechanisms, these nanoparticles are poised to reshape the landscape of immunotherapy, promising innovative strategies for combating diseases and enhancing patient outcomes.

REFERENCES

Akkın, S., Varan, G., and Bilensoy, E. (2021). *Molecules* **26**, 3382.
Baker, R. E., Mahmud, A. S., Miller, I. F. and Rajeev, M. (2022). *Nat. Rev. Microbiol.* **20**, 193.
Cai, X., Prominski, A., Lin, Y. and Ankenbruck, N. (2020). *biorxiv*, 11(30), 404624.
Chen, Q., Chen, J., Yang, Z. and Xu, J. (2019). *Adv. Mater.* **31**, 1802228.
Das, R., Curry, E. J., Le, T. T. and Awale, G. (2020). *Nano Energy* **76**, 105028.
Esfahani, K., Roudaia, L., Buhlaiga, N. and Del Rincon, S. (2020). *Current Oncology* **27**, 87.
Feng, R. M., Zong, Y. N., Cao, S. M. and Xu, R. H. (2019). *Cancer Commun.* **39**, 1
Fu, L., Ma, X., Liu, Y., Xu, Z. and Sun, Z. Chin. (2022). *Chem. Lett.* **33**, 1718.
Gao, S., Yang, X., Xu, J., Qiu, N. and Zhai, G. (2021). *ACS Nano* **15**, 12567.
Genchi, G. G., Marino, A., Rocca, A., Mattoli, V. and Ciofani, G. (2016). *Nanotechnology* **27**, 232001.
Gu, P., Zhang, Y., Cai, G. and Liu, Z. (2021). *Molecular Pharmaceutics* **18**, 2274.
Huang, Z., Callmann, C. E., Wang, S. and Vasher, M. K. (2022). *ACS Cent. Sci.* **8**, 692.
Jahan, S. T., Sadat, S., Walliser, M. and Haddadi, A. (2017). *J. Drug Delivery* **2017** .
Jeremiah, S. S., Miyakawa, K., Morita, T., Yamaoka, Y. and Ryo, A. (2020). *Biochem. Biophys. Res. Commun.* **533**, 195.
Khan, I., Saeed, K. and Khan, I. (2019). *Arabian J. Chem.* **12**, 908.
Liu, Q., Duo, Y., Fu, J. and Qiu, M. (2021). *Nano Today* **36**, 101023.
Ray, A., Das, D. S., Song, Y. and Hideshima, T. (2018). *Leukemia* **32**, 843.
Sarkar, P. K. and Das Mukhopadhyay, C. (2021). *Int. Nano Lett.*, 1.
Siegel, R. L., Miller, K. D., Fedewa, S. A. and Ahnen, D. J. *CA.* (2017). *Cancer J. Clin.* **67**, 177.
Siegel, R. L., Miller, K. D., Wagle, N. S. and Jemal, A. (2023). *Ca Cancer J Clin* **73**, 17.
Takaki, H., Cornelis, F., Kako, Y. and Kobayashi, K. (2017). *Diagn. Interventional Imaging* **98**, 651.
Wang, X., Meng, F., Yen, Y. T., Li, R. and Liu, B. *Adv. Funct. Mater.* **31**, 2004713 (2021).
Wei, H., Wang, H., Xia, Y. and Cui, D. (2018). *J. Mater. Chem. C* **6**, 12446.
Wu, W., Luo, L., Wang, Y. and Wu, Q. (2018). *Theranostics* **8**, 3038.
Yan, S., Zhao, P., Yu, T. and Gu, N. (2019). *Cancer Biology & Medicine* **16**, 486.
Zhang, Y., Wang, R., He, C. and Zhang, Y.-F. (2022). *Nano Today* **43**, 101393.
Zhao, Y., Liao, Q., Zhang, G. and Zhang, Z. (2015). *Nano Energy* **11**, 719.
Zhu, W., Wei, Z., Han, C. and Weng, X. (2021). *Nanomaterials* **11**, 3346.

Biological Sciences and Environmental Health – Gao (Ed.)
© 2025 the Author(s), ISBN: 978-1-032-96016-6

Oral vaccines: Advantages, challenges, and delivery platform

Mingyang Liu
College of Life Science, Sichuan Agricultural University, Ya'an, China

ABSTRACT: Compared with traditional vaccines, oral vaccines provide higher immunological effects, better patient compliance, easier storage, and a lower risk of needlestick injuries. However, due to the gastrointestinal immune system, which includes the mucosal immune system, the low pH environment of the gastrointestinal tract, and the effects of various digestive enzymes, oral vaccines frequently fail to be directly recognized by the immune system and elicit an immune response. Researchers must employ a number of delivery platforms for the antigenic components carried by oral vaccines to trigger the immune system. This article analyzes the benefits and drawbacks of oral vaccines and introduces cutting-edge platforms for oral vaccine delivery, which include acid-resistant biomaterial delivery platform, nanoparticle-based delivery platform, microparticle-based delivery platform, and liposomal delivery platform. Recommendations for future applications and research directions are provided.

1 INTRODUCTION

Vaccination is one of the most successful public health measures for preventing the spread of deadly illnesses and saving countless lives. Traditionally, vaccines have been administered by injection, which comes with certain drawbacks such as the need for trained medical personnel, concerns about needle use, and logistical difficulties. The emergence of oral vaccines in recent years is a ground-breaking approach with the potential to revolutionize vaccination strategies.

Designing an oral vaccine administration system is essential to addressing the myriad issues posed by the gastrointestinal tract. The stability and effectiveness of vaccinations are significantly hampered by the acidic environment in the stomach. Additionally, the presence of digestive enzymes and bile salts can degrade the vaccine antigens, reducing their immunogenicity (Zhu and Berzofsky 2013). To overcome these challenges, researchers have developed innovative strategies to protect the vaccine antigens during their journey through the digestive system. One approach involves encapsulating the antigens within biocompatible materials, such as nanoparticles or liposomes, which can shield them from the harsh gastric environment (Durán-Lobato *et al.* 2020). These protective carriers also facilitate the controlled release of the antigens, ensuring optimal exposure to the immune cells in the gut. Moreover, the oral vaccine delivery platform must also consider the immune barrier posed by the intestinal mucosa. The mucosal immune system plays a crucial role in preventing pathogen invasion and initiating immunological reactions. Therefore, boosting the immunological response at this location is crucial. This can be achieved by incorporating adjuvants or immunomodulatory agents into the vaccine formulation, which can activate and stimulate the mucosal immune cells, leading to a robust and long-lasting immune response. Furthermore, the design of an effective oral vaccine delivery platform should consider factors such as stability, scalability, cost-effectiveness, and ease of administration. It should be able to withstand storage conditions and transportation without compromising vaccine integrity. Additionally, it should be scalable for large-scale production to meet global

DOI: 10.1201/9781003587590-55

vaccination demands. Moreover, a user-friendly administration method should be employed to ensure widespread acceptance and accessibility.

This study provides an overview of oral vaccinations, their benefits over conventional injectable vaccines, and the present difficulties in developing and implementing them. By exploring the developments in oral vaccine technology and comprehending the challenges to overcome, we can pave the way for a new era of immunization that is more widely available, convenient, and effective.

2 DIFFERENT TYPES OF VACCINATION AND ANTIGENS OF VACCINE

2.1 *Traditional vaccination*

Traditional vaccination has been a pivotal tool for disease prevention and control throughout history. By harnessing the power of the immune system, traditional vaccines have successfully protected individuals and communities from a wide range of infectious diseases.

The foundation of traditional vaccines lies in the administration of antigens, which are substances that can trigger an immune response. These antigens can be derived from various sources, including weakened or inactivated forms of pathogens, as well as their components, such as proteins or polysaccharides (Wang *et al.* 2015). These antigens prompt the immune system to identify and initiate an attack against particular infections when they are introduced into the body.

The immune response initiated by traditional vaccines involves several key steps. First, antigen-presenting cells, such as dendritic cells, seize and undergo the processing of antigens. These cells then present the processed antigens to T cells, which are specialized immune cells responsible for coordinating immune responses. This interaction between antigen-presenting cells and T cells initiates a series of events that stimulate the generation of antibodies by B cells and the activation of cytotoxic T cells (Chaplin 2010).

Antibodies play a crucial role in traditional vaccination by binding to pathogens and neutralizing their harmful effects (Bordeaux *et al.* 2010). These cells have the ability to hinder the entry of pathogens into host cells or designate them for elimination by other constituents of the immune system. At the same time, cytotoxic T cells identify and eradicate infected host cells, guaranteeing that the infection is confined and eradicated.

The protective immunity induced by traditional vaccines is characterized by memory immune responses. Following exposure to an antigen, the immune system establishes immunological memory, enabling a quicker and more efficient response during subsequent encounters with the same pathogen. This ability to retain information about previously encountered pathogens forms the basis for long-term protection against infectious diseases.

Traditional vaccination primarily involves injecting the vaccine into the body using a needle. These vaccines contain inactivated or attenuated strains of disease-causing organisms, which act as antigens to stimulate the immune system and provide long-term immunity (Deal and Balazs 2015).

2.2 *Oral vaccination*

Oral vaccination involves administering the vaccine orally, typically in the form of drops or tablets. The vaccine contains live, weakened strains of the pathogen or specific components of it. Moreover, in addition to stimulating the immune system to produce a systemic immune response, oral vaccination can also induce the secretion of protective antigen-specific IgA (sIgA) in the intestinal mucosa, directly preventing the invasion of pathogens (Zhang *et al.* 2021).

2.3 *Antigens of vaccine*

The main components of vaccines are antigens, which are utilized to create immunological memories unique to certain antigens. At present, different categories of antigens exist, which comprise: (1) inactivated pathogens or combinations thereof; (2) live organisms that are weakened; (3) vector-based recombinant vaccines; and (4) subunit vaccines comprising genetic materials like DNA and RNA, as well as isolated or recombinant proteins, glycoproteins, and carbohydrates. Most of the vaccines currently on the market primarily belong to the first and second categories, which involve the inclusion of genetic materials from pathogens. However, there are a few exceptions where protein-based subunits such as virus-like particles, detoxified toxoids/toxins, and polysaccharide-protein conjugates are employed (Wang *et al.* 2015). As a new type of antigen, recombinant protein has some advantages. For instance, recombinant protein technology is well-developed and capable of producing sufficient quantities of the target protein. Moreover, unlike live viruses, recombinant proteins are non-replicating and are characterized by the absence of any infectious components found even in attenuated viral particles (Pollet, Chen, and Strych 2021). In general, recombinant proteins alone tend to generate a relatively weak immune response unless they are combined and arranged into large-size particles (Soler and Houdebine 2007). Thus, it is important to design a proper adjuvant to enhance the immune response of oral vaccines.

3 ADVANTAGES AND CHALLENGES OF ORAL VACCINES

3.1 *Advantages of oral vaccines*

As discussed above, a large volume of published studies demonstrates that oral vaccines offer several advantages compared to traditional vaccines:

(1) **Better compliance**: Needle-free vaccination enhances patient compliance, especially among children and individuals with a fear of needles, due to its painless administration.
(2) **Ease of administration**: Oral vaccines offer a non-invasive and needle-free method of vaccine delivery, reducing the reliance on medical professionals. This accessibility is particularly beneficial for people in resource-poor areas, such as developing countries and remote areas.
(3) **Stronger immune response**: In addition to providing systemic immunity like that of traditional vaccinations, oral vaccinations can stimulate the intestinal mucosa to secrete antigen-specific secretory IgA (sIgA), which offers immediate protection against pathogens. This helps to prevent infections that primarily enter through these routes, such as rotavirus or poliovirus (Davitt and Lavelle 2015).
(4) **Lower cost**: Many oral vaccines do not need stringent storage and transportation conditions. In contrast, some injectable vaccines require refrigeration or cold chain storage during transportation and distribution, driving up vaccination costs (Zhang *et al.* 2021).
(5) **Less risk of needlestick injuries**: Needlestick injuries present as a serious occupational hazard faced by healthcare workers. As a needle-free vaccination approach, oral vaccines can reduce the risk of infections caused by injections, making them safer for both recipients and healthcare providers involved in administering them (Koh 2010).

Overall, oral vaccines possess various advantages compared to traditional injectable vaccines.

3.2 *Challenges of oral vaccine*

Despite the attractive features of oral vaccines mentioned above, the number of approved oral vaccines is limited due to several challenges.

The immunological barrier is one of the most important aspects of antigen delivery. Key barriers to oral vaccines include degradation of acids and enzymes, diffusion layer of mucus, immune tolerance, and epithelial absorption barrier (Zang *et al.* 2021). The gastrointestinal tract provides a pH gradient to withstand exogenous pathogens, with pH levels ranging from about 1.5–3.5 in the stomach to about 5.5–6.9 in the small intestine and about 7.0 in the large intestine (Zhu and Berzofsky 2013). The pH gradient can dissolve the antigen chemically. In addition to the acid degradation, there are various enzymes in the gastrointestinal tract that can decompose the biomolecules, such as proteins, carbohydrates, and lipids.

Once the oral vaccine survives the acidic and enzymatic degradation, it must confront the mucosal immune system, which determines whether the antigen is harmful or innocuous. The well-trained gastrointestinal mucosal system prevents the passage of vaccines, as large particles can be blocked by the mesh structure of the mucosal membrane (Cone 2009). Mucus has a relatively intricate chemical composition, characterized by a highly negative surface and abundant hydrophobic groups that create a barrier that is difficult to penetrate (Thakur and Foged 2020), which is another challenge of vaccine delivery. Mucus, a viscoelastic gel, consists of mucins, antibodies, cellular waste, inorganic ions, and water. The viscoelastic properties of mucus are primarily governed by its macromolecular constituent, which is the mucin (Ensign *et al.* 2012).

Additionally, oral vaccines may require specific adjuvants (additives incorporated into vaccines to augment the immune response) that can activate the immune system without causing adverse effects or interfering with the vaccine's stability or delivery mechanisms (Ou *et al.* 2023).

Furthermore, the safety of vaccines, particularly oral vaccines, is a crucial aspect that requires careful consideration. The materials used in the production of oral vaccines should not pose any harmful side effects or adverse reactions. This is particularly important as these vaccines are directly ingested and enter the gastrointestinal tract. Ensuring the safety of oral vaccines is paramount to protecting individuals from any potential harm or negative health consequences.

In summary, there are several key considerations when it comes to oral vaccines. First, the acidic environment of the gastrointestinal tract can pose a challenge in maintaining the stability and effectiveness of the vaccine. Second, the mucosal immune system plays a crucial role in defending against pathogens that enter through the mucous membranes. Finally, the materials used in oral vaccines must be carefully selected to ensure they are harmless to the human body. Addressing these issues is vital in developing safe and effective oral vaccines that can provide optimal protection against infectious diseases while minimizing potential risks to individuals' health.

4 ADVANCED DELIVERY PLATFORM OF ORAL VACCINES

4.1 *Oral vaccine delivery platforms*

Given the diverse immunological responses, various platforms have been developed to enhance oral vaccination delivery. While some platforms utilize live carriers, most focus on non-living particles, which are the primary focus of this study.

4.2 *Types of oral vaccine delivery platforms*

4.2.1 *Acid-resistant biomaterials delivery platform*

Most studies aimed at enhancing immunity through oral vaccination have focused on improving poor gastrointestinal stability. Consequently, acid-resistant biomaterials are essential components of the oral delivery process. Benn *et al.* (2020), in their research about an oral anthrax microencapsulated vaccine, found that when Sterne spore stability at different pH levels was examined in vitro, it was discovered that the production of an oral vaccination must prioritize safeguarding against the stomach environment since spore exposure to pH 2 causes spore death. To protect the Sterne spores, they coated them with alginate and found that this effectively improved acid resistance. The result shows that alginate microcapsules, as an acid-resistant biomaterial, likely provided essential protection for spores to survive in the stomach environment.

4.2.2 *Nanoparticle-based delivery platform*

Nanotechnology facilitates the modification of the solubility, stability, and surface characteristics of vaccine antigens or adjuvants. Recently, there has been significant interest in nanotechnology-based oral vaccines.

The advantages of nanoparticles compared to other methods include (1) the improvement of antigen presentation and processing; (2) higher concentration of mucosal antigen; (3) localized and targeted delivery of antigen; and (4) better bioavailability (Thakur and Foed 2020).

4.2.3 *Microparticle-based delivery platform*

Microparticle-based oral vaccine delivery platforms are an innovative approach to enhance the efficacy and convenience of vaccine administration. Smet et al. (2013) utilized β-glucan particle (GP)-antigen microparticles as the model antigènes and conduites an oral GP-ovalbumin experiment. The results showed that the GP-antigen microparticles are highly efficient and are effectively internalized by the intestinal epithelial–mucosal interface, suggesting that microparticles could serve as an effective delivery platform for oral vaccines.

4.2.4 *Liposomal delivery platform*

Liposomes and their derivatives are hollow spherical vesicles with one or more lipid bilayers. Hydrophobic medications travel to the lipid bilayer, while hydrophilic drugs can be absorbed by the liposomes in the water-filled core along with antigens, DNA, and RNA (Kang *et al.* 2018). Several benefits of the liposomal delivery technology include antigen/immunomodulator protection, good biocompatibility, and minimal immunogenicity (Irvine *et al.* 2015). Ma *et al.* (2014) used PLGA (poly D, L-lactide-co-glycolide) coupled with lipid nanoparticles as the delivery platform able to controllably release the model antigen ovalbumin, which is trapped while preventing exposure to the gastrointestinal tract. The results indicate that the monophosphoryl lipid A-containing M-cell targeted lipid nanoparticles have the potential to be a reliable oral vaccination delivery strategy for all populations.

5 CONCLUSION

This article emphasizes the significant challenges involved in formulating and stabilizing oral vaccinations. A crucial barrier is the acidic environment of the stomach, which can lead to the breakdown of the vaccine before it reaches its target site. Additionally, the susceptibility of the vaccination is further increased by the presence of numerous digestive enzymes. Another obstacle is the well-trained gastrointestinal mucosal system, which serves as a robust immune barrier, preventing the entry of exogenous substances such as vaccines. The mucosal system is designed to recognize and eliminate foreign agents, making it difficult for oral vaccines to penetrate and elicit an immune response.

Furthermore, the majority of oral vaccinations for humans are still in the experimental stage rather than being tested in clinical research phases. This indicates a lack of sufficient data regarding their safety and efficacy in humans. The experimental nature of these vaccines underscores the need for more research and development before they can be widely implemented.

Despite these challenges, recombinant protein-based and nucleic acid oral vaccines hold research value. However, a significant issue is the weak immune response. To enhance the immune reaction, the mucosal adjuvants provide a potential way to increase the effectiveness of oral vaccinations without introducing oral tolerance (Deal and Balazs 2015). At present, there are three main types of adjuvants utilized to stimulate immune responses at mucosal sites: cytokines, Toll-like receptor agonists, and toxins. However, most of them are not suitable for human oral vaccine delivery, posing a substantial challenge for researchers to develop new adjuvants that can enhance the efficiency of oral vaccines.

Additionally, many mechanisms involved in oral delivery and gastrointestinal immune barriers remain poorly understood. Investigating these complex mechanisms presents a meaningful research direction to figure out complex mechanisms.

Regulatory organizations such as the Food and Drug Administration and the World Health Organization enforce stringent safety and efficacy standards for oral vaccinations. Numerous preclinical and clinical studies are carried out to evaluate their immunogenicity, safety profile, and ability to prevent illness. These studies often entail extensive trials across diverse populations to ensure the vaccine's effectiveness in various age groups and geographic locations, which may prolong the timeline for researchers to develop new vaccines for the disease.

REFERENCES

Benn J. S., Chaki S. P., Xu Y., Ficht T. A., Rice-Ficht A. C. and Cook W. E., (2020). *npj Vaccines*, **5**, 1.

Bordeaux J., Welsh A.W., Agarwal S., Killiam E., Baquero M.T., Hanna J.A., Anagnostou V.K. and Rimm D.L., (2010). *Biotechniques*,**48** 3.

Chaplin D.D., (2010). *Journal of Allergy and Clinical Immunology*, **125** 2.

Cone R.A., (2009). *Advanced drug delivery reviews*,**61** 2.

Davitt C. J. and Lavelle E. C., (2015). *Advanced Drug Delivery Reviews*,**91**.

De Smet R., Demoor T., Verschuere S., Dullaers M., Ostroff G.R., Leclercq G., Allais L., Pilette C., Dierendonck M. and De Geest B.G., (2013). *Journal of Controlled Release*, **172**,3.

Deal C.E. and Balazs A.B., (2015). *Current Opinion in Immunology*, **35**.

Durán-Lobato M., Niu Z. and Alonso M. J., (2020). *Advanced Materials*, **32**, 13.

Ensign L.M., Cone R. and Hanes J., (2012). *Advanced drug delivery reviews*, **64**, 6.

Irvine D. J., Hanson M. C., Rakhra K. and Tokatlian T., (2015). *Chemical Reviews*,**115** 19.

Kang S. H., Hong S. J., Lee Y.-K. and Cho S. (2018). Polymers,**1**, 9

Koh A., (2010). *Masui The Japanese Journal of Anesthesiology*, **59** 1.

Ma T., Wang L., Yang T., Ma G. and Wang S. (2014). *International Journal of Pharmaceutics*, **473** 1–2.

Ou B., Yang Y., Lv H., Lin X. and Zhang M., (2023). *BioDrugs*, **37**, 2.

Pollet J., Chen W.-H. and Strych U. (2021). *Advanced Drug Delivery Reviews*,**170**.

Soler E. and Houdebine L.-M., (2007). *Biotechnology Annual Review*,**13**.

Thakur A. and Foged C., (2020). Nanoparticles for mucosal vaccine delivery, Nanoengineered biomaterials for advanced drug delivery, *Elsevier*, pp. 603–646.

Wang S., Liu H., Zhang X. and Qian F., (2015). *Protein & Cell*, **6**, 7.

Zhang Y., Li M., Du G., Chen X. and Sun X., (2021). *Advanced Drug Delivery Reviews*, **177**.

Zhu Q. and Berzofsky J. A., (2013). *Gut Microbes*,**4**, 3

Biological Sciences and Environmental Health – Gao (Ed.)
© 2025 the Author(s), ISBN: 978-1-032-96016-6

Research progress on melatonin inhibiting the growth and spread of breast cancer cells

Yihan Bai
Nanjing Foreign Language School, Nanjing, China

Zijie Shen
School of Laboratory Medicine and Life Science, Wenzhou Medical University, Wenzhou, China

Ke Yang
Tianjin Wuqing Yinghua Experimental School, Tianjin, China

ABSTRACT: Of all the malignant tumors, breast cancer (BC) is a commonly occurring type of cancer among women and poses an important threat to women's health. In recent years, melatonin, as a hormone naturally produced by the pineal gland, has been widely used to treat sleep disorders and regulate the biological clock. At the same time, studies have shown that melatonin has an obstruction to the expansion and spread of malignant tumor cells such as breast cancer. Here is a review, it first highlighted the dangers of malignant breast cancer, explained the function of melatonin and the mechanism of inhibiting the development and spread of BC, and finally discussed the combined effects of the different drugs and melatonin. This article aims to provide a brief overview of how melatonin inhibits the growth of breast cancer cells and the potential treatment options associated with it. Although it has begun to take shape, there are still deficiencies and unexplained places, such as the specific mechanism of affecting cancer cells, etc., which need to be further studied.

1 INTRODUCTION

Breast cancer (BC) is one of the most common cancers among women worldwide and also it is responsible for the highest number of cancer-related deaths in. The survival rates for breast cancer vary significantly across different regions, withs developed countries reporting a 5-year survival rate of around 80%, while developing countries report less than 40% (Coleman 2008). In the US, approximately1 in 8 women are affected by breast cancer, while in Asia, the prevalence is lower at 1 in 35 women. In Iran, 10 cases per 100,000 population, 7,000 new cases are reported each year (Haghighat 2012).

However, the cause of BC is still unclear, and there are some differences and connections between different subtypes. It is a tricky disease. At present, there are many treatment methods, such as chemotherapy, targeted therapy, surgery, etc., but the prognosis is often poor, with high recurrence rate and a significant decline in the life quality. The search for alternatives to BC treatments is often driven by the desire to reduce the unpleasant side effects associated with these treatments.

The pineal gland excretes the meth-oxy indole melatonin (N-acetyl-5-methoxytryptamine) during night. Melatonin has been shown to have a wide range of beneficial benefits, including those on sleep, immunity, antioxidants, and wound healing. Melatonin is a mammalian hormone that has been shown to target a wide range of molecules and signaling pathways, including angiogenesis, remodeling of the extracellular matrix, migration, and

DOI: 10.1201/9781003587590-56

epithelial-to-mesenchymal transition (EMT), in many cancer types, including breast cancer (Talib 2021). In animal models containing human breast cancer xenografts, melatonin administration throughout the daytime controlled plasma metabolites, which in turn reduced the aggressiveness of breast cancer at an early stage (Junior 2022).

Therefore, melatonin has been shown to inhibit breast cancer cells in recent years, and this article will also elaborate some specific mechanisms and the benefits of combined treatment with other drugs.

2 THE HARM OF MALIGNANT BREAST CANCER

Worldwide, approximately 2 million people were diagnosed with breast cancer worldwide in 2018, about 46 out of every 100,000 people developed breast cancer (Huang 2021). According to statistics, the continents with the highest incidence are Australia, Europe, America and Western countries and developed countries, as well as countries with high HDI (Huang 2021). Timely detection of the illness can result in a favorable outlook and a significant chance of survival.

Meanwhile, breast cancer is divided into the invasive breast cancer and the non-invasive breast cancer. At the same time, there are many subtypes of breast cancer, which are more or less insensitive to chemotherapy drugs, targeted therapy, and conventional therapy, so they cannot achieve the expected effect (Hallett 2012). As an instance, for individuals diagnosed with triple-negative breast cancer, the examination outcomes indicate breast tumors that lack estrogen receptor (ER), progesterone receptor (PR), and the Her-2 proto-oncogene. Their prognosis is generally poor, with more than 50% of patients relapsing within the first 3 to 5 years after diagnosis (Hallett 2012).

In addition, breast cancer has a profound impact on society. From the perspective of patients' families, according to the survey, almost 99% of patients have the support of their families, while about 43% of patients are forced to accept an unfair fate (Alexander 2019). At the same time, financial burden is the primary concern of patients' families. About 57 percent of patients were able to raise the full cost and receive treatment, 30 percent had to sell their assets to fund their own treatment, and 3 percent were unable to get treatment due to lack of financial support (Alexander 2019). Among patients but also among breast cancer survivors, they take their health more seriously than they did before the disease and have regular checkups. According to the survey, most breast cancer patients are socially affected, the hair loss from cancer treatment makes them feel embarrassed, and the pain caused by the treatment makes them emotionally uncontrollable (Alexander 2019). Therefore, breast cancer is not only harmful to the patient's body, but also affects the patient's mind and family.

3 THE FUNCTION OF MELATONIN

Melatonin usually plays a role in sleep, immunity, and scavenging free radicals. One of the most common effects of melatonin is to affect sleep. It promotes night sleep, and controls the body's wake up during the day. Some studies indicate that, Plasma melatonin is essentially an intrinsic circadian rhythm with a single peak, which peaks at night. Furthermore, darkness does not directly cause the melatonin production, in fact, the increase of plasma melatonin at night is related to circadian rhythm (Qian 2022). Melatonin's powerful anti-inflammatory and analgesic properties are due to its specific binding to G protein-coupled receptors. For the expressing location, CNS and peripheral organs are the most commonly used expressed region of these receptors (Pivonello 2022). In addition, TLR may be related to melatonin circadian rhythm. TLR is a protein that cells recognize, of which TLR9 belongs to a receptor of the innate immune system. The daily changes of TLR9 can regulate the auxiliary immunity of ODN, so melatonin's circadian rhythm is closely related to the circadian rhythm regulation of innate immunity (Pivonello 2022). Melatonin affects the scavenging of free radicals, thanks to the direct antioxidant capacity of melatonin. Melatonin's antioxidant properties are due to its high lipophilic properties and its ability to penetrate organic membranes. In addition, melatonin can also promote the activity and expression of antioxidant enzymes, promote enzyme antioxidant. Most of the free radicals are reactive oxygen species and active nitrogen, which have the ability to oxidize and destroy bystander molecules (Fischer 2008).

4 MECHANISM AND EFFECT OF MELATONIN

4.1 *Molecular mechanisms*

Melatonin reduces the development and proliferation of breast cancer cells through a number of mechanisms. (as shown in Figure 1, original).

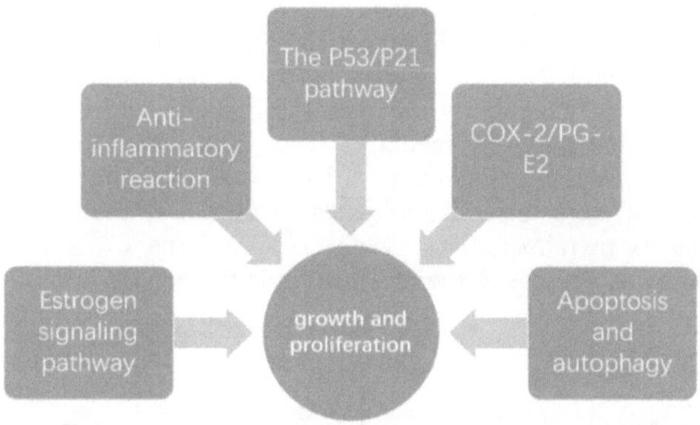

Figure 1. Melatonin inhibits the growth and proliferation of breast cancer cells in multiple way (Original).

4.1.1 *Estrogen signaling pathway*

The estrogen signaling pathway is generally considered to have two pathways: "nuclear-initiated steroid signaling" and "membrane-initiated steroid signaling". In the first pathway, the ER binds to estrogen in the first pathway, moving to the nucleus where it binds to the DNA on ERE sites and triggers the production of the ERE-dependent genes. Estrogens may operate via a new G protein-coupled E2 receptor (GPER) or a subset of ER (mER) on the plasma membrane in the "membrane" route. After these receptors are active, numerous signaling pathways (such as Ca2+, cAMP, and protein kinase cascade) are quickly activated, which in turn affects downstream transcription factors (Hill 2011). Melatonin inhibits the growth of BC cells mainly through acting on molecules involved in the estrogen signaling pathway.

The prevailing consensus is that melatonin can reduce the body's circulating levels of gonadal steroids and so block the systemic effects of estrogen (Sanchez-Barcelo 2012). In addition, melatonin can also interact with Erα, and ERα positivity is often used as a marker for the BC diagnosis; in ER-positive human BC cells, melatonin induces G protein through melatonin receptor 1 (MT1) Signal activation and reduction of cAMP levels inhibit ERα expression of ERα mRNA and estrogen-induced transcriptional activity (Hill 2011). In order to control the estrogen signaling pathway, melatonin also reduces the activity of the several enzymes, including aromatase and soon. By reducing the expression of aromatase mRNA, melatonin can enhance the inhibitory effect of aminoglutathiamine on aromatase activity in BC cells (Martinez-Campa 2005).

4.1.2 *Anti-inflammatory reaction*

Tumor incidence and numbers of the pro- and anti-inflammatory cytokines are strongly connected. The gene expression of pro-inflammatory cytokines is higher in BC cells, and some inflammatory markers also promote the growth of cells (Samanta 2022). IL-6 is an inflammatory response promoter and takes part in the body's immunological response. In addition to promoting the proliferation of breast cancer cells, IL-8 can increase the differentiation of neutrophils, T lymphocytes, and eosinophils. TNF- stimulates the proliferation of breast tumor cells via the NF-B-dependent pathway and is the earliest and most significant inflammatory mediator in the inflammatory response. Melatonin has an anti-inflammatory effect by reducing the expression of anti-adipokine and desmoplastic response, which in turn reduces the production of these inflammatory markers (Amin 2019).

4.1.3 *The P53/P21 pathway inhibits proliferation*

The P53/P21 pathway plays a huge role on the G1 checkpoint of the cell cycle. Cells containing unrepaired damaged DNA cannot pass this checkpoint. Melatonin's ability to inhibit the growth of MCF-7 cell lines mainly relies on the P53/P21 pathway to control the G1-S phase transition, which is ultimately mediated through the TGF-β pathway. The TNF-β pathway is an important regulatory pathway for breast cancer tumorigenesis. TNF-β upregulates the expression of metastasis-related genes, promotes epithelial-mesenchymal transition, and stimulates its own expression. After blocking the G1-S phase transition, the expression of this pathway decreases, thereby inhibiting the proliferation of BC cells (Proietti 2014).

4.1.4 *COX-2/PG-E2*

Cyclooxygenase 2 (COX-2) mediates arachidonic acid to produce PGs and thromboxane; Prostaglandin E2 (PG-E2), through its receptor and the COX-2 pathway, is a tumor promoter. Proliferation, apoptosis, and angiogenesis of cancer cells all entail different signaling pathways (Wang 2012). Melatonin can inhibit the growth and spread of BC cells through two pathways. One is by reducing the activity of p300 histone acetyltransferase to inhibit the coupling of p300 and COX-2 promoting factors; the other is by interfering with NF-κB binding by inhibiting p300-mediated NF-κB acetylation. Both pathways ultimately lead to a reduction in PG-E2 synthesis (Wang 2012).

4.1.5 *Apoptosis and autophagy*

Apoptosis is a normal cell death pathway, which is the formation of apoptotic bodies by the invagination of the cell membrane and is triggered by the Caspase pathway (Samanta 2022). Bcl-2 and Bax proteins are the main regulators of the apoptosis. Through a mitochondria-dependent process, the ratio of the proteins Bax and Bcl2 controls the start of apoptosis. Breast cancer cells that have been exposed to melatonin in the early stages of the process do not rely on proteases and instead primarily activate the Apaf-1-dependent apoptotic pathway. In postapoptotic period, cytochrome C is released, activating Caspase-3 and Caspase-9, and at the same time, the Bcl-2/Bax ratio is downregulated (Bagheri 2020).

Autophagy is a cellular emergency mechanism in which autophagic vacuoles fuse with lysosomes to digest their contents and are triggered by the mTOR pathway. Recent studies have found that melatonin can also induce autophagy to eliminate breast cancer cells. It induces autophagy in the MCF-7 and MDA-MB-231 cell lines by increasing the expression of Beclin-1, LC3, and p62 (Onder 2022).

4.2 *Combined chemotherapy effect*

Chemotherapy will bring many negative effects to breast cancer patients. Free radicals generated by ionizing radiation can cause DNA damage and even cell necrosis. A series of emergency reactions may also lead to the suppression of cellular antioxidant defenses, leading to more oxidative stress, DNA breakage, and cell death. A study involving ten men and women with breast cancer showed that MLT enhanced the effect of chemotherapy regardless of tumor type and chemotherapy regimen (Gurunathan,2021). The levels utilized in randomized controlled studies have shown that when the dosage used is 10-20 mg/day, melatonin is helpful at lowering chemotherapy-induced toxicity and when 20 mg/day, it improve the tumor regression; however, additional study is needed to establish the most suitable dose for human use (Ramos 2023). Studies have also found that 18 mg/day of melatonin intervention in BC patients during chemotherapy can reduce fatigue related to the malignant disease and its treatment.

4.2.1 *Chemoprotectant*

Melatonin can be used as a chemoprotective agent, directly scavenging free radicals such as reactive the oxygen species, or inhibiting the activity of ROS-producing enzymes, thereby preventing excessive DNA damage (Sanchez-Barcelo 2012). At the same time, studies have shown that melatonin can alleviate the toxic effects of IR by regulating DNA damage response, thereby reducing cell death. Melatonin has the ability to change genes implicated in apoptosis in addition to regulating DNA repair, with overexpression of Bax and down-regulation of Bcl-2 favoring apoptosis. An essential signaling mechanism involved in the release of IL-1 and inflammatory mediators during radiation is the NF-B/ NLRP3 inflammasome pathway. Numerous investigations on animals have demonstrated that melatonin inhibits this pathway to reduce inflammatory reactions (Amin 2019).

4.2.2 *Chemosensitizer*

On the other hand, melatonin can also act as a chemotherapy sensitizer. Melatonin and chemotherapy can have a synergistic effect to further inhibit the proliferation and metastasis of BC cells (Samanta 2022). Studies proved that melatonin may reduce DNA repair in BC cells, change the energy supply form of cells from glycolysis-dependent to oxidative phosphorylation-dependent, so that to make BC cells more resistant to chemotherapy by synthesizing estrogen. sensitive. At the same time, under the radiation exposure of chemotherapy, melatonin can also promote the occurrence of the P53 pathway and induce accelerated apoptosis of tumor cells (Amin 2019).

5 COMBINED ACTION OF DIFFERENT DRUGS WITH MELATONIN

Melatonin, being a hormone naturally produced by the body, has various functions such as regulating the body's circadian rhythm, controlling the endocrine system, and modulating the immune system.Therefore, it will also affect the occurrence, development, and managing breast cancer cells. A study involving ten men and women with breast cancer showed that MLT enhanced the effect of chemotherapy regardless of tumor type and chemotherapy regimen (Gurunathan 2021). MLT can inhibit the pituitary-ovarian axis in combination with the synthetic progesterone norethindrone, thereby reducing LH levels and at the same time inhibiting the development of cancer cells and the risk of recurrence.

Rewritten: Research has indicated that the combined use of melatonin and paclitaxel not only hinders the metastasis of breast cancer, but also amplifies the antiproliferative and apoptotic reactions of low-dose paclitaxel towards cancerous cells, as well as modifies the gene expression patterns (Gurunathan 2021). Paclitaxel modulates multiple genes and melatonin counteracts these modulations. Melatonin stimulates the expression of pro-apoptotic genes and enhances paclitaxel-induced repression of anti-apoptotic genes.None of the above have provided rigorous clinical trial data. Through the use of breast cancer cell cultures and treatment techniques, a separate study discovered that the simultaneous application of melatonin and ligand 2-(3,5-diphenylpyrazol-1-yl)-2-thiazoline (DPhPzTn), referred to as PtDPhPzTn, to Triple-negative breast cancer (TNBC) cells notably intensified apoptosis and enhanced the anti-migration effects in comparison to the effects of PtDPhPzTn alone (Estirado 2022). demonstrated that these two substances can exert powerful effects when synergistically treating breast cancer.However, relevant data from some clinical trials are still lacking.

6 CONCLUSION

This article illustrates the heterogeneous biology and complexity of macromolecular of breast cancer, which make significant advances in prevention and diagnosis while complicating treatment. Its development involves multiple molecules and distinct signaling pathways, as well as genetics, inflammation, apoptosis, etc. Most of researches suggest that multiple molecular mechanisms of melatonin can ensure the inhibition of tumor occurrence, progression and metastasis. Since melatonin has multiple potential characteristics, including anti-inflammatory, oxidation resistance, and apoptosis induction, it is recognized as a potential therapeutic drug for cancers such as breast cancer. Furthermore, the synergistic effect of melatonin with other anticancer therapies weakens each other's side effects. Therefore, someone predict melatonin will be a promising drug. However, at present, Melatonin acts on breast cancer, and promotes autophagy of breast cancer cells and reduces various inflammatory responses remain to be studied. It is hoped that in the future, there will be more complete results and treatments.

AUTHORS CONTRIBUTION

All the authors contributed equally and their names were listed in alphabetical order.

REFERENCES

Alexander A. (2019). *Indian J Palliat Care.***25**, 66–72 .

Amin N. (2019). *J Cell Biochem.***120**,12208–12215.

Bagheri M. (2020). *Fundam Clin Pharmacol.***34**,51–64

Coleman P. (2008). *Lancet Oncol.* **9**,730–56.

Estirado S. (2022). *Antioxidants (Basel).***11**.

Fischer T. W. (2008). *Exp Dermatol.* **17**,713–30.

Gurunathan S. (2021). *Onco Targets Ther.* **14**,2019–2052.

Haghighat S. (2012). *Asian Pac J Cancer Prev.* **13**, 5525–8.

Hallett R. M. (2012). *Sci Rep.* **2**,227.

Hill S. M. (2011). *J Mammary Gland Biol Neoplasia.* **16**,235–45.

Huang J. (2021). *Aging (Albany NY)* **13**, 5748–5803.

Junior R.P. (2022). *Int J Mol Sci.* **23**.

Martinez-Campa C. (2005). *Breast Cancer Res Treat* **94**,249–54.

Onder G. O. (2022). *Fundam Clin Pharmacol* **36**,1038–1056.

Pivonello C. (2022). *Obes Rev* **23**,e13390.

Proietti S. (2014). *J Pineal Res.* **57**,120–9

Qian J. (2022). *J Pineal Res.* **72**,e12791.

Ramos E. (2023). *Pharmaceutics.* **15**.

Samanta S. (2022). *J Environ Pathol Toxicol Oncol.* **41**,55–84.

Sanchez-Barcelo E. J. (2012). *Recent Pat Endocr Metab Immune Drug Discov.* **6**,108–16.

Talib W.H. (2021). *Molecules.* **26**.

Wang J. (2012). *J Pineal Res.* **53**,77–90.

Biological Sciences and Environmental Health – Gao (Ed.)

The sky roses never fall—based on the investigation of various common occupational diseases in female flight attendants

Huasong Wang
School of Safety Engineering, North China of Science and Technology, Yanjiao East of Beijing, China

ABSTRACT: Civil aviation air crews are an important part of civil aviation staffs, and also one of the important positions in the field of civil aviation in China, shouldering the responsibility of cabin security and passenger service. Due to the long-term standing work, with irregular work and rest, and working for a long time, flight attendants are affected by various kinds of occupational diseases that are more serious compared to other occupations. Most of the flight attendants in China are young women. When they get older, the negative effects of these occupational diseases in women will affect their pregnancy preparation and family life in a later stage, which is not conducive to the healthy life and family harmony of the employees of civil aviation enterprises, and thus affect the normal safe production orders of the company. Therefore, ensuring the occupational health of female crew is an important measure to indirectly guarantee the safety of civil aviation passenger transport.

1 INTRODUCTION

Civil aviation industry is an important part of China's transportation industry, shouldering the important task of national transportation power and regional personnel exchange (Yu and Yao 2006). Civil aviation passenger transport is an important way of travelling for the middle- and high-class social groups in China, and also an important way of travelling for the heads of states to go out and for domestic inspection. As a kind of airline members in direct contact with passengers and providing services, flight attendants are an important part of the display window of airline impression and service, and are also a direct impression of the airline image. In some international flight cabins, the flight crew is just the image of China's civil aviation and airlines. Air crews belong to the kind of special types of work in the national labor post, and the job belongs to specific high-risk occupation. At the same time, in view of the historical development of the civil aviation industry and the service group class attribution, the civil aviation air crew for young women, whose average ages are between 20 and 35 years, flight attendant groups in the airline post distribution because of the nature of their work. Often in vulnerable groups, their labor rights cannot be protected (Tang 2014). At the same time, due to the average age of employment and gender issues, the flight attendants lack a voice in the workplace, and some flight attendants will experience unfair treatment and disrespect in the workplace, especially female attendants. As a high-risk occupation and a special type of work, the air crew itself is a high-incidence group of all kinds of common occupational diseases and especially occupational diseases in the air crews (Qiu 2015). However, due to the problems of the airline management system, the occupational health of female air crews may not be paid due attention, and the right to occupational health cannot be maintained. The occupational health and occupational disease of flight attendants have become a prominent labor protection problem in the field of civil aviation service, an important professional factor affecting the quality of civil aviation passenger transport service and a potential factor affecting the safety of civil aviation passenger transport in the future.

DOI: 10.1201/9781003587590-57

This paper will re-examine the occupational health and occupational diseases and will discuss the qualitative relationship between the occupational health of flight attendants and the civil aviation passenger safety. The government, the airline and the society should take some measures to ensure the safety of civil aviation female flight attendants.

2 A BASIC OVERVIEW OF THE POST STRUCTURE AND PROPORTION OF CIVIL AVIATION FLIGHT PERSONNEL IN CHINA

Under the current civil aviation transport system in China, the corresponding post structure of different airlines and air operators is different, and the structure of each airline is slightly different. In general, from the perspective of aircrafts, the crews of 330 and 787 (usually on the international route) are equipped with 1 pilot and 1–2 co-pilots for aircrafts with a duration less than 8 hours, plus a pilot for aircrafts of 8–10 hours, and aircrafts of more than 10 hours are generally equipped with a crew lounge on the plane and the crew has more than 3 pilots (Gao and Wang 2012). Flight attendants and the above configuration, according to the ratio of economy class passengers, less than 50 people as 50 people added to match. Taking the narrow-body 320 and 737 as an example, the crew has one captain, one co-pilot and three crew members (that is, one flight attendant for 50 additional passengers in the cabin).

The second is the basic situation that an aircraft should be equipped with crew numbers. The principle of the airline is that the staffs rest, but the planes still work, in order to maximize the economic benefits. CAAC has restrictions on the total flight time and individual flight time of the crew. The basic situation is that a pilot shall fly no more than 8 or 9 hours a day (depending on the ratio of the segment and the crew), not more than 60 hours a week, no more than 100 hours per month, and no more than 1000 hours a year; the crew shall fly no more than 80 hours a week, no more than 100 hours a month, and no more than 1100 hours a year. At the same time, it is stipulated that, for international flights, a time difference of more than 6 hours should be arranged for 48 hours. According to these provisions, an aircraft generally needs to have 1–2 crew members for domestic flights and 2 or more crew members for international flights. For the overall situation of air staffs, the proportion of airline staffs accounts for about 70%–80% of the total number of airline staffs, and the man–machine ratio of air staffs is about 80:1 (Song *et al.* 2014).

The above is the overall situation of the number of air staffs and posts of each airlines in China under the provisions of CAAC. On the whole, the General Administration of China has relatively perfect regulations on the safety flight time and crew configuration of civil aviation practitioners. The flight attendants of each airline company are obviously the backbone of the airline position. And according to the configuration of the flight crew members, the number of flight attendants is more than that of the flight attendants. The regulation of CAAC on the allocation of air crew members and the duration of flight work is an important guarantee to ensure the safety of civil aviation passenger transport in China. According to the statistical data, among the flight attendants in China, women are the main group. As the main body of the flight attendants, the occupational health problems, chronic occupational diseases and sequelae of the female flight attendants have become the key objects of research in the field of civil aviation safety and occupational health. The occupational health problems of female crew members (including the chief steward and ordinary flight attendants) are also directly related to the safety problems of civil aviation passenger transport. Solving the occupational health problems of female flight attendants is an important task to ensure the safe operation of airlines (Chen 2017).

3 REVIEW OF OCCUPATIONAL HEALTH PROBLEMS AND COMMON OCCUPATIONAL DISEASES IN FEMALE FLIGHT ATTENDANTS

According to the relevant data of the National Civil Aviation Administration and the National Health Commission, the common occupational health problems of female flight attendants include varicose veins of the lower limbs, hearing loss, stomach disease, reproductive system diseases, skin cancer, vascular diseases and so on (Qiu *et al.* 2014). The occupational health problems of young women are the main body of the occupational health problems of flight attendants. The following is a classified discussion of the various major occupational health problems and occupational diseases in female flight attendants.

3.1 *Varicosity*

Varicose veins refer to the venous osity and expansion due to blood stasis, a weak venous wall and other factors. Varicose veins can occur in many parts of the body; for example, hemorrhoids are actually a kind of varicose veins, and those that are clinically visible are esophageal and gastric fundus varices, varicocele, abdominal wall varices and so on. The most common site of varicose veins is the lower limbs. It is worth emphasizing that varicose veins are a secondary manifestation of other lesions (Gao and Chen 2011). The above is the etiology principle of varicose veins.

Considering the nature of their work, female flight attendants need to stand for a long time, resulting in insufficient venous blood supply to the lower limbs and thus causing varicose veins. In real life, varicose veins more commonly occur in people with occupations that require standing for a long time during working hours, such as teachers, nurses, car salesmen, flight attendants, etc. These occupations are mainly females. As the occupation of female flight attendants, it is naturally the high-incidence area of female varicose veins.

3.2 *Endocrine system disorders*

A healthy human body regulates its metabolic and physiological functions through various hormones and the nervous system in the endocrine system. The endocrine system is composed of endocrine glands, scattered endocrine cells and their hormones, involved in regulating the metabolism of the human body, growth and development, reproductive endowment, and many other physiological activities and life phenomena, together with various enzymes (biochemical enzymes) to maintain the relative stability of the body's environment and to adapt to the complex changes in vitro and those caused by external factors (Xia, Wang and Zhu 2013). Hormones are the information transmitters of the endocrine system, which is transmitted through the body fluid to the target cells to exert stimulating or inhibitory effects to regulate the function of the target cells. Normal hormones maintain balance through feedback regulation mechanisms, and if the balance is broken for some reasons (too much, too little or hormone resistance), it leads to endocrine disorders (endocrine dyscrasia). When a disorder occurs in the human endocrine system, there will be various signs, and especially in women, the symptoms are more obvious. Due to the presence of a large number of women in flight crews, endocrine disorders have become one of the most important factors affecting the work status. After the interview and investigation of a female crew aged 20–25 of an airline, it was reported that the work and rest were generally irregular due to flight shift, early sleep shortage, and flight check-in, which led to endocrine disorders in most of the employees during the physical examination (Lu 2014).

3.3 *Gastrosia*

Stomach disease is also one of the common occupational diseases in flight attendants due to the perennial flight scheduling problem, plane timing problems, etc. Considering the flight crews generally have no fixed time to eat and have to reduce the normal meal time due to work or miss the suitable time to eat because of the flight delay, long past will eventually lead to the occurrence of stomach diseases (Zeng 2013). Stomach disease is a common occupational disease caused by irregular diet, which has sequelae and will evolve into a lifelong disease. In a later stage, it will become an important occupational disease troubling the normal diet. Severe stomach ache will even affect high-quality sleep, and stomach diseases at a young age may lead to chronic gastric cancers in old ages.

3.4 *High-altitude radiation*

Because the flight area of civil aviation aircrafts is basically the stratosphere or the upper part of the troposphere, the high-altitude radiation is large, so the flight attendants directly face the occupational hazard of perennial exposure to high-altitude radiation exceeding the standard (Marsden and Green 2019). High-altitude radiation is generally difficult to contact with the ground occupation, so this kind of occupational disease is a unique type of occupational disease occurring in flight attendants.

3.5 *Multiple types of cancer*

A previous study found that flight attendants are prone to various types of occupational diseases, and the occupational diseases are generally serious. Compared with ordinary women, the probability of female flight attendants suffering from more common cancers of various young groups is significantly higher than that of ordinary women (Xu *et al.* 2003) (Harvard University study). These cancers include endometrial cancer, gastrointestinal cancer, thyroid cancer and cervical cancer, and female flight attendants are more likely to be affected than ordinary women of the same age group. The study showed that 3.4% of female flight attendants had breast cancer compared with 2.3% of women in the general population group, 2.2% had melanoma skin cancer compared to 0.98%, and 7.4% had non-melanoma skin cancer compared to 1.8%, and that those with a longer working time had higher rates of non-melanoma skin cancer. According to a study published by the American Medical Association in *JAMA Dermatology*, pilots and flight attendants are at a high risk of skin cancer, and melanoma is twice more common than in the general population.

3.6 *Infertility, miscarriage, preterm birth, and fetal abnormalities*

An association between working hours and infertility, miscarriage, preterm birth and fetal deformities was observed in female flight attendants in the Harvard Flight Health Study (FAHS). Another study showed an association of high abortion rates with circadian disturbances, exposure to cosmic ionizing radiation, and intense work in flight attendants (Liu *et al.* 2010).

3.7 *Occupational mechanical trauma*

Stewardesses are at risk of bone disease because they often lift weight, carry luggage and so on (Liu, Qiu and Liu 2021). When working in a confined space, the waist and hand muscles are prone to sprain. In addition, the turbulence into the atmosphere or the sudden movement of the plane is also the cause of frequent mechanical injuries to flight attendants.

3.8 *Fatigue, poor sleep quality, and mental health*

Related studies have found that flight attendants generally have insufficient rest because of flight scheduling, which leads to fatigue and reduced work efficiency. Continuous lack of rest can lead to poor psychological states of anxiety and depression. At the same time, the indirect nature of airline work culture leads to psychological work pressure, such as prolonged and irregular working hours, sexual harassment, insufficient support from bosses and dissatisfaction with work (Xue 2017).

This indicates that female flight attendants are prone to occupational diseases and common occupational health problems in the workplace and at work. Such occupational health problems and occupational diseases seriously affect the working status and physical and mental health of female flight attendants. From a macro point of view, such problems, which have plagued the female flight attendants for a long time, will indirectly affect the safety of civil aviation passenger transport, so it is urgent to solve these problems.

4 EXPLORING THE PREVENTION MECHANISM OF OCCUPATIONAL DISEASES IN FLIGHT ATTENDANTS FROM THE PERSPECTIVE OF OCCUPATIONAL HEALTH AND SAFETY

In view of all kinds of occupational diseases in female flight attendants, corresponding occupational health protection measures and occupational disease prevention mechanisms should be established. For occupational diseases in a certain type of work in a certain industry, it should be analyzed from macro to micro levels and the corresponding preventive measures and mechanisms should be established ranging from engineering technology through medical diets to legal norms.

4.1 *Macro policies and laws and regulations*

At the government level, CAAC has issued relevant laws and regulations to strictly protect the labor rights and interests of female air workers (Zhu 2008). Legislation and the legal system are the best way to protect the rights and interests of workers. At the airline level, each airline shall reasonably specify routes and scheduling planning according to the flight scheduling regulations and the number of crew attendants. At the same time, all airlines should rectify the corporate culture of the company, establish an internal protection mechanism for female flight attendants, create a good atmosphere of respect for female flight attendants within the company, and reduce the work pressure of women, especially young female flight attendants.

At the same time, corresponding monitoring measures should be established for the common and high incidence of mass occupational diseases, such as regular physical examination for international flight crew, and early detection and treatment of occupational health problems. In addition, a reasonable maternity leave system should be established for female flight attendants, and psychological counselors of the airline department should be introduced to carry out regular psychological diagnosis and treatment for the flight crew, so as to timely grasp the psychological state of the flight crew.

4.2 *Engineering and technical measures level*

In view of all kinds of mechanical injuries during check-in, all kinds of mechanical injuries are prevented from the perspective of cabin design. For example, in the front and back of the cabin set up special air staff seats and mechanical reinforcement, and configuration seat belt protection air personnel, at the same time according to the safety ergonomics principle, the air seat back set to humanized seat, increase the crew short time on comfort, protect the female air staffs' back and waist bones (Kong and Ma 2019). Airlines should not blindly seek economic benefits and increase the cabin seats without limitations. They should collect data on the average height and leg length of female flight attendants, formulate reasonable seating space, and reduce the leg fatigue of flight attendants. This kind of engineering technology can effectively reduce the occupational leg sex diseases in flight attendants.

Air circulation and toxic and harmful gases in the aircraft cabin are also important topics in the research on civil aviation occupational health, and also important environmental factors leading to skin diseases and respiratory diseases in flight attendants (Zhang *et al.* 2012). The ventilation design of the aircraft cabin is also very important. Probable and reasonable cabin ventilation engineering transformation is an important technical means to change the toxic and harmful gas composition in the cabin, and also a fundamental measure to solve the problem of respiratory occupational diseases in the stewardess group from the root.

4.3 *Medical treatment (physiological level)*

According to the definition of occupational health engineering and occupational medicine, the occupational diseases or the occupational health problems.

According to the different occupational diseases in flight attendants, the corresponding medical treatment method is appropriate. For example, for the common varicose vein problem, general treatment or drug treatment can be used. The general treatment for female flight attendants includes customized tights with better leg elasticity and measures to avoid sitting and standing for a long time at work (Wan 2004). Drug treatments include choosing drugs that increase venous tone, reduce vascular permeability, and promote lymphatic and venous return, and are generally suitable for younger patients. The commonly used drugs include horse chestnut seed extract tablets, flavonoids, aesinins, coumarins, etc. In addition, some fibrin breakdown drugs and non-steroidal anti-inflammatory drugs can also be used as an effective means to treat varicose veins. There are two main ways to treat endocrine disorders: the first is diet conditioning, it is recommended that flight attendants should develop good eating habits, like eating fresh fruits and vegetables rich in high quality protein, and reducing spicy, cold and other stimulating foods and pickled foods. The second is to stewardess group life and rest, emotional conditioning, long-term late, fatigue and emotional difficulties, mental pressure and other factors may lead to physical metabolic dysfunction, causing endocrine disorders. It is suggested that the flight attendants should ensure adequate rest, reduce staying up late, reduce overwork, adjust flight scheduling, and ensure regular life and rest. At the same time, the airline air service team establishes the corporate culture of off-work sports, conducts appropriate exercise, enhances physical fitness, and tries to keep a happy mood. For high-altitude radiation, air staff should take corresponding mechanical protection measures, such as wearing anti-radiation sunglasses and clothing blocking high-altitude ultraviolet light, and the airline should conduct regular occupational health examination for each crew. These are the main medical means of occupational disease prevention for the stewardess attendants, and medical treatment is one of the best rehabilitation means for the sick groups who have had occupational diseases.

4.4 *Psychological support (psychological level)*

Due to the nature of the work of the flight staff, their working place is the closed cabin space, and the landing place is uncertain, for a long time with their family, and the scope of interpersonal communication in the working environment is narrow, which is easy to cause negative and depressed emotions.

Based on this situation, it is suggested that airlines establish a psychological support system for the crews and establish resident psychological counselors in the airlines and branch bases, responsible for the psychological counseling of the crew after landing (Ma *et al.* 2003). At the same time, the crew chief and two cabin attendants are trained as random psychological counselors, responsible for the psychological counseling work with the team, especially the psychological state of newly hired young stewardesses, so as to create a better crew cabin culture in the company. This kind of psychological consultant system can effectively alleviate the psychological anxiety and depression of the flight attendants, timely grasp their psychological state, and early detection and treatment of psychological and occupational health disorders (Wang and Jing 2009).

4.5 *Dietary conditioning (nutritional level)*

As mentioned above, stomach disease is also one of the most common occupational diseases among female flight attendants, and it is usually caused by irregular worktime and irregular diets. Therefore, through dietary conditioning (dietary conditioning) is also an important means of prevention and treatment of occupational stomach disease (Zeng 2013). Dietary treatment is mainly divided into two aspects. One is from the perspective of individual stewardess, to formulate reasonable diet recipes, and the diet in the overseas accommodation meets the standards of health and nutrition. Second, at the airline level, the food and beverage department of the airline strengthens the management of food safety and formulates reasonable working meal standards according to the corresponding nutrition standards to ensure the most basic nutritional supply for flight attendants. At the same time, according to some flight attendants entering pregnancy, the company can set up a special pregnancy nutrition meal formulation group and specify some separate reasonable meal plans for pregnant female flight attendants.

5 CONCLUSION

This paper analyzes in detail the present Chinese female air crews occupational health and occupational disease status and prevention means, female air crew as the backbone of civil aviation service industry, completes the corresponding occupational health protection system and occupational disease prevention and control and detection system is an effective means to protect female crews, also is the airline practice of important means of female worker labor protection. For various reasons, female flight attendants have a small voice in the airlines, and some airlines will damage the legal rights of female flight attendants on the premise of considering economic interests. Female crew members often suffer from workplace PUA or sexual harassment and unfair treatment, and they are still flying high-intensity flights during pregnancy. Such problems seriously affect the moods during working and the physical and mental health of flight attendants, which is not conducive to the normal development of cabin service, and indirectly affect the safety of civil aviation passenger transport and the economic benefits of airlines. It is urgent to solve these problems. This paper mainly discusses such issues from the perspectives of occupational health protection, occupational health engineering and occupational medicine and obtains the relevant qualitative analysis results and the system management analysis at the macro level. Future civil aviation passenger transport will become the main way of middle income groups, the expansion of airport routes and the establishment of regional airport routes will introduce a large number of civil aviation air crews complement route service gap, so the key node in the development of the civil aviation industry, establish the civil aviation system for female crews of occupational health review mechanism and occupational disease prevention mechanism is an important content of civil aviation labor protection, is the practice of people-oriented, protect female group workers' important safety in production.

REFERENCES

Chen S. S. (2017). (Doctoral dissertation, Tsinghua University).
Gao X. and Chen S.W. (2011). *Hebei Education: Teaching version* (6), 2.
Gao Y. and Wang Y.X. (2012). *China Safety Production Science and Technology*, 8 (12), 7.
Kong X. F. and Ma C.Y. (2019). *Mechanical Design* (9), 6.
Liu T. B., Qiu B. and Liu Z. H. (2021). *Chinese Occupational Medicine*, 48 (1), 7.
Liu Y., Yao Y.X., Zhou L. and Ren T.S. (2010). *Chinese Journal of Aerospace Medicine* (3), 4.
Lu S. (2014). *Tourism Overview* (second half of the month) (02), 357.
Ma W. J., Wang Y. L., Lai H. Z., Sun L. and Miao Z. S. (2003). *Chinese General Practice*, 6 (9), 3.
Marsden J. and Green A.C. (2019). *British Journal of Dermatology*, 181(1), e19–e19.
Qiu B., Bai G.Y., Fan J. H., Li L. L. and Liu T. B. (2014). *The National Academic Conference on Labor Health and Occupational Diseases.*
Qiu Q. M. (2015). *Everybody Health* (late edition), 000 (003), 768–768,769.
Song G., Sun R. S., Li J. Q., ia M. H. J. (2014). Occupational and Health (5), 5.
Tang S. W. (2014). (Doctoral dissertation, Sichuan Normal University).
Wan D. (2004). *Journal of Tianjin Polytechnic University*, 23 (5), 3.
Wang J. and Jing J. (2009). *Modern Hospital*, 9 (10), 2.
Xia S.Y., Wang A.M. and Zhu Z. M. (2013). *Journal of Naval Medicine*, 34 (003), 167–169.
Xu S.X., Wang S.W., Zheng J., Liu H.J. and Xia T.Y. (2003). *The Chinese Journal of Aerospace Medicine.*
Xue C. J. (2017). *Charming China*, 000 (0z1), 259.
Yu L. C. and Yao L. (2006). *Industrial Economy Research* (2), 7.
Zeng D. (2013). (Doctoral dissertation, Guiyang Medical College).
Zeng D. (2013). (Doctoral dissertation, Guiyang Medical College).
Zhang Q. X., Ji J. and Yang Y.N. (2012). *Fire Protection Science and Technology* (10), 4.
Zhu J. Z. (2008). *The Civil Aviation of China* (10), 2.

Biological Sciences and Environmental Health – Gao (Ed.)

Unconditional cash and children's sleep, health, and nutrition: Gender comparison

Changyuan Zhou
School of Public Health, Shanghai Jiao Tong University, Shanghai, PR China

ABSTRACT: Poverty is associated with poorer sleep, health, and nutrition in children. However, research on poverty interventions in healthy US toddlers, particularly regarding gender differences, is limited. This study focuses on the effects of financial aid on the sleep, health, and nutritional outcomes of US children from economically disadvantaged households, with particular emphasis on gender disparities. This study analyzed data from the Baby's First Years project, involving 1,000 women from 12 US hospitals. Participants were split into low-cash (60%) and high-cash (40%) groups. Surveys during the Wave 2 follow-up assessed child health, sleep, and nutrition using pre-registered measures. A total of 922 mothers participated in Wave 2 data collection. Regression analyses revealed no significant differences in sleep disturbance but did show significant differences in overall child health (adjusted P = 0.009) and nutrition. Unhealthy food consumption was lower in the high-cash group (adjusted P = 0.001), indicating a significant interaction between the cash gift and unhealthy food consumption. Gender subgroup analysis showed significant differences in child overall poor health and nutrition in the male subgroup but not in the female subgroup. Interventional approaches for children's nutrition and health in different gender groups should be taken into consideration to promote child health.

1 INTRODUCTION

Poor child sleep and nutrition are significant causes of ill physical and mental health worldwide. Children with low-quality sleep are at a higher risk of adiposity and cardiometabolic ill health (Saunders *et al.* 2016). By providing children with access to high-quality nutrients, malnourished children are less likely to experience physical and mental illness in adulthood (Feng *et al.* 2015).

Girls and boys tend to have differences in fitness due to parental or cultural factors (Morawska 2020). Evidence from China suggests a connection between parents' preference for boys while their children are young and the health of elderly people, with a positive impact on boys and a negative impact on girls (Liu *et al.*2022). In rural India, boys are likely to have a lower hemoglobin level, which is an important indicator of anemia (Pasricha *et al.* 2010).

Child sleep, health, and nutrition have been found to be at risk in cases of poverty. Children from economically struggling families tend to have poorer sleep patterns and bedtime behaviors (Williamson *et al.* 2021), experience acute and chronic illness (Lee *et al.* 2023), and are diagnosed with malnutrition (Shahid *et al.* 2022). Interventions that address child health should take poverty into consideration to achieve more effective outcomes.

Income support policies that address child poverty correlate with child health and well-being, among which money transfers have become widespread in underdeveloped and developing countries over the past two decades, including conditional cash transfers and unconditional cash transfers (Pilkauskas 2023). Some programs of New York City encourage the usage of preventative dental care and medical insurance (Courtin *et al.* 2018). However, unconditional cash transfers do not constitute the primary component of US income support policies.

 DOI: 10.1201/9781003587590-58

Previous trials in undeveloped and developing countries suggest the effect of cash-based assistance on many aspects of child health. For instance, the MAM'Out project using seasonal cash-based assistance increases the intake of high-quality food (Tonguet-Papucci *et al.* 2018). For children in Zimbabwe, unconditional cash transfer is beneficial for their health, as demonstrated by the proportion of up-to-date vaccinations (Robertson *et al.* 2013). Yet trials focusing on the impact of cash-based assistance for American healthy toddlers are relatively uncommon, especially among different gender groups.

To shed light on the gender comparison of the effects of cash-based assistance policies on children in the United States, the current study intends to assess the effect of cash-based approaches on children's sleep, health, and nutritional status in the early years of life and compare the results of boys and girls.

2 METHOD

2.1 *Data and participants*

The data from the Baby's First Years (BFY) project are the focus of the present study's secondary analysis. In the BFY project, 1,000 impoverished women from 12 hospitals dispersed across several American cities participated in a randomized control trial to examine the impact of monetary payment on poverty in early childhood. The participants were enrolled immediately after the birth of their infants. To be eligible, mothers had to meet certain criteria, including age, household income below the federal poverty threshold, healthy full-term birth, proximity to the hospital, and proficiency in English or Spanish.

Within hospitals, participants were randomly assigned, with 40% receiving high payments and others receiving modest monetary gifts every month, with a total of 4000 and 240 dollars per year, respectively. Importantly, the receipt of these cash gifts did not affect mothers' eligibility for public benefits. During the recruitment phase, interviewers were not masked to participants' group assignments. However, during follow-up assessments, interviewers remained uninformed about participants' treatment status.

The present study used data from 2-year-olds (hereafter referred to as the Wave 2 follow-up) with an overall 92.2% completion rate. For more information on the study design, inclusion criteria, and other details, see www.babysfirstyears.com.

2.2 *Measures*

Surveys of outcome variables of concern in this study were completed in the Wave 2 follow-up, which were all preregistered at clinicaltrials.gov (ID: NCT03593356). The examination of the interaction effect between gender and cash gift and gender subgroup analysis was also performed, though these analyses were not preregistered.

2.2.1 *Sleep disturbance*

The PROMIS sleep disturbance-short form was used to assess sleep disturbance, with four items on a five-point Likert scale (1-Never to 5-Always) (Yu *et al.* 2011). Increased scores are indicative of more sleep-related problems.

2.2.2 *Overall poor health*

The child's general health was assessed using an additive index of six health-related factors. A lower health status is indicated by higher scores. The options for each item were 0-1 times, 2-5 times, and 6 or more times.

2.2.3 *Nutrition*

Mothers were asked how frequently the focus child consumes plain cow's milk, drinks sugared beverages, eats fruits, eats vegetables, and eats sweets on a usual day, with responses ranging from 0 (never) to 5 (more than 5 times per day) (Los Angeles County WIC Survey, 2017). Healthy food consumption was assessed using an additive index of two items (consumption of fruits and vegetables), while unhealthy food consumption was evaluated based on the combined consumption of sweet drinks and sweets.

2.3 *Statistical analysis*

The statistical software used for analyses was R Studio (R version 4.3.1). A descriptive analysis of baseline control variables was performed to evaluate the comparability of the two cash-based assistance groups, with significance set at the 0.05 level. Additionally, a series of OLS regression models, adjusted for covariates, were employed to assess the effect of different monetary assistance on various health outcomes. The interaction effect between gender and cash transfers, as well as gender subgroup analysis, was examined to explore potential differences in the impact of cash-based poverty alleviation on outcomes between different gender groups.

3 RESULTS

3.1 *Variable description statistics*

Baseline demographic characteristics are shown in Table 1. Overall, 922 participants were interviewed for age 2 data collection. Statistically, no significant differences could be observed between demographic characteristics between two different payment groups. All children were healthy at birth as per the study design. Most children were more than two years old during the period of the interview. The regional, racial, and ethnic origins of the participants were diverse, with the majority being black or Hispanic. Mothers gave birth at around 27 years of age. Most mothers had a high school diploma or GED or less. Mothers indicated an average household income of slightly above $20,000 in the year before giving birth with no difference between the two groups.

Table 1. Descriptive statistics of Wave 2 sample that completes the full interview (N = 922).

Variable	Low monetary gift group N = 545	N	High monetary gift group N = 377	N	P-value of group difference
CHILD					
Female (%)	50.5	545	47.7	377	0.457
Weight at birth (pounds)	7.15 (1.06)	532	7.09 (1.03)	367	0.447
Gestational age (weeks)	39.1 (1.25)	541	39.0 (1.19)	377	0.442
Age at visit < 2 years old (%)	42.2	545	39.8	377	0.507
MOTHER					
Age at birth (years)	26.9 (5.83)	545	27.5 (5.79)	377	0.155
Site (%)					0.990
– Los Angeles	29.9	545	29.4	377	
– Minnesota	12.1	545	12.5	377	
– The Twin Cities	28.4	545	29.2	377	
– New York City	29.5	545	28.9	377	
Race/Ethnicity (%)					0.274
– White	10.5	543	8.49	377	
– Black	40.3	543	44	377	
– Other	4.42	543	2.39	377	
– Multiple or unknown	4.05	543	2.92	377	
– Hispanic	40.7	543	42.2	377	

(continued)

Table 1. Continued

Variable	Low monetary gift group N = 545	N	High monetary gift group N = 377	N	P-value of group difference
Educational level (%)					0.946
– Junior high school or lower	23.5	544	21.4	374	
– High school diploma or General Educational Development	50.2	544	52.1	374	
– College without degree	17.5	544	17.4	374	
– Associate's degree	3.31	544	3.74	374	
– Bachelor's degree or higher	5.51	544	5.35	374	
Marital status (%)					0.134
– Never married	42.9	539	50.4	371	
– Single, living with partner	26.2	539	21.3	371	
– Married	22.1	539	22.1	371	
– Separated/Divorced	4.64	539	2.96	371	
– Other	4.27	539	3.23	371	
Optimal or good health (%)	88.6	545	92.6	377	0.245
Depression (mean ± SD)	6.69 (4.43)	539	6.78 (4.41)	373	0.765
Weekly cigarette consumption during pregnancy	4.71(20.3)	542	3.28 (11.4)	375	0.175
Weekly alcohol consumption during pregnancy	0.15 (1.67)	543	0.03 (0.39)	376	0.091
Number of adults in household	2.09 (0.98)	545	2.03 (0.98)	377	0.341
Number of children in household	2.68 (1.39)	545	2.81 (1.42)	377	0.156
Household combined income	23793 (44593)	545	21567 (16901)	377	0.289
Biological father lives in household (%)	40	545	34.5	377	0.103

Notes. Data is presented as means (standard deviations) or percentages. Reported p-values for mean differences have not been adjusted.

3.2 Intent-to-treat analyses

To compare age-2 child health in the high and low-cash gift groups, regression analyses were conducted on three subsections: sleep disturbance, overall health, and nutrition. Table 2 shows the intent-to-treat (ITT) estimates both before and after adjustments for baseline covariates and multiple hypothesis testing (Sidak adjustment). Apart from baseline covariates, the regression-adjusted model also includes the child age category (more than two years or not) during the age 2 survey. Full regression details are provided in Table 2. Although there were minor imbalances in baseline characteristics between the different cash groups, as shown in Table 1, it is important to note that incorporating covariates into the models significantly alters the specific ITT estimates.

In the case of sleep disturbance, the cash-rich gift group showed a higher score but both the P levels before and after adjustment were above the 0.05 threshold. Statistically significant differences in overall health were found in the Overall Poor Health Index (effect size = -0.020, β = -0.038, P = 0.007, adjusted P = 0.009). Differences in nutrition varied between healthy and unhealthy food consumption, with the high-cash gift group showing lower consumption of unhealthy food (effect size = -0.025, β = -0.055, P = 0.000, adjusted P = 0.001), but not differing significantly from the low cash-gift group in terms of consumption of healthy foods (effect size = -0.008, β = -0.018, P = 0.239, adjusted P = 0.708).

Table 2. Cash-gift treatment effects on child health and interaction effects by gender.

Variable	Low monetary gift group (Mean ± SD)	High monetary gift group (Mean ± SD)	Coefficient without covariates (SE)	Coefficient with covariates (SE)	Effect size	P-value (unadjusted)	Sidak adjusted P-value	N	P-value for interaction
SLEEP									
PROMIS-Sleep disturbance scale	7.488 (3,467)	7.606 (3.349)	0.118 (0.229)	−0.047 (0.024)	−0.014	0.048	0.198	919	0.620
HEALTH									
Child poor health	4.912 (1.908)	4.928 (1.978)	0.017 (0.130)	−0.038 (0.014)	−0.020	0.007	0.009	919	0.156
NUTRITION									
Index of healthy food consumption	4.180 (2.124)	4.499 (2.160)	0.318 (0.145)	−0.018 (0.015)	−0.008	0.239	0.708	901	0.408
Index of Unhealthy Food Consumption	3.446 (2.215)	3.484 (2.147)	0.038 (0.148)	−0.055 (0.014)	−0.025	0.000	0.001	903	0.006

Notes. The covariate-adjusted treatment impact was divided by the standard deviation of the low-cash group to determine the effect size. Covariates from BFY baseline survey included the variables listed in Table 1.

3.3 *Interaction analyses*

The results revealed a significant interaction effect of gender, indicating that the relationship between cash gifts and unhealthy food consumption differs between boys and girls. Subgroup analysis by gender revealed notable differences in unhealthy food consumption and poor health in the boys' subgroup, while no significant differences in the girls' subgroup were observed (Table 3).

Table 3. Cash-gift treatment effects on child health based on gender subgroup analysis.

Variable	Low monetary gift group (Mean ± SD)	High monetary gift group (Mean ± SD)	Coefficient without covariates (SE)	Coefficient with covariates (SE)	Effect size	P-value (unadjusted)	Sidak adjusted P-value	N
MALE								
SLEEP								
PROMIS-Sleep disturbance scale	7.374 (3.405)	7.515 (3.287)	0.168 (0.315)	−0.041 (0.035)	−0.012	0.248	0.723	464
HEALTH								
Child poor health	5.037 (1.973)	4.857 (1.889)	−0.180 (0.182)	−0.057 (0.020)	−0.029	0.004	0.017	464
NUTRITION								
Index of healthy food consumption	4.094 (2.129)	4.570 (2.150)	0.476 (0.202)	−0.027 (0.022)	−0.013	0.223	0.679	458
Index of unhealthy food consumption	3.513 (2.231)	3.155 (2.130)	−0.358 (0.207)	−0.064 (0.021)	−0.029	0.003	0.014	456
FEMALE								
SLEEP								

(*continued*)

Table 3. Continued

Variable	Low monetary gift group (Mean ± SD)	High monetary gift group (Mean ± SD)	Coefficient without covariates (SE)	Coefficient with covariates (SE)	Effect size	P-value (unadjusted)	Sidak adjusted P-value	N
PROMIS-Sleep disturbance scale	7.625 (3.527)	7.706 (3.421)	0.080 (0.334)	−0.045 (0.033)	−0.013	0.170	0.567	455
HEALTH								
Child poor health	4.789 (1.838)	5.006 (2.073)	0.216 (0.185)	−0.026 (0.019)	−0.014	0.177	0.584	455
NUTRITION								
Index of healthy food consumption	4.266 (2.119)	4.420 (2.174)	0.155 (0.208)	−0.003 (0.021)	−0.002	0.877	1.000	443
Index of unhealthy food consumption	3.381 (2.201)	3.838 (2.115)	0.457 (0.209)	−0.041 (0.020)	−0.018	0.040	0.166	447

4 DISCUSSION

The study examined the baseline characteristics of 922 participants, demonstrating no statistically significant differences in demographics between different cash-based assistance groups. ITT analyses showed that although minor baseline imbalances exist, significant differences emerged in overall child health and nutrition, with the high-cash gift group consuming less unhealthy food. Importantly, a gender interaction effect was observed, highlighting the distinct impacts of cash gifts on unhealthy food consumption between boys and girls. Boys exhibited significant differences in the consumption of unhealthy foods and poor health, while girls did not show significant differences.

The findings of the present study differ from those of a related paper using the same database, which reported significantly higher consumption of fruits and vegetables in high-cash groups (Sperber *et al.* 2023). In contrast, the present study found that the high-cash groups exhibited lower consumption of unhealthy food ($P<0.05$) and a lower poor health index. Previous work has found a positive effect of cash-based assistance on the consumption of high-nutrition-value foods and vitamin A or iron supplementation in low-income countries (Tonguet-Papucci *et al.* 2017). Therefore, the results of the present study warrant further research and follow-up investigations on the same population to confirm these findings.

The present study found a significant interaction effect between gender and the consumption of unhealthy food, with a notable effect on boys but not on girls. Similarly, the receipt of cash gifts promoted boys' health but not girls,' and the interaction effect was not significant ($P>0.05$). Gender bias among parents is associated with some differences in parenting styles, such as using different social interaction strategies and play activities with children (Morawska 2020). Previous research indicates that boys are less likely to develop anemia in rural India (Pasricha *et al.* 2010). However, few trials compare outcomes by gender, highlighting the need for further research to verify the results of the current study.

The present study has several limitations. First, step-down resampling methods as described by Westfall and Young were not used for multiple comparisons. However, the Sidak method can also effectively manage the potential for false positives while minimizing the decline in statistical power. Another limitation is the discrepancies between the results of the current study and those of a previous similar study, which may be due to the differences in covariates and statistical methods (Sperber *et al.* 2023). It is also important to continue follow-up to detect possible adverse health outcomes later in life (Sperber *et al.* 2023).

5 CONCLUSION

In conclusion, cash gifts were found to have an effect on child nutrition and health outcomes in the US preschool population. The present study identified a negative impact of cash gifts on the consumption of unhealthy food and poor health in children. Furthermore, from a gender comparison perspective, the effect of cash gifts differed between girls and boys, with a significant effect observed in boys but not in girls. The present highlights the need for interventional approaches to improve children's nutrition and health across different gender groups.

REFERENCES

Courtin E., Muennig P., Verma N., et al. (2018). Conditional cash transfers and health of low-income families in the us: evaluating the family rewards experiment [J]. *Health Aff (Millwood)*, **37**(3): 438–46.

Feng A., Wang L., Chen X., et al. (2015). Developmental origins of health and disease (DOHaD): Implications for health and nutritional issues among rural children in China [J]. *Biosci Trends*, 2015, **9**(2): 82–7.

Lee A. R., Kingdon C. C., Davie M., et al. (2023). Child poverty and health inequalities in the UK: a guide for paediatricians [J]. *Arch Dis Child,* **108**(2).

Liu Y., Su Y. and Yin Y. (2022). Parental preference for boys in childhood and the health of the elderly: Evidence from China [J]. *Soc Sci Med,* **302**: 114986.

Los Angeles County WIC Survey. Published online 2017. http://lawicdata.org/wp-content/uploads/2014/09/WIC-Parents-Quex-English-FINAL.pdf

Morawska A. (2020). The effects of gendered parenting on child development outcomes: A systematic review [J]. *Clin Child Fam Psychol Rev*, , **23**(4): 553–76.

Pasricha S-R, Black J., Muthayya S., et al. (2010). Determinants of anemia among young children in rural India [J]. *Pediatrics*, **126**(1): e140–e9.

Pilkauskas N. V. (2023). Child Poverty and Health: The Role of Income Support Policies [J]. *Milbank Q*, **101** (S1): 379–95.

Robertson L., Mushati P., Eaton J. W., et al. (2013). Effects of unconditional and conditional cash transfers on child health and development in Zimbabwe: A cluster-randomised trial [J]. *Lancet*, 2013, **381**(9874): 1283–92.

Saunders T. J., Gray C. E., Poitras V. J., et al. (2016). Combinations of physical activity, sedentary behaviour and sleep: relationships with health indicators in school-aged children and youth [J]. *Appl Physiol Nutr Metab*, 2016, **41**(6 Suppl 3): S283–S93.

Shahid M., Ahmed F., Ameer W., et al. (2022). Prevalence of child malnutrition and household socioeconomic deprivation: A case study of marginalized district in Punjab, Pakistan [J]. *PLoS One*, **17**(3): e0263470.

Sperber J. F., Gennetian L. A., Hart E. R., et al. (2023). The effect of a us poverty reduction intervention on maternal assessments of young children's health, nutrition, and sleep: A randomized control trial [J]. *medRxiv*.

Tonguet-Papucci A., Houngbe F., Huybregts L., et al. (2017). unconditional seasonal cash transfer increases intake of high-nutritional-value foods in young burkinabe children: Results of 24-hour dietary recall surveys within the moderate acute malnutrition out (MAM'Out) randomized controlled trial [J]. *The Journal of Nutrition*, **147**(7): 1418–25.

Williamson A. A., Gould R., Leichman E. S., et al. (2021). Socioeconomic disadvantage and sleep in early childhood: Real-world data from a mobile health application [J]. *Sleep Health*, **7**(2): 143–52.

Yu L., Buysse D. J., Germain A., *et al.* (2011). Development of short forms from the PROMIS^{TM} sleep disturbance and Sleep-Related Impairment item banks [J]. *Behav Sleep Med.*, **10**(1).

Biological Sciences and Environmental Health – Gao (Ed.)

Effect of microbial composition on Kombucha and its applications

Ziyi Ye
School of Life Sciences, Shanghai Normal University, Shanghai, China

ABSTRACT: In 2000 years ago, Kombucha was first produced in China. Then it has become increasingly popular in Europe and the United States in recent years. It is a fermented tea beverage that contains a symbiotic consortium of bacteria and yeast (SCOBY). It has risen to prominence in the beverage market with its potential benefits for long-term regulation of intestinal flora, antimicrobial and anticancer properties, and health benefits. Based on the research of existing scholars on the fermentation methods, conditions, sensory properties, bioactivities, and health effects of kombucha tea, this research paper presents a current study and problem analysis of the production process and food value of kombucha tea. It was found that kombucha has good sensory properties, multi-disciplinary applications, and desirable bioactivities such as antibacterial and antioxidant. Kombucha tea is fermented under a wide variety of conditions, all of which affect the fermented flavor, nutritional and health benefits. Therefore, the issue of process optimization and product safety of kombucha is also crucial.

1 INTRODUCTION

Fermentation has a long history as a way to preserve food. Additionally, this low-cost, energy-efficient approach is critical to safeguarding the shelf life and safety of food products. Numerous changes in biochemistry that occur throughout the fermentation process might have an effect on the nutrient content and, as a result, the characteristics of the end product. In recent years, this technology has been increasingly applied to the extraction of natural beneficial substances and product development in the food and beverage industry (Villarreal-Soto *et al.* 2018).

The use of kombucha, a traditional fermented beverage that was first enjoyed in China and is now made both industrially and artisanally, has been rising in Western nations as a result of the beverage's expanding market and purported health advantages. Today, kombucha comes in a variety of tastes and is available in stores all over the world (Bortolomedi).

Using a kombucha culture made of bacteria and yeast, a solution of sweetened tea is fermented to create kombucha tea, a naturally carbonated, non-alcoholic beverage (Nyhan *et al.* 2022). Depending on the metabolic pathway taken, a variety of fermentation methods can be realized to yield different products. Due to the coexistence of many yeasts and bacteria in the medium, the three forms of production—alcoholic, lactic, and acetic—are combined in the fermentation of kombucha. being initiated by osmotolerant bacteria and being eventually regulated by species resistant to acid (Villarreal-Soto *et al.* 2018).

With the increase in consumer awareness, additive-free, nutritional supplementation and health benefits have become the trend in the development of food processes. Due to its probiotic properties, consumers and scholars have recently become interested in traditional kombucha tea. However, for industrial production, it is crucial to take into account the physical and chemical indicators, production processes, microbiological composition and

DOI: 10.1201/9781003587590-59

by-products (Villarreal-Soto *et al.* 2018). Kombucha deserves continued research on process upgrading, optimization of nutritional value and safety.

2 MICROBIOLOGICAL COMPOSITION

There is a wide variety of microorganisms in kombucha. When kombucha is fermenting, the two main species are bacteria and yeasts. However, the origin, substrates, and production circumstances of kombucha can all affect its microbial composition. Therefore, it is unclear what microorganisms exist in kombucha, and it is generally recognized as belonging to a complex microbial symbiotic system. However, according to current research, Figure 1 shows that kombucha will commonly contain the following bacteria and yeast (Coelho *et al.* 2020).

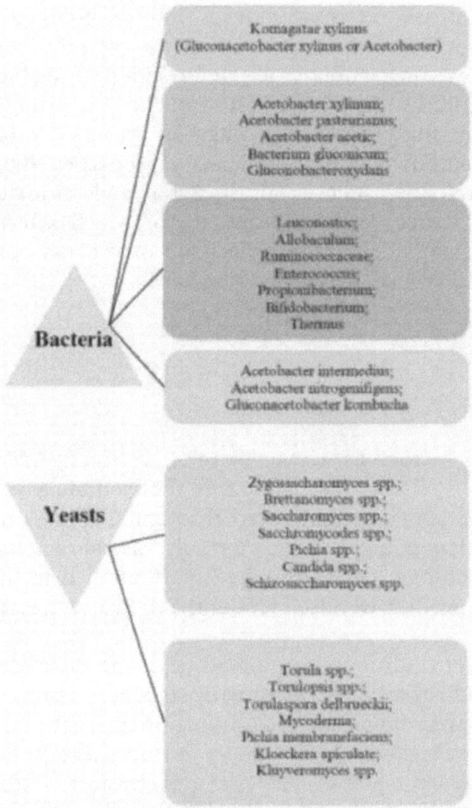

Figure 1. Microorganisms in Kombucha (Coelho *et al.* 2020).

2.1 *Bacteria*

Among the bacteria contained in kombucha, Acetobacter and Gluconobacter spp. are the most essential and abundant (Jayabalan *et al.* 2014). The Acetobacter genus contains strains that convert ethanol into acetic acid. This process can be accomplished by enzymes that produce acetic acid, which enters the Krebs cycle and the end products are water and carbon dioxide, carry out this activity (Leal *et al.* 2018). Lacking the oxidizing enzymes succinate dehydrogenase and alpha-ketoglutarate dehydrogenase, the genus Gluconobacter cannot oxidize acetate through the Krebs cycle, causing a buildup of compounds like gluconate in the medium (Leal *et al.* 2018). However, Gluconacetobacter sp. A4 has a terrific ability to produce D-saccharic acid-1,4-lactone (Jayabalan *et al.* 2014).

2.2 *Yeasts*

A wide range of yeast species (Coelho *et al.* 2020). On the one hand, sucrose is hydrolyzed to glucose and fructose catalyzed by the enzyme converting enzyme of yeast, and ethanol is produced through the glycolysis pathway. Meanwhile, Gluconobacter and Acetobacter utilize the acetic acid produced by ethanol and the gluconic acid produced by glucose to inhibit the growth of pathogenic bacteria in kombucha (Leal *et al.* 2018).

2.3 *Lactobacillus(LAB)*

Nowadays, lactobacillus are incorporated into a variety of food products to provide a distinctive flavor and provide health advantages. Despite the fact that it is now well acknowledged that LAB are not necessary for the creation of kombucha. When LAB is present, the fermentation of Kombucha can produce more D-saccharic acid, 1,4 lactone (DSL), and glucuronic acid. In addition, the antioxidant and antimicrobial activities of kombucha are also enhanced (Wang *et al.* 2022)

3 ROLE OF MICROORGANISMS IN KOMBUCHA

3.1 *Active components in kombucha*

Kombucha contains a wide range of active ingredients, but they are variable in quantity and quality. This depends largely on the fermentation temperature and time, the substrate, and the type of tea (Leal *et al.* 2018). For example, acetic acid is the chemical component that gives vinegar in kombucha its acidic flavor and scent. After 30 days of fermentation, it reaches a concentration of 11 g/L in the beverage. After 60 days of fermentation, the concentration gradually declines to 8 g/L. This reduction occurs as a result of bacteria using acetic acid as a carbon source once their supply of sugar and ethanol has run out. In addition, green tea preparations contain higher levels of lactic acid than other teas (Coelho *et al.* 2020). Active ingredients usually include vitamins, organic acids, minerals, ethanol, sucrose, and so on (Leal *et al.* 2018).

3.2 *Role of microorganisms on kombucha in sensory aspects*

Customers who routinely consume kombucha feel as though they are drinking a healthy beverage that will aid their digestion because of its pleasant flavor. It is often thought to have unique and piquant flavor. Some would even go so far as to call it "unprecedented (Bishop *et al.* 2022)."

The researchers placed different concentrations of black tea, green tea and sugar in certain proportions at 20, 25, and 30 °C, and then evaluate their sensory. The sensory analysis was performed in terms of five specific sensations: visual, gustatory, auditory, olfactory and tactile. Figure 2 shows the final results of the sensory evaluation obtained by the 16 inexperienced tasters who scored the tasting (Tran *et al.* 2020).

From the data in the graph, it follows that, the highest scoring visually related characteristics were color intensity and clarity; the highest scoring olfactory characteristics could be considered the fragrant aroma of tea and the light sweet and sour scent of lemon; and the flavor characteristics could be interpreted as the mellow aroma of tea and the lemon-like sensation of slight acidity, sweetness, and astringency. Even though residual sugar levels varied from 27 to 70 g/L, the adjective "sweetness" was not assessed. In addition, the ratings for "yeastiness" and "acetic acidity" were low, and the bitter flavor and pungent odor were not noticeable (Tran *et al.* 2020).

Although this sensory analysis is not comprehensive and needs to be studied in a more precise and standardized way, we can analyze the reasons for the above sensory analysis results. First, in appearance, kombucha is either clear or cloudy, depending on whether or not the suspended colloidal material is filtered out (Tran *et al.* 2020). Researchers believe that the colloids are made up of fibers made from cellulose, polymerized proteins, and polyphenols that are created by acetic acid bacteria (Bishop *et al.* 2022). The pigmented polyphenols extracted from the tea leaves are the main source of kombucha's hue. For example, the oxidation of tea polyphenol oxidase gives black tea its distinctive color. In addition, air bubbles are an important visual sensory characteristic, as evidenced by the size and abundance of the bubbles, which can be produced by natural fermentation or artificially injected with carbon dioxide, depending on sensory needs (Tran *et al.* 2020).

Second, odor. The odor of kombucha is often described as "sour". Similar to other fermented drinks, the overall fragrance profile of tea is influenced by both the microbes (bacteria and yeasts) and the raw materials (tea). Damascenone, 2-phenylethanol, geraniol, linalool, three-hexanol are only a few of the many volatile organic compounds (VOCs) found in tea. The conventional scent profile of tea does not, however, seem to contribute significantly to the distinctive aroma profile of kombucha. Instead, acetic acid and yeast-produced VOCs predominate in the scent profile (Bishop *et al.* 2022). Third, the flavor. The flavor of Kombucha is generally sweet, sour, bitter these kinds of taste (Tran *et al.* 2020). The main source of sweetness is sucrose broken down into glucose and fructose through fermentation using converting enzymes; sourness comes from organic acids such as acetic acid produced by acetic acid bacteria, yeast, and lactobacilli, which often accompanies a small amount of bitterness and astringency while providing a sour taste; and bitterness is mainly determined by caffeine and tea polyphenols in the tea, which are often masked by increased sweetness in the production process in order to improve the taste (Bishop *et al.* 2022).

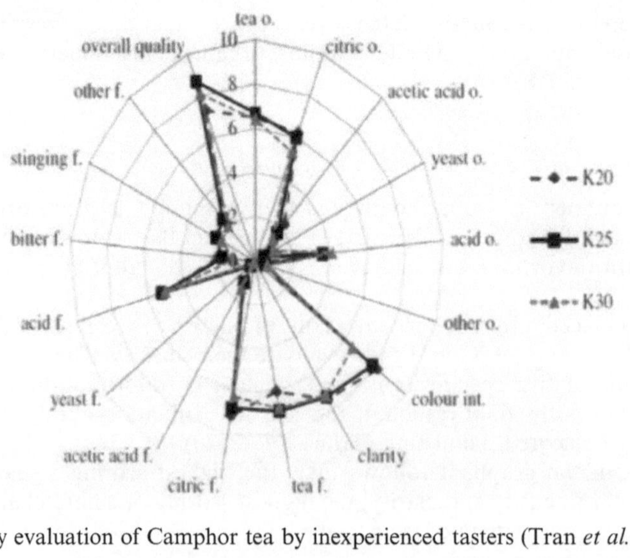

Figure 2. Sensory evaluation of Camphor tea by inexperienced tasters (Tran *et al.* 2020).

3.3 *Role of microorganisms on kombucha in human health*

Natural product kombucha, which is categorized as a nutraceutical, was created to promote both physical and mental wellness in people. It has the effect of regulating immunity, lowering blood sugar, lowering blood lipids and so on. The health advantages of kombucha are attributed to the inclusion of D-saccharic acid-1,4-lactone, gluconic acid, glucuronic acid, tea polyphenols, vitamins, amino acids, other minerals, and antibiotics (Ojo and Smidt 2023). For example, due to GlcUA in kombucha, it can participate in glucuronidation, which improves the bioavailability of polyphenols and prevents the oxidation of polyunsaturated fatty acids in the human body (Leal *et al.* 2018). During the fermentation process, microorganisms produce one of the most important detoxifying agents for the human body, glucuronic acid, through the oxidation of glucose, which can bind toxic substances in the liver and thus excrete them efficiently through the kidneys, while at the same time it is a precursor for the biosynthesis of vitamin C (Coelho *et al.* 2020). In addition, kombucha tea contains a large number of probiotic bacteria, which have hypoglycemic and hypolipidemic properties and can better inhibit the high blood glucose levels (Ojo and Smidt 2023).

4 FERMENTATION MECHANISM AND APPLICATION OF KOMBUCHA

4.1 *Fermentation mode and mechanism of kombucha*

The symbiotic interaction between bacteria and yeast is mainly exploited during the fermentation process. Through kombucha symbiosis, sweetened tea can become a lightly carbonated, energetic drink when it grows aerobically. At the same time, LAB converts carbohydrates, i.e., some sugars, into lactic acid, while acetic acid bacteria convert glucose into gluconic acid and ethanol is oxidized to acetic acid. Yeast hydrolyzes sucrose to produce glucose and fructose, which in turn produces carbon dioxide and ethanol (Nyhan *et al.* 2022).

Specifically, for the typical kombucha preparation and fermentation process: First, the tea or tea leaves must be steeped for the prescribed time (5-10 minutes). Next, steep the tea leaves, which takes about 8-10 minutes. Then, add about 50-150 grams of sugar to the hot water and stir well until it is all dissolved in the water. And inoculate the new tea and wait for the sugar-tea mixture to cool down to room temperature, which is around 18-30 °C, and start adding SCOBY and the kombucha or vinegar that has been fermented for about 100-200 mL. This step enables the pH of the solution to drop, and inhibits the growth and reproduction of substances such as pathogenic microorganisms and spoilage bacteria by changing the acidity and alkalinity. Finally, fermentation, completely cover the fermentation vessel of kombucha with a clean towel or other fabric and place it at room temperature for 1-2 weeks to isolate it from air and prevent contamination (Bishop *et al.* 2022).

In addition, for the fermentation of kombucha, there are some influencing factors. Kombucha recipes vary widely. Substrate, tea type, pH, fermentation time and temperature are the main factors affecting the diversity of microbial composition of kombucha (Ojo and Smidt 2023). Any modification in these variables can have an impact on the product's physicochemical composition, pace of fermentation, spectrum, performance, organoleptic qualities, and nutritional value (Villarreal-Soto 2018). Research on how fermentation conditions affect the synthesis of bioactive chemicals in kombucha extracts has shown, for instance, that the use of various vessel geometries may result in the production of various fermentation metabolites and bioactive compounds. Additionally, utilizing the kombucha consortium for black tea fermentation increases the beverage's bioactive potential and promotes the synergistic interactions between microbes and fermentation metabolites, which results in the production of intriguing compounds (Villarreal-Soto *et al.*

2019). First, about substrate. The kombucha microbiota's growing medium has to have supplies of carbon and nitrogen such as sucrose, fructose, glucose, etc. obtained from tea extracts. The growth of nearly all microorganisms depends critically on substrates like carbon and nitrogen sources. Secondly, type of tea. This will mainly affect the production of microorganisms, for example, green tea leaves have a higher production of bacteria and yeast symbiotic communities than black tea and tea wastes. Third, pH, the growth of acetic acid bacteria is inhibited at tea concentrations above 6 g L-1, then high sugar concentrations inhibit microbial growth, the optimal sugar concentration for kombucha bacteria and yeast symbiotic communities ranges from 6 to 12 g L-1. Fourth, fermentation time, the optimal time for fermentation is between 6 and 14 days, while longer fermentation time reduces the amount of yeast surviving to the end of the fermentation, and the biomass will also decrease. Fifth, fermentation temperature, temperature has a great influence on microbial enzyme activity, so the optimal temperature should be maintained during the fermentation process (Ojo and Smidt 2023).

4.2 *Applications of kombucha*

Kombucha is often used in the development of various types of food products, mainly in beverages, vinegars, wines, yogurts, breads, kimchi, sesame seed ganache, coffee and other food products (Liu, Zhang and Sun 2021). In addition to its nutritional value, cellulose fibers produced by bacteria and yeast in kombucha create a special type of substance. Due to its broad technological range of uses, more scholarly research has focused on the use of kombucha, and microbial symbiotic cultures therein, as well as the use of tea in industrial applications such as skin care products, textiles, and innovative beverages (Soares, Lima and Schmidt 2021).

5 EXISTING PROBLEMS AND PROSPECTS OF KOMBUCHA

5.1 *Safety concerns of kombucha*

The safety talked about here mainly includes the safety of the production process, the safety of the serving size and the applicable population. First, for the production of kombucha.

Kombucha, as a probiotic beverage, is crucial in terms of production and storage, which is related to the quality of the product and the assurance of its efficacy. Generally, there are several major factors that may ultimately lead to safety issues during the production process: poor hygiene during preparation (this is often related to the fact that some people make kombucha in a homemade way without good control of hygiene, such as inappropriate containers, preservation methods, or contaminated ingredients, etc.); incorrect fermentation (e.g., time, pH, etc.); inclusion of non-beneficial microorganisms or inaccurate selection of raw materials (Batista *et al.* 2022). Next, is the serving size. According to CDC, 110 mL of kombucha per day for healthy people has no health risks. However, excessive drinking or consumption by people with pre-existing medical conditions may pose dangers. In addition, the applicable population. Although kombucha has been shown to have some therapeutic effects, some people are skeptical about its adverse effects and safety (Miranda *et al.* 2022). Dizziness and nausea have been recorded as side effects of various Kombucha products, and some people have also experienced anaphylactic reactions and headache, but in almost all cases of toxicity related to kombucha consumption, the patients had suffered from a disease or had some predisposing factor, such as having AIDS, asthma, diabetes, etc (Mousavi *et al.* 2020). Kombucha is not recommended for use by nursing mothers, pregnant women, children under the age of 4, people with renal insufficiency, or people living with HIV since it may cause hazardous reactions in some people (Miranda *et al.* 2022).

5.2 *Sensory deficiencies of products and new market need*

Due to the increasing sensory requirements of food products, new processes, and new product development are inevitable, therefore, standardization of physical and chemical features is required since they have a direct impact on the consumer's sensory perception. For instance, the kinetics of kombucha's fermentation are significantly affected by the sugars utilized as a carbon source. Balancing the right carbon source with optimal metabolic efficiency is a complex task that requires adjusting the fermentation time and temperature according to the carbon source added to the process to prevent severe acetic acid buildup and sensory property loss. It can even affect its safety, since without pasteurization, the sugar remaining in the finished package will continue to ferment, increasing the production of gas and alcohol throughout the storage, distribution, and shelf life of the product, and affecting the quality of final beverage. Then again, kombucha from various origins also exhibits varying antioxidant activity and polyphenol contents, on account of different starting culture microbiota, temperatures and fermentation intervals, which also have a greater impact on sensory attributes. Of course, pH value, alcohol content and Bailey's sugar level are also important indicators that affect sensory attributes.

As a result, future research should focus on three separate fronts: omics study, which broadly considers metabolic and genomic dynamics with the goal of identifying novel sites of significance in the fermentation kernel of kombucha besides the relationships between acetobacter and yeast; Secondly, in conducting research on large-scale kombucha production, physicochemical variables in several fermentation methods were compared, including fermentation batch, mode, and vessel, such as the differences between batch-fed fermentation, single-batch fermentation, and continuous fermentation, the spatial effects of different design layouts of fermenters, and the possible effects of liquid column height and surface area of gas-liquid interactions in response to the oxygen-requiring phase of kombucha fermentation; beyond this, there is a need for research into the real benefits that can be gained from drinking it, and in particular how these benefits are retained and manifested by the different microbiota that make up kombucha around the world (Oliveira *et al.* 2022).

5.3 *Improvement of the nutritional value of Kombucha*

There is a growing demand for its nutritional value, which can also be enhanced from a process perspective. For example, a new product can be formed by combining a certain tea with a food that contains a specific function. It was suggested that drinking fermented black tea with wheatgrass added will have better and more constant antioxidant activity than drinking standard kombucha (Oliveira *et al.* 2022).

In addition, the Kombucha application products currently on the market are basically dead bacteria-type products, although they also have certain health care functions. Future research and development should be directed towards live bacteria-type development, while ensuring the effective content of efficacy components, and developing products with real health benefits (Liu *et al.* 2021).

6 CONCLUSION

In the present study, it was found that there is a wide variety of microorganisms in kombucha, but the exact composition is not certain. The growing popularity of kombucha in Europe and the United States stems from its richness in biologically active substances, pleasant organoleptic properties, and nutritional and health care functions, and it is even expanding into various other areas of application. Kombucha is made by adding bacteria and yeast to sugar and tea and then allowing the mixture to ferment. The fermentation method is not complicated, but there are a wide variety of conditions, such as temperature, type of tea, substrate and other conditions, which will greatly affect the product once changed. At the same time, some chemicals and physiologically active molecules may deteriorate or disappear over time or in different environments.

Suggestions for future research include: safety of the production process, serving size, and applicable population for kombucha; some adjustment of the fermentation method and production process as needed for optimization of sensory attributes; and development of the product from a dead bacterial product to a live bacterial product in order to enhance or strengthen its nutritional value.

Therefore, this study concludes that kombucha has certain nutritional, health care and medicinal values, but nowadays its lack of sensory characteristics, food safety and stability of nutritional value still need to be further optimized and upgraded.

REFERENCES

Batista P., Penas M. R., Pintado M. and Oliveira-Silva P., (2022). *Foods*, **11(13)**, 1977.

Bishop P., Pitts E. R., Budner D. and Thompson-Witrick K. A., (2022). *Food Chem Adv*, **1**, 100025.

Bortolomedi B. M., Paglarini C. S. and Brod F. C. A., (2022). *Food Chem*, **385**, 132719.

Coelho R. M. D., de Almeida A. L., do Amaral R. Q. G., da Mota R. N. and de Sousa P. H. M., (2020). *Int J Gastron Food S*, **22**, 100272.

de Miranda J. F., Ruiz L. F., Silva C. B., Uekane T. M., Silva K. A., Gonzalez A. G. M., Fernandes F. F. and Lima A. R., (2022). *J Food Sci*, **87(2)**, 503–527.

Jayabalan R., Malbasa R. V., Loncar E. S., Vitas J. S. and Sathishkumar M., (2014). *Compr Rev Food Sci F*, **13(4)**, 538–550.

Leal J. M., Suarez L. V., Jayabalan R., Oros J. H. and Escalante-Aburto A., (2018). *CyTA-J Food*, **16(1)**, 390–399.

Liu X., Zhang Y. and Sun T., (2021). *Food Ind*, **42(09)**, 227–230.

Mousavi S. M., Hashemi S. A., Zarei M., Gholami A., Lai C. W., Chiang W. H., Omidifar N. S. and Bahrani, S. (2020). *Mazraedoost, Evid-Based Compl Alt*, **2020**, 4397543.

Nyhan L. M., Lynch K. M., Sahin A. W. and Arendt E. K., (2022). *Applied Microbiology*, **2(1)**, 73–103.

Ojo A. O. and de Smidt O., (2023). *Fermentation*, **9(5)**, 472.

Oliveira Í. A. C. L. d., Rolim V. A. d. O., Gaspar R. P. L., Rossini D. Q., de Souza R. and Bogsan C. S. B., (2022). *Fermentation*, **8(4)**, 185.

Soares M. G., de Lima M. and Schmidt V. C. R., (2021). *Trends Food Sci Tech*, **110**, 539–550.

Tran T., Grandvalet C., Verdier F., Martin A., Alexandre H. and Tourdot-Maréchal R., (2020). *Compr Rev Food Sci F*, **19(4)**, 2050–2070.

Villarreal-Soto S. A., Beaufort S., Bouajila J., Souchard J. P. and Taillandier P., (2018). *J Food Sci*, **83(3)**, 580–588.

Villarreal-Soto S. A., Beaufort S., Bouajila J., Souchard J.-P., Renard T., Rollan S. and Taillandier P., (2019). *Process Biochem*, **83**, 44–54.

Wang B., Rutherfurd-Markwick K., Zhang X.-X. and Mutukumira A. N., (2022). *Foods*, **11(21)**, 3456.

Biological Sciences and Environmental Health – Gao (Ed.)
© 2025 the Author(s), ISBN: 978-1-032-96016-6

Impact of lactic acid bacteria on coffee fermentation

Wenxin Tao
St. John's Kilmarnock School, Breslau Ontario, Canada

ABSTRACT: Lactic acid bacteria (LAB) used in coffee processing are sourced from water and indigenous soil. They flourish by consuming coffee pulp, converting carbon and nitrogen into lactic acid. Coffee producers employ this natural fermentation process to eliminate the mucilage layer from coffee beans before their storage and transportation. LAB metabolism generates numerous compounds in addition to lactic acid through the breakdown of citrate and the metabolism of amino acids. Recent research has shown that metabolites in coffee production not only affect the taste of coffee but also play a vital role in the creation of precursor substances. Nevertheless, the extent to which the application of LAB can improve coffee quality has yet to be determined. This study provides a comprehensive analysis of the significance of LAB in the production of coffee and investigates the influence that the variety of microorganisms and metabolic processes have on the product's overall quality. Additional research is required to determine the suitable LAB strains and their integration with yeast cultures. This has the potential to generate new insights and perspectives on enhancing the overall quality of coffee.

1 INTRODUCTION

Lactic acid bacteria (LAB) are a prominent category of microorganisms that are widely employed in the production of fermented food. These organisms are distinguished by their capacity to generate over 50% lactic acid through the utilization of carbohydrates. They are identified by their gram-positive, non-motile, and non-spore-forming characteristics, typically appearing as coccobacilli or rods. The order *Lactobacillales* consists of 6 families and 40 genera, which have been classified based on their 16S rRNA gene sequences (Holzapfel and Wood 2014).

Although LAB is often linked to dairy products, it is believed that industrial strains of LAB actually come from plant material. These microorganisms are widely distributed in nature and frequently contaminate food under favorable circumstances. During coffee processing, LAB thrives in the coffee pulp, consuming sugars and other substances and producing lactic acid, thereby reducing the pH (Wang *et al.* 2019). Lactic acid facilitates the decomposition of pectin, a polysaccharide found in large quantities in coffee pulp. These metabolisms facilitate the elimination of coffee mucilage components and decrease the duration of the after-harvesting procedures from 7 to 21 days (Carvalho Neto *et al.* 2018).

LAB is involved in the process of removing mucilage as well as producing bioactive compounds that have an effect on the quality of the coffee. Because of their ability to impart a wide variety of aromas to coffee, the use of LAB cultures in the fermentation process of coffee has attracted a lot of attention recently. Specific metabolites produced by LAB, such as aldehydes, higher alcohols, ketones, and esters, can significantly influence the sensory characteristics of coffee. These metabolites contribute to the fruity, floral, and bitter flavors in the coffee (Carvalho Neto *et al.* 2018). This paper presents some novel approaches that

DOI: 10.1201/9781003587590-60

utilize LAB's capabilities in coffee fermentation, exploring their variety, ecological functions, metabolic processes, and significant impact on coffee quality.

2 COFFEE PROCESSING

Caffeine is consumed in large quantities all over the world due to the distinctive flavor profile and sensory qualities that it possesses, which have made it extremely popular. Brazil is widely recognized as the primary producer of coffee beans, boasting an annual yield of 54 million bags (USDA Foreign Agricultural Service 2021).

The processing of coffee cherries after they have been brought to market has a significant impact on both the flavor and quality of coffee; however, the specific mechanisms responsible for these effects are not well understood. The coffee industry is working to improve this understanding. Dry processing and wet processing are the two primary methods that are used to process coffee. The goal is to remove the pulp from the coffee cherries and then improve the quality of the coffee beans by maintaining their moisture content at a level of approximately 12% throughout the roasting process. This takes place after the pulp has been removed from the coffee cherries. In the semi-dry process, the cherries are allowed to dry without being broken up, whereas in the wet process, machines are used to remove the pulp from the cherries, leaving behind a sticky substance called mucilage on the outer skin of the coffee beans. This mucilage can be removed either through the process of wet fermentation or through the use of machinery (Ferreira *et al.* 2023).

During the wet fermentation process, the coffee beans, after being peeled, are typically submerged in water for a period of 6 to 72 hours before they are dried (Ferreira *et al.* 2023). Diverse microorganisms have been extracted from moist coffee fermentations in various geographical areas. The coffee fermentation process in various regions may involve certain shared species of microorganisms as well as distinct microorganisms that are specific to each region. The microorganisms, which consist of yeasts and bacteria, aid in the decomposition of complex molecules, such as carbohydrates, proteins, and polyphenols, found in coffee mucilage. They achieve this by generating enzymes and organic acids, resulting in the formation of aroma precursors like reducing sugars and amino acids (Bruyne *et al.* 2007). These metabolites have the potential to directly or indirectly influence the fragrance and flavor of coffee. Novel microbial species have been discovered in the research field of coffee and coffee fermentation. De Bruyne *et al.* (2007) discovered a new type of LAB species called *Leuconostoc holzapfelii*. In 2001, Fuentes-Ramirez and colleagues discovered two new species of AAB, namely *Gluconacetobacter azotocaptans* and *Gluconacetobacter johannae*, in coffee fermentation processes. Moreover, new filamentous fungi have arisen from coffee-associated ecosystems. In 2003, Peterson and colleagues discovered *Penicillium brocae* in the coffee berry borer in Mexico (Peterson *et al.* 2003). In 2008, Nooim and colleagues reported that Thai coffee beans contained *Aspergillus aculeatinus* and *Aspergillus sclerotiicarbonarius*. Wet fermentation is often a traditional, uncontrolled process that relies on the natural growth of native microorganisms and can, therefore, lead to inconsistencies in coffee yield and quality. However, with well-defined starter cultures, the fermentation process can be transformed into a more efficient and stable industrial process (USDA Foreign Agricultural Service 2021). Furthermore, LAB isolated from natural ecosystems of wet fermentation may become a good source for potential functional starter cultures.

3 ECOLOGICAL ASPECTS AND LAB VARIETY IN PROCESSING COFFEE

Traditionally, LAB has been linked to the processing of coffee for a significant period of time, as evidenced by records dating back 73 years. The laboratory research pertaining to coffee can be categorized into seven distinct groups according to their genetic relationships (Holzapfel and Wood 2014). These are the different types of LAB that exist in coffee. LAB initially established a presence on the surface of coffee fruits. Nevertheless, they can also be acquired from the soil, water utilized in the processing, coffee apparatus, and even insects. During the processing of coffee, LAB can undergo rapid proliferation, resulting in populations that surpass 100 million cells per milliliter in just 20 hours. Despite facing challenges, such as varying acidity, sugar reachability, and competition, compared to other microbes, their ability to adapt to the coffee processing environment enables them to thrive (Velmourougane 2013).

The genus *Leuconostoc* is one of the most common types of LAB that can be found in coffee processing in a variety of countries, such as Brazil, Cameroon, and Colombia. This interaction is fascinating because yeast provides nutrients for the growth of LAB, while LABs create an environment that is conducive to the growth of yeast. It is interesting that it is frequently associated with yeast because of this interaction. This interaction can have a significant impact on the flavor and quality of coffee, despite the fact that the precise mechanisms by which it operates in coffee are not yet completely understood (Avallone *et al.* 2002; Leong *et al.* 2014). Similar to the way in which soil and climate have an effect on wine, the various regions where coffee is grown are home to their own distinct species of LAB, such as *Lactobacillus hordei* and *Lactococcus hircilactis*, which contribute to the diversity of LAB and influence the flavors and characteristics of coffee (Pereira *et al.* 2019). Due to the high concentration of sugar in coffee pulp, LAB is able to thrive in the ecological niche created during the processing of coffee. This is especially true during the wet fermentation stage. The fact that LAB populations can reach over 108 cells/mL in coffee pulp demonstrates how common these organisms are in this ecosystem (Avallone *et al.* 2002). The geographic region and specific processing methods that are used can both have an effect on the composition of the LAB communities that are present during coffee processing (Pereira *et al.* 2019). A variety of LAB species, such as *Leuconostoc*, *Lactobacillus*, and *Pediococcus*, have been discovered to be present in the ecosystems that are utilized in the coffee processing industry. These labs contribute to the development of bioactive compounds that have an effect on the overall quality as well as the flavor of coffee (Endo and Salminen 2013; Pereira *et al.* 2019). The LAB demonstrates a wide variety of metabolic diversity, which results in variations in the production of organic acids and other metabolites while the LAB is fermenting. The chemical properties of coffee beans can be changed as a result of metabolic processes, which also affect how microbial metabolites are transported to the endosperm of the bean. Environmental factors, such as temperature and oxygen levels, have the potential to influence the activity and diversity of LAB during the processing of coffee (Cavanagh, Fitzgerald, and Mcauliffe, 2015). There may be variations in the results of fermentation due to the fact that particular microbial species may flourish under particular conditions. The identification of new LAB species and the investigation of the roles these organisms play in the fermentation of coffee continue to be primary areas of focus for research. A comprehensive investigation of the coffee-making process could lead to novel approaches in coffee production and improvements in flavor.

4 METABOLIC PROCESSES OF LAB DURING COFFEE FERMENTATION

LAB thrives on sugars such as pentoses, which can be found in abundance and richness in coffee pulp. Coffee pulp is an ideal environment for LAB to grow and reproduce. During the fermentation of coffee, the sugars serve as the primary sources of carbon and energy, which enables the rapid growth of LAB. The fermentation of sugars by homofermentative LAB species, such as *Lactococcus lactis*, *Pediococcus pentosaceus*, *Enterococcus faecalis*, and *Lactobacillus hordei*, takes place via the *Embden-Meyerhoff-Parnas* pathway. As a result of the process, lactic acid is produced, and the enzyme lactate dehydrogenase is responsible for transforming sugars into lactic acid (Mayo *et al.* 2010; Silva *et al.* 2013; Zhang *et al.* 2019). However, if the coffee processing is subjected to harsh conditions, such as an acidic environment and carbon deficiency, the species involved in fermentation may shift to a metabolic process that results in the production of various acids. This occurs because harsh conditions force the species to produce acids in response to carbon deficiency, which can happen if coffee processing is subjected to onerous conditions.

In coffee fermentations, heterofermentative LAB, including *Leuconostoc mesenteroides*, *Leuconostoc citreum*, and *Lactobacillus brevis*, are commonly found (Holzapfel and Wood 2014). The LAB species are capable of metabolizing both the pentoses and the hexoses that are present in the coffee pulp, resulting in the production of various end products, including lactate, acetate, and ethanol. Pathways, such as phosphoketolase and pentose phosphate, are utilized by them to accomplish this goal (Pereira *et al.* 2016). In addition, LAB makes it easier to break down complex carbohydrates by producing a number of hydrolytic enzymes, such as pectin lyase, pectin methylesterase, and exo-polygalacturonase, in addition to causing acidification (Avallone *et al.* 2002; Pereira *et al.* 2016). These enzymes include pectin lyase, pectin methylesterase, and exo-polygalacturonase. Pectin hydrolysis results in the release of monosaccharides, which are utilized by lactic acid bacteria as additional sources of carbon for their metabolic processes (Pereira *et al.* 2016).

In addition to the sugars, LAB species have the ability to metabolize citrate, which is a compound that is found in significant amounts in coffee pulp. Citrate transport, the conversion of citrate to oxaloacetate, and the subsequent conversion of oxaloacetate to pyruvate and CO2 are the three essential processes in citrate metabolism (Pereira *et al.* 2016). This metabolic pathway results in the production of flavor-active compounds that each contain four carbon atoms. Some examples of these compounds include diacetyl, acetoin, and 2,3-butanediol. The accumulation of pyruvate in acidic conditions in coffee pulp stimulates the production of acetolactate, which is a precursor for 4-carbon compounds. This occurs because pyruvate is a source of energy. During the fermentation of coffee, certain LAB strains, such as *Leuconostoc* and *Lactococcus* species, are present. These strains are well-known for their significant ability to metabolize citrate (Pereira *et al.* 2016, 2019).

The breakdown of amino acids is an essential part of LAB physiology, particularly for preserving the pH balance in conditions where nutrients are in short supply (Vermeulen *et al.* 2006). The presence of amino acids in coffee pulp, such as leucine, valine, phenylalanine, threonine, and isoleucine, creates a favorable environment for the proliferation of lactic acid bacteria (LAB). The decomposition of amino acids can result in the production of a wide variety of small organic compounds, such as higher alcohols, esters, carboxylic acids, and aldehydes. By degrading phenylalanine, certain strains of LAB, such as *Lactobacillus plantarum*, are able to produce compounds such as phenylacetaldehyde, phenylacetate, and phenylethanol. Other strains of LAB are unable to do so. *Lactococcus lactis* strains, on the other hand, have the ability to convert leucine into a variety of different substances, including 3-methylbutanal, 3-methylbutanol, and 3-methylbutyric acid. During fermentation, these metabolic processes have an effect on the myriad flavor profiles and qualities of coffee beverages.

5 IMPACT ON BEVERAGE QUALITY

The synthesis of metabolites results in alterations in flavor, intensifying the robust taste and aroma of the coffee. Chlorogenic acid, a biologically active compound, increases coffee bitterness and helps in improving human health (Muynarsk *et al.* 2019). The presence of numerous beneficial aromas in coffee can be attributed to the low concentrations of organic acids. The taste of coffee is intricately connected to a range of organic acids. The green coffee bean contains the highest concentration of citric acid, followed by quinic acid and malic acid in descending order of prevalence. The brightness of coffee is attributed to citric acid, which gradually degrades during the roasting process. Medium-roasted coffee contains significant levels of citric acid, which is reduced by approximately 50% during the roasting process, leading to a distinct acidity and precise flavor. Additionally, quinic acid, a chemical compound found in organic acids, also contributes to the bitterness of coffee. The volatile nature of the beverage can be traced to the presence of sugars as well as proteins and amino acids in the coffee bean. Pyrazines are the second most prevalent aromatic compound in coffee, and they are responsible for the toasted flavor and roasted nut aroma that coffee has. Ketones have a tendency to generate acids with fruity, floral, and honey flavors, along with dicarbonyl compounds. These compounds are formed through amino reactions in a process called Strecker degradation. They can be linked to the presence of green coffee during the initial fermentation process (Pereira *et al.* 2019; Vermeulen *et al.* 2006). A qualified taste panel evaluated starter fermentation samples using cup measurement scales to assess flavor characteristics. Sensory scores showed a negative correlation with undesirable flavors such as astringency and burnt notes. A reduction of these flavors was also observed in the starter fermentation samples (Pereira *et al.* 2019).

6 IMPACT OF OTHER MICROORGANISMS

The fermentation of coffee pulp involves the proliferation of yeast and LAB, which metabolize the sugars (glucose and fructose) present in the pectin and convert them into organic acids. The primary metabolite observed was lactic acid, with a concentration of 3.28 g/L after 48 hours of fermentation. This was followed by acetic acid and succinic acid, with concentrations of 1.27 g/L and 0.30 g/L, respectively. The limited production of acetic acid (<1.5 g/L) and the absence of butyric and propionic acids help reduce the occurrence of undesirable flavors in the coffee beverage. Conversely, the generation of lactic acid aids in the acidification of the coffee pulp without compromising the excellence of the end product. The synthesis of this organic acid is primarily associated with the metabolic processes of LAB, although yeast may contribute a minor portion of the organic acids found in coffee pulp (Pereira *et al.* 2016).

In the antagonism test, LPBY11B and Lactobacillus LPBB03 were found to have the greatest inhibitory activity against *Aspergillus ochratogens* and were selected for further characterization. Lactic acid and ethanol are products of fermentation. These concentrations remain low during the early stages of fermentation and then increase rapidly toward completion. Since lactic acid is produced in large quantities by LAB and ethanol is produced by yeast in the presence of glucose, exponential growth of either substance indicates that the corresponding microorganism is multiplying. Lactic acid concentrations increased rapidly upon completion, suggesting that the growth of LAB may dominate these sites. Similarly, ethanol concentration increases rapidly upon completion. These differences suggest that the nature of the dominant processes at the completion of the fermentation batch may be different (Pereira *et al.* 2016).

Despite the development and utilization of numerous LAB strains in the food industry, it is currently not feasible to directly employ commercially available LAB starter cultures in coffee bean fermentation processes, primarily due to the unique physical and chemical characteristics of this process. Consequently, recent research has examined bacteria in natural environments to identify LAB strains that are appropriate for the fermentation of coffee. LPBR01, obtained from natural coffee fermentation, has the ability to enhance the acidification process of coffee pulp and reduce the time needed for mucus clearance. Another study chose Lcb. rhamnose HN001, which also facilitated the effective utilization of the pulp matrix. The discovery offers fresh possibilities for enhancing the coffee fermentation procedure (Pereira *et al.* 2016).

7 FUNCTIONAL GENOMICS

In recent years, significant strides have been made in the area of high-throughput sequencing technology, which is an essential method for conducting scientific research. Our comprehension of LAB's metabolic capacity and their proficiency in biological processing has been significantly bolstered as a result of this study. However, it was only recently discovered that a LAB strain (*Pediococcus acidilactici* LPBC101) derived from coffee fermentation has a complete genome sequence. Genome sequencing has made it possible to understand how LAB adapts and metabolizes in the unique environment of coffee processing (Prabhurajeshwar and Chandrakanth 2017). This understanding will help improve coffee quality.

The fermentation of coffee resulted in the production of the bacterium *P. acidilactici* LPBC10, which possesses a number of unique genes that are necessary for using the sugars in coffee pulp. This particular LAB strain also contains a variety of stress-related proteins, such as thiol peroxidase, glutathione reductases, NADH-oxidases, and alkaline-shock proteins. Because of its genetic characteristics, it is extraordinarily well-suited to thrive in the environmental conditions of coffee processing. This coffee-associated LAB strain possesses all of the essential enzymes for the glycolysis, phosphoketolase, and pentose-phosphate pathways, which is another factor that contributes to its remarkable phenotypic diversity (Muynarsk *et al.* 2019).

Although the existence of these genes shows potential, it is essential to acknowledge that genomic data only provides a predictive model at most. The manifestation of genes is intricately interconnected with the current environmental conditions. Thus, to enhance the reliability of these discoveries, it is crucial to verify genomic insights by conducting transcriptome, proteome, and metabolome profiling. These comprehensive methodologies enable researchers to acquire a more profound comprehension of the functions and impacts of specific LAB strains during the processing of coffee. To fully exploit their potential in the coffee industry, it is essential to thoroughly assess their practical usefulness under real-world field conditions.

8 CONCLUSION

LAB cultures have significant potential for attaining accurate control, replicability, and uniform quality in coffee processing. Their metabolic functions, specifically related to carbohydrates, citrate, and amino acids, are essential in processing coffee. LAB aids in the acidification of coffee pulp, helping in the easy removal of mucilage from coffee fruits. Additionally, LAB generates metabolites that augment the taste of the coffee, enhancing the overall quality of the end products. Surprisingly, the application of LAB in the production of coffee has not been the subject of extensive research. At this time, evaluations of real-world environments have only been conducted on two species: Lcb. plantarum LPBR01 and Lcb. rhamnosus HN001. However, this only accounts for a small portion of the vast variety of species that are involved in natural fermentations. It has not yet been determined whether or not Leuconostoc sp. will live up to its full potential as a starter culture. Without a doubt, the complete range of abilities of LAB strains in relation to coffee processing remains to be fully revealed. Many challenges need to be further investigated before they can be applied in industry. Future research should focus on investigating novel LAB strains and assessing the viability of developing adaptable mixed cultures that integrate yeast strains. As mentioned earlier, various factors impact the activities of LAB during the process of coffee fermentation. To fully comprehend the interactions between LAB in inoculated fermentations, it is necessary to develop and implement a well-planned approach that utilizes "omics" methodologies. Moreover, the developing discipline of synthetic biology presents opportunities for understanding and regulating the interactions between cells and the stability of LAB in the microbial communities that participate in coffee fermentation.

REFERENCES

Avallone S., Brillouet J. M., Guyot B., Olguin E. and Guiraud J. P., (2002). *Int J Food Sci Technol*, **37**, 191–198

Bruyne K. D., Schillinger U., Caroline L., Boehringer B., Cleenwerck I., Vancanneyt M., Vuyst L. D., Franz C. M. A. P. and Vandamme P, (2007). *Int J Syst Evol Micr*, **57**, 2952–2959

Carvalho Neto D. P., Pereira G. V. M., Finco A. M. O., Letti L. A. J., Silva B. J. G., Vandenberghe L. P. S. and Soccol C. R., (2018). *Food Biosci*, **26**, 80–87

Cavanagh D., Fitzgerald G. F. and Mcauliffe O., (2015). *Food Microbiol*, **47**, 45–61

Endo A. and Salminen S., (2013). *Syst Appl Microbiol*, **36**, 444–448

Ferreira L. J. C., Gomes M. D. S., Oliveira L. M. D. and Santos L. D, (2023). *Food Res Int*, **169**, 112793.

Fuentes-Ramírez L. E., Bustillos-Cristales R., Tapia-Hernández A., Jiménez-Salgado T., Wang E.T., Martínez-Romero E. and Caballero-Mellado J., (2001). *Int J Syst Evol Micr*, **51**, 1305–1314

Holzapfel W. H. and Wood B. J. B., (2014). *Introduction to the LAB, Lactic Acid Bacteria: Biodiversity and Taxonomy* (John Wiley & Sons)

Leong K. H., Chen Y. S., Pan S. F., Chen J. J., Wu C. H., Chang Y.C. and Yanagida F., (2014). *Curr Microbiol*, **68**, 440–447

Mayo B., Aleksandrzak-Piekarczyk T., Fernández M., Kowalczyk M., Álvarez-Martín P. and Bardowski J., (2010). *Updates in the metabolism of lactic acid bacteria, Biotechnology of Lactic Acid Bacteria: Novel Applications* (Blackwell)

Muynarsk E. S. M., Pereira G. V. M., Mesa D., Thomaz-soccol V., Carvalho J.C., Pagnoncelli M. G. B. and Soccol C. R., (2019). *Microbiol Resour*, **8**, e00332–19

Pereira G. V. M., Beux M., Pagnoncelli M. G., Soccol V. T., Rodrigues C. and Soccol C.R., (2016). *Lett Appl Microbiol*, **62**, 96–101

Pereira G. V. M., Carvalho Neto D. P., Júnior A. I. M., Vásquez Z. S., Medeiros A. B. P., Vandenberghe L. P. S. and Soccol C. R., (2019). *Food Chem*, **272**, 441–452

Pereira G. V. M., Carvalho Neto D. P., Medeiros A. B. P., Soccol V. T., Neto E., Woiciechowski A. L. and Soccol C. R., (2016). *Int J Food Sci Technol*, **51**, 1689–1695

Petersen L. M., Frisvad J. C., Knudsen P.B., Rohlfs M., Gotfredsen C.H. and Larsen T.O., (2015). *J Antibiot*, **68**, 603–608

Peterson S. W., Pérez J., Vega F.E. and Infante F., (2003). *Mycologia*, **95**, 141–147

Prabhurajeshwar C. and Chandrakanth R. K., (2017). *Biomed J*, **40**, 270–283.

Silva C. F., Vilela D. M., Cordeiro C. D. S., Duarte W. F., Dias D. R. and Schwan R. F., (2013). *World J Microb Biot*, **29**, 235–247.

USDA Foreign Agricultural Service, (2021). *Brazil: Coffee Annual* (USDA)

Velmourougane K., (2013). *Proc Natl Acad Sci India Sect B - Biol Sci*, **83** 233–239

Vermeulen N., Gánzle M. G. and Vogel R. F., (2006). *J Agric Food Chem*, **54**, 3832–3839

Wang C., Sun J., Lassabliere B., Yu B., Zhao F., Chen Y. and Liu S.Q., (2019). *J Sci Food Agric*, **99**, 409–420

Zhang S. J., Bruyn F. D., Pothakos V., Torres J., Falconi C., Moccand C., Weckx S. and Vuyst L. D., (2019). *Appl Environ Microbiol*, **85**, 1–22

Author index